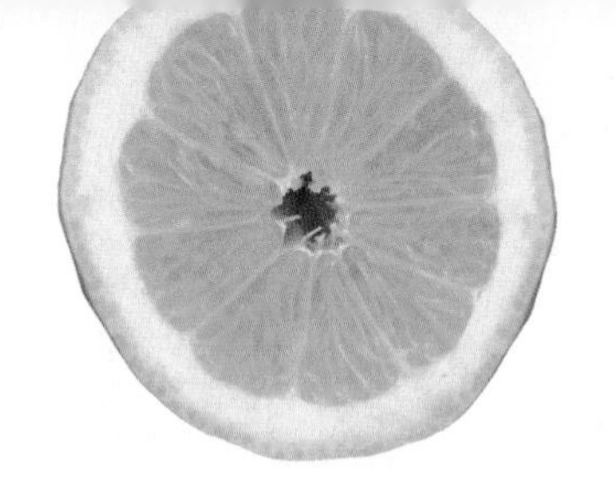

FIFTH EDITION, REVISED REPRINT

NUTRITION ESSENTIALS *for* NURSING PRACTICE

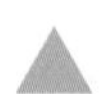

Susan G. Dudek, RD, CDN, BS

Assistant Professor, Dietetic Technology Program
Erie Community College
Williamsville, New York

Consultant Dietitian for Employee Assistance
Program of Child and Family Services
Buffalo, New York

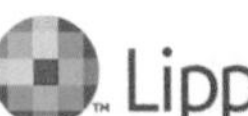
Lippincott Williams & Wilkins
a Wolters Kluwer business

Philadelphia • Baltimore • New York • London
Buenos Aires • Hong Kong • Sydney • Tokyo

Acquisitions Editor: Pete Darcy
Managing Editor: Dana Irwin/Betsy Gentzler
Director of Nursing Production: Helen Ewan
Managing Editor / Production: Erika Kors
Senior Production Editor: Tom Gibbons
Art Director: Carolyn O'Brien
Interior Design: BJ Crim
Senior Manufacturing Manager: William Alberti
Indexer: Ann Cassar
Compositor: Circle Graphics
Printer: R. R. Donnelley-Crawfordsville

5th Edition, Revised Reprint

9 8 7 6 5 4 3 2 1

Library of Congress Cataloging-in-Publication Data
Dudek, Susan G.
Nutrition essentials for nursing practice / Susan G. Dudek.—5th ed., revised reprint
p. ; cm.
Includes bibliographical references and index.
ISBN 0-7817-6651-6 (pbk. : alk. paper)
1. Diet therapy. 2. Nutrition. 3. Nursing. I. Title.
[DNLM: 1. Diet Therapy—Handbooks. 2. Diet Therapy—Nurses' Instruction. 3. Nutrition—Handbooks. 4. Nutrition—Nurses' Instruction. WB 39 D845n 2006]
RM216. D8627 2006
615.8'54—dc22

2004020115

To my son "Fwis" and my dad "Bop"—for everything beautiful you brought to my life. May you find joy with each other until I find you again.

REVIEWERS

Donna Brodski, RN, MSN
Assistant Professor, Nursing
Cuyahoga Community College
Parma, Ohio

Freda Kilburn, RN, DSN
Professor of Nursing
Morehead State University
Morehead, Kentucky

Patricia B. Lisk
Instructor
Augusta Technical College
Augusta, Georgia

Pamela Y. Mahon, PhD, RN
Associate Professor of Nursing
Kingsborough Community College
of the City University of New York
Brooklyn, New York

Donna Nayduch, RN-CS, MSN, ACNP
Regional Trauma Director
Banner Health
Greeley, Colorado

Marsha L. Ray, RN, MSN
Associate Degree Nursing Faculty
Shasta Community College
Redding, California

Mary Margaret Spica, RN, BSN, MSN, CSE
Faculty Instructor
Christ Hospital School of Nursing
Cincinnati, Ohio

PREFACE

Nutrition is a basic human need, ever-changing throughout the life cycle and along the wellness–illness continuum. It is a vital and integral component of nursing care. Knowledge of nutrition principles and the ability to apply that knowledge are required of nurses, whether they are involved in home health, community wellness, outpatient settings, or acute or long-term care.

Today, more than ever, health care providers are expected to do more with less. Often the constraints of time and resources challenge nurses to be all things to all people. With the movement of health care toward wellness and primary prevention, the significance of nutrition becomes more evident.

The guiding theme for the evolution of the fifth edition of *Nutrition Essentials for Nursing Practice* was to change the question potential users ask from "Can I afford to buy this book?" to "Can I afford NOT to buy this book?" My goal was to fuel the reader's interest in nutrition on a personal level as well as illuminate how nutrition is intimately intertwined with the practice of nursing. Popular features of the fourth edition have been retained, such as Nursing Process Care Plans, Questions You May Hear (which are now titled How Do You Respond?), True/False questions at the beginning of each chapter, and Key Concepts summarized at the end of each chapter. The feature Focus on Critical Thinking has been expanded to every chapter and asks the student to respond to controversial statements related to the chapter content. A more valuable fifth edition has been created by:

- Updating and streamlining the content to reflect the latest science-based practice. I am always surprised by how much the science and art of nutrition changes between editions. Updates to this edition include new Dietary Reference Intakes for all macronutrients, micronutrients, and water; Nutrition Facts labeling changes incorporating trans fat content; and revised nutrition recommendations from the American Heart Association, the National Cholesterol Education Program, and the American Diabetes Association. The newly revised Exchange Lists for Meal Planning appear in Chapter 19.
- Defining key terms in the margins.
- Spotlighting "Quick Bites," a new feature that provides a snapshot view of food or nutrition details.
- Introducing "Career Connection," a new feature designed to answer the student's question of "How will I use this information in my career?" In essence, Career Connection is a bridge between theory and professional practice.
- Incorporating a list of appropriate and reliable websites in each chapter.
- Adding a chapter entitled "Consumer Issues," which deals with nutrition information and misinformation, including understanding nutrition labels; the use of dietary supplements; food quality concerns, such as functional foods, nutraceuti-

cals, and organically grown foods; and food safety issues, including foodborne illness, biotechnology, and food irradiation.
- Using a Connection website to provide additional instructor and student resources.
- Offering a comprehensive IRCD that features an instructor's manual, test generator, image bank, WebCT/Blackboard-ready files, and PowerPoint presentation.

Unit One is entitled "Principles of Nutrition." It begins with Chapter 1, "Nutrition in Nursing," which focuses on why and how nutrition is important to nurses in all settings. Chapters that address carbohydrates, protein, lipids, vitamins, fluids and minerals, and energy metabolism present a foundation for wellness. The second part of each chapter highlights health promotion topics and demonstrates practical application of essential information, such as criteria to consider when buying a vitamin supplement, the lowdown on vegetarian diets, and the advantages of a Mediterranean diet.

Unit Two, "Nutrition in Health Promotion," begins with Chapter 8, "Guidelines for Healthy Eating." This chapter features the Dietary Guidelines for Americans and MyPyramid. Because these icons of America's national food and nutrition policy were being revised while the first printing of this edition was taking place, this book was revised in 2006 to incorporate the newest versions of these tools. It was striking to me personally to discover how many changes were needed throughout the book to reflect the new pyramid and its recommendations. I am grateful that Betsy Gentzler, the Managing Editor for the revised reprint, is so meticulous and conscientious. Other chapters in this unit are Chapter 9, "Consumer Issues," and Chapter 10, "Cultural, Ethnic, and Religious Influences on Food and Nutrition." The nutritional needs associated with the life cycle are discussed in chapters devoted to pregnant and lactating women, children and adolescents, and adults and older adults.

Unit Three, "Nutrition in Clinical Practice," presents nutrition therapy for obesity and eating disorders, enteral and parenteral nutrition, critical illness and hypermetabolic conditions, gastrointestinal disorders, cardiovascular disorders, diabetes, renal disorders, and cancer and HIV/AIDS. Pathophysiology is tightly focused within the context of nutrition.

My sincere hope is that this text provides the impetus to improve nutrition on both a personal and professional level.

ACKNOWLEDGMENTS

This book is the product of combined efforts by many dedicated and creative professionals at Lippincott Williams & Wilkins. I humbly acknowledge that because of their support and talents, I am able to do what I love—write, create, teach, and learn. I especially thank:

- Quincy McDonald, Senior Acquisitions Editor, who provided the spark to ignite the project. His vision and energy shaped the direction and set the tone.
- Dana Irwin, Managing Editor, for her meticulous attention to detail. I am grateful that she saw things I didn't notice and asked questions I didn't think of.
- Tom Gibbons, Senior Production Editor, and the production staff for their creative and artistic genius.
- The reviewers of the fifth edition chapters, whose thoughtful comments and suggestions helped guide the evolution of this text into a new and improved edition.
- My friends, who gave me the space and time to focus on the all-consuming task of writing.
- My children, who made sacrifices so I could "work on the book": Chris, Kait (my pink princess of power), and Kara (aka Moochie), the collective sunshine of my life.
- And most especially my husband, Joe. Thanks for being here—literally and figuratively.

CONTENTS

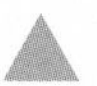

UNIT ONE
Principles of Nutrition 1

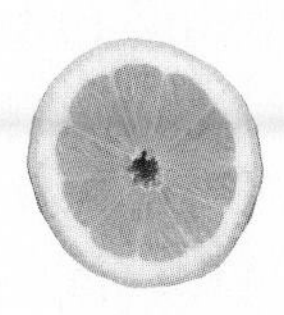

1 Nutrition in Nursing 3
2 Carbohydrates 19
3 Protein 45
4 Lipids 66
5 Vitamins 94
6 Water and Minerals 127
7 Energy Metabolism 155

UNIT TWO
Nutrition in Health Promotion 177

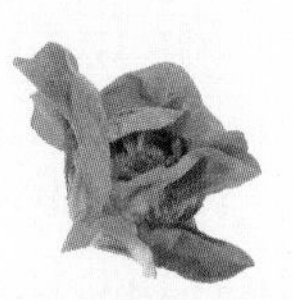

8 Guidelines for Healthy Eating 179
9 Consumer Issues 208
10 Cultural, Ethnic, and Religious Influences on Food and Nutrition 243
11 Healthy Eating for Healthy Babies 271
12 Nutrition for Infants, Children, and Adolescents 312
13 Nutrition for Adults and Older Adults 347

UNIT THREE
Nutrition in Clinical Practice 373

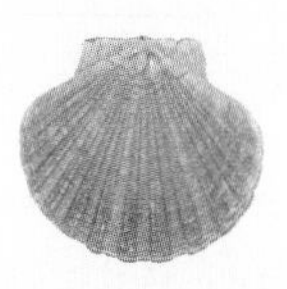

14 Obesity and Eating Disorders 375
15 Feeding Patients: Hospital Food and Enteral and Parenteral Nutrition 417
16 Critical Illness and Hypermetabolic Conditions 457
17 Nutrition for Patients With Gastrointestinal Disorders 477
18 Nutrition for Patients With Cardiovascular Disorders 529
19 Nutrition for Patients With Diabetes Mellitus 570
20 Nutrition for Patients With Renal Disorders 605
21 Nutrition for Patients With Cancer or HIV/AIDS 634

APPENDICES

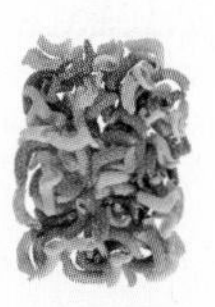

1 Dietary Reference Intakes (DRIs): Recommended Intakes for Individuals, Vitamins 667
2 Dietary Reference Intakes (DRIs): Recommended Intakes for Individuals, Elements 670
3 Dietary Reference Intakes (DRIs): Recommended Intakes for Individuals, Macronutrients 672
4 Acceptable Macronutrient Distribution Ranges 674
5 Growth Charts 675
6 Diet and Drugs 686

Index 699

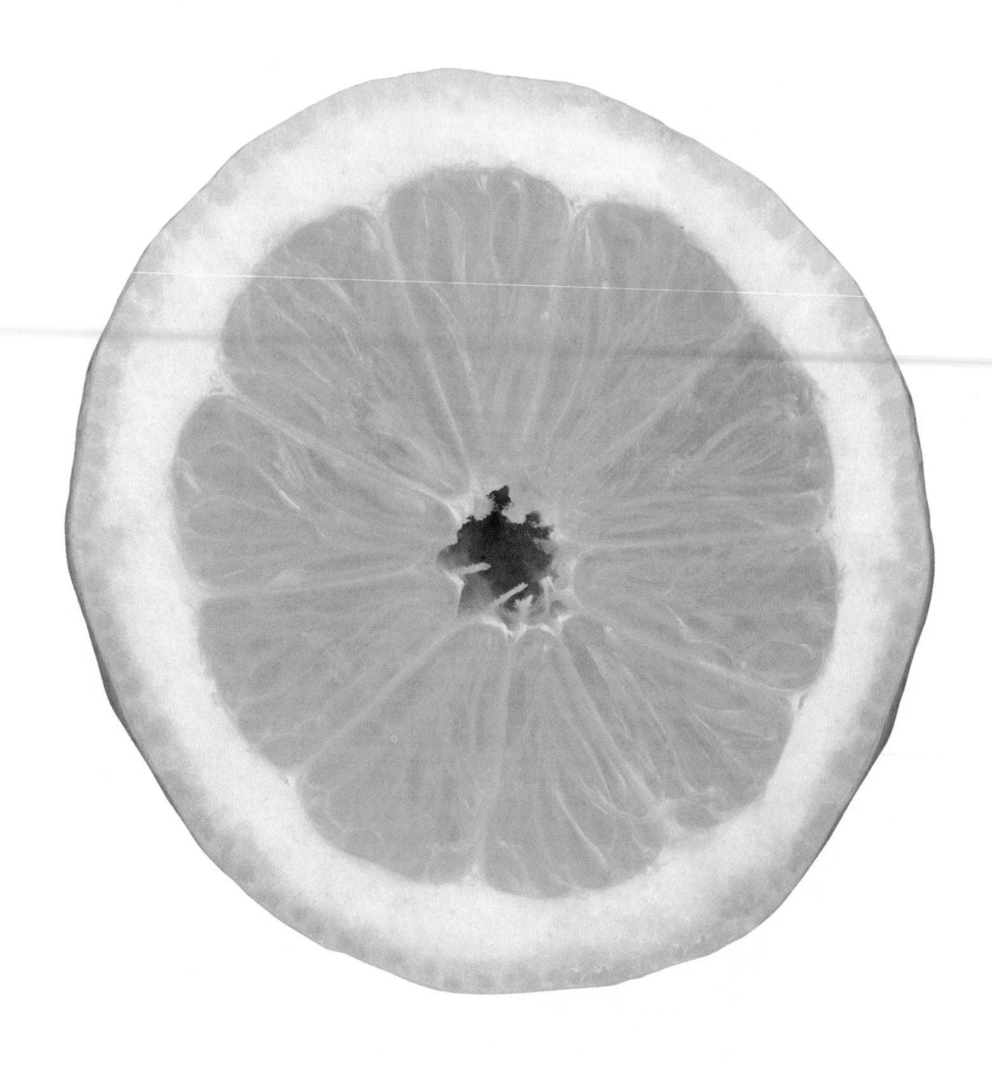

UNIT ONE

Principles of Nutrition

1

Nutrition in Nursing

TRUE	FALSE	
○	○	1 The nurse's role in nutrition is to call the dietitian.
○	○	2 Nutritional status is the balance between nutrient intake and requirements.
○	○	3 Asking a client if he/she is on a diet may not be of much value in determining usual intake.
○	○	4 Changes in weight reflect acute changes in nutritional status.
○	○	5 A person can be malnourished without being underweight.
○	○	6 The only cause of a low serum albumin concentration is protein malnutrition.
○	○	7 "Significant" weight loss is 5% of body weight in 1 month.
○	○	8 People who take five or more prescription or over-the-counter medications or dietary supplements are at risk for nutritional problems.
○	○	9 Written handouts that list "foods to avoid" and "foods to choose" are valuable teaching tools because they provide explicit dos and don'ts.
○	○	10 Physical signs and symptoms of malnutrition develop only after other signs of malnutrition are apparent (e.g., abnormal lab values, weight change).

UPON COMPLETION OF THIS CHAPTER, YOU WILL BE ABLE TO

- Describe how nutritional care can be approached using the nursing care process.
- Describe the "rule of thumb" formula for calculating ideal body weight for men and women based on height.
- Discuss disadvantages of using albumin as an indicator of nutritional status.
- Discuss alternatives to the term "diet."
- Explain why an alternative term to "diet" is useful.

Based on Maslow's Hierarchy of Needs, food and nutrition rank on the same level as air in the basic necessities of life. Obviously, death eventually occurs without food. But unlike air, food does so much more than simply sustain life. Food is loaded with personal, social, and cultural meanings that define our food values, beliefs, and customs. That food nourishes the mind as well as the body broadens nutrition to an art as well as a science. For most people, nutrition is not simply a matter of food or no food but rather a question of what kind, how much, and how often. Merging want with need and pleasure with health are key to achieving optimal nutritional status.

Nutritional Status: the state of balance between nutrient supply (intake) and demand (requirement). An imbalance between intake and requirement can result in overnutrition or undernutrition.

To achieve optimal nutritional status, intake may need to be adjusted upward or downward. For instance, when the goal is recovery from illness or surgery, nutrition therapy focuses on meeting increased needs for calories, protein, and other nutrients. Clients who fail to meet their nutritional needs may experience prolonged or complicated recovery from illness, and their responses to medical treatments and drug therapies may be diminished. In wellness settings, when optimal nutritional status means disease prevention, the nutritional focus is frequently to ensure that intake does not exceed requirement. The emphasis is on avoiding excesses of calories, fat, saturated fat, cholesterol, and sodium to reduce the risk of chronic diseases such as heart disease, hypertension, diabetes, and obesity. However, these settings do not have mutually exclusive nutritional priorities. Some hospital patients require restrictive diets (e.g., low-sodium diet), and some wellness clients have nutrient intakes below their requirements (e.g., not enough calcium or fiber). Therefore, a priority for all clients is to consume or obtain an adequate and appropriate intake of calories and nutrients based on their own individual needs.

Just what is an adequate and appropriate intake of calories and nutrients and how to achieve that intake is determined by analyzing data to identify actual or potential nutritional problems. The decision-making process continues with goal setting, implementing a plan, and evaluation. While the dietitian or diet technician may shoulder most of the responsibility for the nutritional care of hospitalized patients deemed to be at moderate to high nutritional risk, low-risk hospitalized patients and clients in other settings (e.g., home health, corporate wellness, parish nursing) may be relegated to the nurse. In addition, it may be the nurse who screens clients to determine the existing level of risk and who reinforces diet counseling. As such, nurses are intimately involved in all aspects of nutritional care.

This chapter focuses on the importance of nutrition in nursing practice. The *nursing process* is used to illustrate how nutrition is integrated into nursing in the real world. Real-life situations are described to show practical application.

NUTRITIONAL CARE PROCESS

What does the client need? What can you or others do to effectively and efficiently help the client meet his or her needs? What criteria will you use to judge success? These and similar questions are the foundation of the decision-making process, whether the focus is on general nursing or specifically on nutrition.

 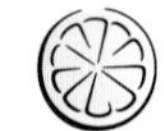

Career Connection

What is the nurse's role in facilitating nutritional care?

- Communicate with the registered dietitian (RD).
- Serve as a liaison between the physician and the RD.
- Identify clients who may benefit from programs such as Meals on Wheels.
- Request a referral to a speech therapist.
- Confer with the discharge planner, social services worker, and physical or occupational therapist.

Assessment

Nutritional Assessment: an in-depth analysis of a person's nutritional status. In the clinical setting, nutritional assessments focus on moderate- to high-risk patients with suspected or confirmed protein-energy malnutrition.

In all settings, it is appropriate to evaluate the client's nutritional status so that appropriate goals and interventions can be devised to correct actual or potential imbalances. Nutritional status can be assessed by looking at a few or many criteria. Exactly which criteria are evaluated and how the results are interpreted depend on the particular population and setting as well as the availability of time and resources. Although everyone agrees that it is important to identify actual and potential nutritional problems, there is no universally accepted, definitive tool to do so. Often professional judgment is as important as objective criteria.

The process of assessment involves gathering and analyzing data. Nurses are in an ideal position to screen clients for nutritional problems through an initial nursing history and physical examination. Clients deemed at low or no risk for nutritional problems may need only to be monitored for any deterioration in nutritional status. Clients found to be at moderate or high risk are usually referred to a dietitian for a comprehensive nutritional assessment (see **Connection** website for in-depth assessment criteria). It is important to remember that nutritional risks may exist that simply were not evaluated and that a person's relative risk can change. Here are some key questions to consider.

Is the Client at Nutritional Risk Because of Health Problems?

A positive response to any of these questions may indicate the need for nutrition intervention:

Does the client have a medical condition that may benefit from nutrition therapy such as diabetes or hypertension?

Do physical complaints interfere with the client's intake such as difficulty chewing and swallowing, anorexia, heartburn, nausea, vomiting, or pain?

Does the client have increased needs? For instance, nutritional needs increase in response to pregnancy, fever, sepsis, thermal injuries, skin breakdown, cancer, acquired immunodeficiency syndrome (AIDS), major surgery, and trauma.

Is the client losing nutrients as in the case of malabsorption, diarrhea, and certain renal diseases?

Is the Client at Nutritional Risk Because of Intake?

Obtaining reliable and accurate information on what the client usually eats is far more difficult than it sounds. Eating is highly personal and people often get defensive when questioned about their eating habits. Although the nurse may only be required to fill in a blank space next to the word "diet," simply asking the client "Are you on a diet?" will probably not give accurate or sufficient information to determine what the client eats. First of all, a client may interpret that leading question as "You should be on a diet. If you're a good patient you'll tell me you follow a diet." A better question would be, "Do you avoid any particular foods?" or "Do you watch you eat in any way?" Even the term "meal" may elicit a stereotypical mental picture. Questions to consider include

How many meals and snacks do you eat in a 24-hour period? This question helps to establish the pattern of eating and identifies unusual food habits such as pica, food faddism, eating disorders, and meal skipping.

Do you have any food allergies or intolerances, and, if so, what are they? The greater the number of foods restricted or eliminated in the diet, the greater the likelihood of nutritional deficiencies. This question may also shed light on the client's need for nutrition counseling. For instance, clients with hiatal hernia who are intolerant of citrus fruits and juices may benefit from counseling on how to ensure an adequate intake of vitamin C.

What types of vitamin, mineral, herbal, or other supplements do you use and why? A multivitamin, multimineral supplement that provides 100% or less of the Daily Value offers some protection against less than optimal food choices. Folic acid in supplements or fortified food is recommended for women of childbearing age; people over age 50 are encouraged to obtain vitamin B_{12} from fortified foods or supplements. However, potential problems may arise from other types or amounts of supplements. For instance, large doses of vitamin A, B_6, and D have the potential to cause toxicity symptoms. Iron supplements may decrease zinc absorption and negatively impact zinc status over time.

What concerns do you have about what or how you eat? This question places the responsibility of healthy eating with the client, where it should be. A client who may benefit from nutrition intervention and counseling *in theory* may not be a candidate for such *in practice* depending on her or his level of interest and motivation. This question may also shed light on whether or not the client understands what he or she should be eating and if the client is willing to make changes in eating habits.

For clients who are acutely ill, how has illness affected your choice or tolerance of food?

Who prepares the meals? This person may need nutritional counseling.

Do you have enough food to eat? Be aware that pride and an unwillingness to admit inability to afford an adequate diet may prevent some clients and families from answering this question. For hospitalized clients, it may be more useful to ask the client to compare the size of the meals they are served in the hospital to the size of meals they normally eat.

How much alcohol to you drink daily? Risk begins at more than one drink daily for women and more than two drinks daily for men.

 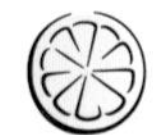

Does the Client's Weight Indicate a Health Risk?

Body Mass Index: an index of weight in relation to height that is calculated mathematically by dividing weight in kilograms by the square of height in meters.

Height and weight are used to indirectly assess undernutrition and overnutrition in adults. Measuring height and weight is relatively quick and easy and requires little skill; therefore, *measures* not *estimates* should be used whenever possible to ensure accuracy and reliability. After height and weight are obtained, they can be used to calculate body mass index (BMI) from which relative risk of health problems related to weight can be estimated. "Healthy" or "normal" BMI is defined as 18.5 to 24.9. Values above and below this range are associated with increased health risks. Keep in mind that a person can have a high BMI and still be undernourished in one or more nutrients if intake is unbalanced or if nutritional needs are high and intake is low. See chapter 14 for more on BMI.

A different, quick, and easy rule-of-thumb method of assessing weight is to calculate "ideal" body weight using the Hamwi method, then analyze the client's weight as a percent of ideal (Table 1.1). Keep in mind that neither method measures body fatness or evaluates distribution of body fat, both of which impact health risk. Also, edema or dehydration skews accurate weight measurements.

"Ideal" Body Weight: the formula given here is a universally used standard in clinical practice to quickly estimate a person's reasonable weight based on height, even though it and all other methods are not absolute.

TABLE 1.1 **CALCULATIONS AND ANALYSIS OF WEIGHT FOR HEIGHT**

	Body Mass Index		Hamwi Method	
Calculate	$\text{BMI} = \frac{\text{weight (kg)}}{\text{Height squared}}$		1. "Ideal" weight based on height: Men: 106 pounds for the first 5 feet of height and 6 pounds for each additional inch Women: 100 pounds for the first 5 feet of height and 5 pounds for each additional inch Add or subtract 10% depending on body frame size 2. Use current weight and "ideal" weight to determine percent ideal body weight: $\%\text{IBW} = \frac{\text{current weight}}{\text{ideal weight}} \times 100$	
Analyze	<18.5	may ↑ health risk	>200%	morbid obesity
	18.5–24.9	healthy weight	120–199%	obese
	25.0–26.9	may ↑ health risk in some	110–119%	overweight
			90–110%	within normal range
	>27.0	↑ health risk	89–90%	mild malnutrition
			70–79%	moderate malnutrition
			<69%	severe malnutrition

Has the Client Experienced Significant Weight Change?

Significant weight change is determined by how much weight is lost per specified unit of time, usually in terms of months (Box 1.1). Regardless of whether the change was intentional (e.g., dieting) or unintentional (e.g., related to illness), significant weight loss increases the risk of poor nutritional status. However, because changes in weight may be slow to occur, they are more reflective of chronic, not acute, changes in nutritional status.

Do Medications or Nutritional Supplements Warrant a Closer Look for Their Impact on Nutrition or Food Interactions?

Both prescription and over-the-counter drugs have the potential to affect and be affected by nutritional status. Sometimes drug-nutrient interactions are the intended action of the drug. At other times, alterations in nutrient intake, metabolism, or excretion may be an unwanted side effect of drug therapy. Although well-nourished individuals on short-term drug therapy may easily withstand the negative effects of drug–nutrient interactions, malnourished clients and those on long-term drug regimens may experience significant nutrient deficiencies and decreased tolerance to drug therapy. Clients at greatest risk for development of drug-induced nutrient deficiencies include those who

- Habitually consume fewer calories and nutrients than they need
- Have increased nutrient requirements including infants, adolescents, and pregnant and lactating women
- Are elderly
- Have chronic illnesses
- Take large numbers of drugs (five or more), whether prescription drugs, over-the-counter medications, or dietary supplements
- Are receiving long-term drug therapy
- Self-medicate
- Are substance abusers

Does the Client Look Malnourished?

Subclinical: asymptomatic.

The problem with relying on physical appearance to reveal nutritional problems is that most signs cannot be considered diagnostic; rather, they must be viewed as suggestive of malnutrition because evaluation of "normal" versus "abnormal" findings is subjec-

BOX 1.1 **EVALUATING WEIGHT CHANGE**

Calculate percent weight change:
(usual weight – present weight) ÷ usual weight × 100

The following guidelines indicate significant weight loss:
1% to 2% in 1 week
5% in 1 month
7.5% in 3 months
10% in 6 months

 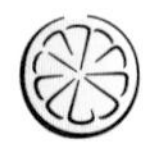

tive and the signs of malnutrition may be nonspecific. For instance, dull, dry hair may be related to severe protein deficiency or to overexposure to the sun. In addition, physical signs and symptoms of malnutrition can vary in intensity among population groups because of genetic and environmental differences. Lastly, physical findings occur only with overt malnutrition, not subclinical malnutrition. Physical signs and symptoms suggestive of malnutrition appear in Box 1.2.

Are There Social Factors That Impact Nutrition?

Social factors that may influence intake, nutritional requirements, or nutrition counseling needs include a history or evidence of

- Illiteracy
- Language barriers
- Limited knowledge of nutrition and food safety
- Altered or impaired intake related to culture
- Altered or impaired intake related to religion
- Lack of caregiver or social support system
- Social isolation
- Lack of or inadequate cooking arrangements
- Limited or low income
- Limited access to transportation to obtain food
- Advanced age (>80 years)
- Lack of or extreme physical activity
- Use of tobacco or recreational drugs
- Limited use or knowledge of community resources

Do Lab Values Suggest Nutritional Problems?

A wide variety of serum and urine laboratory values can be examined to assess a person's health status or response to treatment. For a quick look at protein status, albumin is the measurement most commonly used. Normal albumin levels range from 3.5 to 5.4 g/dL;

BOX 1.2 **PHYSICAL SIGNS AND SYMPTOMS SUGGESTIVE OF MALNUTRITION**

- Hair that is dull, brittle, dry, or falls out easily
- Swollen glands of the neck and cheeks
- Dry, rough, or spotty skin that may have a sandpaper feel
- Poor or delayed wound healing or sores
- Thin appearance with lack of subcutaneous fat
- Muscle wasting (decreased size and strength)
- Edema of the lower extremities
- Weakened hand grasp
- Depressed mood
- Abnormal heart rate, heart rhythm, or blood pressure
- Enlarged liver or spleen
- Loss of balance and coordination

TABLE 1.2 **GENERAL GUIDELINES FOR INTERPRETING ALBUMIN AND PREALBUMIN LEVELS**

	Albumin (g/dL)	Prealbumin (mg/dL)
Normal	3.5–5.5	23–43
Mild depletion	2.8–3.4	10–15
Moderate depletion	2.1–2.7	5–9
Severe depletion	<2.1	<5

values less than normal may indicate protein malnutrition. Unfortunately, albumin is not specific for nutritional status; other non-nutritional factors such as injury, infection, dehydration, liver disease, renal disease, and congestive heart failure, impact serum levels. Nor is albumin sensitive to acute changes in nutrition because it is degraded slowly (half-life: 14 to 21 days) so changes are slow to develop. The body's large extravascular pool of albumin can be mobilized to maintain serum levels until malnutrition is in a chronic stage.

Prealbumin, also known as thyroxin-binding protein, is a more sensitive indicator of protein status than albumin but it is also more expensive and less frequently ordered. Prealbumin is often used to assess protein status in critically ill patients at high risk for malnutrition. See Table 1.2 for general guidelines for interpreting albumin and prealbumin levels.

Nursing Diagnosis

Based on the data collected and interpreted, actual or potential nutritional problems are stated in nursing diagnoses. Nursing diagnoses in hospitals and long-term care facilities provide written documentation of the client's status and serve as a framework for the plan of care that follows. The diagnoses relate directly to nutrition when altered nutrition is the problem or indirectly when a change in intake will help to manage a nonnutritional problem. See Box 1.3 for some nursing diagnoses with nutritional relevance.

In wellness settings, documentation may be informal or nonexistent as in the case of a one-time-only opportunity such as a community health fair. In those instances, nursing diagnoses may be mentally noted but physically unwritten.

Planning and Implementation

The steps in planning and implementation include setting priorities, formulating goals, and determining what nursing actions are needed to help the client achieve those goals. Although planning for high-risk clients is the dietitian's responsibility, the nurse may plan for healthy clients and for those at low or mild risk for nutritional problems.

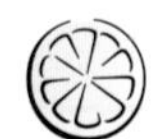

BOX 1.3

SOME NURSING DIAGNOSES WITH NUTRITIONAL RELEVANCE

- Altered nutrition: more than body requirements
- Altered nutrition: less than body requirements
- Altered nutrition: risk for more than body requirements
- Constipation
- Diarrhea
- Fluid volume excess
- Fluid volume deficit
- Risk for aspiration
- Altered oral mucous membrane
- Altered dentition
- Impaired skin integrity
- Noncompliance (with prescribed diet)
- Impaired swallowing
- Knowledge deficit (about nutrition therapy)
- Pain
- Nausea

Setting Priorities

What is the individual's most pressing health problem and how can nutrition help in its treatment? Does the client need more calories and protein to meet increased needs or a restricted intake to treat chronic disease? For instance, the priority for a nursing home resident with heart disease who is experiencing significant weight loss is not to maintain a low-fat diet but to increase calories (even with more fat) so as to halt or reverse the weight loss. Equally important is that those calories and nutrients must be in a usable form: clients get little benefit from food they cannot digest and absorb. Finally, whenever possible it is a priority to provide calories and nutrients through foods that are familiar to and liked by the client.

It is also essential to prioritize what the client needs to learn about nutrition. The client who is a newly diagnosed type 2 diabetic with irregular eating habits, a high cholesterol level, obesity, and osteoporosis has many nutritional concerns. Rather than suggest that he or she avoid sugar, time meals consistently, cut fat, limit red meat intake, switch to soft margarine, eat more vegetables, use canola oil, eat oatmeal, and drink more milk, it is better to prioritize: establishing a regular eating pattern and simply reducing portions are the most important first steps.

Formulating Goals

Goals should be measurable, attainable, specific, and client-centered. How do you measure success against a vague goal of "gain weight by eating better"? Is "eating better" achieved by adding butter to foods to increase calories or by substituting 1% milk for whole milk because it is heart-healthy? Is a 1-pound weight gain in 1 month acceptable or is 1 pound/week preferable? Is 1 pound/week attainable if the client has accelerated metabolism and catabolism caused by third-degree burns?

Client-centered goals place the focus on the client not the health care provider; they specify where the client is heading. Whenever possible, give the client the opportunity to actively participate in goal setting, even if the client's perception of need differs from yours. In matters that do not involve life or death, it is best to first address the client's concerns. Your primary consideration may be the patient's significant weight loss during the last 6 months of chemotherapy; the patient's major concern may be fatigue. The two issues are undoubtedly related but your effectiveness as a change agent is greater if you approach the problem from the client's perspective. Commitment to achieving the goal is greatly increased when the client "owns" the goal.

Keep in mind that the goal for all clients is to maintain or restore optimal nutritional status using foods they like and tolerate as appropriate. If possible, additional short-term goals may be to alleviate symptoms or side effects of disease or treatments and to prevent complications or recurrences if appropriate. After short-term goals are met, attention can center on promoting healthy eating to reduce the risk of chronic diet-related diseases such as obesity, diabetes, hypertension, and atherosclerosis.

Examples of client-centered goals in a community-based weight management program are

- Eat breakfast every day.
- On 3 days/week, replace the usual mid-morning snack of soda and a doughnut with sugar-free soda and a piece of fruit.
- Switch from regular margarine to diet margarine.
- Switch from whole milk to 2% milk.

Nursing Interventions

What can you or others do to effectively and efficiently help the client achieve his or her goals? Interventions may take the form of promoting an adequate and appropriate intake, teaching the client about nutrition, and monitoring the client's response.

Promoting an Adequate and Appropriate Intake

Throughout this book, the heading Nutrition Therapy is used in place of Diet because among clients, *diet* is a four-letter word with negative connotations such as counting calories, deprivation, sacrifice, and misery. A diet is viewed as a short-term punishment to endure until a normal pattern of eating can resume. Clients respond better to newer terminology that is less emotionally charged. Use terms such as *eating pattern, food intake, eating style,* or *the food you eat* to keep the lines of communication open.

Nutrition therapy recommendations are usually general suggestions to increase/decrease, limit/avoid, reduce/encourage, or modify/maintain aspects of the diet because exact nutrient requirements are determined on an individual basis. Where more precise amounts of nutrients are specified, consider them as a starting point and monitor the client's response.

Keep in mind that nutrition theory may not apply to practice. Factors such as the client's prognosis, outside support systems, level of intelligence and motivation, willingness to comply, emotional health, financial status, religious or ethnic background,

 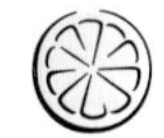

Career Connection

How can I promote an adequate intake?

- Reassure clients who are apprehensive about eating.
- Encourage a big breakfast if appetite deteriorates throughout the day.
- Advocate discontinuation of intravenous therapy as soon as feasible.
- Replace meals withheld for diagnostic tests.
- Promote congregate dining if appropriate.
- Question diet orders that appear inappropriate.
- Display a positive attitude when serving food or discussing nutrition.
- Order snacks and nutritional supplements.
- Request assistance with feeding or meal setup.
- Get the patient out of bed to eat if possible.
- Encourage good oral hygiene.
- Solicit information on food preferences.

and other medical conditions may cause the optimal diet to be impractical in either the clinical or the home setting. Generalizations do not apply to all individuals at all times. Also, comfort foods (e.g., chicken soup, mashed potatoes, ice cream) are valuable for their emotional benefits if not nutritional ones. Honor clients' requests for individual comfort foods whenever possible.

Client Teaching

Compared with "well" clients, patients in a clinical setting may be more receptive to nutritional advice especially if they feel better by doing so or are fearful of a relapse or complications. But hospitalized patients are also prone to confusion about nutrition messages. Time spent with a dietitian or diet technician learning about a "diet" may be brief or interrupted. Even if the "diet" represents a whole new eating style that is best achieved by making sequential changes, nutrition counseling in the hospital is often limited to one or two sessions with the dietitian. The patient may not even know what questions to ask until long after the dietitian is gone. The patient's ability to assimilate new information may be compromised by pain, medication, anxiety, or a distracting setting. Hospital menus or diets that differ from discharge orders add to the confusion.

Nutrition counseling by nurses *and* dietitians is more effective and efficient than that done by nurses *or* dietitians. First, the nurse is often available as a nutrition resource when dietitians are not, such as when trays are passed, during the evening, on weekends, and when the client is sitting on the edge of the bed fully dressed and waiting for transport home. In home care and wellness settings, dietitians may be available only on a consultative basis. Secondly, nurses reinforce nutrition counseling performed by dietitians: the more the message is repeated and the more people tell it, the more likely the message will stick. Finally, nurses initiate basic nutrition counseling for hospitalized clients with low to mild risk who may not have contact with a dietitian. The nurse has greatest con-

Career Connection

What can I do to facilitate client and family teaching?

- Listen to the client's concerns and ideas.
- Encourage family involvement if appropriate.
- Reinforce the importance of obtaining adequate nutrition.
- Help the client to select appropriate foods.
- Counsel the client about drug–nutrient interactions.
- Avoid using the term "diet."
- Emphasize things "to do" instead of things "not to do."
- Keep the message simple.
- Review written handouts with the client.
- Advise the client to avoid any foods that are not tolerated.

tact with the client, family, and other members of the health care team; the dietitian has nutrition and food expertise. Together, the nurse and dietitian form a strong alliance.

Nutritional Screen: a quick look at a few variables to judge a client's relative risk for nutritional problems. Can be custom designed for a particular population (e.g., pregnant women) or for a specific disorder (e.g., cardiac disease).

As an example, consider a male client of normal weight who is admitted to the hospital because of difficulty breathing. According to nutritional screening data, he is not at nutritional risk. You find that although his weight is within the normal range, he experienced progressive weight loss before admission because of shortness of breath and fatigue that interfered with eating. You seize the opportunity to suggest protein- and calorie-dense foods that are easy to prepare and consume such as instant breakfast made with whole milk, yogurt with cereal, whole-milk fruit smoothies, and cottage cheese with canned fruit. You also suggest that the client eat or drink every 2 hours. He admits that he considered this idea before but rejected it because he thought it would interfere with his appetite. You reassure him that planned nutritious snacks will add to rather than detract from his eating plan. You ask the dietitian to see the client in case there are other concerns or misconceptions. Without your intervention, his weight loss probably would have continued, increasing the risk of future health problems.

Monitoring

Think of monitoring as a precursor to evaluation in which you watch and document the impact of interventions on the client on an ongoing basis so that immediate concerns can be quickly addressed.

For example, after counseling a female employee at a worksite on how to manage mild hypertension through food choices and exercise, you suggest she stop by the health office every day during her lunch break so that you can take her blood pressure. During those visits you ask her specific questions: How many meatballs did you eat with your spaghetti last night? Was the sauce labeled "reduced sodium"? Did you double your normal portion of vegetables? What kind of milk are you drinking? How much exercise did you do yesterday? Her answers help you determine how well she understands the counseling information and how successfully she is implementing the strate-

 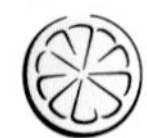

Career Connection

How do I stay on top of the client's nutrition?

- Observe intake whenever possible to judge the adequacy.
- Document appetite and take action when the client does not eat.
- Order supplements if intake is low or needs are high.
- Request a nutritional consult.
- Assess tolerance (i.e., absence of side effects).
- Monitor progress (e.g., weight gain).
- Monitor progression of restrictive diets. Clients who are receiving nothing by mouth (NPO), who are restricted to a clear liquid diet, or who are receiving enteral or parenteral nutrition are at risk for nutritional problems.
- Monitor the client's grasp of the information and motivation to change.

gies to achieve her goals. Talking about specific foods is likely to stimulate discussion that provides the client with more information, more options, or revised goals.

Ideally, behavior change occurs gradually and sequentially to become part of the client's new normal way of eating. In a less than perfect, time-challenged world, it is necessary to prioritize the client's needs and address the most important ones.

Evaluation

The optimal outcome of interventions is that the client's goals are completely met on a timely basis. But goals may be only partially met or not achieved at all; in those instances it is important to determine why the outcome was less than ideal. Were the goals realistic for this particular client? Were the interventions appropriate and consistently implemented? Evaluation includes deciding whether to continue, change, or abolish the plan.

Consider a male client admitted to the hospital for chronic diarrhea. During the 3 weeks before admission, the client experienced significant weight loss due to malabsorption secondary to diarrhea. Your goal is for the client to maintain his admission weight. Your interventions are to provide small meals of low-residue foods as ordered, to eliminate lactose because of the likelihood of intolerance, to increase protein and calories with appropriate nutrient-dense supplements, and to explain the nutrition therapy recommendations to the client to ease his concerns about eating. You find that the client's intake is poor because of lack of appetite and a fear that consumption of foods and fluids will promote diarrhea. You notify the dietitian, who counsels the client about low-residue foods, obtains likes and dislikes, and urges the client to think of the supplements as part of the medical treatment not as a food eaten for taste or pleasure. You document intake and diligently encourage the client to eat and drink everything served. However, the client's weight continues to drop. You attribute this to his reluctance to eat and to the slow resolution of diarrhea due to inflammation. You determine that the goal is still realistic and appropriate but that the client is not willing or able to consume foods orally. You consult with the physician and dietitian about the client's refusal to eat and the plan changes from an oral diet to tube feeding.

How Do You Respond?

Should I save my menus from the hospital to help me plan meals at home? This is not a bad idea if the in-house and discharge food plans are the same, but the menus should serve as a guide, not a gospel. Just because shrimp was never on the menu doesn't mean it is taboo. Likewise, if the client hated the orange juice served every morning, he or she shouldn't feel compelled to continue drinking it. By necessity, hospital menus are more rigid than at-home eating plans.

Can you just tell me what to eat and I'll do it? A black-and-white approach should be used only when absolutely necessary such as for food allergies or for clients who insist on a rigid plan rather than the flexibility of being able to decide for themselves. In most cases, advice should be as flexible as possible, even if the client insists it is not necessary to individualize the eating plan for his or her particular eating pattern. Individualization requires more work, but it is worth the effort for the flexibility it provides. Impress on the client that foods are not inherently good or bad except in special conditions. What matters more is how much, what kind, and how often a food is eaten.

▲ Focus on Critical Thinking

Respond to the following statements:

1. Nurses should not have to deal with nutrition.
2. "Ideal" weight is a misnomer.
3. It is possible to be overweight yet undernourished.
4. In the acute care setting, nutritional status is less important than medical treatments.

Key Concepts

- Through a routine history and physical, nurses can identify who may be at nutritional risk.
- Chronic or acute changes in health can impact nutritional status by altering intake, digestion, metabolism, or excretion of nutrients.
- A client may be at nutritional risk because of what he or she does or does not eat. Ask open-ended, non-leading questions to ascertain usual intake.
- Neither BMI nor "ideal" body weight may reliably assess health risk related to weight if muscle mass is large or edema is present. Nor does either method take into account where body fat is deposited.

 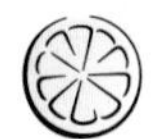

- Significant weight loss increases the risk of poor nutrition even if the weight loss was intentional.
- Medications and nutritional supplements should be evaluated for their potential impact on nutrient intake, absorption, utilization, or excretion.
- Physical signs and symptoms of malnutrition are nonspecific, subjective, and develop slowly. They can be considered suggestive of malnutrition but not diagnostic.
- Nursing diagnoses relate directly to nutrition when the client's intake of nutrients is too much or too little for body requirements. Many other nursing diagnoses, including constipation, impaired skin integrity, health-seeking behaviors, noncompliance, and risk for infection, relate indirectly to nutrition because nutrition contributes to the problem or solution.
- A nutrition priority for all clients is to obtain adequate calories and nutrients based on individual needs. Sometimes it is necessary to prioritize nutrient needs. Other priorities are to provide calories and nutrients in a form the client can use and, if possible, through foods familiar to and liked by the client. The client's nutrition priorities may be completely different from yours.
- Short-term nutrition goals are to attain or maintain adequate weight and nutritional status and (as appropriate) to avoid nutrition-related symptoms and complications of illness. Long-term goals are to promote healthy eating so as to avoid chronic diet-related diseases such as heart disease, hypertension, obesity, and type 2 diabetes. Help the client to formulate nutrition goals that are measurable, attainable, and specific.
- The term *diet* inspires negative feelings in most people. Replace it with *eating pattern, eating style,* or *foods you normally eat* to avoid negative connotations.
- Keep in mind that intake recommendations are not always appropriate for all persons, that clients' needs change, that what is recommended in theory may not work for an individual, and that clients may revert to comfort foods during periods of illness or stress.
- The term *counseling* means teaching plus brainstorming to help the client understand *and implement* intake recommendations. Nurses can reinforce nutrition counseling done by the dietitian and initiate counseling for clients with low or mild risk.
- Use preprinted lists of "do's and don'ts" only if absolutely necessary such as in the case of celiac disease. For most people, actual food choices should be considered in view of how much and how often they are eaten rather than as foods that "must" or "must not" be consumed.

ANSWER KEY

1. **FALSE** The nurse is in an ideal position to provide nutrition information to patients and their families since he or she is the one with the greatest client contact.
2. **TRUE** Nutritional status is loosely defined as the state of balance between nutrient supply and demand.
3. **TRUE** Clients may respond to the buzzword diet with an answer they think you expect. Asking if they avoid any particular foods or "watch" what they eat may be more revealing.

4. **FALSE** Changes in weight may be slow to occur. Weight changes are more reflective of chronic, not acute, changes in nutritional status.
5. **TRUE** A person can be malnourished without being underweight. Weight does not provide qualitative information about body composition.
6. **FALSE** Low serum albumin levels may be caused by problems other than protein malnutrition such as injury, infection, overhydration, and liver disease.
7. **TRUE** Weight loss is judged significant if there is a 5% loss over the course of 1 month.
8. **TRUE** People who take five or more prescription drugs, over-the-counter drugs, or dietary supplements are at increased risk for developing drug-induced nutrient deficiencies.
9. **FALSE** Specific lists of foods to choose and foods to avoid should be used only if absolutely necessary. It is important to focus on the quantity and frequency of foods consumed rather than absolute "do's" and "don'ts."
10. **TRUE** Physical signs and symptoms of malnutrition develop only after other signs of malnutrition, such as laboratory and weight changes, are observed.

WEBSITES

For Dietary Analysis and Intake Calculators, a variety of Dietary Assessment Tools, and Resource Information, go to "Dietary Assessment" Under Topics A-Z at the Food and Nutrition Information Center at **www.nal.usda.gov/fnic.html**

REFERENCES

American Dietetic Association. (2002). Position of the American Dietetic Association: Total diet approach to communicating food and nutrition information. *Journal of the American Dietetic Association, 102*(1), 100–108.

Chicago Dietetic Association, The South Suburban Dietetic Association, Dietitians of Canada. (2000). *Manual of clinical dietetics* (6th ed.). Chicago: American Dietetic Association.

Duyff, R. (2002). *The American Dietetic Association's complete food and nutrition guide* (2nd ed.). New York: John Wiley.

For information on the new dietary guidelines 2005 and MyPyramid, visit **http://connection.lww.com/go/dudek**

2

Carbohydrates

TRUE	FALSE	
⬭	⬭	**1** Starch is made from glucose molecules.
⬭	⬭	**2** Sugar is higher in calories than starch.
⬭	⬭	**3** The sugar in fruit is better for you than the sugar in candy.
⬭	⬭	**4** Most commonly consumed American foods provide adequate fiber to enable people to meet the recommended intake.
⬭	⬭	**5** Enriched bread is nutritionally equivalent to whole wheat bread.
⬭	⬭	**6** Soft drinks contribute more added sugars to the typical American diet than any other food or beverage.
⬭	⬭	**7** Bread is just as likely as candy to cause cavities.
⬭	⬭	**8** The sugar content on food labels refers only to added sugars, not those naturally present in the food.
⬭	⬭	**9** Artificial sweeteners are dangerous for most people.
⬭	⬭	**10** Sugar causes hyperactivity in kids.

UPON COMPLETION OF THIS CHAPTER, YOU WILL BE ABLE TO

- Name the types of carbohydrates and sources of each.
- Discuss the differences between refined and whole grains.
- Discuss the Nutrition Facts label as it applies to carbohydrates.
- Explain ways to limit sugar intake.
- Describe ways to increase fiber intake.
- Discuss the benefits and disadvantages of using sugar alternatives.

CARBOHYDRATES

"Sugar" and "starch" come to mind when people hear the word carbohydrates. But carbohydrates are so much more than just granulated sugar and bread. Chemically carbohydrates are monosaccharides, disaccharides, and polysaccharides; they differ in the number of sugar molecules they contain. From a nutritional standpoint, foods containing carbohydrates can be simply empty calories, nutritional powerhouses, or something in between. Globally, carbohydrates provide the majority of calories in almost all human diets. For dieters and diabetics, carbohydrates may be counted, coveted, or cursed.

This chapter describes what carbohydrates are, where they are found in the diet, and how they are handled in the body. The role of carbohydrates in health and recommendations regarding intake are presented.

Carbohydrate Classifications

Carbohydrates are classified as either simple carbohydrates or complex carbohydrates based on the number of single sugar molecules they contain.

Simple Carbohydrates

Simple carbohydrates include monosaccharides and disaccharides.

Monosaccharides

Fructose, galactose, and glucose are the simplest of all sugars; they are composed of just one (mono) sugar (saccharide) molecule. As basic units, these sugar molecules are absorbed "as is" without undergoing digestion.

Carbohydrates: a class of energy-yielding nutrients that contain only carbon, hydrogen, and oxygen, hence the common abbreviation of CHO.

Glucose (dextrose). Glucose is the sugar of greatest distinction: it circulates through the blood to provide energy for body cells; it is a component of all disaccharides and is virtually the sole constituent of complex carbohydrates; and it is the sugar the body converts all other digestible carbohydrates to. In foods, glucose is found in fruit, vegetables, honey, corn syrup, and cornstarch.

Fructose. Fructose ("fruit sugar") is found naturally in fruit and honey and is the sweetest of all natural sugars. High-fructose corn syrup (HFCS) is commercially made from the dextrose in cornstarch. Because it is much sweeter than sucrose, less fructose can be used to sweeten foods so the cost is less. HFCS is used extensively in soft drinks, fruit drinks, baked foods, and other products. Americans' intake of fructose as a proportion of total sugars is rising.

Simple Carbohydrates: a classification of carbohydrates that includes monosaccharides and disaccharides; commonly referred to as sugars.

Galactose. Galactose does not occur in appreciable amounts in foods; it is significant only as it combines with glucose to form the disaccharide lactose.

Disaccharides

Disaccharides are composed of two linked monosaccharides, at least one of which is glucose. Disaccharides are split into their component monosaccharides before being absorbed. Sucrose, maltose, and lactose are disaccharides.

Monosaccharide: single (mono) molecules of sugar (saccharide).

Sucrose. Sucrose, composed of glucose and fructose, is what is commonly called "sugar" or table sugar. It is produced when sucrose from sugarcane and sugar beets is refined

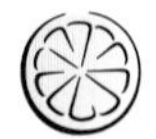

Disaccharide: "double sugar" composed of two (di) mono-saccharides.

and granulated. The differences among brown, white, confectioner's, and turbinado sugars have to do with the degree of refining. Sucrose also occurs naturally in some fruits and vegetables. Sucrose is sweeter than glucose but not as sweet as fructose.

Maltose. Maltose is composed of two joined glucose molecules. Maltose is not found naturally in foods, but it occurs as an intermediate in starch digestion.

Lactose. Lactose ("milk sugar") is composed of glucose and galactose. It is the carbohydrate found naturally in milk and is used as an additive in many foods and drugs. Lactose enhances the absorption of calcium and promotes the growth of friendly intestinal bacteria that produce vitamin K.

Complex Carbohydrates

Polysaccharide: carbohydrates consisting of many (poly) sugar molecules.

Complex carbohydrates are polysaccharides that include starch, glycogen, and fiber. Although they are composed of glucose molecules, polysaccharides do not taste sweet because their molecules are too large to fit on the tongue's taste bud receptors that sense sweetness.

Starch

Complex Carbohydrates: a group name for starch, glycogen, and fiber; composed of long chains of glucose molecules.

Plants synthesize glucose through the process of photosynthesis. Glucose not used by the plant for immediate energy is stored in the seeds, roots, stems, or tubers in the form of starch composed of hundreds to thousands of glucose molecules. When people eat plant foods, the resulting digestion reduces starch back to glucose.

Glycogen

Starch: the storage form of glucose in plants.

Glycogen is the animal (including human) version of starch: a stored carbohydrate available for energy as needed. Humans have a limited supply of glycogen stored in the liver and muscles. Liver glycogen breaks down and releases glucose into the bloodstream between meals to maintain normal blood glucose levels and provide fuel for tissues. Muscles do not share their supply of glycogen but use it for their own energy needs. There is virtually no dietary source of glycogen because any glycogen stored in animal tissue is quickly converted to lactic acid at the time of slaughter.

Fiber

Glycogen: storage form of glucose in animals and humans.

Dietary Fiber: carbohydrates and lignin that are natural and intact components of plants that cannot be digested by human enzymes.

Fiber is generally a mixture of nondigestible polysaccharides that are part of the plant cell wall or intercellular structure. Although nondigestible, fibers have important physiologic functions and provide significant health benefits.

Historically, fibers have been categorized as soluble or insoluble. Insoluble fibers include cellulose, many hemicelluloses, and lignins. They give texture to plant foods and are found in the skin of fruits, the shell of corn kernels, the covering of seeds, and the bran (outer layer) of grains. Insoluble fibers increase stool weight and thereby promote normal laxation. The richest sources of insoluble fiber are wheat bran, whole grains, dried peas and beans, and vegetables.

Soluble fibers include gums, pectins, some hemicelluloses, and mucilages. Apples, barley, dried peas and beans, fruits, vegetables, oatmeal, oat bran and rice hulls are rich in soluble fibers. Soluble fibers are credited with lowering serum cholesterol levels and improving glucose control in diabetics.

The National Academy of Sciences recommends that the terms insoluble and soluble be phased out in favor of ascribing specific physiologic benefits to a particular fiber. The rationale for discontinuing that terminology is that the amounts of soluble and insoluble fibers measured in a mixed diet are dependent on methods of analysis that are not able to exactly replicate human digestion. Also, although fibers are labeled as either soluble or insoluble, particular foods may have functional properties of both soluble and insoluble types of fiber. For instance, oats and oat bran function as a soluble fiber to lower cholesterol levels but also act like insoluble fiber to promote laxation. All sources of fiber provide a blend of both water-insoluble and water-soluble fibers.

How the Body Handles Carbohydrates

Digestion

Functional Fiber: as proposed by the Food and Nutrition Board, functional fiber consists of extracted or isolated nondigestible carbohydrates that have beneficial physiological effects in humans.

Total Fiber: total fiber = dietary fiber + added fiber.

Insoluble Fiber: nondigestible carbohydrates that do not dissolve in water.

Monosaccharides are the only form of carbohydrates the body is able to absorb intact and the form all other digestible carbohydrates must be reduced to before they can be absorbed (Fig. 2.1). For disaccharides, digestion is accomplished by simply splitting the double sugars into single molecules. For starches, digestion proceeds step by step as the long glucose chains are ultimately reduced to single glucose units. The human gastrointestinal tract lacks the enzymes needed to digest fibers.

Cooked starch begins to undergo digestion in the mouth by the action of salivary amylase, but the overall effect is small because food is not held in the mouth for a long time. The stomach serves to churn and mix its contents, but its acid medium halts any residual effect of the swallowed amylase. Most carbohydrate digestion occurs in the small intestine, where pancreatic amylase works to reduce complex carbohydrates into shorter chains and disaccharides. Disaccharidase enzymes (maltase, sucrase, and lactase) on the surface of the cells of the small intestine finish the process of digestion by splitting maltose, sucrose, and lactose respectively into monosaccharides. Normally 95% of starch is digested usually within 1 to 4 hours after eating.

Fibers are not digested but they influence the speed of digestion. Soluble fibers delay gastric emptying, which contributes to a feeling of satiety or fullness. Although they are not truly digested by enzymes, most fibers are fermented by bacteria in the colon to produce water, gas, other compounds, and short-chain fatty acids. These short-chain fatty acids are a source of energy for the mucosal lining of the colon.

Absorption

Soluble Fiber: nondigestible carbohydrates that dissolve to a gummy, viscous texture.

Glucose, fructose, and galactose, which are the end products of digestion, are absorbed through intestinal mucosa cells and travel to the liver via the portal vein. Small amounts of starch that have not been fully digested pass into the colon with fiber and are excreted in the stools. Fibers may impair the absorption of some minerals—namely calcium, zinc, and iron—by binding with them in the small intestine. Soluble fiber slows the absorption of glucose, thereby delaying and stifling the rise in serum glucose that occurs after eating.

Metabolism

Glucose, fructose, and galactose arrive at the liver via the portal vein where fructose and galactose are converted to glucose. The liver releases glucose into the bloodstream, where its level is held fairly constant by the action of hormones. A rise in blood

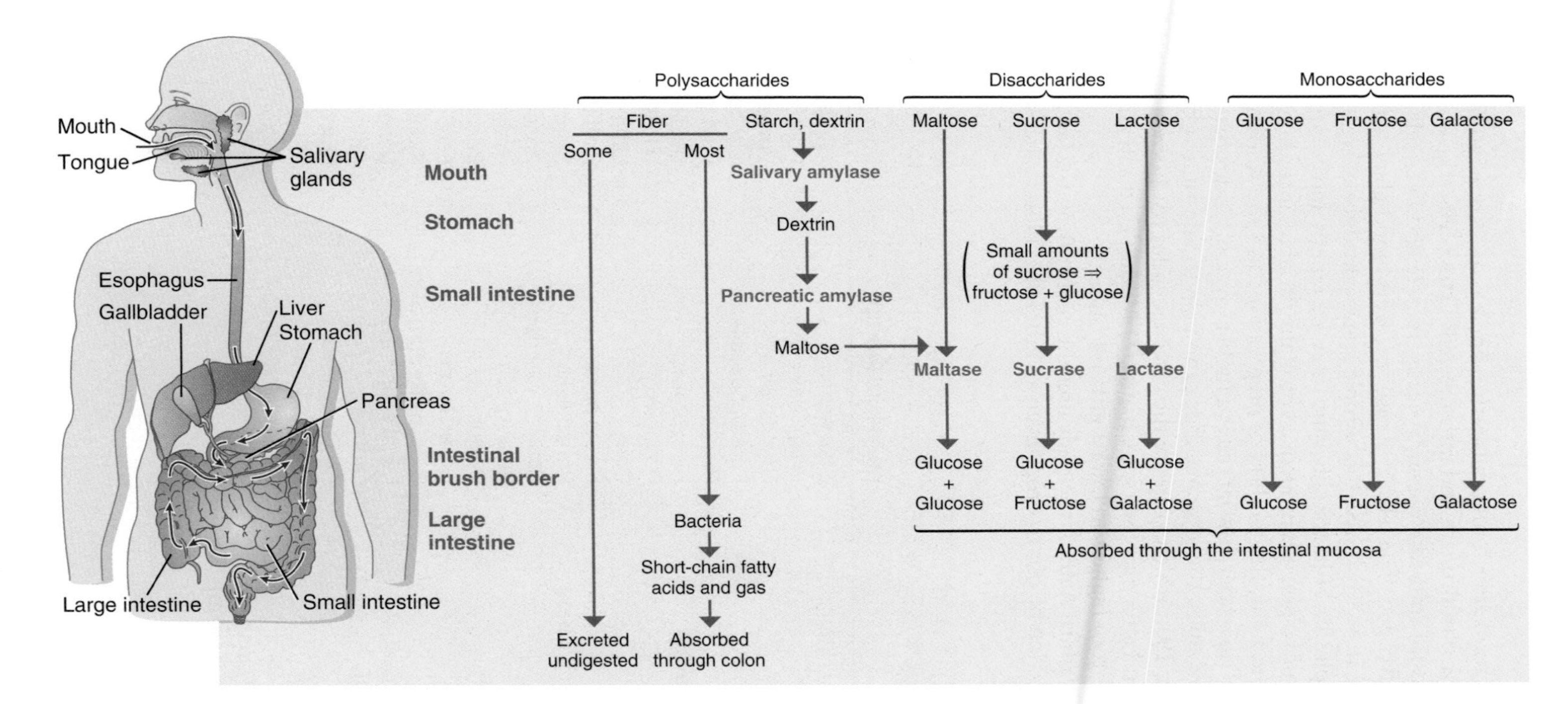

FIGURE 2.1 Carbohydrate digestion. Dietary carbohydrates include the polysaccharides or complex carbohydrates (fiber, starch, dextrin), the disaccharides (maltose, sucrose, lactose), and the monosaccharides (glucose, fructose, and galactose). Digestion begins in the *mouth,* where food is chewed into pieces and salivary amylase begins the process of chemical digestion. The *stomach* churns and mixes the carbohydrate, but stomach acids halt residual action of the salivary amylase. The *small intestine* is the site of most carbohydrate digestion, and pancreatic amylase reduces complex carbohydrates into disaccharides. Disaccharide enzymes (maltase, sucrase, and lactase) on the surface of the small intestine cells split maltose, sucrose, and lactose into monosaccharides, thus completing the process of carbohydrate digestion. Fiber is not digested per se, but most is fermented by bacteria in the *large intestine* to yield gas, water, and short-chain fatty acids.

Glycemic Response: the effect a food has on the blood glucose concentration: how quickly the glucose level rises, how high it goes, and how long it takes to return to normal.

glucose concentration after eating causes the pancreas to secrete insulin, which moves glucose out of the bloodstream and into the cells. Most cells take only as much glucose as they need for immediate energy needs; muscle and liver cells take extra glucose to store as glycogen. The release of insulin lowers blood glucose to normal levels.

Traditionally it was believed that simple sugars produce a greater glycemic response than complex carbohydrates because they are rapidly and completely absorbed. However, glycemic response is influenced by many variables including the amounts of fat and fiber in the food, the method of preparation, and the amount eaten. For instance, cornflakes (low fiber, low fat) have a higher glycemic index than does ice cream (high fat). For diabetics, the glycemic index can help to fine-tune optimal meal planning (see Chapter 19). Athletes can use the glycemic index to choose optimal fuels for before, during, and after exercise (see Chapter 7). Within each category in Table 2.1, foods are ranked from highest to lowest glycemic index.

In the postprandial state, as the body uses the energy from the last meal, the blood glucose concentration begins to drop. Even a slight fall in blood glucose stimulates the

TABLE 2.1 **GLYCEMIC INDICES OF SELECTED FOODS**

High (>60)	Moderate (40–60)	Low (<40)
Glucose	Bran muffin	Apple
Gatorade	Bran Chex	Pear
Potato, baked	Orange juice	PowerBar
Cornflakes	Potato, boiled	Chocolate milk
Rice cakes	Rice, white	Fruit yogurt, low-fat
Potato, microwaved	Rice, brown	Chickpeas
Jelly beans	Popcorn	P R Bar
Vanilla Wafers	Corn	Lima beans
Cheerios	Sweet potato	Split peas, yellow
Cream of Wheat (instant)	Pound cake	Skim milk
Graham crackers	Banana, overripe	Apricots, dried
Honey	Peas, green	Green beans
Watermelon	Bulgur	Banana, underripe
Bagel	Baked beans	Lentils
Bread, white	Rice, white parboiled	Kidney beans
Bread, whole wheat	Lentil soup	Barley
Shredded wheat	Orange	Grapefruit
Soft drink	All-Bran cereal	Fructose
Mars Bar	Spaghetti (no sauce)	
Grape-Nuts cereal	Pumpernickel bread	
Stoned Wheat Thins	Apple juice	
Cream of Wheat (regular)		
Table sugar		
Raisins		
Oatmeal		
Ice cream		

Glycemic Index: a numeric measure of the glycemic response of 50 g of a food sample; the higher the number, the higher the glycemic response.

 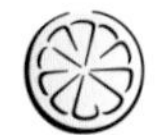

Career Connection

The types of carbohydrate eaten before, during, and after prolonged exercise influences an athlete's endurance. **Generally, athletes are advised to eat low glycemic index carbohydrates before prolonged exercise and moderate to high glycemic index carbohydrate foods during long distance events to ensure adequate glucose availability. After exercise, high glycemic index foods appear to enhance glycogen repletion compared to low glycemic index carbohydrates. While these recommendations have the potential to enhance an athlete's endurance, there is no way to estimate a food's glycemic index with the information available on the Nutrition Facts label. Products with similar total carbohydrate content and even similar ingredients on their labels can produce dramatically different glycemic responses. Data are needed to elucidate what kind, how much, and when carbohydrate foods should be consumed for optimal exercise endurance.**

pancreas to release glucagon, which causes the liver to release glucose from its supply of glycogen. The result is that blood glucose levels increase to normal.

Another hormone that influences blood glucose concentration is epinephrine, the "stress hormone" secreted by the adrenal gland. Epinephrine is quickly released during times of stress to make extra energy available for the "fight or flight" response. It works by stimulating the release of glucose from glycogen and inhibiting the secretion of insulin.

Functions of Carbohydrates

Glucose metabolism is a dynamic state of balance between burning glucose for energy (*catabolism*) and using glucose to build other compounds (*anabolism*). This process is a continuous response to the supply of glucose from food and the demand for glucose for energy needs.

Glucose for Energy

The primary function of carbohydrates is to provide energy for cells. Glucose is burned more efficiently and more completely than either protein or fat, and it does not leave an end product that the body must excrete. Although muscles use a mixture of fat and glucose for energy, the brain is totally dependent on glucose for energy. All digestible carbohydrates provide 4 cal/g consumed. (See Chapter 7 for details on how the body extracts energy from carbohydrates.)

As a primary source of energy, carbohydrates also spare protein and prevent ketosis.

Protein Sparing

Although protein provides 4 cal/g just like carbohydrates, it has other specialized functions that only protein can perform, such as replenishing enzymes, hormones, antibodies, and blood cells. Consuming adequate carbohydrate to meet energy needs has the effect of "sparing protein" from being used for energy, leaving it available to do its special functions. An adequate carbohydrate intake is especially important whenever protein needs are high such as for wound healing and during pregnancy and lactation.

Preventing Ketosis

Ketone Bodies: intermediate, acidic compounds formed from the incomplete breakdown of fat when adequate glucose is not available.

Fat normally supplies about half of the body's energy requirement. To efficiently and completely burn fat for energy, however, glucose fragments are needed. Without adequate glucose, fat oxidation prematurely stops at the intermediate step of ketone body formation. Although muscles and other tissues can use ketone bodies for energy, they are normally produced only in small quantities. An increased production of ketone bodies and their accumulation in the bloodstream causes nausea, fatigue, loss of appetite, and ketoacidosis. Dehydration and sodium depletion may follow as the body tries to excrete ketones in the urine. A minimum of 50 to 100 g of carbohydrates is needed daily to prevent ketosis.

Using Glucose to Make Other Compounds

After energy needs are met, excess glucose can be converted to glycogen, be used to make nonessential amino acids and specific body compounds, or be converted to fat and stored.

Glycogen

The body's backup supply of glucose is liver glycogen. Liver and muscle cells pick up extra glucose molecules during times of plenty and join them together to form glycogen, which can quickly release glucose in time of need. Typically one-third of the body's glycogen reserve is in the liver and can be released into circulation for all body cells to use and two-thirds is in muscle, which is available only for use by muscles. Unlike fat, glycogen storage is limited and may provide only enough calories for about a half-day of moderate activity.

Nonessential Amino Acids

If an adequate supply of essential amino acids is available, the body can use them and glucose to make nonessential amino acids.

Carbohydrate-Containing Compounds

The body can convert glucose to other essential carbohydrates such as ribose, a component of ribonucleic acid (RNA) and deoxyribonucleic acid (DNA), keratin sulfate (in fingernails), and hyaluronic acid (found in the fluid that lubricates the joints and vitreous humor of the eyeball).

Fat

Any glucose remaining at this point—after energy needs are met, glycogen stores are saturated, and other specific compounds are made—is converted by liver cells to triglycerides and stored in the body's fat tissue. The body does this by combining acetate molecules to form fatty acids, which then are combined with glycerol to make triglycerides. Although it sounds easy for excess carbohydrates to be converted to fat, it is not a primary pathway; the body prefers to make body fat from dietary fat, not carbohydrates.

Sources of Carbohydrates

Carbohydrates in food appear in the form of natural sugars, added sugars, starch, and fiber. One or more forms of carbohydrates are found in every MyPyramid group (Fig 2.2), with the exception of the Oils group. The amounts and types of carbohydrates vary considerably between food groups and among selections within each group.

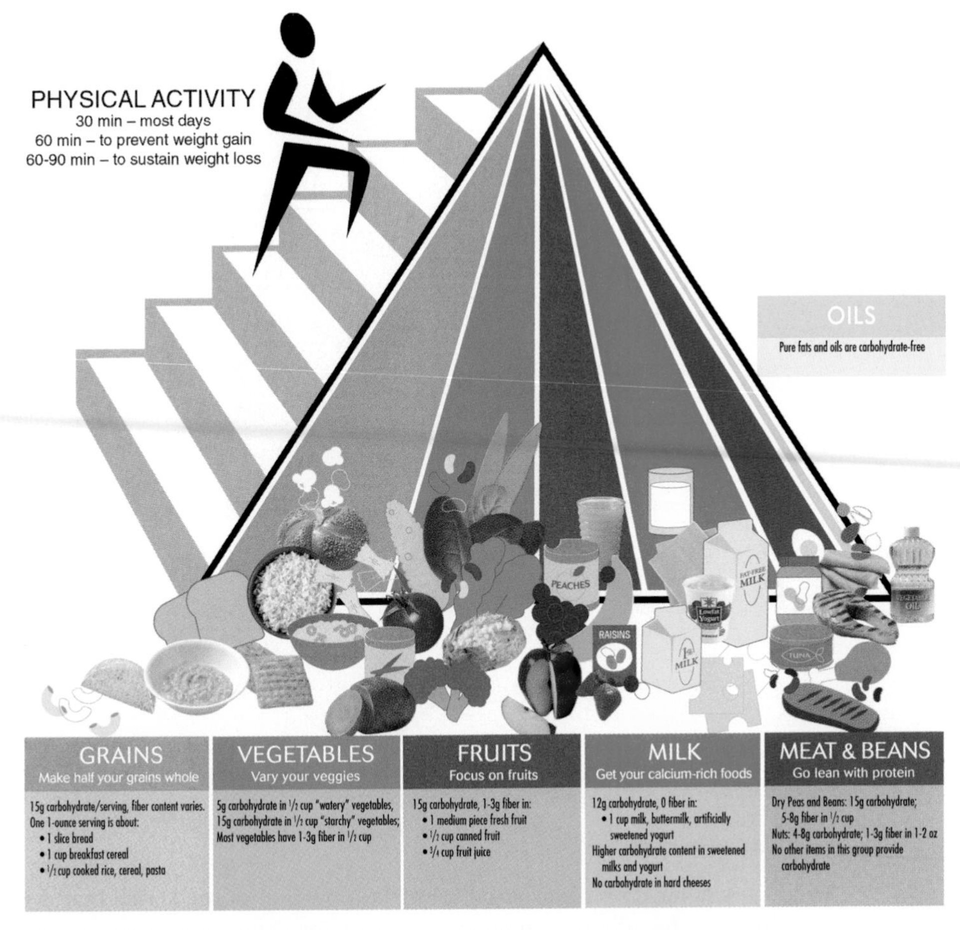

FIGURE 2.2 Carbohydrate content of MyPyramid groups.

Grains

Refined Grains and Refined Flours: consist of only the endosperm (middle part) of the grain and therefore do not contain the bran and germ portions.

This group is synonymous with "carbs" and consists of grains (e.g., wheat, barley, oats, rye, corn, and rice) and products made with flours from grains (e.g., items made with wheat flour, such as bread, crackers, pasta, and tortillas). Grains are classified as "whole" or "refined" (Fig 2.3).

"Whole" grains consist of the entire kernel of a grain, such as oatmeal, brown rice, whole wheat flour, and a whole kernel of corn. Whole grains, regardless of the variety, are composed of three parts:

- The bran, or tough outer coating, which is an excellent source of fiber and minerals.
- The endosperm, the largest portion of the kernel, which supplies all of the grain's starch. The endosperm is the basis of all flours.

Whole Grains and Whole Grain Flours: contain the entire grain, or seed, which includes the endosperm, bran, and germ.

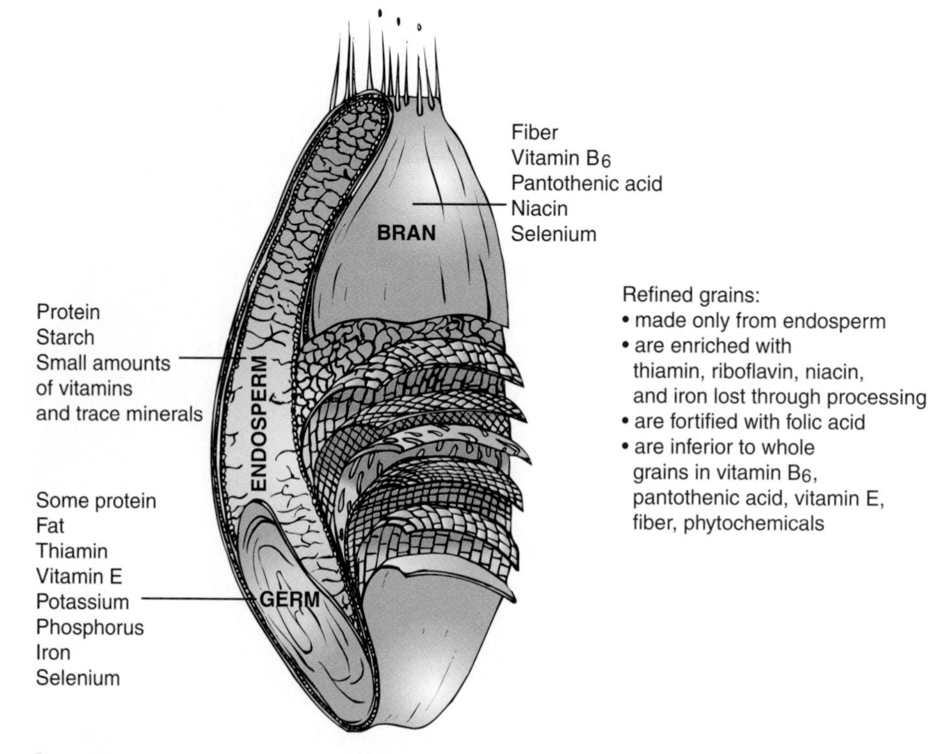

FIGURE 2.3 Whole wheat kernel. The components of the whole wheat kernel are the *bran*, the *germ*, and the *endosperm*.

- The germ (embryo), the smallest portion of the kernel that is rich in fat and provides vitamins, minerals, and some protein.

"Refined" grains consist only of the endosperm. They are rich in starch, but lack the fiber, vitamins, minerals, and phytochemicals found in whole grains. Enrichment is the process of adding back some of the nutrients that are lost in the milling process, namely thiamin, riboflavin, niacin, folate, and iron. Other substances that are lost, such as vitamin E and fiber, are not replaced by enrichment. Examples of refined grains include white flour, white bread, white rice, and refined cornmeal.

It is recommended that at least half of a person's grain choices be whole grain products, such as whole wheat bread, oatmeal, and whole wheat cereals. Many grain products, especially breads, are made from a combination of whole wheat flour and "enriched wheat flour" or "enriched flour," which mean white flour. Bran cereals are not truly whole grain because they are made only from the bran, but they are rich sources of fiber and other nutrients and thus are a healthy choice. Likewise, wheat germ is not a whole grain but is also nutritious.

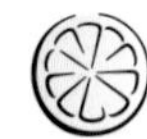

Vegetables

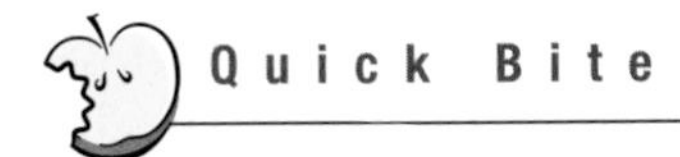

Dietary fiber content of various vegetables (per ½ cup serving unless otherwise noted)

	Fiber (g)		Fiber (g)
Starchy Vegetables		*Watery Vegetables*	
Split peas	8.1	Brussels sprouts	2
Lentils	7.8	Carrots	1.8
Kidney beans	4.5	Celery	1
Green peas	3.5	Iceberg lettuce	0.4
Corn	3	Alfalfa sprouts	0.4
Potato (boiled)	1.6		

Starch and some sugars provide the majority of calories in vegetables, but the content varies widely among individual vegetables. A serving of "starchy" vegetables provides approximately 15 g carbohydrate, the same amount as found in a slice of bread, whereas "watery" vegetables provide 5 g of carbohydrate or less per serving. The average fiber content is 1 to 3 g/serving. Vegetables provide insignificant amounts of fat and varying amounts of protein.

Fruits

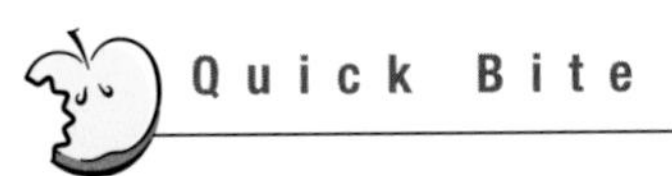

The effect of processing on fiber content

	Fiber, g/serving
Unpeeled fresh apple (1)	3.0
Peeled fresh apple (1)	1.9
Applesauce (½ cup)	1.5
Apple juice (¾ cup)	Negligible

Fruits contain mostly sugars with small amounts of starch and minute quantities of protein. Avocado, olives, and coconut are the only fruits that provide fat. Generally a serving of fruit, defined as ¾ cup of juice, 1 piece of fresh fruit, ½ cup of canned fruit, or ¼ cup dried fruit, provides 15 g of carbohydrate. On average, fruits provide approximately 1–3 g fiber/serving. Because fiber is located in the skin of fruits, fresh whole fruits provide more fiber than do fresh peeled fruits, canned fruits, or fruit juices.

Milk

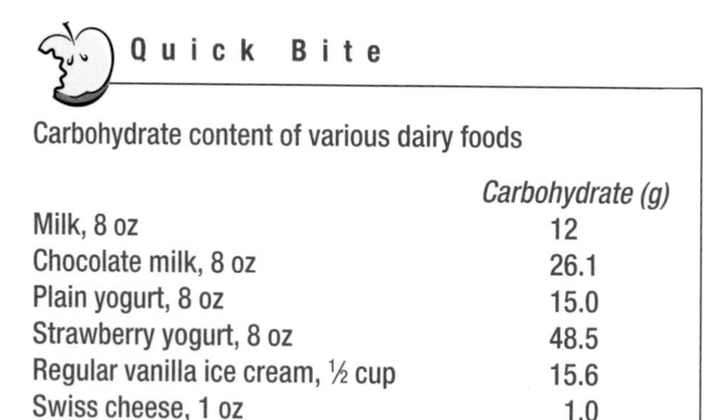

Quick Bite

Carbohydrate content of various dairy foods

	Carbohydrate (g)
Milk, 8 oz	12
Chocolate milk, 8 oz	26.1
Plain yogurt, 8 oz	15.0
Strawberry yogurt, 8 oz	48.5
Regular vanilla ice cream, ½ cup	15.6
Swiss cheese, 1 oz	1.0

Lactose is the carbohydrate found naturally in milk. One cup of milk, regardless of the fat content, provides 12 g of carbohydrate. Flavored milk and yogurt have added sugars, as do ice cream, ice milk, and frozen yogurt. With the exception of cottage cheese, which has about 6 g carbohydrate per cup, cheese is virtually lactose-free because it is converted to lactic acid during production. Because fiber is found only in plants, all items in this group are fiber free. The fat content of these products ranges from negligible to high.

Meat and Beans

This group is synonymous with *protein,* yet the plants in this group, namely nuts and dried peas and beans, also provide starch and fiber. Although the majority of calories in nuts are from fat, most varieties of nuts have 4 to 8 g of carbohydrates per 1-ounce serving. Dry peas and beans, which are technically vegetables, are considered part of this group because they are excellent sources of vegetable protein. One-half cup of dried peas and beans provides approximately 15 g of carbohydrate with 5 to 8 g of fiber.

Oils

Pure fats and oils, such as olive oil and butter, are carbohydrate-free. Other foods in this group that are mainly oil, such as mayonnaise and margarine, are also considered carbohydrate-free.

Discretionary Calories

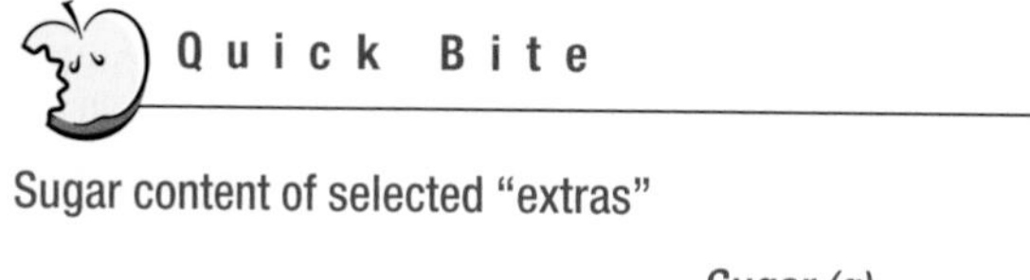

Quick Bite

Sugar content of selected "extras"

	Sugar (g)
White sugar, 1 tsp	4.0
Brown sugar, 1 tsp	4.5
Jelly, 1 tsp	4.5
Gelatin, ½ cup	19.0
Cola drink, 12 oz	40.0

Discretionary calories refer to the "extras" that may be added to the diet after the minimum calories to meet nutrient requirements have been consumed. Because it is a "catch-all" group, the carbohydrate content varies considerably, from none in items like whole milk and sausage to 100% of the calories in syrup, sweetened sodas, and hard candies.

 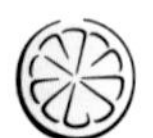

Career Connection

Although leading health authorities recommend that the majority of calories in the diet come from carbohydrate, they don't mean just ANY carbohydrate. Specifically, the recommendation is to eat a diet based on whole grain breads and cereals, with plenty of fruits, vegetables, and dried peas and beans—not an ad lib intake of products made with white flour and white sugar. A fat-free coffee cake *is* high in carbohydrates but fails to deliver the nutrient dense package of vitamins, minerals, and phytochemicals important for disease prevention. Emphasize to clients that "high carbohydrate" is only half the story: high carbohydrate should be achieved with wholesome, unprocessed foods for optimum health benefits and weight management.

Intake Recommendations

The Recommended Dietary Allowance (RDA) for carbohydrate is set at 130 g for both adults and children, the average minimum amount needed to fuel the brain. However, at this level, total energy needs are not met unless protein and fat intakes exceed levels considered healthy. The median carbohydrate intake among adult men is 200 to 330 g/day and among women, 180 to 230 g/day. The Acceptable Macronutrient Distribution range for carbohydrates is 45% to 65% of calories.

An Adequate Intake for total fiber is set at 25 g/day for women and 38 g/day for men, which is approximately double the median intake of approximately 12 to 14 g/day for women and 16.5 to 18 g/day for men.

Most leading health authorities recommend that carbohydrates provide the majority of calories in the diet, mostly in the form of complex carbohydrates. At least half of all grain choices should be whole grain products. The Nutrition Facts label uses 60% of total calories to arrive at the Daily Value for carbohydrate (Table 2.2).

TABLE 2.2 **DAILY VALUE FOR CARBOHYDRATES ON THE NUTRITION FACTS LABEL**

	Daily Value Based on a Total Calorie Intake of	
	2000 Calories	**2500 Calories**
Total carbohydrate	300 g	375 g
Fiber	25 g	30 g
Sugar	no daily value	no daily value

CARBOHYDRATES IN HEALTH PROMOTION

Regarding carbohydrate intake, Americans are urged to increase their intake of fiber and limit consumption of added sugars.

Getting Enough Fiber

The Health Benefits of Fiber

Fiber is important for maintaining health and preventing disease. Generally, foods high in fiber are lower in calories than refined and processed foods. Because of their bulk and the feeling of fullness they provide, high-fiber foods may aid weight management. High-fiber foods such as whole grains, legumes, vegetables, and fruits are also major sources of micronutrients and phytochemicals that may be protective against chronic disease. Clearly there are benefits to consuming adequate amounts of fiber, particularly in preventing or treating constipation, diverticular disease, obesity, cardiovascular disease, and type 2 diabetes. Fiber may also be protective against colon and breast cancers.

Constipation

The most consistent benefit of consuming adequate fiber is to relieve or prevent constipation. Fibers in dried peas and beans, whole grains, and bran increase stool weight; the large, soft stool mass stimulates the colon to contract, propelling the contents toward excretion. The increase in stool weight is attributed to the fiber content in the stool, the water the fiber holds, and the increase in the amount of bacteria in the stool from fermentation of fiber in the colon.

Diverticular Disease

Diverticula, pouches that protrude outward from the muscular wall of the intestine, are caused by increased pressure within the intestinal lumen as the bowel uses strong contractions to move a small stool mass through the gut. A high-fiber diet prevents formation of diverticula by providing adequate bulk, which requires less forceful contractions. Once diverticula have formed, a high-fiber diet is used to prevent additional diverticula from forming but it cannot reverse existing diverticula.

Obesity

Studies show weight gain is inversely related to the intake of high-fiber, whole-grain foods but positively related to the intake of refined-grain foods. Adequate fiber may help to prevent or treat obesity because high-fiber foods

- Are generally less calorically dense that refined foods, which may bring about a natural decrease in calories
- Are high in bulk, which means they may take longer to consume and may promote a quicker feeling of fullness
- Delay gastric emptying, leaving a person fuller over a longer period of time

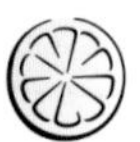

Cardiovascular Disease

Viscous fibers, such as those found in oatmeal, oat bran, dried peas and beans, apples, barley, fruits, and vegetables, lower blood cholesterol levels, specifically LDL-cholesterol (the "bad" cholesterol). It appears that bile acids become trapped in the viscous fiber–food mixture in the intestines and are excreted. To replace these bile acids lost in the stool, LDL-cholesterol is removed from the blood and sent to the liver where it is synthesized into bile acids. It is also speculated that changes in the bile acid pool related to the intake of viscous fibers may lower blood cholesterol levels by inhibiting endogenous cholesterol synthesis. By lowering cholesterol levels, fiber decreases the risk of cardiovascular disease. Studies focusing on breakfast cereals show an inverse relationship between whole-grain cereal intake and both total mortality and CVD-specific mortality that is not observed when refined-grain breakfast cereals are consumed.

Type 2 Diabetes

Although it is not entirely clear how fiber affects insulin requirements or sensitivity, viscous fibers slow gastric emptying rates, digestion, and the absorption of glucose to delay and stifle the rise in postprandial glucose in diabetics. Studies with type 2 diabetics suggest that high-fiber intakes lower the need for insulin.

In terms of diabetes prevention, diets high in whole grains are associated with a decreased risk of diabetes related to the fiber content but also perhaps from the action of nutrients provided in whole grains such as vitamin E and magnesium.

Breast and Colon Cancers

Although results of studies are inconsistent, it appears that fiber protects against colon cancer. Colon cancer risk appears to be inversely related to stool weight: the greater the stool weight (the result of a high-fiber diet), the lower the risk of colon cancer. Although studies on the role of fiber in preventing breast cancer are conflicting, international comparisons show an inverse relationship between breast cancer death rates and the intake of high-fiber foods.

Increasing Fiber Intake

The recommendation to eat more fiber—25 to 38 g/day—is not qualified as to how much of which types of fiber. In the first place, fiber does not fit the definition of an essential nutrient that must be consumed through food in order to prevent a deficiency disease; the need for fiber is based on its physiologic effects in the body. For instance, people who are prone to constipation benefit from eating more fiber, whereas people with rapid transit times do not "need" more fiber. Likewise, someone with a high blood cholesterol concentration may experience a drop in the cholesterol level from eating more high-fiber foods, whereas a person with a normal level may see no change from eating more fiber. Secondly, fiber is the carbohydrate that remains after digestion. Because digestion is difficult to replicate in a laboratory, methods for measuring dietary fiber may not be valid. Finally, it is difficult to calculate fiber intake because (1) current data on fiber content may not be accurate, (2) data on total fiber content are not available for all food sources, and (3) data on the amount of specific types of fiber (e.g., cellulose, hemicellulose, pectin) are even more scarce. Inherent in the general recommendation to eat more fiber are the following points: individual tolerance to fiber must be considered, and it is important to consume a variety of fiber sources because different sources provide different types and proportions of specific fibers.

Currently the usual intake of fiber among Americans is approximately one-half the recommended level for both men and women. That is because most popular American foods are not high in fiber: grains, vegetables, and fruits commonly eaten provide only 1 to 3 g/serving. Richer sources of fiber, namely dried peas and beans, whole grain breads, and high-fiber cereals, are not routinely eaten. To increase the intake of fiber, encourage clients to

Replace refined grains with whole grains. Examples of whole grains appear in Table 2.3. Ideally all grain choices should be whole grain—but if not all, then at least half. Whole-grain breads have "whole wheat flour," "100 percent whole wheat flour," or "stone ground whole wheat flour" listed as the first ingredient.

Choose a ready-to-eat cereal with 5 grams of fiber or more per serving. Whole-grain and bran cereals offer variety, convenience, fiber, and lots of nutrition in a low-fat package. Without a high-fiber cereal in the diet, it is difficult to consistently consume adequate fiber in the typical American diet.

Eat dried peas and beans two to three times/week. Dried peas and beans are excellent sources of both insoluble and soluble fibers and are a fat-free alternative to meat. Try meatless entrees featuring beans such as bean burritos, minestrone soup, hummus on pita bread, or meatless chili.

Eat at least five servings of fruits and vegetables daily. Do not peel fruits or vegetables. Peeling cuts the fiber content of potatoes in half and reduces fiber from fruits by 25%. Edible seeds, such as those found in strawberries, kiwifruit, tomatoes, and

TABLE 2.3 **SOURCES OF REFINED AND WHOLE GRAINS**

	Refined	Whole Grain
Wheat	white flour, wheat flour (except "whole wheat" flour), white pasta, Cream of Wheat, puffed wheat, flour tortillas, pretzels	whole wheat flour; bread with whole wheat, 100% whole wheat, or stone ground wheat flour listed as the first ingredient on the label; whole wheat pasta; shredded wheat, Wheaties, wheat berries, bulgur, cracked wheat
Oats	oat flour	oatmeal, Cheerios
Corn	cornstarch, cornflakes, grits, hominy	corn
Rice	white rice, Rice Krispies, Cream of Rice, puffed rice	brown rice
Barley	pearl barley	whole grain barley
Other		amaranth, millet, quinoa, sorghum, triticale

 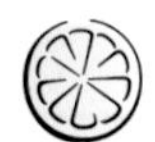

cucumbers, contribute significant fiber. Whole and fresh fruits and vegetables have more fiber than canned ones. Juices have negligible fiber.

Eat a variety of plant foods daily. The types and amounts of fiber in strawberries differ from those in kidney beans, which differ from those in bran cereal, which differ from those in oatmeal. However, there do not seem to be differences in fiber content among different varieties of the same foodstuff; for instance, the fiber content of apples is consistent among Granny Smith, Macintosh, Cortland, and Delicious varieties. Eating a variety of plant foods means choosing different foods, not different varieties of the same food.

Increase fiber intake gradually to avoid GI intolerance. Cramping, increased gas, and diarrhea can occur in some people when fiber intake is increased too quickly. Clients should be urged to increase fiber as individual tolerance allows.

Consume adequate fluid. Fiber functions by holding water. Recommend at least 8 to 10 glasses of fluid daily.

Sugar: Too Much of a Good Thing

In foods, sugar adds flavor and interest. Few would question the value brown sugar adds to a bowl of hot oatmeal. Besides its sweet taste, sugar has important functions in baked goods. In yeast breads, sugar promotes fermentation by serving as food for the yeast. Sugar in cakes promotes tenderness and a smooth crumb texture. Cookies owe their crisp texture and light-brown color to sugar. In jams and jellies sugar inhibits the growth of mold; in candy it influences texture. Sugar has many functional roles in foods including taste, physical properties, antimicrobial purposes, and chemical properties.

In the body, sugar is frequently blamed for a variety of health problems, including

Behavioral problems in children. However, evidence that sugar causes hyperactivity is lacking, even among children who are reported to be sensitive to sugar.

Obesity. Obesity is a complex problem that cannot simply be blamed on one factor. Total calorie intake is important as are activity patterns, reasons for eating, fat grams, and sugar grams. However, sugar-sweetened beverages in particular have been suggested to promote obesity. It appears that when extra calories are consumed in solid form, people tend to eat less at subsequent meals to compensate for those calories but when extra calories are consumed in liquid form, compensation is incomplete or absent. The consumption of soft drinks correlates to an increase in calorie intake.

Diabetes mellitus. For type 2 diabetes, too many calories and too much body weight are the problem, not specifically too much sugar.

Heart disease. Diets very low in fat (<20% total calories) and high in carbohydrate may alter lipoprotein levels, specifically lipoproteins that cause atherosclerosis. High sugar diets in particular are linked to increased triglyceride levels and increased risk of coronary heart disease.

The Downside of Sugar

Avoiding too much sugar is prudent because sugar promotes dental caries and provides empty calories that may make it difficult to consume adequate levels of nutrients without exceeding calorie needs.

Dental Caries

Feeding from sugars and starches, bacteria residing in the mouth produce an acid that erodes tooth enamel. Although whole-grain crackers and orange juice are more nutritious than caramels and soft drinks, their potential damage to teeth is the same. How often carbohydrates are consumed, what they are eaten with, and how long after eating brushing occurs may be more important than whether or not they are "sticky." Anticavity strategies include the following:

- Choose between-meal snacks that are healthy and teeth-friendly such as fresh vegetables, apples, cheese, and popcorn.
- Limit between-meal carbohydrate snacking including drinking soft drinks.
- Avoid high-sugar items that stay in the mouth a long time such as hard candy, suckers, and cough drops.
- Brush promptly after eating.
- After eating, chew gum sweetened with sugar alcohols (e.g., sorbitol, mannitol, xylitol) or with nonnutritive sweeteners. This may reduce the risk of cavities by stimulating production of saliva, which helps to rinse the teeth and neutralize plaque acids. Unlike sucrose and other nutritive sweeteners, sugar alcohols and artificial sweeteners are not fermented by bacteria in the mouth so they do not promote cavities.
- Use fluoridated toothpaste.

Empty Calories

Empty-calorie foods provide calories with few or no other nutrients. Consumption of empty-calorie foods *in place of* nutrient-dense foods results in lower levels of nutrients per total calorie intake. For instance, people who eat diets high in sugar consume less calcium, fiber, zinc, iron, folate and vitamins A, C, and E than people with low intakes of added sugar. Empty-calorie foods *added to* a meal plan cause calories to increase while the nutrient intake remains unchanged. With either scenario, the ratio of nutrients to calories decreases; that is, the meal plan becomes less nutrient-dense.

How Much Is Enough?

The *Dietary Guidelines for Americans* (see Chapter 8) recommends that people choose and prepare foods and beverages with little added sugars or caloric sweeteners. Under the theme of "moderation," MyPyramid recommends Americans choose forms of foods that do not have added sugar.

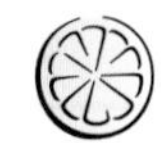

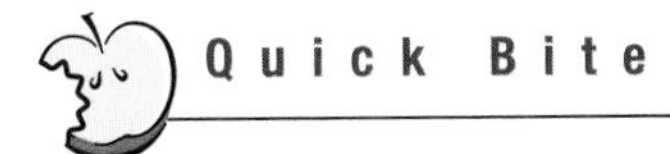

Quick Bite

The most common sources of added sugars in the American diet

Soft drinks
Cakes, cookies, pies
Fruit drinks and punches
Dairy desserts such as ice cream
Candy

According to U.S. Food Supply Data, Americans' per capita consumption of added sugars went from 27 teaspoons/person/day in 1970 to 32 teaspoons/person/day in 1996, far in excess of the FGP recommendations at any calorie level. As food consumption surveys indicate, Americans are eating more calories today than they were 2 decades ago, and the majority of the increase is from carbohydrates, primarily as soft drinks.

To limit the intake of sugar, encourage clients to

Cut back or eliminate sugar-sweetened soft drinks. Because soft drinks are the biggest source of added sugars in many diets, eliminating them can make a big impact on sugar intake. In fact, every 12 oz can of soft drink provides 9 to 10 teaspoons of added sugar. Water, flavored water, and diet sodas are sugar-free alternatives to sweetened soft drinks. Using low fat milk or 100% fruit juice in place of soft drinks may not impact total calorie intake, but vitamin and mineral intake will increase.

Rely on natural sugars in fruit to satisfy a "sweet tooth." Besides being less concentrated in sugars than candy, cookies, pastries, and cakes, fruits boost nutrient and fiber intake.

Cut sugar in home-baked products, if possible. Although reducing the amount of sugar in some foods does not appreciably alter taste or other qualities, in others it can be disastrous. For instance, because sugar in jams and jellies inhibits the growth of mold, less sugar results in a product that supports mold growth.

Check labels. Although Nutrition Facts labels (see Chapter 8) list the amount of total carbohydrates and sugars per serving, they do not include sugar alcohols and do not distinguish between natural and added sugars. People concerned with limiting sugar who confine their focus to the grams of sugar per serving may inappropriately conclude that foods high in natural sugars, such as milk and fruit juice, should be avoided. When judging the value of a food high in sugar, it is important to look beyond sugar grams to the whole package. What other nutrients are provided and are they present in significant amounts? Are the sugars naturally present or are they added? Box 2.1 lists sources of added sugars. The more added sugars on the ingredient label and the closer to the beginning of the list they appear, the higher the content of added sugar in that product.

Consider using sugar alternatives such as sugar alcohols or artificial sweeteners. On the plus side, sugar alternatives are low in calories or calorie-free; they do not produce a rise in blood glucose levels and do not promote tooth decay because they are not fermented by mouth bacteria. On the downside, the use of sugar alternatives does not guarantee lower calorie intake. Sugar-free is not synonymous with calorie-free (see section below on sugar alternatives).

BOX 2.1 **SOURCES OF ADDED SUGARS**

Brown sugar
Cane sugar
Confectioner's sugar
Corn sweeteners
Corn syrup
Crystallized cane sugar
Dextrose
Evaporated cane juice
Fructose
Fruit juice concentrate
Glucose
High-fructose corn syrup (HFCS)
Honey
Invert sugar
Lactose
Malt
Maltose
Molasses
Raw sugar
Sucrose
Turbinado sugar

Sugar Alternatives

Alternatives to sugar arise from Americans' desire to "have their cake and eat it too." People want the taste of sweetness without feeling guilty about the calories. The food industry has responded to this demand by developing numerous low-calorie and calorie-free (nonnutritive) sweeteners.

Sugar Alcohols

Sugar alcohols (e.g., sorbitol, mannitol, xylitol) are natural sweeteners derived from monosaccharides. Sorbitol and mannitol are 50% to 70% as sweet as sucrose; xylitol has the same sweetness as sucrose. Although small amounts of sugar alcohols are found in some fruits and berries, most are commercially synthesized and used as alternatives to sugar. They are considered low-calorie sweeteners because they are incompletely absorbed, so their calorie value ranges from 1.6 to 2.6 cal/g. This slow and incomplete absorption causes them to produce a smaller effect on blood glucose levels and insulin secretion than sucrose does.

Sugar alcohols are approved for use in a variety of products, including candies, chewing gum, jams and jellies, baked goods, and frozen confections. Some people experience a laxative effect (abdominal gas, discomfort, osmotic diarrhea) after consuming sorbitol or mannitol. In small amounts and in products that stay in the mouth a long time, such as chewing gum and breath mints, sugar alcohols offer sweetness without promoting cavities.

Artificial Sweeteners

Artificial Sweeteners: synthetically made sweeteners that do not provide calories.

Artificial sweeteners are virtually calorie-free and hundreds of times sweeter than sugar. Sometimes combinations of artificial sweeteners are used in a food to produce a synergistically sweeter taste, decrease the amount of sweetener needed, and minimize aftertaste. Because they do not raise blood glucose levels, artificial sweeteners appeal to diabetics. The five artificial sweeteners approved by the FDA for use in the United States are featured in Table 2.4.

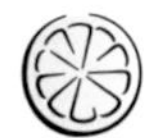

TABLE 2.4

ARTIFICIAL SWEETENERS APPROVED FOR USE IN THE U.S.

Sweetener	Sweetness (Sucrose = 1)	Taste Characteristics	Uses	Comments
Saccharin (Sweet Twin, Sweet 'n Low)	200–700	Persistent aftertaste; bitter at high concentrations	Soft drinks, assorted foods, tabletop sweetener	Potential (weak) carcinogen; the FDA has officially withdrawn its proposed ban so warning labels no longer required
Aspartame (Nutrasweet, Equal, Spoonful)	180	Similar to sucrose; no aftertaste	Tabletop sweeteners, dry beverage mixes, chewing gum, beverages, confections, fruit spreads, toppings, and fillings	Made from the amino acids aspartic acid and phenylalanine; people with PKU (phenylketonuria) must avoid aspartame
Acesulfame K (Sunette, Sweet One)	130–200	Bitter aftertaste like saccharin	Tabletop sweeteners, dry beverage mixes, and chewing gum	Often mixed with other sweeteners to synergize the sweetness and minimize the aftertaste. Not digested; excreted unchanged in the urine
Sucralose (Splenda)	600	Maintains flavor even at high temperatures	Soft drinks, baked goods, chewing gums, and tabletop sweeteners	Poorly absorbed; excreted unchanged in the feces
Neotame	8000	Clean, sugar-like taste; enhances flavors of other ingredients	Approved as general-purpose sweetener	Made from aspartic acid and phenylalanine but is not metabolized to phenylalanine so a warning label is not required

Are They a Good Idea?

At first glance, artificial sweeteners appear to answer Americans' passion for calorie-free sweetness. But do they really help people to manage their weight? Are they appropriate for diabetics? Are they safe for everyone, including pregnant women and children?

Weight management. Nonnutritive sweeteners are not a panacea for weight control. In theory, use of nonnutritive sweeteners in place of sugar can save 16 cal/teaspoon, or 160 cal in a 12-ounce can of cola. Eliminating one regularly sweetened soft drink per day for 22 days (160 cal × 22 days = 3520 cal) translates to a 1-pound loss (3500 calories equals 1 pound of body weight) without any other changes in eating or activity. This is because *all* calories in the regular soft drink have been eliminated. But foods whose calories come from a mixture of sugar, starch, protein, and fat still provide calories after sugar calories are reduced or eliminated. For instance, sugar-free cookies can provide as many or more calories than cookies sweetened with sugar. Many people falsely believe that low sugar means low calories; they, therefore, overeat because they overestimate the calories saved by replacing sugar. Ironically the prevalence of obesity has increased significantly as the intake of nonnutritive sweeteners has increased. Artificial sweeteners may help to manage weight but only when they are used within the context of an otherwise varied, balanced, and calorie-appropriate meal plan.

Diabetes mellitus. Contrary to what was previously believed, regular sugar does not raise blood glucose levels more than complex carbohydrates do; a food's glycemic index is influenced by several factors, not just sugar content. The focus in management of blood glucose levels has shifted from avoiding simple sugars to maintaining a relatively consistent total carbohydrate intake with less emphasis on the source. For that reason, sweets can be included within the context of a nutritious, calorie-appropriate, diabetic diet. However, because most type 2 diabetics are overweight, substitution of calorie-free sweets for calorie-containing ones has the potential to improve blood glucose levels by promoting weight management.

Acceptable Daily Intake (ADI): the estimated amount of artificial sweetener per kilogram of body weight that a person can safely consume every day over a lifetime without risk; usually reflects an amount 100 times less than the maximum level at which no observed adverse effects have occurred in animal studies.

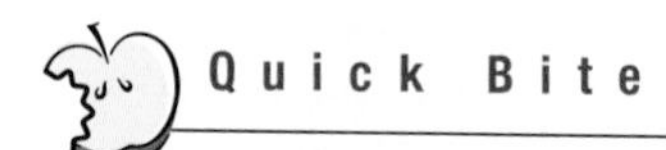

The number of artificially sweetened soft drinks a 130-pound person can consume daily before meeting the ADI for each particular sweetener

Saccharin	1
Aspartame	24
Acesulfame-K	20

Safety. The FDA is responsible for approving the safety of all food additives, including artificial sweeteners. An acceptable daily intake (ADI) is established as a safety limit for each sweetener. For instance, the ADI of aspartame is 50 mg/kg of body weight; currently, aspartame users consume an average of just 3.0 g/kg, or 6% of the safety limit.

For most adults, nonnutritive sweeteners are safe when used within approved guidelines; for pregnant women, the issue is less straightforward. Some physicians recommend that women avoid all artificial sweeteners during pregnancy; others suggest that they may be used in moderation. The position of the American Dietetic Association is that saccharin, aspartame, acesulfame-K, sucralose, and neotame are safe during pregnancy when consumed in amounts within ADI.

Saccharin has not been well studied in children, so caution is advised. Other artificial sweeteners are relatively safe for children with the exception of aspartame for children with PKU. The qualifier *relatively* refers to the fact that any substance becomes toxic at some level, but average consumption of artificial sweeteners among children is less than the ADI set for them. But even if they are relatively safe, are they really necessary? Regular sugar, which is the alternative to artificial sweeteners, is not plagued with safety concerns and can fit within the context of a nutritious and balanced meal plan. One must look at the risk–benefit ratio to decide if use of artificial sweeteners is appropriate for children.

How Do You Respond?

Aren't carbohydrates fattening? At 4 cal/g, carbohydrates are no more fattening than protein and are less than half as fattening as fat at 9 cal/g. Whether or not a food is "fattening" has more to do with portion size and frequency than if the food gets its calories from carbohydrates, protein, or fat.

"Light" breads are high in fiber. Can I use them in place of whole-grain breads? So-called light breads usually have processed fiber from peas or other foods substituted for some starch; the result is a lower-calorie, higher-fiber bread that may help to prevent constipation but lacks the unique "package" of vitamins, minerals, and phytochemicals found in whole grains.

▲ Focus on Critical Thinking

Respond to the following statements:

1. Carbohydrates form the foundation of a healthy diet.
2. Too much sugar increases the risk of obesity.
3. Artificial sweeteners can help people to manage weight.
4. With fiber, the more the better.

Key Concepts

- Carbohydrates, which are found almost exclusively in plants, provide the major source of energy in almost all human diets.
- The two major groups are simple carbohydrates (monosaccharides and disaccharides) and complex carbohydrates (polysaccharides).
- Monosaccharides and disaccharides are composed of one or two sugar molecules respectively. They vary in sweetness.
- Polysaccharides, namely starch, glycogen, and fiber, are made up of many glucose molecules. They do not taste sweet because their molecules are too large to sit on taste buds in the mouth that perceive sweetness.
- Fiber, the nondigestible part of plant cell walls, is commonly classified as either water-soluble or water-insoluble; each type has different physiologic effects.
- The majority of carbohydrate digestion occurs in the small intestine, where disaccharides and starches are digested to monosaccharides. Monosaccharides are absorbed through intestinal mucosal cells and transported to the liver through the portal vein. In the liver, fructose and galactose are converted to glucose. The liver releases glucose into the bloodstream.
- The major function of carbohydrates is to provide energy, which includes sparing protein and preventing ketosis. Glucose can be converted to glycogen, used to make nonessential amino acids, used for specific body compounds, or converted to fat and stored in adipose tissue.
- Carbohydrates are found in every MyPyramid group except Oils. Starches are most abundant in grains, vegetables, and the plant foods found in the meat and bean group; natural sugars occur in fruits and in the milk group. Discretionary calorie items may provide sugar and/or starch, depending on the individual selection.
- The RDA for carbohydrates is set as the minimum amount needed to fuel the brain but not an amount adequate to satisfy typical energy needs. Most experts recommend that 45% to 65% of total calories come from carbohydrates and that added sugars be limited. Twenty-five to 38 g of fiber are recommended daily for adult women and men respectively.
- The most popular American foods do not represent rich sources of fiber. Whole grains, bran cereals, dried peas and beans, and unpeeled fruits and vegetables are the best sources of fiber.
- Sugars—as well as starches—promote dental decay by feeding bacteria in the mouth that produce an acid that damages tooth enamel. Sugar is also a source of empty calories. The higher the intake of empty calories, the greater the risk of an inadequate nutrient intake, an excessive calorie intake, or both. Americans' intake of sugar and artificial sweeteners is rising.
- Sugar alcohols are considered to be low-calorie sweeteners because they are incompletely absorbed and, therefore, provide fewer calories per gram than regular sugar does. Because they do not promote dental decay, they are well suited for use in gum and breath mints that stay in the mouth a long time.
- Artificial sweeteners provide negligible or no calories. Their use as food additives is regulated by the FDA, which sets safety limits known as ADI. The ADI, a level per kilogram of body weight, reflects an amount 100 times less than the maxi-

 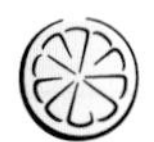

mum level at which no observed adverse effects have occurred in animal studies. Artificial sweeteners have intense sweetening power, ranging from 180 to 8000 times sweeter than that of sucrose.

ANSWER KEY

1. **TRUE** Starch, the storage form of carbohydrates in plants, is made from hundreds to thousands of glucose molecules.
2. **FALSE** All digestible carbohydrates—whether sugars or starch—provide 4 cal/g. Fibers do not provide calories because they are not digested.
3. **FALSE** The body cannot distinguish between the sugar in fruit and the sugar in candy. However, the *package* of nutrients in fruit (vitamins, minerals, fiber, phytochemicals) is better than the package of nutrients in candy (few to no other nutrients with the possible exception of fat.)
4. **FALSE** The most commonly consumed American foods provide 1 to 3 g fiber/serving, which is why most Americans typically eat only about one-half the recommended intake of fiber.
5. **FALSE** Although enrichment returns certain B vitamins and iron lost through processing, other vitamins, minerals, phytochemicals, and fiber are not replaced so whole wheat bread is nutritionally superior to white or "wheat" bread.
6. **TRUE** Soft drinks contribute more added sugar to the average American diet than any other food or beverage.
7. **TRUE** All carbohydrates, whether sweet or not, promote dental decay by feeding bacteria in the mouth that damages tooth enamel.
8. **FALSE** Although Nutrition Facts labels do not distinguish between natural and added sugars, they do list the total sugar content per serving.
9. **FALSE** Alternative sweeteners approved for use in the United States are safe in amounts specified as the Acceptable Daily Intake. The exception is the use of aspartame by people who have phenylketonuria.
10. **FALSE** Sugar has not been proven to cause hyperactivity in children.

WEBSITES

Learn about grains at **www.wheatcouncil.org**

REFERENCES

American Dietetic Association. (2002). Position of the American Dietetic Association: Health implications of dietary fiber. *Journal of the American Dietetic Association, 102,* 993–1000.

American Dietetic Association. (2004). Position of the American Dietetic Association: Use of nutritive and nonnutritive sweeteners. *Journal of the American Dietetic Association,* 104(2), 255–275.

Brown, A. (2004). *Understanding food* (2nd ed.). Belmont, CA: Wadsworth/Thomson Learning.

Coulston, A., & Johnson, R. (2002). Sugar and sugars: Myths and realities. *Journal of the American Dietetic Association, 102,* 351–353.

Fung, T., Hu, F., Pereira, M., Liu, S., Stampfer, M., Colditz, G., & Willett, W. (2002). Whole-grain intake and the risk of type 2 diabetes: A prospective study in men. *American Journal of Clinical Nutrition, 76,* 535–540.

Gretebeck, R., Gretebeck, K. & Tittlebach, T. (2002). Glycemic index of popular sport drinks and energy foods. *Journal of the American Dietetic Association, 102,* 415–417.

Institute of Medicine of the National Academies (2002). *Dietary reference intakes for energy, carbohydrate, fiber, fat, fatty acids, cholesterol, protein, and amino acids.* Washington, DC: National Academies Press.

International Food Information Council Foundation. (March 2002). Sugars & low-calorie sweeteners. Available at www.ific.org/nutrition/sugars/index/cfm. Accessed on 12/5/03.

Liu, S., Sesso, H., Manson, J., Willett, W., & Buring, J. (2003). Is intake of breakfast cereals related to total and cause-specific mortality in men? *American Journal of Clinical Nutrition, 77,* 594–599.

Liu, S., Willett, W., Manson, J., Hu, F., Rosner, B., & Colditz, G. (2003). Relation between changes in intakes of dietary fiber and grain products and changes in weight and development of obesity among middle-aged women. *American Journal of Clinical Nutrition, 78,* 920–927.

Trumbo, P., Schlicker, S., Yates, A., & Poos, M. (2002). Dietary Reference Intakes for energy, carbohydrate, fiber, fat, fatty acids, cholesterol, protein and amino acids. *Journal of the American Dietetic Association, 102,* 1621–1630.

For information on the new dietary guidelines 2005 and MyPyramid, visit
http://connection.lww.com/go/dudek

3

Protein

TRUE	FALSE	
⬭	⬭	**1** Most Americans eat more protein than they need.
⬭	⬭	**2** Protein is the nutrient most likely to be deficient in a purely vegetarian diet.
⬭	⬭	**3** The body stores extra amino acids in muscle tissue.
⬭	⬭	**4** The quality of soy protein is comparable to or greater than that of animal proteins.
⬭	⬭	**5** Nutritionally the limiting factor in building muscle tissue is calorie intake, not protein intake.
⬭	⬭	**6** A protein classified as "high quality" has the majority of calories provided by protein with few fat or carbohydrate calories.
⬭	⬭	**7** Protein is found in all MyPyramid groups.
⬭	⬭	**8** Healthy adults are in a state of positive nitrogen balance.
⬭	⬭	**9** Vegetarian diets are not adequate during pregnancy.
⬭	⬭	**10** There are no risks associated with eating too much protein.

UPON COMPLETION OF THIS CHAPTER, YOU WILL BE ABLE TO

- Explain the difference between complete and incomplete proteins and name sources of each.
- Explain protein "sparing."
- Discuss the Recommended Dietary Allowance (RDA) for protein for adults and compare the RDA with the average American intake for protein.
- Discuss the nutrients that are most likely to be deficient in a vegetarian diet and vegetarian sources for each.
- Discuss how protein is used in the body.
- Describe protein digestion and absorption.

PROTEIN

Proteins: a class of energy-yielding nutrients composed of individual building blocks known as amino acids.

Protein is a component of every living cell. Except for bile and urine, every tissue and fluid in the body contains some protein. In fact, the body may contain as many as 100,000 different proteins that vary in size, shape, and function. Amino acids or proteins are components of or involved in

Body structure and framework. Almost 50% of protein in the body is found in skeletal muscle and approximately 15% is found in the skin and the blood.

Enzymes. Enzymes are proteins that facilitate specific chemical reactions in the body without undergoing change themselves. Some enzymes (e.g., digestive enzymes) break down larger molecules into smaller ones; others (e.g., enzymes involved in protein synthesis in which amino acids are combined) combine molecules to form larger compounds.

Other body secretions and fluids. Hormones (e.g., insulin, thyroxine, epinephrine), neurotransmitters (e.g., serotonin, acetylcholine), and antibodies are all made from amino acids as are breast milk, mucus, sperm, and histamine.

Fluid and electrolyte balance. Proteins help to regulate fluid balance because they attract water, thereby creating osmotic pressure. Circulating proteins, such as albumin, maintain the proper balance of fluid among the intravascular (within veins and arteries), intracellular (within the cells), and interstitial (in the fluid between the cells) compartments of the body. A symptom of low albumin is edema, which is characterized by the swelling of body tissues secondary to accumulation of fluid in the interstitial spaces.

Acid–base balance. Because amino acids contain both an acid (COOH) and a base (NH_2), they can act as either acids or bases depending on the pH of the surrounding fluid. This ability to buffer or neutralize excess acids and bases enables proteins to maintain normal blood pH, which protects body proteins from being denatured (with subsequent loss of function).

Transport molecules. Globular proteins transport other substances through the blood. For instance, lipoproteins transport fats, cholesterol, and fat-soluble vitamins; hemoglobin transports oxygen; and albumin transports free fatty acids and many drugs.

Other compounds. Amino acids are components of numerous body compounds such as opsin, the light-sensitive visual pigment in the eye, and thrombin, a protein necessary for normal blood clotting.

Fueling the body. Like carbohydrates, protein provides 4 cal/g. Although it is not the body's preferred fuel, protein is a source of energy when it is consumed in excess of need or when calorie intake from carbohydrates and fat is inadequate.

Amino Acids

Amino acids are the basic building blocks of all proteins. All amino acids have a carbon atom core with four bonding sites: one site holds a hydrogen atom, one an amino group (NH_2), and one an acid group (COOH) (Fig 3.1). Attached to the fourth bonding site

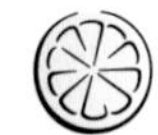

Amino Acids: organic compounds made from carbon, hydrogen, and oxygen atoms plus a nitrogen component, which distinguishes them from the other energy nutrients.

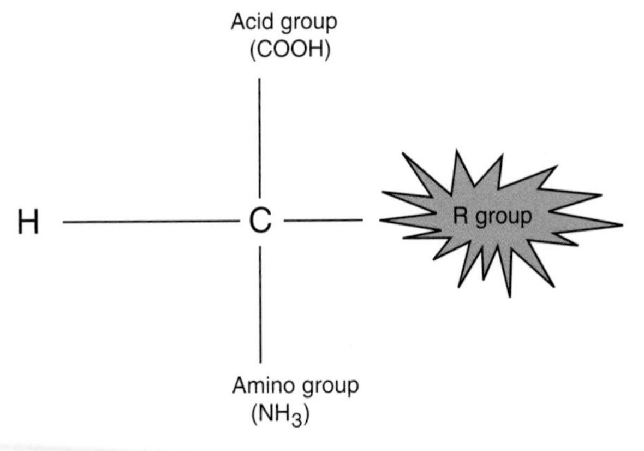

FIGURE 3.1 Amino acid group.

Essential or Indispensable Amino Acids: amino acids that cannot be made by the body; they must be consumed through food.

is a side group (R group), which contains the atoms that give each amino acid its own distinct identity. For instance, the R group of the amino acid glycine is simply one hydrogen atom. Some side groups contain sulfur; some are acidic, and some are basic. The differences in these side groups account for the differences in size, shape, and electrical charge among amino acids.

There are 20 common amino acids, 9 of which are essential (Box 3.1). The body cannot make essential amino acids so they must be supplied through the diet. The remaining 11 amino acids are classified as nonessential because cells can make them as needed through the process of transamination. Note that the terms essential and nonessential refer to whether or not they must be supplied by the diet, not to their relative importance: all 20 amino acids must be available for the body to make proteins.

Protein Structure

Nonessential or Dispensable Amino Acids: amino acids the body can make if nitrogen and other precursors are available.

Transamination: the process of removing the amino group from one amino acid and combining it with carbon fragments of glucose molecules to create a different particular amino acid.

The types and amounts of amino acids and the unique sequence in which they are joined determine a protein's primary structure. Most proteins contain several dozen to several hundred amino acids: just as the 26 letters of the alphabet can be used to form

BOX 3.1 **AMINO ACIDS**

Essential Amino Acids	Nonessential Amino Acids
Histidine	Alanine
Isoleucine	Arginine
Leucine	Asparagine
Lysine	Aspartic acid
Methionine	Cystine (cysteine)
Phenylalanine	Glutamic acid
Threonine	Glutamine
Tryptophan	Glycine
Valine	Proline
	Serine
	Tyrosine

an infinite number of words, so can amino acids be joined in different amounts, proportions, and sequences to form a great variety of proteins.

Another consideration in protein structure is the shape. Amino acids may form proteins that are straight, folded, or coiled along one dimension or they may take on a three-dimensional shape as spheres or globes. Even larger proteins are assembled when two or more three-dimensional polypeptides combine. A protein's shape determines its function.

How the Body Handles Protein

Digestion

Polypeptides: ten or more amino acids bonded together.

Chemical digestion of protein begins in the stomach, where hydrochloric acid denatures protein to make the peptide bonds more available to the actions of enzymes (Fig. 3.2). Hydrochloric acid also converts pepsinogen to the active enzyme pepsin,

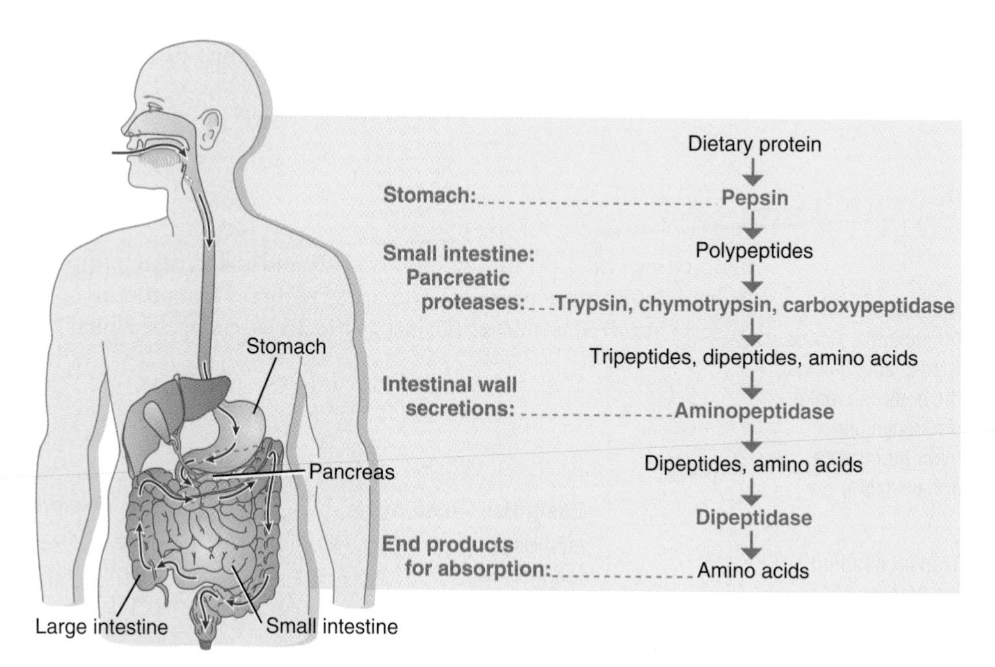

FIGURE 3.2 Protein digestion. Chemical digestion of protein begins in the stomach. Hydrochloric acid converts pepsinogen to the active enzyme pepsin, which begins the process of breaking down proteins into small polypeptides and some amino acids. The majority of protein digestion occurs in the small intestine, where pancreatic proteases reduce polypeptides into shorter chains, tripeptides, dipeptides, and amino acids. Enzymes located on the surface of the cells that line the small intestine complete the digestion: aminopeptidase splits amino acids from the amino ends of short peptides, and dipeptidase reduces dipeptides to amino acids.

 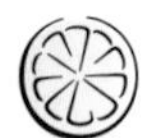

Tripeptides: three amino acids bonded together.

Dipeptides: two amino acids bonded together.

which begins the process of breaking down proteins into smaller polypeptides and some amino acids.

The majority of protein digestion occurs in the small intestine, where pancreatic proteases reduce polypeptides to shorter chains, tripeptides, dipeptides, and amino acids. The enzymes trypsin and chymotrypsin act to break peptide bonds between specific amino acids. Carboxypeptidase breaks off amino acids from the acid (carboxyl) end of polypeptides and dipeptides. Enzymes located on the surface of the cells that line the small intestine complete the digestion: aminopeptidase splits amino acids from the amino ends of short peptides and dipeptidase reduces dipeptides to amino acids.

Absorption

Amino acids, and sometimes a few dipeptides or larger peptides, are absorbed through the mucosa of the small intestine by active transport with the aid of vitamin B_6. Intestinal cells release amino acids into the bloodstream for transport to the liver via the portal vein.

Metabolism

The liver acts as a clearinghouse for the amino acids it receives: it uses the amino acids it needs, releases those needed elsewhere, and handles the extra. For instance, the liver retains amino acids to make liver cells, nonessential amino acids, and plasma proteins such as heparin, prothrombin, and albumin. The liver regulates the release of amino acids into the bloodstream and removes excess amino acids from the circulation. As enzymes are needed, the liver synthesizes specific enzymes to degrade excess amino acids. The liver removes the nitrogen from amino acids so that they can be burned for energy and it converts amino acids to glucose or fat as appropriate. The liver coordinates amino acid metabolism.

Protein Synthesis

Primarily amino acids are used by all body cells to synthesize proteins that are either lost through normal wear and tear or are needed to build new tissue such as during pregnancy or adolescent growth. Protein synthesis is a complicated but efficient process that quickly assembles amino acids to create proteins needed by the body. Part of what makes every individual unique is the minute differences in body proteins, which are caused by variations in the sequencing of amino acids determined by genetics. Genetic codes created at conception hold the instructions for making all of the body's proteins. Cell function and life itself depend on the precise replication of these codes. Some important concepts related to protein synthesis are metabolic pool, nitrogen balance, and protein turnover.

Metabolic Pool: a limited amount of free amino acids available in cells that are given up and accepted as a dynamic reserve.

Metabolic Pool

Unlike glucose and fat, the body is not able to store excess amino acids for later use. However, a limited supply of free amino acids exists within cells in a metabolic pool, which accepts and donates amino acids as needed. This metabolic pool is constantly changing in response to the constant buildup and breakdown of body proteins and the influx of amino acids from food.

Career Connection

Many dieters believe a high-protein diet is superior to a high carbohydrate diet in promoting weight loss. And they may be right. Although the ideal ratio of carbohydrate to protein for overall health weight management is unknown, at least one recent study indicates that women who consume a lower carbohydrate to protein ratio (170 g CHO, 125 g protein/day) while dieting lost more weight, more fat, and had greater satiety than women who had a higher carbohydrate to protein ratio (246 g CHO, 68 g protein/day). While the *amount* of weight loss was not dramatically different between the groups, the protein-eaters lost significantly more fat to muscle tissue than the carbohydrate eaters; obviously the loss of fat tissue is more desirable than the loss of muscle. Both groups had a daily intake of about 1700 calories and 50 g of fat. Also noteworthy is that even the "low" carbohydrate group ate more than the RDA of 130 g for CHO. Although one study is not enough to draw hard and fast conclusions, it clearly demonstrates that much is yet to be learned about the ideal macronutrient composition of weight loss diets. Clients who choose to eat a high-protein diet in an attempt to lose weight should be reminded to choose low-fat sources of protein to keep calories under control:

- Low-fat or skim milk and milk products
- Lean cuts of meat and skinless poultry that are baked, broiled, or roasted
- Egg whites, whole eggs
- Dried peas and beans

(Neutral) Nitrogen Balance: when protein synthesis and protein breakdown occur at the same rate.

Positive Nitrogen Balance: when protein synthesis exceeds protein breakdown.

Negative Nitrogen Balance: an undesirable state that occurs when protein breakdown exceeds protein synthesis.

Nitrogen Balance

Body cells continuously make proteins to replace those that break down from normal wear and tear. For example, red blood cells are replaced every 60 to 90 days, gastrointestinal cells are replaced every 2 to 3 days, and enzymes used in the digestion of food are continuously replenished. The state of nitrogen balance is determined by comparing the rate of protein synthesis to protein breakdown. Healthy adults are in neutral nitrogen balance. A positive nitrogen balance exists during growth, pregnancy, or recovery from injury. A negative nitrogen balance occurs during starvation or the catabolic phase after injury.

In the clinical setting, nitrogen balance is determined by comparing nitrogen intake with nitrogen excretion over a 24-hour period. To calculate nitrogen intake, protein intake is measured for a 24-hour period. The total amount of protein consumed (in grams) is then divided by 6.25 because protein is 16% nitrogen by weight. The result is the grams of nitrogen consumed per 24 hours. Nitrogen excretion is ascertained by having a 24-hour urine sample analyzed for the amount (grams) of urinary urea nitrogen it contains. A coefficient of 4 is added to this number to account for the estimated daily nitrogen loss in feces, hair, nails, and skin. Finally the amount of nitrogen consumed is compared with the total amount of nitrogen excreted to reveal a positive, negative, or neutral nitrogen balance (Box 3.2).

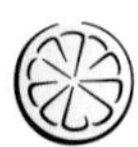

BOX 3.2

CALCULATING NITROGEN BALANCE

Mary is a 25-year-old woman who was admitted to the hospital with multiple fractures and traumatic injuries from a car accident. A nutritional intake study indicated a 24-hour protein intake of 64 g. A 24-hour urinary urea nitrogen (UUN) collection result was 19.8 g.

1. Determine nitrogen intake by dividing protein intake by 6.25:

   $64 \div 6.25 = 10.24$ g of nitrogen

2. Determine total nitrogen output by adding a coefficient of 4 to the UUN:

   $19.8 + 4 = 23.8$ g of nitrogen

3. Calculate nitrogen balance by subtracting nitrogen output from nitrogen intake:

   $10.24 - 23.8 = -13.56$ g in 24 hours

4. Interpret the results.

A negative number indicates that protein breakdown is exceeding protein synthesis. Mary is in a catabolic state.

Protein Turnover: the constant breakdown and synthesis of endogenous protein.

Protein Turnover

The body's supply of amino acids comes from food (exogenous) and from its own protein tissue (endogenous). Amino acids released when body proteins break down may be recycled to build new proteins or stripped of their nitrogen and burned for energy. Body proteins vary in their rate of turnover. For instance, protein turnover in the liver, pancreas, and small intestine is rapid; during times of need, these tissues give up amino acids for protein synthesis or energy. The turnover of muscle proteins is slower; the turnover in the brain and nervous system is negligible.

Other Uses of Amino Acids

Although the primary fate of amino acids is to repair or replace body proteins, amino acids may be used for other functions in the body. For instance, cells use amino acids to synthesize other nitrogen-containing compounds such as the purine bases of DNA. Some amino acids have specific functions within the body. For instance, tryptophan is a precursor of the vitamin niacin and tyrosine is the precursor of melanin, the pigment that colors hair and skin. Amino acids may also be converted to glucose, burned for energy, or converted to fat.

Deamination: the process of stripping amino acids of their amino group (NH_2).

Converted to Glucose

Certain body tissues, such as brain and nervous tissue, rely solely on glucose for energy. When carbohydrate intake is inadequate and glycogen reserves are exhausted, the body resorts to converting glucogenic amino acids into glucose. First these amino acids undergo deamination, which yields a three-carbon atom fragment that is converted to pyruvate. Two of these pyruvate molecules are joined to form the six-carbon atom molecule, glucose. Although only glucogenic amino acids can be converted to glucose,

Glucogenic Amino Acids: amino acids that can be used to synthesize glucose; approximately 58% of the amino acids in proteins are glucogenic.

whole proteins must be broken down to make them available. The protein's remaining amino acids that are not glucogenic are used for energy by other body cells.

The deamination of amino acids yields ammonia (NH_3), which can be used in the synthesis of nonessential amino acids. The remaining ammonia combines with carbon dioxide to make urea, which is released into the blood, circulates to the kidneys, and is excreted in the urine.

Burned for Energy

Normally the body uses very little protein for energy as long as intake and storage of carbohydrate and fat are adequate. If insufficient carbohydrate and fat are available for energy use or if protein is consumed in amounts greater than those needed for protein synthesis, amino acids are broken down for energy. However, the use of protein for energy is a physiologic and economic waste because amino acids used for energy are not available to be used for protein synthesis, a function unique to amino acids. Another disadvantage of using protein for energy is the burden placed on the kidneys to excrete the nitrogenous waste. Thus an adequate supply of energy from carbohydrate and fat is needed to "spare protein" from being burned for calories.

Converted to Fat

Lipogenesis: the formation of fat.

At this point, amino acids that have not been used for specific protein functions have been deaminated, leaving a carbon fragment ready to be burned for energy. But if energy needs are already satisfied, the carbon fragment (initially or eventually acetyl-CoA) undergoes lipogenesis to form fatty acids that combine with glycerol to form triglycerides, the storage form of fat in the body. Protein is converted to fat only when it is consumed in excess of need.

Protein in Food

With the exception of the Fruits and Oils, all groups in MyPyramid have protein—albeit of varying amounts and quality (Fig. 3.3). However, any discussion of protein in food must include the *quality* of protein, not just the *quantity,* because quality influences how much protein is needed.

Just as body proteins contain different quantities and proportions of amino acids, so do the proteins in food. It is this amino acid profile that determines the quality of a food protein (i.e., its ability to support protein synthesis). For most Americans, protein quality is not important because the amounts of protein and calories consumed are more than adequate. But when protein needs are increased or protein intake is marginal, quality becomes a crucial concern. Terms that refer to protein quality are complete and incomplete. The digestibility of a protein is another quality consideration.

Complete Proteins

Complete proteins provide all nine essential amino acids in adequate amounts and proportions needed by the body for tissue growth and maintenance. With the exception of gelatin, all animal sources of protein (meat, fish, poultry, eggs, milk, and dairy products) are complete proteins. Soy protein is the only complete plant protein.

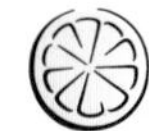

Complete Protein: a protein composed of all essential amino acids in amounts needed by the body to support tissue growth and repair.

Incomplete Protein: a protein that is low in one or more essential amino acids.

Limiting Amino Acid: the essential amino acid that is present in the smallest amount; it limits protein synthesis because if it is not available, protein synthesis cannot occur.

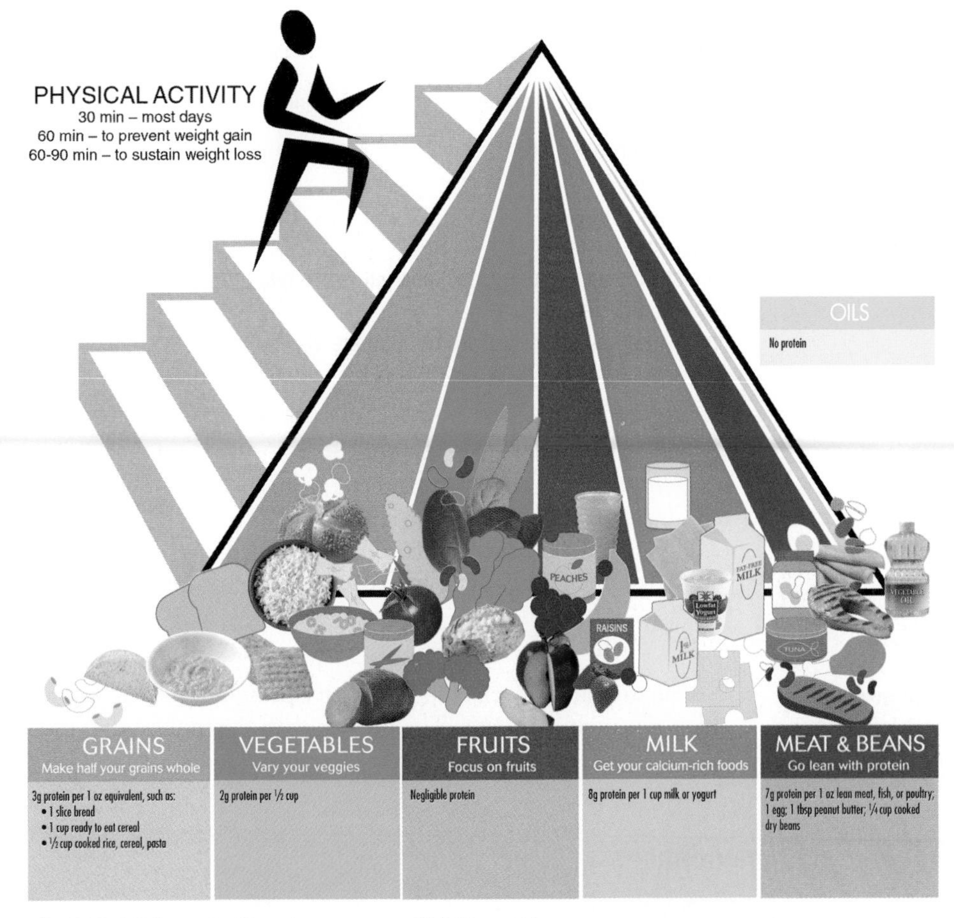

FIGURE 3.3 Protein content of MyPyramid groups.

Incomplete Proteins

Incomplete proteins provide all the essential amino acids but have one or more limiting amino acids that render them incapable of meeting the body's need for normal protein synthesis. With the exception of soybeans, all plant proteins are incomplete. Fortunately limiting amino acids differ among plant proteins. For instance grains are typically low in lysine, legumes are low in methionine and cysteine, and

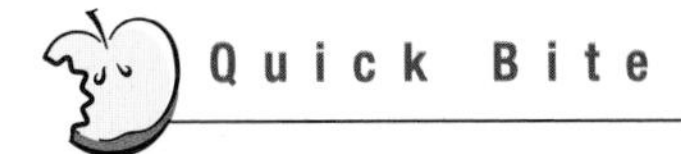

Quick Bite

Examples of a plant protein complemented by a small amount of an animal protein to form a complete protein

- Bread pudding
- Rice pudding
- Corn pudding
- Cereal and milk
- Macaroni and cheese
- Cheese fondue
- French toast
- Cheese sandwich
- Vegetable quiche

Complementary Proteins: two proteins that when combined, provide adequate amounts and proportions of all essential amino acids needed to support protein synthesis.

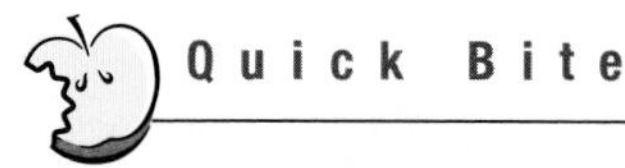

Examples of two complementary plant proteins

Black beans and rice
Bean tacos
Pea soup with toast
Lentil and rice curry
Falafel sandwich (ground chickpea patties on pita bread)
Peanut butter sandwich
Pasta e fagioli (pasta and white bean stew)

nuts are low in lysine and isoleucine. Combining two different incomplete proteins or a small amount of any complete protein with an incomplete protein boosts the overall quality to that of a complete protein. Proteins that can be combined to obtain sufficient quantities and proportions of all essential amino acids are called complementary proteins.

Historically vegetarians were advised to eat complementary proteins at every meal. Experts now contend that it is not necessary to consciously complement proteins at every meal, so long as a variety of proteins is eaten and calorie intake is adequate. Over the course of a day, adequate amounts of all the essential amino acids will be provided if calories are adequate and a variety of grains, legumes, seeds, nuts, and vegetables are consumed.

Protein Digestibility

High-Quality Protein: a complete protein that is highly digestible.

Protein digestibility refers to how well a protein is digested to make amino acids available for protein synthesis. The protein with the highest digestibility is egg.

Intake Recommendations

The Recommended Dietary Allowance (RDA) for protein for a healthy adult is 0.8 g/kg, which is approximately 10% of recommended total calories. This protein allowance is derived from the absolute minimum requirement needed to maintain nitrogen balance plus an additional factor to account for individual variations and the mixed quality of proteins typically consumed and assumes calorie intake is adequate. Thus the RDAs for protein for the "reference man" and "reference woman" are 56 g and 46 g, respectively. Box 3.3 shows how to calculate daily protein intake.

In the United States, the protein intake among adult men during 1994 to 1996 and 1998 ranged from 71 g to 101 g/day; for women, the median ranged from 55 to 62 g/day. For both men and women, protein provided approximately 15% of total calories. The Acceptable Macronutrient Distribution Range for protein for adults is 10 to 35% of total calories.

In addition to body weight, other factors influence how much protein the body needs. Protein needs are increased

- When calorie intake is inadequate because protein required for energy production cannot be used for protein synthesis.

 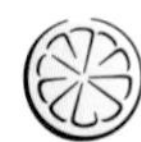

BOX 3.3

CALCULATING DAILY PROTEIN ALLOWANCE

John is a 30-year-old man who weighs 184 pounds. What is his daily protein allowance?

1. Determine the weight in kilograms by dividing the weight in pounds by 2.2:

   $184 \div 2.2 = 83.6$ kg

2. Multiply the weight in kilograms by 0.8 g/kg (the RDA for men 19 years of age and older or women 15 years and older):

   $83.6 \times 0.8 = 66.88$ g

John should consume 67 g of protein per day.

- When the body needs to heal itself, whether from surgery, trauma, or burns. For instance, people with severe burns may require as much as 2.0 g/protein/kg of body weight.
- During periods of normal tissue growth such as during pregnancy, lactation, and infancy through adolescence. The Adequate Intake set for infants through the first 6 months of life is 1.52 g/kg of body weight, almost double the RDA for adults.

Protein restriction is used for people with severe liver disease and those with renal failure who are unable to excrete nitrogenous wastes. It is important to remember that the RDA is intended for healthy people only.

Career Connection

Some people take amino acid capsules or powders, based on the belief that regarding protein, the more the better. However, the average American diet provides approximately 50% more protein than needed. So why take supplements? Many people are under the notion that if a little is good, a lot is better. In truth, more is not better. First, protein eaten in excess of need is not stored; excess amino acids are converted to fat when eaten in excess of need, just as carbohydrates and fat are. Secondly amino acid supplements often provide only one or few particular amino acids, creating a disproportion in amounts of amino acids available. Because protein synthesis in the body uses all amino acids, there is no advantage to having an excess of any of them: protein synthesis cannot continue after the supply of the limiting amino acid has been depleted. Not only is there no good reason *to* take amino acid supplements, the National Academy of Sciences warns against using any single amino acid in quantities significantly above what is normally found in foods. People most vulnerable to adverse effects include

- Pregnant and lactating women
- Infants, children, and adolescents
- The elderly
- People who need to limit their protein intake (e.g., people with liver or renal disease)

Protein intake, per se, is not addressed in the *Dietary Guidelines for Americans* (see Chapter 8); the issue of protein appears to be more an afterthought than a key element among leading health agencies that make diet recommendations. Protein is usually addressed indirectly in terms of choosing lean meats and low-fat dairy products and eating a plant-based diet. What amazes meat-loving Americans is that even *without any* selections from the Meat and Beans group, protein intake is considerable. For instance, choosing the minimum number of servings recommended from all the other food groups provides approximately 40 g of protein. No one recommends eliminating this or any of the MyPyramid groups (vegetarians don't eliminate this group but choose selectively from it); this case simply shows that obtaining enough protein is not a problem for most Americans.

In developing countries, protein deficiency, or protein-energy malnutrition, is a major health concern. In the United States, protein deficiency is rare except among the elderly, fad dieters, and hospitalized patients.

PROTEIN IN HEALTH PROMOTION

Vegetarian Diets

Vegetarianism: loosely defined as the abstinence from animal products; encompasses a variety of eating styles.

Pure Vegetarians or Vegans: people who eat only plants; they form the smallest group of vegetarians.

Lacto-Vegetarians: vegetarians whose diets include milk and milk products.

Lacto-Ovo Vegetarians: vegetarians whose diets include both milk products and eggs.

Vegetarian eating patterns range from complete elimination of all animal products to simply avoiding red meat. Within each defined category of vegetarianism, individuals differ as to how strictly they adhere to their eating style. For instance, some vegans do not eat refried beans that contain lard because lard is an animal product, but other vegans do not avoid animal products so conscientiously. Semi-vegetarians are occasional meat eaters who mostly follow a vegetarian diet or those who eat fish and poultry but less than once a week.

In addition to the political, philosophical, religious, and economic motivations for becoming vegetarian, the potential health benefits are attracting a growing number of recruits. Many leading health organizations recommend eating a plant-based diet including The American Institute for Cancer Research, the World Cancer Research Fund, and the American Cancer Society. The American Heart Association and the Heart and Stroke Foundation of Canada recommend a balanced diet with an emphasis on grains, fruit, and vegetables.

Because they eat fewer or no animal products, vegetarians consume less saturated fat, cholesterol, and animal protein. Their intakes of carbohydrates, fiber, magnesium, boron, folate, antioxidants, carotenoids, and phytochemicals are higher. Health benefits may come from eating less of certain substances, eating more of others, or a combination of the two. Or health benefits may be related to some other lifestyle practice vegetarians may adopt such as participating in regular exercise, abstaining from tobacco, or using alcohol only moderately if at all. Whatever the reasons, the end result is that vegetarians have lower incidences of obesity, cardiovascular disease, hypertension, type 2 diabetes, cancer, and dementia compared with nonvegetarians. Vegetarians may also be at lower risk for renal disease, gallstones, and diverticular disease.

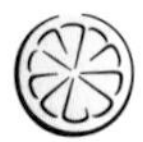

Vegetarian diets are not automatically healthier than nonvegetarian diets. Poorly planned vegetarian diets may lack certain essential nutrients, which endangers health. Also vegetarian diets can be excessive in fat and cholesterol if whole milk, whole-milk cheeses, eggs, and high-fat desserts are used extensively. Whether a vegetarian diet is healthy or detrimental to health depends on the actual food choices made over time.

Nutrients of Concern

A nutrient that does not make this list, even among vegans, is protein. Most vegetarian diets meet or exceed the RDA for protein, even though they contain less protein and lower-quality protein than nonvegetarian diets. Over the course of a day, if a variety of foods are consumed and calories are adequate, sufficient amounts of all essential amino acids can be obtained from plants. In addition, the quality of soy protein is comparable to or exceeds that of animal proteins, so soy products are excellent alternatives to meat (see Box 3.4). Furthermore, avoiding excessive protein offers the benefits of improved calcium retention and decreased renal workload.

Iron, zinc, calcium, vitamin D, and alpha-linolenic acid are nutrients of concern—not because they cannot be obtained in sufficient quantities from plants but because they may not be adequately consumed, depending on an individual's food choices. Vitamin B_{12} is of concern because it does not occur naturally in plants.

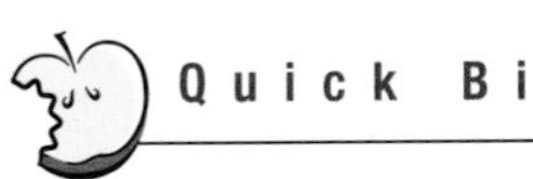

Vegetarian sources of iron

iron-fortified bread and cereals
baked potato with skin
dried peas and beans
cooked soybeans
tofu
veggie "meats"
dried fruit

BOX 3.4

GLOSSARY OF SOY PRODUCTS

Edamame: parboiled fresh soybeans sold refrigerated or frozen usually in the pod
Meat analogs: imitation burgers, hot dogs, bacon, chicken fingers, etc. made from soy, not meat
Miso: fermented soybean paste
Soy cheese: cheese made from soymilk; can substitute for sour cream, cream cheese, or other cheese
Soymilk: the liquid from soaked, ground, strained soybeans. Available plain, chocolate, and vanilla flavors.
Soy nuts: whole soybeans that have been soaked in water then baked
Soy nut butter: soy nuts that are crushed and blended with soy oil to resemble peanut butter
Soy sprouts: spouted soybeans
Tofu: soybean curd
Tempeh: caked fermented soybeans
Textured vegetable protein (TVP): soy flour modified to resemble ground beef when rehydrated

Iron

Iron in plants (nonheme iron) is not as well absorbed as the heme iron in meat. Because of the lower bioavailability of iron from a vegetarian diet, it is recommended that vegetarians consume 1.8 times the normal iron intake. However, vegetarians do not have higher rates of iron deficiency anemia although they have lower stores of iron than nonvegetarians. This may be because vegetarians consume more vitamin C, which enhances the absorption of nonheme iron.

Zinc

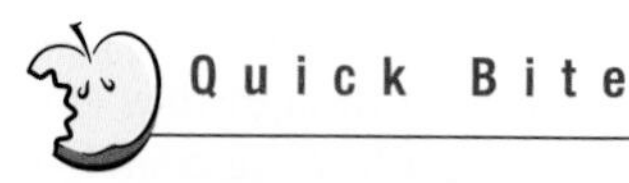

Plant sources of zinc include

whole grains (especially the bran and germ)
dried peas and beans
soybean products
seeds
nuts

Many plants provide zinc, but it is not absorbed as well as the zinc in meats. Some vegetarians may eat significantly less than the recommended amount of zinc; however, overt zinc deficiency has not been seen in Western vegetarians. Still, vegetarians are urged to meet or exceed the RDA for zinc. Lacto-ovo vegetarians obtain zinc from milk, yogurt, and eggs.

Calcium

Calcium intake of lacto-vegetarians and lacto-ovo vegetarians is comparable to or higher than that of nonvegetarians. Vegans, however, often consume less than the recommended intake of calcium and bioavailability of vegetarian sources is a consideration. For instance, calcium absorption is significantly impaired by oxalates; thus the calcium from high oxalate vegetables (spinach, beet greens, Swiss chard) is poorly absorbed. Interestingly the bioavailability of calcium is higher in low-oxalate greens, such as bok choy, broccoli, Chinese/Napa cabbage, collard greens, kale, okra, turnip greens, than it is in cow's milk, fortified juices, and calcium-set tofu.

All vegetarians are advised to consume at least the level of calcium recommended for their age group. The Vegetarian food guide pyramid that appears in Figure 3.4 recommends eight servings of calcium-rich foods daily. These servings also count towards servings from the other food groups in the guide. For people who do not use milk or dairy products, calcium-fortified orange juice, calcium-fortified or calcium-processed soyfoods, calcium-fortified breakfast cereals, legumes, tortillas made from lime-processed corn, and some dark green leafy vegetables can provide adequate calcium. Calcium supplements are recommended for people who do not meet their requirement from food.

Vitamin D

Vitamin D status depends on sunlight exposure and the intake of vitamin D fortified foods or supplements. Light-skinned people have the *potential* to obtain adequate vitamin D from just 5 to 15 minutes of daily sun exposure on the face, hands, and arms during the summer and at the 42nd latitude (Boston) and southward. In practice, sunlight alone is not enough for many people including people with dark skin, people living in northern climates (especially in the winter), people who use sunscreens,

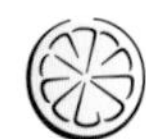

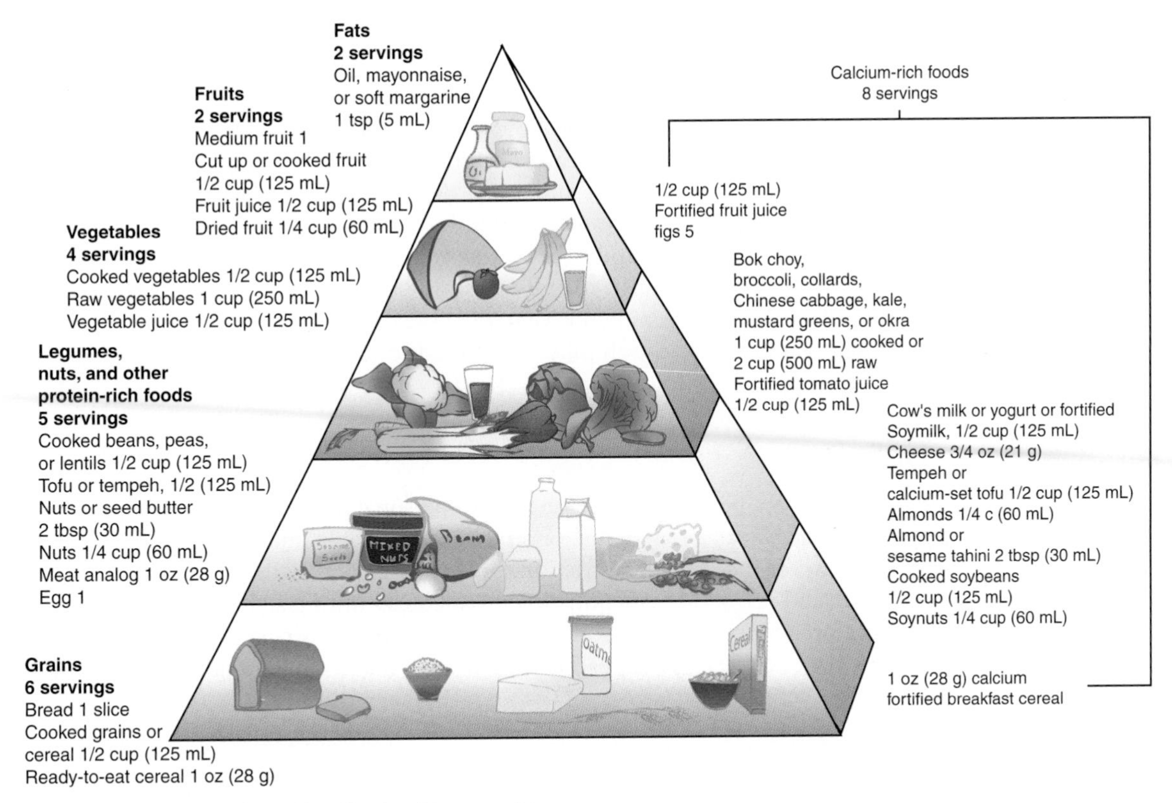

FIGURE 3.4 Vegetarian food guide pyramid.

people who live in smoggy areas, and the elderly (because aging impairs vitamin D synthesis).

Fortified milk is the biggest dietary source of vitamin D. Other sources include fortified ready-to-eat cereals, fortified soymilk, and other fortified nondairy milk products. Supplements are needed if sun exposure and vitamin D intake are inadequate.

Omega-3 Fatty Acids

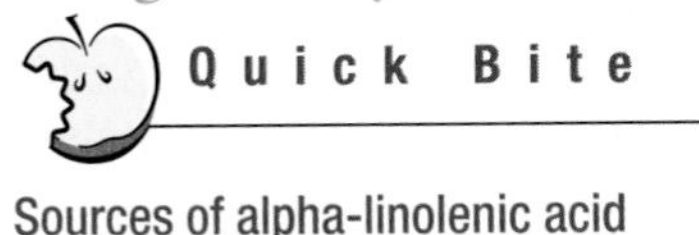

Sources of alpha-linolenic acid

Ground flaxseed
Flaxseed oil
Walnuts
Walnut oil
Canola oil
Soybean oil

Diets that do not include fish, eggs, or generous amounts of sea vegetables do not contain direct sources of the omega-3 fatty acids eicosapentaenoic acid (EPA) and docosahexanoic acid (DHA). Some studies show that vegetarians have low levels of EPA and DHA in their blood but the significance of this is not known. As a safety measure, vegetarians are advised to consume good sources of the essential fatty acid alpha-linolenic acid because the body can convert some alpha-linolenic acid to DHA.

Vitamin B_{12}

Vitamin B_{12} is a concern for vegans because it is naturally found only in animals. Depending on food choices, some lacto-ovo vegetarians may have inadequate intakes also. Vitamin B_{12} from supplements and fortified foods, such as fortified nondairy milks and breakfast cereals, is very well absorbed. Some brands of nutritional yeast contain vitamin B_{12} and some do not (baking yeast does not provide vitamin B_{12}). Products that are *not* reliable for this vitamin are seaweed, algae, spirulina, tempeh, miso, beer, and other fermented foods; they contain a form of vitamin B_{12} that the body cannot use. Because B_{12} absorption declines with age, the Institute of Medicine recommends that all people over the age of 50 consume supplemental vitamin B_{12} through pills or fortified foods regardless of the type of diet they consume.

Is Vegetarianism for Everyone?

Vegetarianism is a personal choice, subject to personal interpretation. Although some view vegetarianism as a way of life, others prefer to simply opt for occasional meatless meals. Whatever the level of restriction, properly planned lacto-vegetarian, lacto-ovo vegetarian, and vegan diets are nutritionally adequate during all phases of the life cycle including pregnancy and lactation. *Proper planning* means paying close attention to the nutrients of concern (listed earlier) and using a vegetarian food guide for planning. Encourage clients to

Eat a variety of foods including whole grains, vegetables, fruits, dried peas and beans, nuts, seeds, and if desired, dairy products and eggs. Vary choices from each of the food groups: the greater the variety, the greater the likelihood that adequate amounts of essential nutrients will be consumed.

Eat enough calories. Adequate calories are necessary to avoid using amino acids for energy, which could lead to a shortage of amino acids for protein synthesis. Remember the serving sizes listed for each food group are minimum intakes; choose more servings from any of the groups to meet calorie needs. But calories should not be eaten just for the sake of calories: focus on sources of calories that also provide nutrients.

Choose grains wisely. Grains are the foundation of a healthy diet for both vegetarians and meat-eaters. Whole grains provide fiber, iron, and zinc; fortified cereals are rich sources of iron and folic acid. Experimenting with a variety of grains—barley, amaranth, buckwheat, bulgur, millet, kasha, quinoa, triticale—can turn familiar meals into exciting new feasts.

Consume a rich source of vitamin C at every meal. Sources of vitamin C include citrus fruits and juices, tomatoes, broccoli, green and red peppers, guava, brussel sprouts, strawberries, and cabbage. Eating a good source of vitamin C at every meal helps to maximize iron absorption from plants.

Choose two servings daily of fats that supply omega-3 fats. A serving is 1 teaspoon flaxseed oil, 1 tablespoon canola or soybean oil, 1 tablespoon ground flaxseed, or ¼ cup walnuts. Olive and canola oil are the best oils to use for cooking. Nuts and seeds may be used as substitutes from the fat group.

 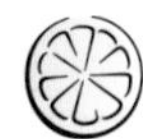

Limit saturated fat. If milk and dairy products are in the meal plan, select low-fat varieties. Limit high-fat and/or high-sugar desserts and snacks that are calorie-rich but nutritionally bankrupt.

Supplement nutrients that are lacking from food. For vegans, that means vitamin B_{12} (unless reliable fortified foods are consumed) and perhaps vitamin D. The adequacy of calcium, iron, and zinc intakes is evaluated on an individual basis.

Protein for Bodybuilders: Not the Limiting Factor

Bodybuilders easily fall prey to advertising claims that protein is the key to building muscle. They forsake starches for mounds of beef, chicken, tuna, and eggs. For extra measure, they take protein or amino acid supplements in pills, powders, and potions. They reason that more protein means more energy, more strength, and more muscles. In truth, high-protein diets—with or without amino acid supplements—are neither beneficial nor harmless.

Building Muscles

Logic would indicate that to increase the size of a muscle, a protein tissue, one must feed it more protein. To some extent this is true; in theory, to gain 1 pound of muscle per week, an extra 14 grams of protein are needed daily (the amount of protein in only 2 ounces of meat). In general, experts recommend that athletes consume 1.0 to 1.5 g of protein per kilogram of body weight, up from the RDA of 0.8 g/kg. Considering that the average American diet contains ample amounts of protein, most people already eat more than enough protein to build muscle. If muscle building were simply a matter of eating enough protein, Americans would be bulging with muscles. Although muscles do take up extra protein as they increase in size, they are not able to simply grab extra amino acids and convert them to muscle. The only way to build and strengthen muscle is through resistance exercises such as weight lifting and pushups. Nutritionally the limiting factor for building muscle is calorie intake, not protein. Although actual calorie requirements vary among individuals and with the frequency and intensity of athletic training, it is recommended that carbohydrates contribute 60% to 65% of total calories, up slightly from the normal recommendation of 50% to 60%. To bulk up, athletes need exercise, enough calories, and adequate protein.

More Is Not Better

Not only are high-protein diets not able to stimulate muscle gain, they are potentially harmful. High-protein diets burden the kidneys to excrete excess nitrogen; some experts believe that a high-protein diet over time leads to loss of renal function with aging. High-protein diets are often high in fat; like the general public, athletes are urged to limit total fat intake to 30% or less of total calories. High-protein diets are proportionately low in carbohydrates; inadequate carbohydrate intake compromises glycogen storage in the liver and muscles, risking fatigue and poor performance that can hinder exercise and muscle building. Finally, protein consumed in excess of need is used for energy or converted to fat and stored; for everyone, health risks increase as the percentage of body fat increases.

Tips for Eating to Build Muscles

Stick to MyPyramid. Athletes need the same balance and proportion of foods as the general public, but they may need to choose the highest number of servings for each food group. Use fats and sugars sparingly.

Eat enough calories. Extra nutrient-dense calories should come from high-carbohydrate, low-fat foods. Depending on calorie requirements, athletes may need more servings, larger portions, or more frequent meals.

Eat protein every day. Because the body cannot store amino acids, they need to be consumed daily. It is not essential to eat meat to obtain adequate protein.

Drink plenty of fluid. Muscle activity generates heat, which is dissipated through evaporation of water on the skin. Water must be replaced faster than it is lost or dehydration will occur.

Think wholesome. The requirements for certain vitamins and minerals increase in response to the increased need for calories. A high-carbohydrate, moderate-protein, low-fat diet featuring a variety of wholesome foods is the best way to meet increased needs.

Be wary of potions and pills that sound too good to be true. Researchers have failed to substantiate claims that ergogenic aids such as bee pollen, glycine, carnitine, lecithin, and gelatin improve strength or endurance.

How Do You Respond?

What is Quorn? Quorn is the brand name for a line of imitation meats approved for use in the United States in 2002. Although the manufacturer claims the products are made from "mycoprotein," a more descriptive term is fungus extract. Quorn is made from a single cell fungus grown in large fermentation vats; eggs and flavorings are added and the product is formed into imitation chicken or ground beef. Quorn has been used in Europe for more than a decade and appears in 90 varieties of foods such as lasagna and chicken-style patties. So far, its availability in the United States has been limited to frozen products "adjusted" to American tastes. The manufacturer claims that reports of adverse reactions are less than what would be expected for soy products; however, consumer advocates contend that adverse effects of Quorn include vomiting for several hours after eating the product, diarrhea, and possibly hives and difficulty eating. Despite the positive nutritional attributes (fiber, high quality protein, polyunsaturated fat), promoting fungus as a healthy alternative to meat is likely to be a hard sell in the United States.

Does "vegetarian" on the label mean the product is also low fat? No, vegetarian is not synonymous with low fat, particularly for items like vegetarian hot dogs, soy cheese, soy yogurt, and refried beans. Advise clients to read the Nutrition Facts label to determine if a vegetarian item is a good nutritional buy.

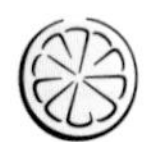

▲ Focus on Critical Thinking

Respond to the following statements:

1. Protein is more important than carbohydrates or fat.
2. Vegetarian diets are healthier than diets containing meat.
3. Special planning is needed for vegetarians to consume adequate high quality protein.

Key Concepts

- Protein is a component of every living cell. Protein in the body provides structure and framework. Amino acids are also components of enzymes, hormones, neurotransmitters, and antibodies. Proteins play a role in fluid balance and acid–base balance and are used to transport substances through the blood. Protein provides 4 cal/g of energy.
- Amino acids, which are composed of carbon, hydrogen, oxygen, and nitrogen atoms, are the building blocks of protein. Of the 20 common amino acids, 9 are considered essential because the body cannot make them. The remaining 11 amino acids are no less important but they are considered nonessential because they can be made by the body if nitrogen is available.
- Amino acids are joined in different amounts, proportions, and sequences to form the thousands of different proteins in the body.
- The small intestine is the principal site of protein digestion; amino acids and some dipeptides are absorbed through the portal bloodstream.
- In the body, amino acids are used to make proteins, nonessential amino acids, and other nitrogen-containing compounds. Some amino acids can be converted to glucose. Amino acids consumed in excess of need are burned for energy or converted to fat and stored.
- Healthy adults are in nitrogen balance, which means that protein synthesis is occurring at the same rate as protein breakdown. Nitrogen balance is determined by comparing the amount of nitrogen consumed with the amount of nitrogen excreted in urine, feces, hair, nails, and skin.
- Except for the Fruits and Oils, all MyPyramid groups provide protein in varying amounts.
- The quality of proteins varies. Complete proteins, those with high biologic value, provide adequate amounts and proportions of all essential amino acids needed for protein synthesis. Animal proteins and soy protein are complete proteins. Incomplete proteins lack adequate amounts of one or more essential amino acids. Except for soy protein, all plants are sources of incomplete proteins. Gelatin is also an incomplete protein.
- The RDA for protein for adults is 0.8 g/kg of body weight. Most experts recommend that protein contribute 10% to 20% of total calories in the diet. Most Americans consume more protein than they need.

- Pure vegans eat no animal products. Most American vegetarians are lacto-vegetarians or lacto-ovo vegetarians, whose diets include respectively milk products or milk products and eggs.
- Most vegetarian diets meet or exceed the RDA for protein and are nutritionally adequate across the life cycle. Pure vegans who do not have reliable sources of vitamin B_{12} and vitamin D need supplements.
- Although bodybuilding requires more than the RDA for protein, the limiting factor in adding muscle mass is energy intake, not protein. Muscle building requires resistance exercise, adequate calories, and moderate protein.

ANSWER KEY

1. **TRUE** Most Americans consume more protein than they need.
2. **FALSE** Over the course of a day, if the food consumed is varied and contains sufficient calories, most vegetarian diets meet or exceed the RDA for protein.
3. **FALSE** Unlike glucose and fat, the body is not able to store excess amino acids for later use.
4. **TRUE** Soy protein is complete, or has high biologic value, protein, and is comparable in quality to animal protein.
5. **TRUE** The limiting factor in muscle building is energy intake (calories), not protein.
6. **FALSE** The quality of a protein is determined by the balance of essential amino acids provided.
7. **FALSE** Fruits generally provide negligible protein, and oils are protein free.
8. **FALSE** Healthy adults are in neutral nitrogen balance: Protein synthesis is occurring at the same rate as protein breakdown.
9. **FALSE** Properly planned vegetarian diets are nutritionally adequate during all phases of pregnancy and lactation.
10. **FALSE** High protein intake may increase the risk of osteoporosis and renal insufficiency. In addition, high intake of animal protein is associated with atherosclerosis and colon and prostate cancers.

WEBSITES FOR INFORMATION ABOUT GENERAL VEGETARIAN NUTRITION

Food and Nutrition Information Center, U.S. Department of Agriculture at **www.nal.usda.gov/fnic/etext/000059.html**
Loma Linda University Vegetarian Nutrition & Health Letter at **www.llu.edu/llu/vegetarian/vegnews.htm**
Vegan Outreach at **www.veganoutreach.org/whyvegan/health.html**
The Vegan Society (vitamin B_{12} information) at **www.vegansociety.com/html/info/b12sheet.htm**
Vegetarian Resource Group at **www.vrg.org**
The Vegetarian Society of the United Kingdom at **www.vegsoc.org/health/**
Seventh-Day Adventist Dietetic Association at **www.sdada.org/facts&fiction.htm**

WEBSITES FOR SOY INFORMATION

www.soyfoods.com
www.soyeveryday.com
www.talksoy.com

WEBSITES FOR QUORN INFORMATION

www.fda.gov
www.cspinet.org

REFERENCES

American Dietetic Association. (2003). Position of the American Dietetic Association and the Dietitians of Canada: Vegetarian diets. *Journal of the American Dietetic Association, 103,* 748–765.

Haddad, E., & Tanzman, J. (2002). What do vegetarians in the United States eat? *American Journal of Clinical Nutrition,* 78, 626S–632S.

Institute of Medicine of the National Academies. (2002) *Dietary reference intakes for energy, carbohydrate, fiber, fat, fatty acids, cholesterol, protein, and amino acids.* Washington, DC: National Academies Press.

Jacobson, M. (Executive Editor). (2002). Center for Science in the Public Interest Newsroom: CSPI calls for recall of "quorn" meat substitute. Available at www.cspinet.org/new/200209212.html. Accessed on 12/9/03.

Layman, D., Boileau, R., Erickson, D., et al. (2003). A reduced ratio of dietary carbohydrate to protein improves body composition and blood lipid profiles during weight loss in adult women. *Journal of Nutrition, 133,* 411–417.

Messina, V., Melina, V., & Mangels, A. (2003). A new food guide for North American vegetarians. *Journal of the American Dietetic Association, 103,* 771–775.

Peregrin, T. (2002). Mycoprotein: Is American ready for a meat substitute derived from a fungus? *Journal of the American Dietetic Association, 102,* 628.

Trumbo, P., Schlicker, S., Yates, A., & Poos, M. (2002). Dietary reference intakes for energy, carbohydrate, fiber, fat, fatty acids, cholesterol, protein and amino acids. *Journal of the American Dietetic Association, 102,* 1621–1630.

U.S. Department of Agriculture, Agricultural Research Service. (1997). Data tables: Results from ISDA's 1996 continuing survey of food intakes by individuals and 1996 diet and health knowledge survey, (online). ARS Food Surveys Research Group. Available (under "Releases"): www.barc.usda.gov/hgnrc/foodsurvey/home.htm. Accessed 12/9/03.

For information on the new dietary guidelines 2005 and MyPyramid, visit
http://connection.lww.com/go/dudek

4

Lipids

TRUE	FALSE	
⬭	⬭	**1** Fat provides more than double the amount of calories as an equivalent amount of carbohydrate or protein.
⬭	⬭	**2** All fats are bad fats.
⬭	⬭	**3** Ground beef is one of the biggest sources of saturated fat in the average American diet.
⬭	⬭	**4** In a "healthy" diet, no foods have more than 30% of their calories from fat.
⬭	⬭	**5** Butter is healthier than margarine.
⬭	⬭	**6** A statement on a label of ground beef that says it is 95% lean means that 5% of the calories in that meat are from fat.
⬭	⬭	**7** Saturated fat is found only in animal products.
⬭	⬭	**8** *Trans* fatty acids raise blood levels of LDL-cholesterol (the "bad" cholesterol).
⬭	⬭	**9** Most Americans limit their fat intake to 30% of total calories or less.
⬭	⬭	**10** Eating less cholesterol is the most effective dietary approach to lowering serum cholesterol levels.

UPON COMPLETION OF THIS CHAPTER, YOU WILL BE ABLE TO

- Discuss the differences between saturated, monounsaturated, and polyunsaturated fats and name sources of each.
- Discuss the digestion and absorption of fat.
- List functions of fat in the body.
- Discuss recommendations regarding fat intake.
- Name strategies for reducing "bad" fat and increasing "good" fat intake.

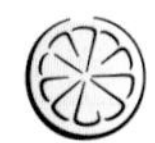

"Eat less fat" has long been a nutritional mantra. But decades of study have shown that the relationship between fat and chronic disease is far more complex than that simple advice implies. While an excess of any type of fat can contribute to obesity, cutting fat intake with low fat and nonfat foods does not guarantee weight loss. And although obesity increases the risk of certain cancers, the risk may come from an excess of calories, not specifically dietary fat. With heart disease and stroke, the type of fat may be more important than the amount of fat. Likewise, people with metabolic syndrome may fare better with a fat intake higher than the average American typically consumes, *if* the fat is predominantly unsaturated. The bottom line is that while all fats are calorically dense and can increase the risk of obesity, some fats are "good" (unsaturated) and should be eaten in moderation and other fats are "bad" (saturated fat and trans fats) and should be limited.

This chapter describes what fats are and the health implications of different fats. Also presented are sources of fats; the digestion, absorption and metabolism of fats; and recommendations regarding fat intake.

LIPIDS

Lipids, commonly referred to as fats, include triglycerides (fats and oils), phospholipids (e.g., lecithin), and sterols (e.g., cholesterol).

Triglycerides

Lipids: a group of water-insoluble, energy-yielding organic compounds composed of carbon, hydrogen, and oxygen atoms.

Triglycerides account for approximately 98% of the lipids in foods and are the major storage form of fat in the body. Just as amino acids can be arranged in limitless combinations to form different proteins, fatty acids can attach to glycerol molecules in various ratios and combinations to form a variety of triglycerides within a single food fat. Fatty acids vary in the length of their carbon chain and in the degree of unsaturation.

Carbon Chain Length

Triglycerides: a class of lipids composed of a glycerol molecule as its backbone with 3 fatty acids attached.

Almost all fatty acids have an even number of carbon atoms in their chain, the range being 2 to 24. Short-chain fatty acids contain 2 to 4 carbon atoms, medium-chain fatty acids contain 6 to 12 carbon atoms, and long-chain fatty acids contain 14 or more carbon atoms. The length of the carbon chain determines how the fatty acid is absorbed. Most food fats contain predominately long-chain fatty acids.

Degree of Unsaturation

As dictated by nature, each carbon atom in a fatty acid chain must have four bonds connecting it to other atoms. When all the carbon atoms in a fatty acid have four single bonds each, the fatty acid is said to be "saturated" with hydrogen atoms. An "unsaturated" fatty acid does not have all the hydrogen atoms it can potentially hold; therefore, one or more double bonds form between carbon atoms in the chain. If one double bond exists between two carbon atoms, the fatty acid is monounsaturated; if there is more than one double bond between carbon atoms, the fatty acid is polyunsaturated. Saturation is an important characteristic because it influences a fat's physical traits and its impact on health.

Triglycerides in Food

All food fats contain a mixture of saturated, monounsaturated, and polyunsaturated fatty acids. The types and proportions of fatty acids present influence the sensory and functional properties of the food fat. For instance, butter tastes and acts differently from corn oil, which tastes and acts differently from lard. When applied to sources of fat in the diet, "unsaturated" and "saturated" are not absolute terms used to describe the only types of fatty acids present; rather they are relative descriptions that indicate which kinds of fatty acids are present in the largest proportion (Table 4.1).

TABLE 4.1

PREDOMINANT TYPES OF FATTY ACIDS IN SELECTED FATS AND OILS

			Polyunsaturated fats		
	Cholesterol (mg/Tbsp)	% mono-unsaturated	% linolenic acid	% alpha-linolenic acid	% saturated
Highest in monounsaturated fat					
Olive oil	0	**77**	8	1	14
Canola oil	0	**62**	22	10	6
Peanut oil	0	**49**	33	0	18
Highest in polyunsaturated fat					
Safflower oil	0	13	**77**	trace	10
Flaxseed oil	0	18	**16**	**57**	9
Sunflower oil	0	20	**69**	**0**	11
Soybean oil	0	24	**54**	**7**	15
Corn oil	0	25	**61**	**1**	13
Cottonseed oil	0	19	**54**	**0**	27
Hydrogenated fat					
Margarine	0	**49**	30	2	19
Vegetable shortening (Crisco)	0	**44**	26	2	28
Highest in saturated fat					
Coconut oil	0	6	2	0	**92**
Palm kernel oil	0	12	2	0	**85**
Butter	33	30	2	2	**66**

All food fats contain a mix of saturated, monounsaturated, and polyunsaturated fatty acids.

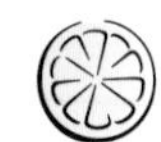

Unsaturated Fats, the "Good" Fats

Fatty Acids: organic compounds composed of a chain of carbon atoms to which hydrogen atoms are attached. An acid group (COOH) is attached at one end and a methyl group (CH_3) at the other end.

Glycerol: a three-carbon atom chain that serves as the backbone of triglycerides.

Saturated Fatty Acids: fatty acids in which all the carbon atoms are bonded to as many hydrogen atoms as they can hold so no double bonds exist between carbon atoms.

Unsaturated Fatty Acids: fatty acids that are not completely saturated with hydrogen atoms, so one or more double bonds form between the carbon atoms.

Unsaturated fats

- Are soft or liquid at room temperature, such as oils and soft margarines.
- Are susceptible to rancidity when exposed to light and oxygen over a prolonged period. Rancidity produces chemical changes that result in an offensive taste and smell and the loss of vitamins A and E (fat-soluble vitamins). Antioxidants added to fats, such as butylated hydroxyanisole (BHA) and butylated hydroxytoluene (BHT), help to extend shelf life as do minimizing storage time and avoiding high temperatures.
- Include monounsaturated fatty acids, which are highest in canola, olive, and peanut oils.
- Include polyunsaturated fatty acids, which come in two types:
  - omega-6 polyunsaturated oils found in plant oils such as safflower, sunflower, corn, soybean, and cottonseed oils
  - omega-3 polyunsaturated oils found in fish oils such as salmon, herring, trout, mackerel, and swordfish and also in some plant oils such canola oil, flaxseeds, flaxseed oil, walnut, and hazelnuts
- Lower LDL-cholesterol, although monounsaturated fats may lower cholesterol only if eaten in place of saturated fat. Omega-3 fats may protect the heart by mechanisms other than lowering cholesterol.

Essential Fatty Acids

Except for two polyunsaturated fatty acids, the body can make all the fatty acids it needs from carbohydrates, protein, and fat. Those two fatty acids, linoleic acid (an n-6 fatty acid) and alpha-linolenic acid (an n-3 fatty acid), are thus considered essential. Linoleic acid is the most common polyunsaturated fatty acid in food and is especially abundant in vegetable oils, nuts, seeds, leafy vegetables, whole grains, and poultry fat. Alpha-linolenic acid, the n-3 fatty acid found in plants, occurs in flaxseed, canola oil, soybean products, walnuts, and hazelnuts.

Essential fatty acids play a role in maintaining healthy skin and promoting normal growth in children. As part of phospholipids, essential fatty acids are a component of cell membranes and are precursors of eicosanoids, a group of hormone like substances involved in inflammation and blood clotting. Prostaglandins, thromboxanes, and leukotrienes are types of eicosanoids. Although the body cannot make essential fatty acids, it does store them so that deficiencies are rare.

Fish Oils

Eicosapentaenoic acid (EPA) and docosahexaenoic acid (DHA) are omega-3 polyunsaturated fatty acids found in animal tissues, primarily in cold-water fish, but not in plants. To a limited extent humans can convert alpha-linolenic acid to EPA and DHA in the body.

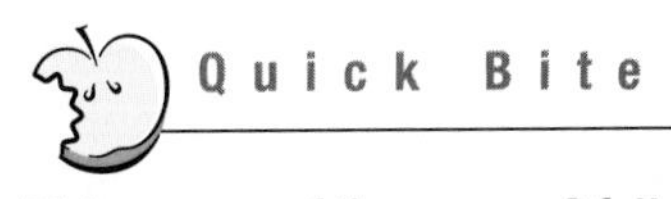

Rich sources of the omega-3 fatty acids EPA and DHA are

Salmon
Sardines
Trout
Herring
Swordfish
Oysters
Mackerel

Omega-6 (n-6) Fatty Acid: an unsaturated fatty acid whose endmost double bond occurs six carbon atoms from the methyl end of its carbon chain.

EPA and DHA have several actions in several body systems. EPA and DHA lower high triglyceride levels; have anti-arrhythmic, anti-inflammatory, and immune-modulating properties; and are beneficial for the musculoskeletal, gastrointestinal, and immune systems. EPA and DHA also play roles in normal blood flow. DHA is involved in normal brain development in the fetus and the infant and for normal brain functioning throughout life. It is abundant in the structural lipids in the brain and may play a role in the maintenance of normal cognition and mood. Both EPA and DHA are vital for normal functioning of rods and cones in the retina.

Over the last 20 years, research has shown that n-3 fatty acids may help to prevent or treat certain diseases. They have been shown to lower serum triglyceride levels, reduce blood pressure, and decrease factors involved in blood clotting and stroke. They also have anti-inflammatory effects that may benefit people with ulcerative colitis, Crohn's disease, and rheumatoid arthritis. Animal studies indicate n-3 fatty acids may inhibit the development of certain cancers. Results of studies on humans, animals, and cell cultures indicate that fish oils prevent arrhythmias and sudden cardiac death.

"Bad" Fats

Omega-3 Fatty Acid (n-3): an unsaturated fatty acid whose endmost double bond occurs three carbon atoms from the methyl end of its carbon chain.

"Bad" fats raise LDL-cholesterol, which is a major cause of coronary heart disease. Saturated fat and trans fats are clearly "bad" fats. Hydrogenated fats are "bad" because they are more saturated than the oil from which they are made and often contain trans fats. Yet lightly hydrogenated fats (e.g., soft margarine) offer a healthier alternative to more naturally saturated fats (e.g., butter) or more partially hydrogenated items (e.g., stick margarine).

Saturated Fats

Saturated fats

Low Density Lipoprotein (LDL)-Cholesterol: the major class of atherogenic lipoproteins that carry cholesterol from the liver to the tissues.

- Are solid at room temperature. Saturated fatty acids have a straight configuration (no double bonds) and so are usually capable of being packed into a solid at room temperature.
- Are stable, meaning less likely to become rancid than unsaturated fats.
- Occur naturally in almost all food fats but are highest in meats, dairy products, and tropical oils such as palm kernel and coconut.
- Raise LDL-cholesterol in the blood more than any other dietary component including dietary cholesterol. Conversely it is well known that eating less saturated fat lowers LDL-cholesterol levels, which in turn reduces the risk of coronary heart disease.

Essential Fatty Acids: fatty acids that cannot be synthesized in the body and so must be consumed through food.

Hydrogenated Fats

Food manufacturers hydrogenate polyunsaturated oils to make them solid at room temperature (e.g., margarine) or to make them less susceptible to rancidity so that products stay fresher longer. As polyunsaturated oils are hydrogenated, the proportion of polyunsaturated fatty acids decreases and the proportion of saturated and monounsaturated fatty acids increases.

The degree of hydrogenation varies from "light" to "partial" according to the desired outcome. For instance, lightly hydrogenated oils are more stable because they have fewer double bonds but are still in liquid form. They would not necessarily be considered "bad" fats because many polyunsaturated fats remain in the product.

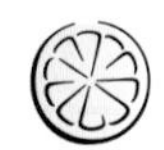

Fish Oils: a common term for the long-chain, polyunsaturated omega-3 fatty acids eicosapentaenoic acid (EPA) and docosahexaenoic acid (DHA) found in the fat of fish, primarily in cold-water fish.

Hydrogenation: a process of adding hydrogen atoms to unsaturated vegetable oils (usually corn, soybean, cottonseed, safflower, or canola oil), which reduces the number of double bonds; the number of saturated and monounsaturated bonds increase as the number of polyunsaturated bonds decreases.

Cis-Fats: unsaturated fatty acids whose hydrogen atoms occur on the same side of the double bond.

Trans-Fats: unsaturated fatty acids that have at least one double bond whose hydrogen atoms are on the opposite sides of the double bond; "trans" means across in Latin.

However, more solid (more saturated) products result from "partially hydrogenated" oils such as stick margarine and shortening. While the physical properties improve with hydrogenation (e.g., compared to the oil from which it was derived, the shortening can be reused more times in deep frying and produces flakier pie crusts and crispier French fries), the potential impact on health is negative (more saturated fat that increases LDL-cholesterol that increases CHD risk). The creation of trans fats additionally qualifies hydrogenated fats for the "bad" fat list.

Trans Fats

Unsaturated fatty acids occur in one of two shapes: either "cis" or "trans" (Fig. 4.1). These shapes are determined by the placement of the hydrogen atoms around the double bond. Most natural unsaturated fatty acids in food occur in the cis position.

Only small amounts of trans fats occur naturally in dairy products and meat. Studies suggest that the naturally occurring trans fats known as conjugated linoleic acid (CLA) may inhibit cancer and atherosclerosis, enhance the immune response, and have a positive effect on growth. Conjugated linoleic acid acts differently than manmade trans fats formed during the process of hydrogenation.

Hydrogenated fats (e.g., margarine, shortening) and processed foods made with hydrogenated fats (e.g., commercially prepared baked goods, crackers, snack foods, fried foods, and microwave popcorn) are the largest contributors of trans fats in the typical American diet. Like saturated fat, these trans fats raise LDL-cholesterol, which increases the risk of developing coronary heart disease. Even worse, trans fats may also lower HDL-cholesterol, the "good" cholesterol that is protective against heart disease. In theory, the effect of trans fat on blood cholesterol may be worse than the effect of saturated fat. However, because we consume so much less trans fat (an average of 2.6% of total calories among American adults) than saturated fat (an average of 13% of total calories), it is inaccurate to assume that cutting trans fat will make a greater impact on heart health than cutting saturated fat.

Because of the clinical evidence that trans fats are as heart unhealthy as saturated fat and because of pressure from consumer groups, the FDA has amended its regulations on nutrition labeling to require trans fatty acids be declared on the Nutrition Facts label. The grams of trans fat in a serving of food or dietary supplement will appear on a separate line immediately under saturated fat. Trans fat does not have to be listed if a food has less than 0.5 g total fat/serving and if no claims are made about fat, fatty acids, or cholesterol content. When trans fat is not listed, a footnote will state that the food is "not a significant source of trans fat." A Daily Value has not been established so that will appear blank. Because amounts less than 0.5 g/serving can be

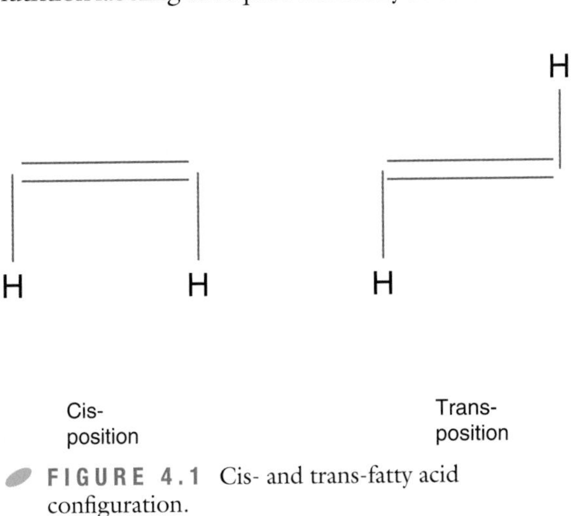

FIGURE 4.1 Cis- and trans-fatty acid configuration.

rounded down to zero, it is possible that the content of trans fat will be zero even if hydrogenated oils or shortenings appear on the ingredient list. These changes are effective January 1, 2006.

Other Lipids

The other 2% of lipids in foods are made up of phospholipids and sterols.

Phospholipids

Phospholipids: a group of compound lipids that is similar to triglycerides in that they contain a glycerol molecule and two fatty acids. In place of the third fatty acid, phospholipids have a phosphate group and a molecule of choline or another nitrogen-containing compound.

Phospholipids are both fat-soluble (because of the fatty acids) and water-soluble (because of the phosphate group), a unique feature that enables them to act as emulsifiers. Because of this, phospholipids are used extensively by the food industry. They occur naturally in almost all foods but make up a very small amount of total lipid intake.

Phospholipids perform many vital functions in the body. As emulsifiers they keep fats suspended in blood and other body fluids. As a component of all cell membranes, phospholipids not only provide structure but help to transport fat-soluble substances across cell membranes. Phospholipids are precursors of prostaglandins.

Lecithin is the best known phospholipid. Claims that it lowers blood cholesterol, improves memory, controls weight, and cures arthritis, hypertension, and gallbladder problems are unfounded. Studies show no benefit from taking supplements because lecithin is digested in the gastrointestinal tract into its component parts and is not absorbed intact to perform super functions. Lecithin is not even an essential nutrient because it is synthesized in the body. Many people who take lecithin supplements do not realize that they provide 9 cal/g, just like all other fats.

Cholesterol

Emulsifier: a stabilizing compound that helps to keep both parts of an emulsion (oil and water mixture) from separating.

Sterols: one of three main classes of lipids that include cholesterol, bile acids, sex hormones, the adrenocortical hormones, and vitamin D.

Cholesterol is a sterol, a waxy substance whose carbon, hydrogen, and oxygen molecules are arranged in a ring. Cholesterol occurs in the tissues of all animals. It is found in all cell membranes and in myelin; brain and nerve cells are especially rich in cholesterol. The body synthesizes bile acids, steroid hormones, and vitamin D from cholesterol. Although cholesterol is made from acetyl-CoA, the body cannot break down cholesterol into CoA molecules to yield energy; so cholesterol does not provide calories.

Quick Bite

Cholesterol content of selected foods

	Cholesterol (mg)		Cholesterol (mg)
Beef brains, 3 oz	1746	Shrimp, 4	37
Beef liver, 3 oz	375	Whole milk, 1 cup	30
Beef kidney, 3 oz	329	2% milk, 1 cup	15
Egg yolk, 1	213	Butter, 1 Tbsp	12
Broiled lobster, 1 cup	110	Nonfat milk, 1 cup	7
Broiled steak, 4 oz	71	Egg whites	0

 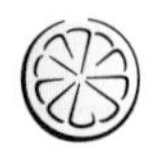

Cholesterol is found exclusively in animals, with meat and egg yolks as the largest sources in the typical American diet. The cholesterol in food is just cholesterol; descriptions of "good" and "bad" cholesterol refer to the lipoprotein packages that move cholesterol through the blood (see Chapter 18). You cannot eat more "good" cholesterol, but you can make lifestyle changes, such as quitting smoking, exercising, and losing weight if overweight, that increase the amount of "good" cholesterol in the blood.

Because all body cells are capable of making enough cholesterol to meet their needs, cholesterol is not an essential nutrient. In fact, daily endogenous cholesterol synthesis is approximately 2 to 3 times more than average cholesterol intake. When dietary cholesterol decreases, endogenous cholesterol production increases to maintain an adequate supply. The body makes cholesterol from acetyl coenzyme A (acetyl-CoA), which can originate from carbohydrates, protein, fat, or alcohol.

Dietary cholesterol increases total and LDL-cholesterol but the effect is lessened when saturated fat intake is low. Dietary cholesterol may have an independent effect on heart disease risk beyond its effect on serum cholesterol.

Functions of Fat in the Body

As already mentioned, specific lipids have specific functions in the body. Phospholipids and cholesterol are vital components of cell membranes, and cholesterol is a precursor of vitamin D, steroid hormones, and bile acids. As a component of phospholipids, essential fatty acids help to maintain cell membrane integrity; they also regulate cholesterol metabolism and are precursors of eicosanoids. Omega-3 fatty acids affect triglyceride metabolism, blood pressure regulation, and blood clotting.

General functions of fat in the body are to provide energy, protect vital organs, insulate against cold environmental temperatures, and facilitate the absorption of fat-soluble vitamins.

Provide Energy

Fat is a major source of energy, providing about 55% of the body's calorie needs at rest. All fat, whether unsaturated or unsaturated, cis- or trans-, provides 9 cal/g, more than double the amount of calories as an equivalent amount of either carbohydrate or protein. Fat metabolism is more complex than that of glucose, and it requires some glucose to be completely oxidized. Although fat is an important energy source, certain cells, such as brain cells and cells of the central nervous system, rely solely on glucose for energy.

Stored fat in adipose cells represents the body's largest and most efficient energy reserve. Unlike glycogen, which can be stored only in limited amounts and is accompanied by water, adipose cells have a virtually limitless capacity to store fat and carry very little additional weight as intracellular water. Each pound of body fat provides 3500 calories. Although normal glycogen reserves may last for half a day of normal activity, fat reserves can last up to 2 months during a complete fast in people of normal weight.

Career Connection

The number of calories needed to produce weight loss can be calculated based on the fact that 1 pound of body fat provides 3500 calories. In theory, to lose 1 pound of weight/week, usual calorie intake needs to decrease by 500 cal/day (3500 calories divided by 7 days/week = 500 cal/day deficit). Likewise, to lose 2 pounds/week, daily intake needs to be lowered by 1000 calories, a significant reduction that may leave many people unable to meet their requirements for nutrients or their basal energy needs, not to mention leaving them hungry. Using math, it is easy to see why health professionals recommend weight loss not exceed 2 pounds/week.

Other Functions of Fat

In the body, fat deposits insulate and cushion internal organs to protect them from mechanical injury. Fat under the skin helps to regulate body temperature by serving as a layer of insulation against the cold. Dietary fat also facilitates the absorption of the fat-soluble vitamins A, D, E, and K when consumed at the same meal.

How the Body Handles Fat

Digestion

A minimal amount of chemical digestion of fat occurs in the mouth and stomach through the action of lingual lipase and gastric lipases respectively (Fig. 4.2).

As fat enters the duodenum, it stimulates the release of the hormone cholecystokinin, which in turn stimulates the gallbladder to release bile. Bile, an emulsifier produced in the liver from bile salts, cholesterol, phospholipids, bilirubin, and electrolytes, prepares fat for digestion by suspending the hydrophobic molecules in the watery intestinal fluid. Emulsified fat particles have enlarged surface areas on which digestive enzymes can work.

Monoglyceride: a glyceride molecule with only one fatty acid attached.

Most fat digestion occurs in the small intestine. Pancreatic lipase, the most important and powerful lipase, splits off one fatty acid at a time from the triglyceride molecule, working from the outside in until two free fatty acids and a monoglyceride remain. Usually the process stops at this point but sometimes digestion continues and the monoglyceride splits into a free fatty acid and a glyceride molecule. The end products of digestion—mostly monoglycerides with free fatty acids and little glycerol—are absorbed into intestinal cells. It is normal for a small amount of fat (4–5 g) to escape digestion and be excreted in the feces.

The digestion of phospholipids is similar with the end products being two free fatty acids and a phospholipid fragment. Cholesterol does not undergo digestion; it is absorbed as is.

Absorption

About 95% of consumed fat is absorbed, mostly in the duodenum and jejunum. Small fat particles, such as short- and medium-chain fatty acids and glycerol, are absorbed

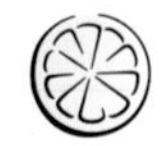

Micelles: fat particles encircled by bile salts to facilitate their diffusion into intestinal cells.

Chylomicrons: lipoproteins that transport absorbed lipids from intestinal cells through the lymph and eventually into the bloodstream.

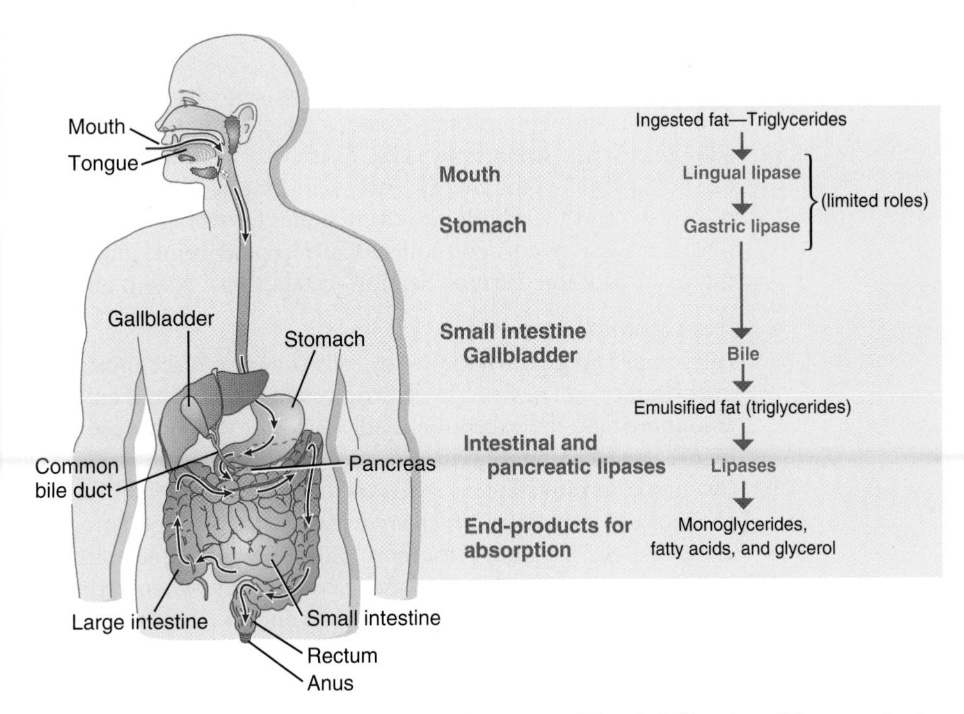

FIGURE 4.2 Fat digestion. A minimal amount of chemical digestion of fat occurs in the mouth and stomach through the action of lingual lipase and gastric lipases respectively. As fat enters the duodenum, it stimulates the release of the hormone cholecystokinin, which in turn stimulates the gallbladder to release bile. Bile prepares fat for digestion by suspending the hydrophobic molecules in the watery intestinal fluid. Most fat digestion occurs in the small intestine. Pancreatic lipase splits off one fatty acid at a time from the triglyceride molecule, working from the outside in until two free fatty acids and a monoglyceride remain. Usually the process stops at this point but sometimes digestion continues and the monoglyceride spits into a free fatty acid and glyceride molecule. The end products of digestion—mostly monoglycerides with free fatty acids and little glycerol—are absorbed into intestinal cells. It is normal for a small amount of fat (4 to 5 g) to escape digestion and be excreted in the feces.

directly through the mucosal cells into capillaries. They bind with albumin and are transported to the liver via the portal vein.

The absorption of larger fat particles, namely monoglycerides and long-chain fatty acids, is more complex. Although they are insoluble in water, monoglycerides and long-chain fatty acids dissolve into micelles, which deliver fat to the intestinal cells. Once inside the intestinal cells, the monoglycerides and long-chain fatty acids combine to form triglycerides. The reformed triglycerides, along with phospholipids and cholesterol, become encased in protein to form chylomicrons. Chylomicrons distribute dietary lipids throughout the body.

Their job done, most of the released bile salts are reabsorbed in the terminal ileum, transported back to the liver, and recycled (enterohepatic circulation). Some bile salts become bound to fiber in the intestine and are excreted in the feces.

Metabolism

In the bloodstream, triglycerides in the chylomicrons are broken down into glycerol and fatty acids by lipoprotein lipase, a fat-digesting enzyme located on the surface of adipose cells and other body cells. These fatty acids and glycerol enter cells where they can be catabolized for energy. Fatty acids not needed for energy are picked up by adipose tissue and are rebuilt into triglycerides for storage. Fat metabolism is regulated by hormones: adrenocorticotropin (ACTH), epinephrine, glucagon, glucocorticoids, and thyroxine promote fat mobilization (catabolism); insulin inhibits the activity of lipase.

Fat Catabolism

Fatty acids and glycerol for use by cells come from the most recent meal (triglycerides in chylomicrons) or from stored triglycerides. Most cells are able to store only minute amounts of fat; the exception is adipose cells, which have a virtually boundless capacity to store fat. Adipose cells give up stored fat when an enzyme within the adipose cell (hormone-sensitive lipase) reacts to the need for energy by splitting triglycerides into glycerol and fatty acids, which are released into the bloodstream and picked up by cells as needed. See Chapter 7 for more on energy metabolism from fat.

During starvation or uncontrolled diabetes, when carbohydrate intake is inadequate or unavailable, the body meets its energy needs by increasing the catabolism of fatty acids. However, in the absence of adequate glucose, fatty acids are incompletely broken down and ketone formation increases. Ketosis and acidosis may result.

Fat Anabolism

Most newly absorbed fatty acids end up stored in adipose tissue in the form of triglycerides. While the body makes triglycerides for storage from any excess calories from any source, the ease and efficiency of doing so varies among nutrients. The steps to convert carbohydrates and protein to fat are complex and numerous; the pathway for dietary fat is quick and easy. For instance, excess glucose (six carbon atoms) must first be split into pyruvate molecules (three carbon atoms) and then into acetyl-CoA (two carbon atoms). Molecules of acetyl-CoA are then joined to form fatty acids, which combine with glycerol to make triglycerides. Each step of this lengthy process requires energy; approximately 23% of the original carbohydrate calories are used to convert glucose to fat. By comparison, the pathway for turning excess dietary fat into body fat is much more direct and efficient: the body simply puts the glycerol and fatty acids back together into triglycerides. The body uses little energy, only about 3% of the original calories, to make fat from fat. That is why an excess of dietary fat is more likely to become body fat than an excess of either carbohydrate or protein.

Fat in Foods

With the exception of most fruits and vegetables, each MyPyramid group has at least some items that contain fat (Fig. 4.3). It is recommended that people choose the lowest-fat selections from each group. When higher-fat choices are made, the extra calories from the fat should be counted as part of a person's discretionary calories for the day. However, most discretionary calorie allowances are very small (between 150

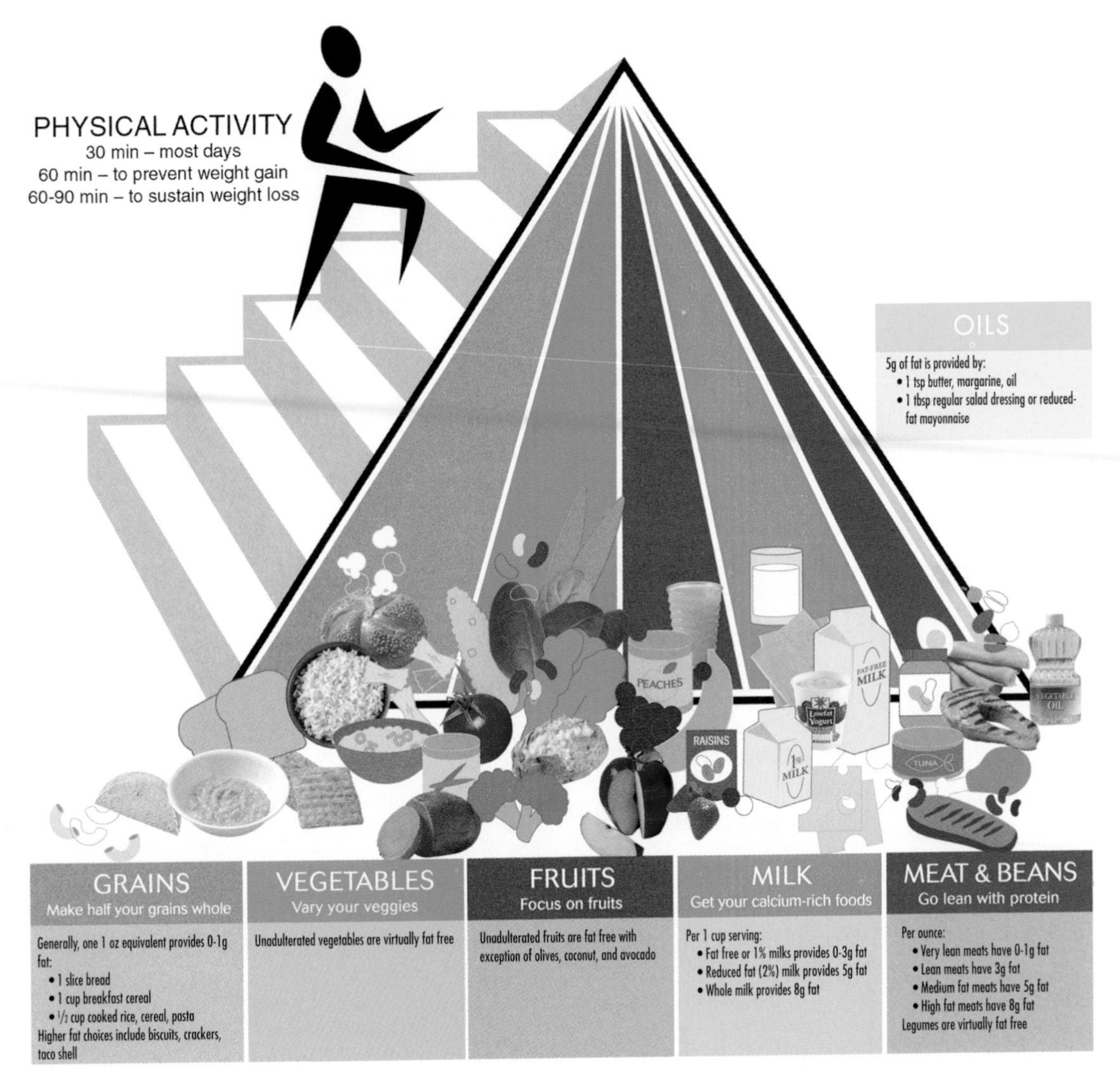

FIGURE 4.3 Fat content of MyPyramid.

and 300 discretionary calories/day, depending on total calorie needs), so the "budget" for higher-fat choices is limited.

Grains

Grains naturally contain very little fat, although prepared items within this group—such as granola cereals, crackers, and biscuits—provide fat.

Vegetables

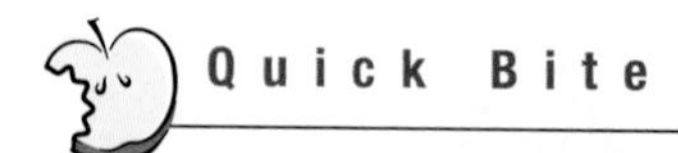

A look at how the method of preparation impacts fat content

	Fat (g)		Fat (g)
Boiled potato, ½ cup	trace	French fries, 10	8
Mashed potatoes, ½ cup	4.4	Potato salad, ½ cup	10.3
Scalloped potatoes, ½ cup	4.5	Homemade hash browns, ½ cup	10.8

Unadulterated vegetables contain little or no fat. Vegetables that are fried, creamed, served with cheese, or mixed with mayonnaise provide significant fat.

Fruits

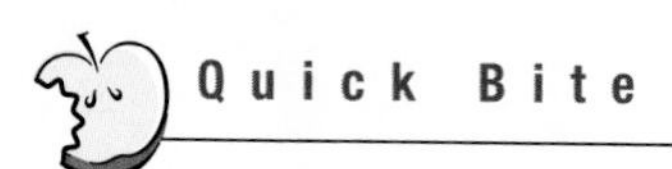

The only fruits with natural fat

	Fat (g)	Saturated fat (g)
Avocado, 1 medium	15	2.3
Coconut, 2 tbsp shredded	4.0	4.0
Coconut milk, 1 cup	48.2	42.7
Olives (green or ripe), 5 large	3.0	0.5

With the exception of avocado, coconut, and olives, fruits are naturally fat-free.

Milk

Saturated fat is the predominate fat in milk. The differences in total fat content between and among items from this group can be significant. For instance, fat free milk provides no fat while whole milk has 8 grams per cup. Likewise, fat free cheddar cheese has no fat while full fat cheddar provides 9 g/oz. Similarly, cholesterol content varies with the amount of fat, ranging from 5 mg cholesterol in a cup of skim milk to 32 mg in a cup of whole milk.

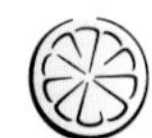

Career Connection

Can you believe 2% milk is 98% fat free? It's true, but it is 98% fat free *by weight,* not by calories. Clients who do not understand that percent fat by weight differs from percent calories from fat may inaccurately assume a product is low in fat. For instance, the 2% fat by weight of 2% milk (which contains a lot of heavy, but calorie-free, water) actually translates to 48% calories from fat. Follow the math found on the label:

1 cup of 2% milk contains 5 g of fat and 120 cal
$5 \text{ g} \times 9 \text{ cal/g} = 45$ cal from fat per cup
45 cal divided by $120 \text{ cal/cup} \times 100 = 37.5\%$ calories from fat

For practical purposes, the fat content claims that appear on packaged meat labels can be used to compare one brand to another but not to determine the percentage of calories from fat. For instance, packaged ham labeled "94% fat free" is lower in fat than ham labeled "92% fat free," but assumptions about the percentage of calories from fat cannot be made.

Meat and Beans

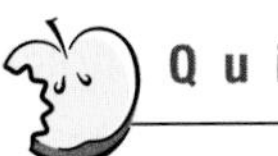

Quick Bite

The majority of calories in nuts come from fat; notice the small portion size.

Per 1 oz dry roasted	*Fat (g)*	*Per 1 oz dry roasted*	*Fat (g)*
Almonds, 24	14	Pine nuts, 157	14
Hazelnuts, 20	17	Pistachios, 47	13
Peanuts, 14	14	Walnuts, 14 halves	18
Pecans, 20 halves	20		

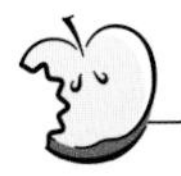

Quick Bite

Wild game is generally low in fat.

3-oz portion with visible fat removed	*Fat (g)*	*3-oz portion with visible fat removed*	*Fat (g)*
Beef, T-bone (for comparison)	10	Ostrich (tenderloin)	3
Bison	2	Pheasant (without skin)	3
Deer (venison)	3	Rabbit (wild)	4
Elk	2	Squirrel	5

Marbling: fat deposited in the muscle of meat.

The type and amount of fat from the meat group vary considerably. Generally, *per ounce,* very lean meats provide 0 to 1 g fat, lean meats have 3 g fat, medium fat meats have 5 g, and high fat meats contain 8 g of fat. A *serving size* of meat may be 3 or 4 ounces, but many people eat much more. Cooking methods can add fat (e.g., frying, basting with fat). Per ounce, nuts provide 13 to 20 g of fat. Also note that

- Untrimmed meats are higher in fat than lean-only portions.
- "Red meats," namely beef, pork, and lamb, are higher in saturated fat than the "white meats" of poultry and seafood.
- White poultry meat is lower in fat than dark meat; removing poultry skin removes significant fat.
- Fat content varies among different cuts of meat. The leanest cuts are beef loin and round; veal and lamb from the loin or leg; and pork tenderloin or center loin chop.
- Beef grades can be used as a guide to fat content because grades are based largely on the amount of marbling. Beef graded "prime," sold mostly to restaurants, is the most heavily marbled grade and thus the fattiest. In retail stores, within any cut "choice" has more marbling and higher fat content than "select."
- Shellfish are very low in fat but have considerable cholesterol.
- Most wild game is low in fat.
- Processed meats, such as sausage and hot dogs, may provide more fat calories than protein calories.
- Egg yolks provide 5 g fat and approximately 213 mg of cholesterol, whereas egg whites are fat- and cholesterol-free.
- Nuts have many healthy attributes; they contain plant protein, fiber, vitamin E, selenium, magnesium, zinc, phosphorus, potassium, in a low–saturated fat, cholesterol-free package. Their high fat content comes mostly from monounsaturated fats and polyunsaturated fats. Walnuts are particularly high in omega-3 fats.
- Dried peas and beans are virtually fat-free.

Oils

Items from this group provide approximately 5 g of fat per serving, whether liquid fat in the form of oils or solid fat in the form of margarine and butter.

Discretionary Calories

Discretionary calories are considered "luxury" choices that are allowed after essential nutrient needs are met *if* all food choices are fat-free or low-fat and with no added sugars. If less than ideal choices are made, the difference in fat and sugar calories is subtracted from the discretionary calorie "budget." Discretionary calories provide fat when they come from higher-fat versions of a food from any group or when they are used for more servings from the Oils group. The fat content varies with the selections made.

Intake Recommendations

Neither an Adequate Intake (AI) nor Recommended Dietary Allowance (RDA) is set for total fat due to insufficient data to define a level of fat intake at which risk of

 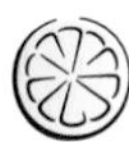

deficiency or prevention of chronic disease occurs. An Acceptable Macronutrient Distribution Range (AMDR) is estimated to be 20 to 35% of total calories for adults.

Adequate Intakes have been set for the essential fatty acids: linoleic acid and linolenic acid (Table 4.2). Both values are based on the median intake in the United States where fatty acid deficiencies do not exist in healthy people. Because the body makes saturated fatty acids and monounsaturated fatty acids, a dietary requirement does not exist. It is recommended that trans fatty acid intake be as low as possible.

An upper limit for linoleic acid is set at 10% of total calories because 1) intakes of linoleic acid greater than 10% of calories are rare, 2) there is insufficient epidemiological evidence to conclude that intakes greater than 10% of calories are safe, and 3) high intakes of linoleic acid produce a pro-oxidant condition that may increase the risk of heart disease and cancer.

Essential fatty acid deficiencies are extremely rare in people eating a mixed diet. Those at risk for deficiency include infants and children consuming low-fat diets (their need for essential fatty acids is proportionately higher than that of adults), clients with anorexia nervosa, and people receiving lipid-free parenteral nutrition for long periods. People with fat malabsorption syndromes are also at risk. Symptoms of essential fatty acid deficiency include growth failure, reproductive failure, scaly dermatitis, and kidney and liver disorders.

Fat Intake Guidelines

The focus of dietary recommendations issued by health authorities is to improve Americans' intake to reduce the risk of chronic disease rather than to avoid nutrient deficiencies. Fat, more than any other nutrient, is singled out as a public health enemy based on the evidence that

- Regardless of the type of fat, high-fat diets are high in calories and increase the risk of obesity. Independently, obesity, especially central obesity, increases the risk of heart disease, hypertension, stroke, insulin resistance, and type 2 diabetes. Obesity is also a risk factor for several types of cancer: namely colon, endometrium,

TABLE 4.2 **FAT INTAKE RECOMMENDATIONS**

	Acceptable Macronutrient Distribution Range—Adequate Intake				
	% of total calories from fat	% of total calories from linoleic acid	% of total calories from alpha-linolenic acid	Linoleic acid (g/day)	Linolenic acid (g/day)
Adult men	20–35%	5–10%	0.6–1.2%	17 g	1.6 g
Adult women	20–35%	5–10%	0.6–1.2%	12 g	1.1 g

esophagus, gallbladder, pancreas, kidney, and breast (among postmenopausal women) cancers.

- High intakes of saturated fat and trans fat increase LDL-cholesterol and so increase the risk of coronary heart disease. Some studies implicate saturated fat as a risk factor for certain cancers.

Total Fat

Although most experts agree that Americans should eat less fat, the recommended percentage of total calories from fat varies. For instance, the Acceptable Macronutrient Distribution Range (AMDR) for adults for fat intake is set at 20% to 35% of total calories, the same range recommended in the Therapeutic Lifestyle Change (TLC) Diet of

Career Connection

Many clients know what they need to do to eat healthier but do no know how to do it. Advise the client who needs or wants to eat less fat to

Think small. Small changes can add up to big results. For instance, someone who drinks 3 cups of whole milk daily can save 9 g of fat per day by switching to 2% milk, 15 g of fat by using 1% milk, or 24 g of fat with skim milk.

Make changes gradually. Gradual changes in food choices are more likely to result in long-lasting lifestyle modifications than are drastic "quick fixes" that are difficult to maintain over the long haul. People who are accustomed to whole milk are much more likely to accept 2% milk than skim milk. After they have become accustomed to 2% milk, they should try 1% then skim milk. Each change makes subsequent changes easier.

Be positive. Focus on all the things the client can eat, not on what should not be eaten. Natural and wholesome plant foods are naturally low in fat and are loaded with essentials for good health such as vitamins, minerals, fiber, and phytochemicals.

Rethink the importance of meat. Meats are a mainstay in the typical American diet but many are high in fat and saturated fat. Ground beef, in particular, is one of the leading contributors of saturated fat in the average American diet. Encourage the client to experiment with meatless entrees. Clients who absolutely must have meat should think of it as a condiment or side dish and focus on fruits, vegetables, and grains.

Use the plate method. Divide the dinner plate into two parts: three-quarters for plant foods and one-quarter for animal foods. This arrangement turns out to be approximately equivalent to 50% to 60% complex carbohydrates, 20% to 30% protein, and 20% to 30% fat, which is right on target.

Be mindful of portion sizes. Three ounces of meat is the size of a deck of cards; 1 teaspoon is about the size of a thumbnail; a tennis ball is approximately 1 cup.

Be careful when eating out. Restaurant portion sizes tend to be much bigger than the recommended serving sizes. Encourage clients to order a regular burger instead of a supersized or specialty burger. Other ideas are to ask for a "doggie bag" and take home part of the meal, to split dessert with a companion, to ask that dressings be served on the side, to forgo gravies and sauces, and to select baked or broiled foods rather than fried foods.

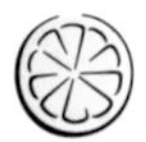

the National Cholesterol Education Program (NCEP) and the 2005 edition of the Dietary Guidelines for Americans. A goal of Healthy People 2010 is to increase the proportion of people aged 2 and older who consume no more than 30% of calories from total fat. The World Health Organization recommends total fat be limited to 15% to 30% of total calories. Dean Ornish's Reversal Diet, which is proven to cause clearing in clogged arteries, and the Pritikin Diet limit fat to approximately 10% of total calories. According to results from the USDA's 1996 Continuing Survey of Food Intakes by Individuals (CFSII), only one-third of Americans aged 2 and older actually consume 30% or less of their total calories from fat. Average fat intake among American adults is approximately 34% of total calories.

In addition to the lack of consensus about the optimal percentage of calories from fat, specifying fat intake as a percentage of total calories is meaningless in practice. Clients often misinterpret the recommendation to "limit total calories from fat to 30%" to mean "do not eat any foods that have more than 30% of their calories coming from fat." However, the guideline of 30% calories from fat pertains to the total diet, not to individual foods. Higher-fat foods such as nuts need not be excluded from the diet because the percentage of total calories from fat is lessened when averaged over an entire day with foods that provide little or no fat (vegetables, fruits, skim milk, and grains).

Therefore, a more effective approach to lowering fat intake is to focus on the types and amounts of food *to* eat—the "total diet approach." For instance, both the American Heart Association and the American Cancer Society urge a plant-based diet, which is inherently lower in total fat, saturated fat, and cholesterol than a typical meat-based diet. Strategies for lowering total fat and "bad" fat as well as increasing "good" fat appear in Box 4.1.

BOX 4.1

STRATEGIES FOR REDUCING AND MODIFYING FAT INTAKE

Eat Less Meat

- Eat occasional meatless meals like bean burritos, meatless chili, vegetable soup with salad, spaghetti with plain sauce.
- Limit meat to 5 oz/day; a recommended portion is size of a deck of cards or smaller.

Eat Lean Meats

- Eat meat, fish, and poultry that are baked, broiled, or roasted instead of fried.
- Remove the skin from chicken before eating.
- Choose "select" grades of beef, which have less marbling than "choice" grades.
- Trim all visible fat from meat.
- Choose ground beef that is at least 90% lean as indicated on the label.
- Choose beef cuts labeled "loin" or "round."
- Limit egg yolks to two per week.

Substitute Low-Fat or Nonfat for Regular Varieties

- Use 1% or nonfat milk.
- Use lowfat or nonfat yogurt.
- Choose cheese with 3 g or less per serving.
- Try sherbet, reduced fat ice cream, nonfat ice cream and yogurt.

BOX 4.1 (continued)

STRATEGIES FOR REDUCING AND MODIFYING FAT INTAKE

- Try low-fat or nonfat salad dressing.
- Use nonstick spray in place of oil, margarine, or butter to sauté foods and "butter" pans.
- Use imitation butter spray to season vegetables and hot air popcorn.

Limit Fat as a Flavoring

- Eat bread, rolls, muffins, or crackers without butter or margarine.
- Season with spice such as picante sauce, salsa, ginger, flavored vinegar, Italian spice blends.
- Eat potatoes and vegetables that are not fried.
- Instead of pouring dressing on salad, have it on the side; dip your fork into the dressing before spearing salad.
- Have desserts without cream or whipped cream toppings.

Reduce Hydrogenated Fat Intake

- Use the soft margarine (liquid or tub) in place of butter or stick margarine. Look for margarine that is "trans fat free," contains no more than 2 g saturated fat/tablespoon, and has liquid vegetable oil as the first ingredient.
- Look for processed foods made with unhydrogenated oil rather than hydrogenated or saturated fat.
- Avoid French fries, doughnuts, cookies, and crackers unless they are labelled fat-free.
- Avoid fried fast foods that are made with hydrogenated shortenings and oils.

Replace Fatty Foods With Fruit and Vegetables

- Eat fruit for dessert.
- Snack on raw vegetables or fresh fruit instead of snack chips.
- Double up on your usual portion of vegetables.

Use "Good" Fats in Moderation

- Make canola or olive oil your oil of choice.
- Eat fatty fish twice a week.
- Eat nuts and nut butters that are rich in monounsaturated fats: walnuts, almonds, hazelnuts, pecans, pistachios, and pine nuts. Walnuts also contain alpha-linolenic acid. Cashews and macadamia nuts are higher in saturated fats.
- Sprinkle flaxseed (1 to 2 tablespoons/day) over cereal or yogurt or use as a fat substitute in many recipes: 3 tablespoons of ground flaxseed can replace 1 tablespoon fat or oil.

Saturated Fat and Trans Fat

Likewise, health experts agree that Americans need to reduce their combined intake of saturated fat and trans fat to 7 to 10% of total calories. Generally as total fat intake increases, the proportion of saturated fat increases; so it is unlikely that a low saturated fat diet can be achieved when total fat intake exceeds 35%. According to results from the USDA's 1996 Continuing Survey of Food Intakes by Individuals (CFSII), only

 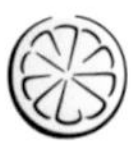

36% of Americans aged 2 and older actually consume less than 10% of total calories from saturated fat. On average, American adults consume approximately 13% of total calories from saturated fat and 2% to 3% from trans fat. Table 4.3 lists the amount of total fat (at 20 to 30% of calories) and saturated/trans fat (at 7 to 10% of calories) recommended at various calorie intakes.

Unsaturated Fats and Omega-3 Fats

Perhaps equally as important as *reducing* saturated fat and trans fat is *substituting* polyunsaturated and monounsaturated fats for saturated fat while keeping total fat intake reasonable. That means using canola or olive oil in dressings and for sautéing and baking and using a tub or liquid margarine in place of stick margarine or butter.

Because omega-3 fats protect against sudden cardiac death, the American Heart Association recommends Americans eat fatty fish twice a week. For people who do not eat seafood, the small amount of DHA and EPA the body makes from the alpha-linolenic acid in flaxseed, canola oil, soybeans, soybean oil, and walnuts is better than nothing. Designer eggs touted to contain omega-3 fats because they come from chickens fed fish oil or flaxseed do not provide any EPA and have only small amounts of DHA. Fish oil pills are an alternative to seafood for omega-3 fats but they have drawbacks. See Supplement Alert: Fish Oils.

Cholesterol

Cholesterol intake becomes less important when saturated fat intake is low. Still because total and LDL-cholesterol are positively related to the intake of saturated fat, trans fat, and cholesterol, the intake of these three lipids should be as low as possible within the context of a nutritionally adequate intake. Many health authorities recommend a daily cholesterol intake of 200 to 300 mg/day or less. The intake of cholesterol among American adults ranges from less than 100 mg/day to slightly less than 800 mg/day with an average intake of 270 mg/day.

TABLE 4.3 **AMOUNT OF TOTAL FAT (AT 20–30% OF TOTAL CALORIES) AND SATURATED/TRANS FAT (AT 7–10% OF TOTAL CALORIES) RECOMMENDED AT VARIOUS CALORIE INTAKES**

Daily Calorie Intake	Total fat (g) at 20–30% of total calories	Saturated fat + trans fat (g) at 7–10% of total calories
1200	27–40	9–13
1500	33–50	12–17
1800	40–60	14–20
2100	47–70	16–23
2400	53–80	19–27
2700	60–90	21–30
3000	67–100	23–33

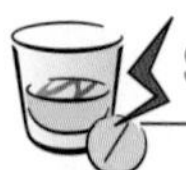

SUPPLEMENT ALERT: FISH OILS

Fish oil supplements are used for a variety of ills. Most often, fish oils are used to lower serum triglyceride levels. Other proposed benefits include decreased blood clotting; lowered blood pressure; improved symptoms of rheumatoid arthritis and ulcerative colitis; mood stabilization in bipolar disorder; and prevention of rejection after renal transplant.

Typically, natural fish oil supplements contain 30% EPA and DHA in a ratio of 1:1.5 (e.g., a 1 g softgel capsule contains 180 mg EPA and 120 mg DHA), although higher and lower ratios are available. Also available is a semisynthetic fish oil supplement concentrated to 85% EPA and DHA that provides 490 mg EPA and 350 mg DHA per 1 g capsule. Enteric-coated capsules of the free fatty acids are available.

Fish oil supplements are best tolerated with meals and should be consumed in divided doses throughout the day. The usual oral dose to lower triglyceride levels is 5 g combined EPA and DHA. For hypertension, rheumatoid arthritis, ulcerative colitis, and Crohn's Disease, the usual dose is 3 g/day. To promote wellness but not to treat illness, some experts recommend limiting intake to 1 g/day of EPA and DHA combined.

But whether or not fish oil supplements are a good idea is controversial. For instance, it is not known if fish oil supplements have the same beneficial effects in the body as eating fish. Also the actual content of fish oils in supplements may be much less than that stated on the label. Furthermore fish oil supplements, like certain fish, may contain high levels of pesticide residues, fat-soluble vitamins, or the heavy metal mercury. Certainly fish oil supplements are contraindicated when other "blood thinners" are used, such as warfarin, aspirin, garlic, and ginkgo, and should not be used prior to surgery. Finally, reported side effects include mild GI upset; "fishy" smelling breath, skin, and urine; nosebleeds; and easy bruising. As with other supplements, self-medicating carries potential risks.

FAT IN HEALTH PROMOTION

Obviously, the fat intake guidelines outlined in the previous section are intended to promote health. The traditional Mediterranean Diet and the use of fat replacers are of further interest in health promotion.

The Mediterranean Diet

The so-called Mediterranean diet reflects the traditional eating style of people living in Greece, parts of Italy, Lebanon, Morocco, Portugal, Spain, Syria, Tunisia, and Turkey (Fig. 4.4). Although high in fat (approximately 40% of calories), it is associated with a long life expectancy and low rates of heart disease, certain cancers, and other diet-related chronic diseases. Granted, its high monounsaturated fat content and very low saturated fat content impart definite health benefits, but they are probably only one piece of the healthy diet and lifestyle puzzle.

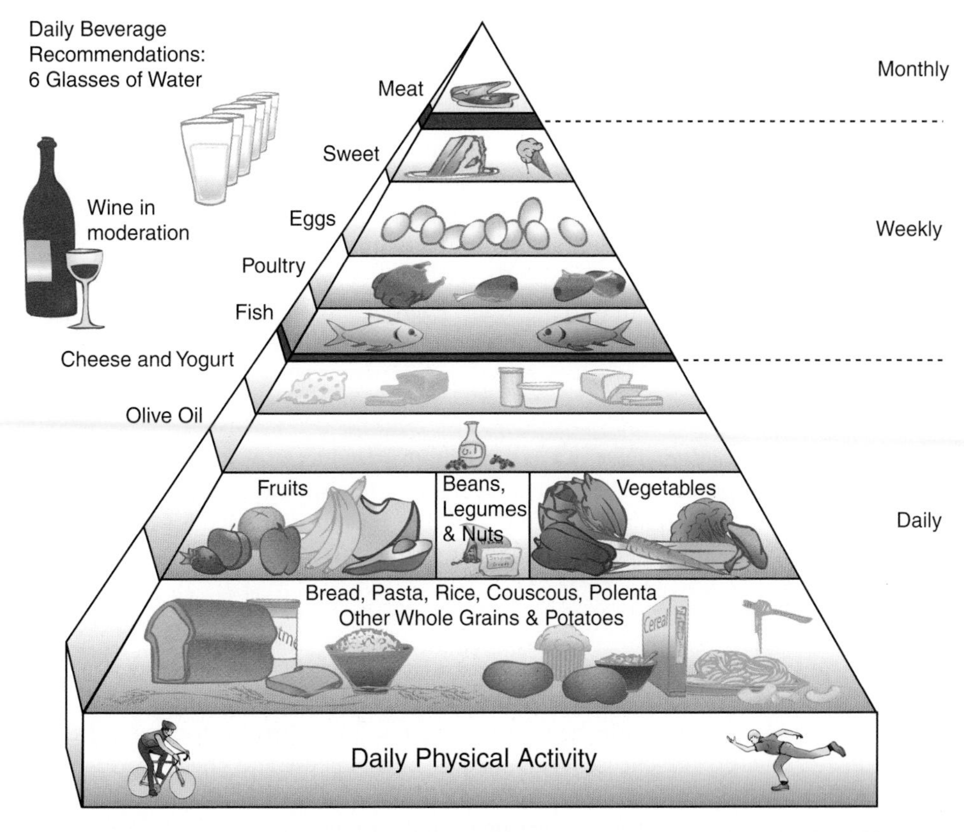

FIGURE 4.4 The traditional healthy Mediterranean diet pyramid. (© 2000 Oldways Preservation & Exchange Trust. www.oldwayspt.org.)

The minimally processed plant-based diet with added nuts and olive oil contains very little meat, eggs, or dairy products. Daily fruit and vegetable intake is approximately 1 pound and moderate amounts of red wine are consumed with meals. High levels of physical activity, a less stressful lifestyle, and lean body weights play a role in disease prevention. The bottom line is that although the Mediterranean diet and lifestyle may be optimal for health and longevity, it cannot be achieved simply by adding olive oil and red wine to the typical American diet. It is not as easy as drizzling olive oil on a cheeseburger.

Reducing Fat With Fat Replacers

Anyone who has tried to eliminate or reduce fat in a recipe knows that fat does more than simply provide calories. Fat provides flavor of its own, from the mild taste of canola oil and corn oil to the distinctive tastes of peanut oil and olive oil. Fat also contributes to the sensory appeal of foods by absorbing flavors and aromas of ingredients to improve overall taste. It has a creamy and smooth "mouth feel," as evident in full fat ice cream. Fats tenderize and add moisture in baked goods such as cookies, pies, and cakes.

Although some foods can be made low fat by simply reducing the fat content (e.g., milk), others use fat replacers to simulate the functional properties of fat while reducing total fat, saturated fat, and calories. Depending on how well they are digested, replacers made from carbohydrates or protein supply 4 cal/g or less compared with 9 cal/g in the fat they replace; the calorie content of replacers made from fats varies from 0 to 5 cal/kg. Each type has its own advantages, disadvantages, and most practical food uses. Three are discussed below.

Lighter Bake

Lighter Bake is a carbohydrate-based fat replacer for consumer use made from prune puree. It offers the advantage of retaining moisture and adding texture when used in place of fat in baked goods, but it cannot be used for frying and can have a laxative effect when consumed in large amounts.

Simplesse

Simplesse is a protein-based fat replacer made from the whey of milk or egg white protein that has been processed to produce a "mouthfeel" similar to fat. It provides only one-seventh the calories of fat and is approved for use in frozen desserts such as ice cream, cheese foods such as cream cheese and cheese spreads, and in other uncooked products. Because it breaks down when heated, it cannot be used for frying or baking. People who are allergic to milk or eggs should not use Simplesse.

Olestra

Olestra (brand name, Olean) was approved by the FDA in 1996. It is a large molecule made from sugar plus fatty acids from vegetable oil. Enzymes in the gastrointestinal tract are not able to split the fatty acids from the sugar molecule, so olestra passes through the body unabsorbed. Because it is not absorbed, it provides no calories. It may cause gastrointestinal upset (abdominal cramping, flatulence, diarrhea) and impair the absorption of fat-soluble vitamins when eaten at the same time as those nutrients. Manufacturers are required to add specified amounts of vitamins A, D, E, and K to products containing olestra to compensate for the potential loss of these nutrients; they must disclose on the product label that vitamins have been added and that potential gastrointestinal side effects may occur. The mouth feel and flavor of olestra are similar to those of fat. Olestra is used as a replacement for up to 100% of the fat in salty snack foods (e.g., potato chips, corn chips, cheese puffs) and crackers.

Do They Work?

According to the American Dietetic Association, "Fat replacers may offer a safe, feasible, and effective means to maintain the palatability of diets with controlled amounts

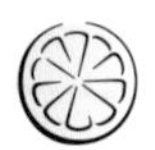

of fat and/or energy." Whether they actually help Americans to eat less fat and fewer calories depends on whether they are used in addition to foods normally eaten or take the place of regular fat foods that would otherwise be eaten. Furthermore, diets low in fat are not guaranteed to be low in calories. For instance, even if the fat content of coffee cake is reduced, there are still considerable calories provided by starch and sugar. People who choose to use fat replacers should do so with the understanding that they are only one component of a total diet and as such they alone cannot transform an "unhealthy" diet into a healthy one. Fat replacers should be consumed only at levels that are well tolerated. Only time will tell if fat replacers will help Americans to eat less fat, maintain healthy body weight, and reduce the risk of chronic diseases.

How Do You Respond?

What is flaxseed? Flaxseed is derived from the flax plant, the same plant used to make linen. It is a nutritional powerhouse, providing essential fatty acids, fiber, and lignans. Specifically, 57% of its fat is from alpha-linolenic acid, the precursor of the omega-3 fats DHA and EPA. The fiber in flaxseed is predominately soluble, which helps to lower cholesterol levels and improves glucose levels in diabetics. Flaxseed contains 100- to 800 times more lignans than other grains; lignans, a group of plant estrogens, may help to reduce the risk of breast and prostate cancers. While flaxseed oil and flaxseed oil pills provide the benefits of alpha-linolenic acid, they lack the fiber found in the whole grain and the lignan content is variable. However, humans are unable to digest the tough outer coating so flaxseeds must be eaten ground, not whole. Because they are high in polyunsaturated fat, they are prone to rancidity. Ground flaxseed should be refrigerated and used within a few weeks.

What is the best type of oil to buy? Soy oil is often the oil of choice in restaurants and in many prepared grocery store items such as mayonnaise, salad dressings, spaghetti sauce, and cookies. In fact, soy oils accounts for more than 80% of all oil used in the United States, about half of which gets partially hydrogenated to make margarine or shortening. To balance that high intake of polyunsaturated fat, which is rich in the omega-6 fat linoleic acid, choose a monounsaturated fat with the omega-3 fat alpha-linolenic acid to use at home in cooking and baking. Even though oil used at home represents only a small part of total fat intake, canola oil may be the best to use: compared to (the other monounsaturated fat) olive oil, canola oil is lower in saturated fat and has much more alpha-linolenic acid for a better n-6:n-3 ratio. However, consider flavor when appropriate. For instance, olive oil may be preferred for homemade salad dressing while canola oil is reliable for routine sautéing and baking.

Is counting fat grams a good way to track fat intake? It's possible but not practical to keep track of fat intake by counting fat grams. To use this method as a reliable means of monitoring fat intake, an individual must know his or her daily fat gram budget as well as the fat content of all foods eaten. The problem in counting fat grams is that not all foods are labeled. The fact that fresh fruits and vegetables are not labeled is inconsequential because they generally provide insignificant amounts of fat. But foods eaten away from home account for an estimated 25% of fat consumed—a significant unknown amount. Comparing labels for fat grams does allow consumers to make informed choices. However, information on grams of polyunsaturated fat and monounsaturated fat is not required on food labels, so tracking the type of fat consumed is almost impossible. Although low-fat diets may be among the best options for promoting weight loss, simply counting fat grams does not guarantee a low-calorie eating plan nor a healthy intake.

▲ Focus on Critical Thinking

Respond to the following statements:

1. Americans should strive to reduce their saturated fat intake to nothing.
2. Hydrogenation is a good thing.
3. The traditional Mediterranean diet is high in fat but healthier than the typical American diet.
4. Fish oil supplements are a safe and effective way to consume fish oils for people who don't eat fish.

Key Concepts

- Ninety-eight percent of lipids consumed in the diet are triglycerides, which are composed of one glyceride molecule and three fatty acids. Phospholipids and sterols are the other two types of dietary lipids.
- Saturation refers to the hydrogen atoms attached to the carbon atoms in the fatty acid chain. Saturated fatty acids do not have any double bonds between carbon atoms; each carbon is "saturated" with as much hydrogen as it can hold. Unsaturated fats have one (monounsaturated) or more than one (polyunsaturated) double bond between carbon atoms. When used to describe food fats, these terms are relative descriptions of the type of fatty acid present in the largest amount. All foods contain a mixture of saturated, monounsaturated, and polyunsaturated fats.
- Omega-3 fatty acids help to lower serum triglyceride levels, may lower blood pressure, and decrease platelet aggregation. They may also have anti-inflammatory effects. The best sources of n-3 fatty acids are fatty cold-water fish such as salmon, trout, herring, swordfish, sardines, and mackerel. Walnuts, soybeans, flaxseed, and canola oil are plant sources of the omega-3 fatty acid alpha-linolenic acid.
- *Trans* fatty acids are produced through the process of hydrogenation. They are chemically unsaturated fats that function like saturated fat in the body.
- Linoleic acid (n-6) and linolenic acid (n-3) are essential fatty acids because they cannot be made by the body. They are important constituents of cell membranes, and they function to maintain healthy skin and promote normal growth. Deficiencies of essential fatty acids are nonexistent in healthy people.
- Phospholipids are structural components of cell membranes that facilitate the transport of fat-soluble substances across cell membranes. They are widespread but appear in small amounts in the diet.

 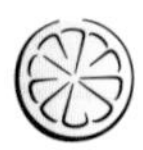

- Cholesterol, a sterol, is a constituent of all cell membranes and is used to make bile acids, steroid hormones, and vitamin D. Cholesterol is found in all foods of animal origin except egg whites. Most Americans eat about half as much cholesterol as the body makes each day.
- Fat digestion occurs mostly in the small intestine. Short-chain and medium-chain fatty acids and glycerol are absorbed through mucosal cells into capillaries leading to the portal vein. Larger fat molecules—namely cholesterol, phospholipids, and reformed triglycerides made from monoglycerides and long-chain fatty acids—are absorbed in chylomicrons and transported through the lymph system.
- The major function of fat is to provide energy; 1 g of fat supplies 9 cal of energy. Fat also provides insulation, protects internal organs from mechanical damage, and promotes absorption of the fat-soluble vitamins. The essential fatty acids are important for cell membrane integrity and eicosanoid synthesis.
- All MyPyramid food groups provide fat except the Fruits and Vegetables. The type and quantity of fat varies considerably among items within each group.
- Most leading health authorities recommend that Americans limit total fat intake to approximately 30% of total calories or less, saturated fat and trans fat intake to less than 10% of total calories, and cholesterol intake to 200 to 300 mg/day. The majority of Americans fail to meet these guidelines.
- High-fat diets are linked to heart disease and obesity. Obesity is an independent risk factor for type 2 diabetes, hypertension, certain cancers, and heart disease.
- Generally saturated fats and trans fats are "bad" because they raise LDL-cholesterol. Unsaturated fats are "good" because when they lower LDL-cholesterol. However, monounsaturated fats may lower LDL-cholesterol only when substituted for saturated fat.
- Population studies show that the higher-fat Mediterranean diet (approximately 40% of calories from fat with most from monounsaturated fats) may actually be optimal for disease prevention. Other lifestyle differences (exercise, normal body weight, less stress) contribute to the diet's positive effect on health.
- Fat replacers are safe and may help Americans to reduce their fat and calorie intake if they are used to replace high-fat foods normally eaten. Their use does not guarantee a low-calorie or healthy diet. Because olestra is not absorbed, it may cause abdominal cramping, flatulence, and diarrhea.

ANSWER KEY

1. **TRUE** All fats, whether saturated or unsaturated, provide 9 cal/g compared to 4 calories/g from carbohydrates and protein.
2. **FALSE** "Good" fats, namely polyunsaturated and monounsaturated fats, may help to lower LDL-cholesterol when used in place of saturated fat. Omega-3 fish oils are also "good": they lower triglyceride levels, decrease platelet aggregation, and may decrease inflammation in rheumatoid arthritis, Crohn's disease, and ulcerative colitis.
3. **TRUE** Ground beef is one of the biggest sources of total fat and saturated fat in the typical American diet.

4. **FALSE** The 30% guideline refers to the total diet, not individual foods. Over the course of the day, high fat items (e.g., canola oil, peanut butter) are balanced by low-fat and fat-free items (nonfat milk, grains, vegetables, and fruit).
5. **FALSE** Even though some margarines contain more *trans* fats than butter, the combined amount of "bad" fat (saturated fat plus trans fat) is higher in butter than in margarine, even stick margarine. In addition, butter contains cholesterol; margarine generally does not.
6. **FALSE** 95% lean refers to weight, not calories. Three ounces of 95% lean ground beef provide 6 g of fat and 145 calories. That translates to 37% of calories from fat (6 g fat × 9 cal/g = 54 cal. 54 cal divided by 145 cal × 100 = 37% fat calories) even though only 5% of the meat is fat by weight.
7. **FALSE** Cholesterol is found only in animal products. Saturated fat is found in animal products (meat and full fat dairy items) as well as coconut, palm kernel, and palm oils.
8. **TRUE** Trans fatty acids act like saturated fatty acids to raise blood levels of LDL-cholesterol (the "bad" cholesterol). Trans fat also lowers HDL-cholesterol (the "good" cholesterol).
9. **FALSE** Only about one-third of Americans consume 30% or less of their total calories from fat.
10. **FALSE** Eating less saturated fat has a greater impact on lowering serum cholesterol than does simply limiting cholesterol intake.

WEBSITES

American Heart Association at **www.americanheart.org**
American Oil Chemist's Society at **www.aocs.org**
Calorie Control Council's glossary of fat replacers at **www.caloriecontrol.org/frgloss.html**
Lower dietary fat intake at **www.nalusda.gov/fnic/dga/dga95/lowfat.html**
International Tree Nut Council at **www.treenuts.org**
Institute of Shortening and Edible Oils at **www.iseo.org**
International Food Information Council at **www.ificinfo.org**
National Heart, Lung and Blood Institute at **www.nhlbi.nih.gov**

REFERENCES

American Cancer Society. (2002). Prevention and early detection. The complete guide-nutrition and physical activity. Available at www.cancer.org.docroot/PED/content/PED_3_2X_Diet_and_Activity_Factors_Tha. . . . Accessed on 12/17/03.

American Heart Association. (2002). Know your fats. Available at www.americanheart.org/presenter.jhtml?identifier=532. Accessed on 12/18/03.

American Heart Association. (2000). Journal Report. American Heart Association dietary recommendations dish out a more individualized approach. Available at www.americanheart.org/presenter.jhtml?identifier=3296. Accessed on 12/16/03.

American Heart Association Conference Proceedings. (2001). Summary of the scientific conference on dietary fatty acids and cardiovascular health. Available at http://circ.ahajournals.org/cgi/content/full/103/7/1034?eaf. Accessed on 4/9/03.

Belury, M. (2002). Not all trans fatty acids are alike: What consumers may lose when we oversimplify nutrition facts. *Journal of the American Dietetic Association, 102,* 1606.

Brown, A., (2004). *Understanding food* (2nd ed.). Belmont CA: Wadsworth/Thomson Learning.

Chanmugam, P., Guthrie, J., Cecilio, S., et al. (2003). Did fat intake in the United States really decline between 1989–1991 and 1994–1996? *Journal of the American Dietetic Association, 103,* 867–872.

Federal Register, July 11, 2003. Vol. 68, No. 133, pp. 41433–41516. Available at www.cfsan.fda/gov/~lrd/fr03711a.html. Accessed on 12/16/03.

Gentry, M. (Ed.) (2003). Fat and fiction. *American Institute for Cancer Research Newsletter on Diet, Nutrition and Cancer Prevention, 76,* 1–3.

Healthy People 2010. Nutrition goals. Available at www.healthypeople.gov. Accessed on 12/18/03.

Hendler, S., & Rorvik, D. (Eds.). (2001). PDR for nutritional supplements. Montvale, NJ: Thomson PDR.

Liebman, B. (2002). Face the fats. *Nutrition Action Health Letter, 29*(6), 1, 3–7.

National Cholesterol Education Program, National Heart, Lung, and Blood Institute, National Institutes of Health. (2001). *Third report of the National Cholesterol Education Program (NCEP) expert panel on detection, evaluation, and treatment of high blood cholesterol in adults (Adult Treatment Panel III).* (Executive Summary. NIH Publication No. 01-3670).

Rosenberg, I. (Ed.) (2003). Ground beef by the numbers. *Tufts University Health & Nutrition Letter, 21*(10), 8.

Rosenberg, I. (Ed.) (2003). How to make leaner choices at the meat counter. *Tufts University Health & Nutrition Letter, 21*(9), 8.

Schaefer, E. (2002). Lipoproteins, nutrition, and heart disease. *American Journal of Clinical Nutrition, 75,* 191–212.

Trumbo, P., Schlicker, S., Yates, A., & Poos, M. (2002). Dietary Reference Intakes for energy, carbohydrate, fiber, fat, fatty acids, cholesterol, protein and amino acids. *Journal of the American Dietetic Association, 102,* 1621–1630.

U.S. Food and Drug Administration, Center for Food Safety and Applied Nutrition. (2003). Questions and answers about trans fat nutrition labeling. Available at www.cfsan.fda.gov/~dms/qatrans2.html. Accessed on 12/16/03.

For information on the new dietary guidelines 2005 and MyPyramid, visit **http://connection.lww.com/go/dudek**

5

Vitamins

TRUE	FALSE	
⬭	⬭	**1** Most people need a daily multivitamin supplement.
⬭	⬭	**2** Vitamins provide energy.
⬭	⬭	**3** Taking large doses of water-soluble vitamins is harmless.
⬭	⬭	**4** Most Americans eat less than the recommended amount of vitamin C.
⬭	⬭	**5** With vitamin supplements, the higher the price, the better the quality.
⬭	⬭	**6** "Natural" vitamins are superior to "synthetic" ones.
⬭	⬭	**7** Under optimal conditions, vitamin D is not an essential nutrient because the body can make all it needs from sunlight on the skin.
⬭	⬭	**8** Natural folate in foods is better absorbed than synthetic folic acid added to foods.
⬭	⬭	**9** USP on a label of vitamin supplements means that the product is safe.
⬭	⬭	**10** On any given day, 75% of Americans do not consume the recommended five or more servings of fruit and vegetables.

UPON COMPLETION OF THIS CHAPTER, YOU WILL BE ABLE TO

- Compare and contrast fat- and water-soluble vitamins.
- Describe general functions and uses of vitamins.
- Name certain population groups who need to obtain certain vitamins through supplements.
- Discuss what to look for in choosing a vitamin supplement.
- Discuss why it is better to obtain vitamins from food than supplements.
- Discuss why the adage "If a little is good, a lot is better" does not apply to vitamins.

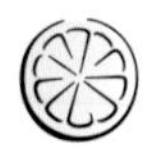

Enrich: to add nutrients back that were lost during processing, e.g., white flour is enriched with B vitamins lost when the bran and germ layers are removed.

Vitamins were discovered a mere 100 years ago as scientists searched to identify what components in food prevented the development of deficiency diseases such as scurvy. As knowledge of vitamin functions and requirements grew, policies were enacted to enrich and fortify foods. Because of those policies, vitamin deficiency diseases have been virtually eliminated in the general American population. Today the focus of vitamin research has evolved from preventing deficiencies to reducing the risk of chronic diseases such as heart disease and cancer. Somewhere between the brink of deficiency and the point of toxicity lies the optimal dosage for optimal health.

UNDERSTANDING VITAMINS

Fortify: to add nutrients that are not naturally found in the food, e.g., milk is fortified with vitamin D and some breakfast cereals are fortified with vitamin B_{12}.

Vitamins are organic compounds made of carbon, hydrogen, oxygen, and sometimes nitrogen or other elements. Vitamins facilitate biochemical reactions within cells to help regulate body processes such as growth and metabolism. They are essential to life. Unlike the organic compounds covered previously in this unit (carbohydrates, protein, and fat), vitamins

- Are individual molecules, not long chains of molecules linked together.
- Do not provide energy but are needed for metabolism of energy.
- Are needed in microgram or milligram quantities, not gram quantities. Because they are needed in such small amounts, they are referred to as micronutrients (Fig. 5.1).

1 large paperclip weighs approximately 1 gram
RDA for protein for adult female is 46 grams

If you divide 1 large paperclip into 1000 equal portions, each piece weighs 1 milligram
RDA for thiamin for adult female is 1.1 mg

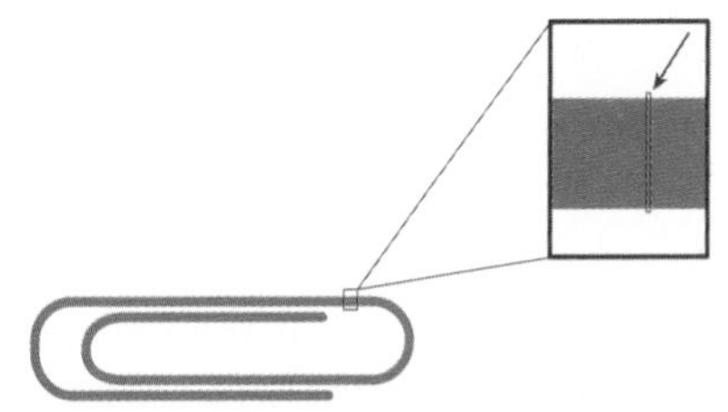

If you divide a 1 mg piece into 1000 equal portions, each piece weighs 1 microgram
RDA for vitamin B_{12} for adult female is 2.4 µg

FIGURE 5.1 Representative sizes of 1 g, 1 mg, and 1 µg.

Vitamins Are Chemically Defined

Vitamins are extremely complex chemical substances that differ widely in their structures. Because vitamins are defined chemically, the body cannot distinguish between natural vitamins extracted from food and synthetic vitamins produced in a laboratory. However, the absorption rates of natural and synthetic vitamins sometimes differ because of different chemical forms of the same vitamin (e.g., synthetic folic acid is better absorbed than natural folate in foods) or because the synthetic vitamins are "free," not "bound" to other components in food (e.g., synthetic vitamin B_{12} is not bound to small peptides, as natural vitamin B_{12} is).

Vitamins Are Susceptible to Destruction

As organic substances, vitamins in food are susceptible to destruction and subsequent loss of function. Individual vitamins differ in vulnerability to heat, light, oxidation, acid, and alkalis. For instance, thiamin is heat sensitive and is easily destroyed by high temperatures and long cooking times. Riboflavin is resistant to heat, acid, and oxidation but is quickly destroyed by light. That is why riboflavin-rich milk is sold in opaque, not transparent, containers. Baking soda (an alkali) added during cooking, a practice used by some cooks to retain the color of beets and red cabbage, destroys thiamin. Fifty percent to 90% of folate in foods may be lost during preparation, processing, and storage. Vitamin C is destroyed by heat, air, and alkalis.

Vitamins May Exist in More Than One Form

Provitamins: precursors of vitamins.

Many vitamins exist in more than one active form. Different forms perform different functions in the body. For instance, vitamin A exists as retinol (important for reproduction), retinal (needed for vision), and retinoic acid (which acts as a hormone to regulate growth). Some vitamins have provitamins, an inactive form found in food that the body converts to the active form. For instance, beta-carotene is a provitamin of vitamin A. Recommended allowances take into account the biologic activity of vitamins as they exist in different forms.

Vitamins Are Essential

Vitamins are essential in the diet because, with few exceptions, the body cannot make vitamins. The body can make vitamin A, vitamin D, and niacin if the appropriate precursors are available. Microorganisms in the gastrointestinal tract synthesize vitamin K and vitamin B_{12} but not in amounts sufficient to meet the body's needs.

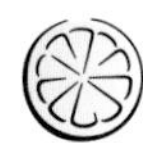

Some Vitamins Are Coenzymes

Enzymes: proteins produced by cells that catalyze chemical reactions within the body without undergoing change themselves.

Many enzymes cannot function without a coenzyme, and many coenzymes are vitamins. In addition to other functions, all B vitamins work as coenzymes to facilitate thousands of chemical conversions. For instance, thiamin, riboflavin, niacin, and biotin participate in enzymatic reactions that extract energy from glucose, amino acids, and fat. Folacin facilitates both amino acid metabolism and nucleic acid synthesis; without adequate folacin, protein synthesis and cell division are impaired. An adequate and continuous supply of B vitamins in every cell is vital for normal metabolism.

Some Vitamins Are Antioxidants

Coenzymes: an organic molecule that activates an enzyme.

Free Radicals: highly unstable, highly reactive molecular fragments with one or more unpaired electrons.

Oxidation: a chemical reaction in which a substance combines with oxygen; the loss of electrons in an atom.

Antioxidants: substances that donate electrons to free radicals to prevent oxidation.

Free radicals are produced continuously in cells as they burn oxygen during normal metabolism. Ultraviolet radiation, air pollution, ozone, and smoking can also generate free radicals in the body. The problem with free radicals is that they oxidize body cells and DNA in their quest to gain an electron and become stable. These structurally and functionally damaged cells are believed to contribute to aging and various health problems such as cancer, heart disease, and cataracts. Polyunsaturated fatty acids in cell membranes are particularly vulnerable to damage by free radicals.

Antioxidants protect body cells from being oxidized (destroyed) by free radicals by undergoing oxidation themselves, which renders free radicals harmless. In the body, vitamin C, vitamin E, and beta-carotene are major antioxidants. Each has a slightly different role, so one cannot completely substitute for another. For instance, water-soluble vitamin C works within cells to disable free radicals and fat-soluble vitamin E functions within fat tissue. Because antioxidants complement each other, an excess or deficiency of one may impair the action of other antioxidants.

Headlines and advertisements often tout antioxidants as "magic bullets" to prevent aging and chronic disease. Although population studies show that diets rich in fruits and vegetables appear to be protective against heart disease and cancer, it is not known whether this effect is caused by antioxidants, other vitamins, phytochemicals, or (most likely) a combination of substances in those foods. A study in which large doses of beta-carotene supplements were given to smokers to reduce their risk of lung cancer was aborted when it became apparent that the supplements actually increased the risk of lung cancer in the study subjects. Fruits and vegetables are safe and protective; research has yet to prove if the same is true for antioxidant supplements.

Some Vitamins Are Used as Food Additives

Food Additive: a substance added intentionally or unintentionally to food that affects its character.

Some foods have vitamins added to them simply to boost their nutritional content; examples include vitamin C-enriched fruit drinks, fortified ready-to-eat cereals, and enriched flour and breads. Other foods have certain vitamins added to them to help preserve quality. For instance, added vitamin C helps to prevent rancidity in frozen fish and stabilizes the red color of luncheon meats and other cured foods. Small amounts of vitamin E added to vegetable oils retard rancidity. Beta-carotene adds color to margarine.

Vitamins as Drugs

Megadoses: amounts at least 10 times greater than the RDA.

In megadoses vitamins function like drugs, not nutrients. Large doses of niacin are used to lower cholesterol, LDL-cholesterol, and triglycerides in people with hyperlipidemia who do not respond to diet and exercise. Tretinoin (retinoic acid, a form of vitamin A) is used as a topical treatment for acne vulgaris and orally for acute promyelocytic leukemia. Gram quantities of vitamin C promote wound healing in patients with thermal injuries.

VITAMIN CLASSIFICATIONS BASED ON SOLUBILITY

Vitamins are classified according to their solubility. Vitamins A, D, E, and K are fat-soluble. Vitamin C and the B vitamins (thiamin, riboflavin, niacin, folate, B_6, B_{12}, biotin, and pantothenic acid) are water-soluble. Solubility determines vitamin absorption, transportation, storage, and excretion.

Fat-Soluble Vitamins

Table 5.1 highlights sources, functions, deficiency symptoms, and toxicity symptoms of each fat-soluble vitamin. Recommended intakes, median intakes, and tolerable upper limit values appear in Table 5.2. As a group, fat-soluble vitamins

- Are absorbed with fat in chylomicrons that enter the lymphatic system before circulating in the bloodstream. Whenever fat absorption is impaired, such as in the case of cystic fibrosis or pancreatic insufficiency, secondary deficiencies of the fat-soluble vitamins can develop.
- Attach to protein carriers to be transported through the blood because fat is not soluble in watery blood. For instance, most circulating vitamin E is found in low-density lipoprotein (LDL)-cholesterol.
- Are stored, not excreted, when consumed in excess of need. The liver and adipose tissue are the primary storage sites. Because these vitamins are stored, deficiency symptoms can take months or years to develop when intake is less than adequate.
- Can be toxic when consumed in large doses over a prolonged period. This applies primarily to vitamins A and D; large doses of vitamins E and K are considered relatively nontoxic. Vitamin toxicities are not likely to be caused by food; inappropriate use of supplements is usually to blame.
- Do not have to be eaten every day because the body can retrieve them from storage as needed.
- Are found in the fat and oil portion of foods.

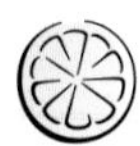

TABLE 5.1

SUMMARY OF FAT-SOLUBLE VITAMINS

Vitamin and Sources	Functions	Deficiency/Toxicity Signs and Symptoms
Vitamin A • Retinol: Liver, milk, butter, cheese, cream, egg yolk, fortified milk, margarine, and ready-to-eat cereals • Beta-Carotene: Green leafy vegetables, broccoli, carrots, peaches, pumpkin, red peppers, sweet potatoes, winter squash, mango, watermelon, apricots, cantaloupe	The formation of visual purple, which enables the eye to adapt to dim light Normal growth and development of bones and teeth The formation and maintenance of mucosal epithelium to maintain healthy functioning of skin and membranes, hair, gums, and various glands Important role in immune function	*Deficiency* Night blindness, or the slow recovery of vision after flashes of bright light at night Bone growth ceases; bone shape changes; enamel-forming cells in the teeth malfunction; teeth crack and tend to decay. Skin becomes dry, scaly, rough, and cracked; keratinization or hyperkeratosis develops; mucous membrane cells flatten and harden: Eyes become dry (xerosis); irreversible drying and hardening of the cornea can result in blindness Decreased saliva secretion → difficulty chewing, swallowing → anorexia Decreased mucous secretion of the stomach and intestines → impaired digestion and absorption → diarrhea, increased excretion of nutrients Susceptibility to respiratory, urinary tract, and vaginal infections increases. *Toxicity* Headaches, vomiting, double vision, hair loss, bone abnormalities, liver damage Can cause birth defects during pregnancy
Vitamin D • Sunlight on the skin • Liver, fatty fish, egg yolks, fortified milk, some ready-to-eat cereals, and margarine	Maintains serum calcium concentrations by: Stimulating GI absorption Stimulating the release of calcium from the bones Stimulating calcium reabsorption from the kidneys	*Deficiency* Rickets (in infants and children) Retarded bone growth Bone malformations (bowed legs) Enlargement of ends of long bones (knock-knees) Deformities of the ribs (bowed, with beads or knobs) Delayed closing of the fontanel → rapid enlargement of the head
Vitamin E		

(table continues on page 100)

TABLE 5.1
(continued)

SUMMARY OF FAT-SOLUBLE VITAMINS

Vitamin and Sources	Functions	Deficiency/Toxicity Signs and Symptoms
		Decreased serum calcium and/or phosphorus Malformed teeth; decayed teeth Protrusion of the abdomen related to relaxation of the abdominal muscles Increased secretion of parathyroid hormone Osteomalacia (in adults) Softening of the bones → deformities, pain, and easy fracture Decreased serum calcium and/or phosphorus, increased alkaline phosphatase Involuntary muscle twitching and spasms *Toxicity* Kidney stones, irreversible kidney damage, muscle and bone weakness, excessive bleeding, loss of appetite, headache, excessive thirst, calcification of soft tissues (blood vessels, kidneys, heart, lungs), death
• Vegetable oils, margarine, salad dressing, other foods made with vegetable oil, nuts, seeds, wheat germ, dark green vegetables, whole grains, fortified cereals	Acts as an antioxidant to protect vitamin A and PUFA from being destroyed Protects cell membranes	*Deficiency* Increased RBC hemolysis In infants, anemia, edema, and skin lesions *Toxicity* Relatively nontoxic High doses enhance action of anticoagulant medications
Vitamin K • Bacterial synthesis • Green leafy vegetables, liver, eggs, vegetables of the cabbage family	Synthesis of blood clotting proteins and a bone protein that regulates blood calcium	*Deficiency* Hemorrhaging *Toxicity* No symptoms have been observed from excessive vitamin K

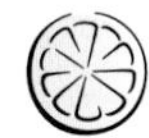

TABLE 5.2

COMPARISON BETWEEN ACTUAL AVERAGE INTAKE, RECOMMENDED INTAKE, AND TOLERABLE UPPER LIMITS FOR SELECTED VITAMINS IN MEN AND WOMEN

	Men		Women		
Vitamin	**Actual Intake (age 20 and older)**	**Recommended Intake (ages 19–30)**	**Actual Intake (age 20 and older)**	**Recommended Intake (ages 19–30)**	**Tolerable upper level (for men and women ages 19–70)**
Vit A (micrograms RE)	1087	900	904	700	3000
Vit E (mg)	9.8	15	7.2	15	1000
Vit C (mg)	106	90	94	75	2000
Thiamin (mg)	1.87	1.2	1.35	1.1	ND
Riboflavin (mg)	2.17	1.3	1.56	1.1	ND
Niacin (mg)	26.9	16	18.5	14	35
Vit B_6 (mg)	2.12	1.3	1.5	1.3	100
Folate (micrograms)	303	400	228	400*	1000
Vit B_{12} (micrograms)	6.55	2.4	3.92	2.4	ND

*It is recommended that women capable of becoming pregnant consume 400 micrograms of folic acid through supplements or fortified foods in addition to natural folate in a normal mixed diet.

Intake data from: USDA, Agricultural Research Service. 1997. Data Tables: Results from USDA's 1996 Continuing Survey of Food Intakes by Individuals and 1996 Diet and Health Knowledge Survey (Online). ARS Food Surveys Research Group. Available (under "Releases"): www.barc.usda.gov/bhnrc/foodsurvey/home.htm. Accessed on 10/10/03.

Vitamin A

Preformed Vitamin A: the active form of vitamin A.

Carotenoids: a group name of retinol precursors found in plants.

In its preformed state, vitamin A exists as either an alcohol (retinol), aldehyde (retinaldehyde) or acid (retinoic acid). Preformed vitamin A is found only in animal sources such as liver, whole milk, and fish. Low-fat milk, skim milk, margarine, and ready-to-eat cereals are fortified with vitamin A.

Provitamin A carotenoids are found in plants. Carotenoids, of which beta-carotene, lutein, and lycopene are among the most common, are found in deep yellow and orange fruits and vegetables and most dark-green leafy vegetables. Carrots, cantaloupe, broccoli, winter squash, peas, and spinach are major contributors to beta-carotene intake. Carotenoids account for about one-quarter to one-third of the usual intake of vitamin A.

Vitamin A is best known for its roles in normal vision, gene expression, reproduction, embryonic development, growth, and immune system functioning. Because carotenes are important antioxidants in the body (by comparison, vitamin A is a relatively poor antioxidant), there is much interest in their possible role in the prevention of heart disease and cancer. To date, results of studies are conflicting, and widespread supplementation is not recommended.

The body can store up to a year's supply of vitamin A, 90% of which is in the liver. Because deficiency symptoms do not develop until body stores are exhausted, it may

Retinol Equivalents (RE): the unit of measure for active vitamin A that includes preformed vitamin A and retinol derived from beta-carotene.

take 1 to 2 years for them to appear. Severe vitamin A deficiency is rare in the United States. However, although they are not clinically deficient, a large percentage of adults may have suboptimal liver stores of vitamin A. Worldwide, vitamin A deficiency is a major health problem and is the major cause of childhood blindness.

Only preformed vitamin A is toxic in high doses. Although high intakes of naturally occurring and fortified preformed vitamin A can produce toxicity, the risk of toxicity is much more likely when supplements of vitamin A are consumed. Acute

Career Connection

If a little is good, is more better? Usually not, and sometimes more can be dangerous, as in the case of vitamin A. In 2001, the Institute of Medicine lowered the RDA for vitamin A from 1000 micrograms to 900 micrograms RE/day for men and from 800 micrograms to 700 micrograms/day for women. However, the Daily Reference Value used to calculate the percent Daily Value (DV) on food and supplement labels is 5000 IU (approximately 1500 micrograms RE), which is the 1968 Recommended Dietary Allowance. That means that food and supplement labels underreport the percentage of vitamin A provided according to current recommendations. For instance, a vitamin supplement that supplies 100% of the Daily Value, with all of it in the form of preformed vitamin A, is actually providing 1500 micrograms RE, not 700 or 900 micrograms as one would expect. With one vitamin supplement, the intake of vitamin A is above recommended intake.

But that may be only half the problem. Because food manufacturers are free to decide which foods to fortify with vitamin A, which form of vitamin A to add, and at what level, the variety of foods fortified with preformed vitamin A is increasing. No longer limited to milk, some margarines, and some ready-to-eat cereals, preformed vitamin A can now be found in cereal bars, energy bars, and even candy. Look how quickly the UL of 3000 micrograms/day is approached:

	Micrograms vit A
1 vitamin supplement with 100% DV for vitamin A	1500
1 meal replacement bar	750
2 cups milk	300
1 cup ready to eat cereal	215
Total	2765 micrograms

While 2765 micrograms seems like a long way from the levels known to actually produce toxicity symptoms (e.g., 30,000 micrograms/day for months), recent epidemiological studies suggest that intakes as low as 1500 to 2000 micrograms/day of retinol increase the risk of hip fractures.

- Dispel the myth that more is better.
- Advise clients that %DV and current RDAs are not consistent.
- Point out that a better choice than fortified foods and vitamin supplements may be fortified foods OR vitamin supplements, the exception being milk because vitamin A is present naturally in whole milk and added to lowfat milks.

 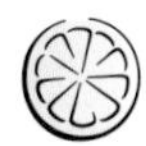

symptoms can occur after a single or short-term dose of 150,000 micrograms or more in adults. Symptoms are usually transient and may include nausea, vomiting, headache, increased cerebrospinal fluid pressure, vertigo, blurred vision, and muscular incoordination. An adult who consumes at least 30,000 micrograms/day for months or years may develop nonspecific symptoms from hypervitaminosis A: CNS changes, liver abnormalities, and bone and skin changes. At high doses during pregnancy, such as three to four times the recommended intake, vitamin A is teratogenic. Supplementation is not recommended during the first trimester of pregnancy unless there is specific evidence of vitamin A deficiency.

The body can make only 1 unit of retinol from about 12 units of beta-carotene. The conversion is not rapid enough to cause hypervitaminosis A. Instead, carotene is stored primarily in adipose tissue and may accumulate under the skin to the extent that it causes the skin color to turn yellowish-orange, a harmless condition known as hypercarotenemia.

Vitamin D

Vitamin D is unique in that under optimal conditions the body can synthesize all the vitamin D it needs. Sunlight on the skin converts a precursor (7-dehydrocholesterol) into vitamin D, which becomes 25-hydroxyvitamin D in the liver and is then activated to 1, 25-dihydroxyvitamin D in the kidneys. A light-skinned Caucasian living in Boston may need only 5 to 10 minutes of exposure on the hands, face, and arms between 11 AM and 2 PM to fulfill daily vitamin D requirement. For that same person living in Florida, the exposure time may be only 2 to 3 minutes. In reality, a dietary source is considered essential because few people meet optimal conditions. For instance, only people living south of Los Angeles and Atlanta make vitamin D in the winter. Dense clouds, heavy smog, sunscreen, clothing, window glass, and dark-colored skin block vitamin D synthesis. Also, the ability to produce vitamin D decreases with aging.

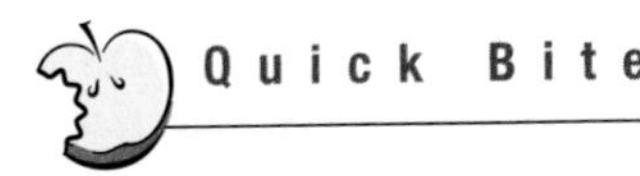

Vitamin D content of selected items

	Micrograms vitamin D
Cod liver oil, 1 Tbsp	34
Halibut, 3 oz	17
Catfish, 3 oz	14
Most multivitamin/mineral supplements	100
Canned tuna, 1/4 cup	3.25
Milk, 1 cup	2.45
Minute maid calcium + Vit D orange juice, 8 oz	2.5
Viactive soft calcium chews, 1 chew	2.5
Egg, 1	0.65

Very few foods provide vitamin D naturally: liver, fatty fish, and egg yolks. Fortified foods are important sources: all milks and most ready-to-eat cereals are fortified but only a few brands of orange juice, yogurt, margarine, and hot cereals are.

Another unique feature of vitamin D is that it is considered to be a hormone rather than a vitamin because it is synthesized in one part of the body and stimulates functional activity elsewhere as mediated by a vitamin D receptor. Vitamin D maintains normal blood concentrations of calcium and phosphorus by

- Increasing calcium and phosphorus absorption from the GI tract
- Mobilizing calcium and phosphorus from the bone as needed
- Stimulating the kidneys to retain calcium and phosphorus

The role of vitamin D in maintaining bone strength and integrity is well known; by enhancing GI absorption, vitamin D helps to ensure adequate calcium is available in the blood so that bone cells can incorporate it into the bone matrix. What is less well known is how adequate vitamin D may help to protect against type 1 diabetes, multiple sclerosis, congestive heart failure, and some cancers. Vitamin D may also help to protect against high blood pressure: the active form of vitamin D suppresses renal production of renin, a hormone that increases the risk of hypertension.

Rickets: vitamin D deficiency disease in children most prominently characterized by bowed legs.

Without vitamin D, only 10 to 15% of calcium consumed is absorbed. Combined with normal daily calcium losses of 100 to 200 mg in the urine and 100 to 200 mg from the GI tract, a calcium deficit occurs. Blood calcium levels fall, causing bones to forfeit calcium to raise blood level to normal range. In children, vitamin D deficiency causes rickets. Vitamin D deficiency in adults precipitates and exacerbates osteoporosis and leads to osteomalacia.

Osteoporosis: porous bones due to the loss of bone density.

Osteomalacia: adult rickets characterized by inadequate bone mineralization due to the lack of vitamin D.

Elderly persons are particularly at risk for vitamin D deficiency because of various risk factors: inadequate intake, limited sun exposure, reduced skin thickness, impaired GI absorption, and impaired activation by the liver and kidneys. Older adults with borderline or overt vitamin D deficiency may appear asymptomatic. At one time, vitamin D-fortified milk was credited with eliminating vitamin D deficiency in American children. Today vitamin D deficiency appears to be making a comeback in some segments of the pediatric population, particularly breastfed infants who do not receive vitamin D supplements, toddlers given unfortified soy and rice beverages in place of milk, and children who replace milk with soft drinks. The use of sunscreens also impacts vitamin D status.

IU: International Units, the former unit of measure of vitamin D that has been replaced by micrograms of cholecalciferol, the active form of vitamin D.

In the absence of adequate sunlight exposure, the Institute of Medicine recommends 10 micrograms of cholecalciferol (400 IU) for people over 50 and 15 micrograms cholecalciferol (600 IU) for people over 70. Even though the committee had (as of then) unpublished evidence that much higher levels were needed, they were obligated to limit their data to published studies and thus set the recommendations at levels they believed to be suboptimal. Many experts agree that, on average and without sun exposure, 25 micrograms (1000 IU) of vitamin D are needed daily.

An excess of vitamin D is toxic, but large amounts are needed over a long period of time before toxicity symptoms appear. Too much vitamin D causes excessive calcium absorption, which can lead to hypercalcemia, kidney stones, kidney calcification, kidney failure, soft-tissue calcification, and blood vessel calcification that can be fatal. Although the upper limit for vitamin D is set at 50 micrograms (2000 IU), many experts agree that much larger doses are needed before toxicity symptoms develop. It is virtually impossible to consume that much vitamin D from food, and excessive consumption is unlikely from supplements. Because the body destroys excess vitamin D produced from overexposure to the sun, there has never been a reported case of vitamin D toxicity from too much sun.

Vitamin E

Vitamin E is a generic term that describes a group of at least eight naturally-occurring compounds. However, only alpha-tocopherol is considered the active form of vitamin E so the RDA for vitamin E is based only on alpha-tocopherol. Unfortunately, most nutrient databases and nutrition labels include all eight naturally occurring forms of vitamin E when they represent the vitamin E content of food.

Vitamin E functions primary as an antioxidant in the body, protecting polyunsaturated fatty acids (PUFAs) and other lipid molecules from oxidative damage. By doing so, it helps to maintain the integrity of PUFA-rich cell membranes; protects red blood cells against hemolysis; and protects vitamin A from oxidation.

Because of its antioxidant properties, vitamin E is believed to help prevent diseases associated with oxidative stress such as cardiovascular disease, cancer, chronic inflammation, and neurologic disorders. So far, however, the results of clinical trials have been inconsistent, confirming the need for additional research. Specifically, vitamin E is being investigated for its role in

- Preventing the oxidation of LDL cholesterol to prevent atherosclerosis. Other mechanisms by which vitamin E may lower heart disease risk are also under study such as its ability to inhibit smooth muscle proliferation, inhibit platelet aggregation, and inhibit thrombin formation. Although evidence suggests that high intakes of vitamin E may reduce the risk of heart disease, at this time there is insufficient data to recommend vitamin E supplements to prevent heart disease in the general public.
- Cancer prevention. Although the link between vitamin E and cancer is not as strong as the relationship between vitamin E and heart disease, study results suggest that vitamin E may help to prevent prostate cancer.
- Reversing some aspects of age-related immune system decline at least in some individuals.
- Treating Alzheimer's disease. Results of a 2-year, double-blind, placebo-controlled, randomized, multicenter trial indicate that 2000 IU/day of vitamin E significantly slowed the progression of Alzheimer's disease in moderately severely impaired patients.

Doctors often recommend large doses of vitamin E to help to relieve the pain of fibrocystic disease. Vitamin E therapy may also be useful in the treatment of intermittent claudication. Although vitamin E is vital for maintaining health, it is not a miracle nutrient. There is no evidence to support claims that vitamin E cures infertility, diabetes, ulcers, skin disorders, shortness of breath, and muscular dystrophy. Nor does vitamin E increase physical performance and sexual potency, protect against air pollution, reverse gray hair and wrinkles, or slow the aging process.

As indicated in Table 5.2, median vitamin E intake for men and women aged 19 to 30 is less than the RDA; however, this may not actually be true. For one thing, calorie intake is known to be under-reported in national food consumption surveys and fat intake is likely to be more under-reported than calorie intake. Also, the amount of fats and oils used in food preparation is difficult to determine from diet recalls, yet would contribute substantially to vitamin E intake. Likewise, because different vegetable oils vary widely in their content of alpha-tocopherol, accurate vitamin E content cannot be obtained from foods that have the type of oil vaguely listed as "may contain one or more of the following oils. . . ." Because vitamin E deficiency symptoms have never been reported in normal people eating a low vitamin E diet, it is assumed that typical American diets provide sufficient vitamin E.

Vitamin E deficiency can occur in very specific instances. Premature infants who have not benefited from the transfer of vitamin E from mother to fetus in the last weeks of pregnancy are at risk for red blood cell hemolysis. The breaking of their red blood cell membranes is caused by oxidation; vitamin E corrects red blood cell hemolysis by preventing oxidation. Other cases of vitamin E deficiency are rare and occur secondary to a genetic abnormality, malabsorption syndromes, or protein-energy malnutrition.

The need for vitamin E increases as the intake of PUFA increases. Fortunately, vitamin E and PUFA share many of the same food sources, particularly vegetable oils and products made from oil such as margarine, salad dressings, and other prepared foods. However, not all oils are rich in alpha tocopherol, the active form of vitamin E. Soybean oil, the most commonly used oil in food processing, ranks low in alpha-tocopherol content.

Large amounts of vitamin E are relatively nontoxic but can interfere with vitamin K action (blood clotting) by decreasing platelet aggregation. Large doses may also potentiate the effects of blood-thinning drugs, increasing the risk of hemorrhage. The UL is 66 times higher than the RDA.

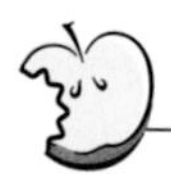

Quick Bite

Oils containing the active form of vitamin E in descending order

Wheat germ oil
Walnut oil
Sunflower oil
Cottonseed oil
Safflower oil
Palm oil
Canola oil
Sesame oil
Peanut oil
Olive oil
Corn oil
Soybean oil
Coconut oil

Vitamin K

Vitamin K occurs naturally in two forms: phylloquinone, which is found in plants such as green leafy vegetables, and menaquinones, which are synthesized in the intestinal tract by bacteria. Animal sources, such as liver and milk, provide both forms of vitamin K.

Approximately one-half of vitamin K requirements are met through food sources, the other half through bacterial synthesis. Unlike other fat-soluble vitamins, stores of vitamin K are quickly depleted when requirements are not obtained.

Vitamin K is a coenzyme essential for the synthesis of prothrombin and at least six other proteins required for normal blood clotting. Without adequate vitamin K, life is threatened: even a small wound can cause someone deficient in vitamin K to bleed to death. Vitamin K also activates at least three proteins involved in building and maintaining bone. A large study with women showed that those with a high intake of vitamin K rich green vegetables had fewer hip fractures than those who ate fewer green vegetables.

Newborns are prone to vitamin K deficiency because their sterile gastrointestinal tracts cannot synthesize vitamin K and it may take weeks for bacteria to establish themselves in the newborn's intestines. To prevent hemorrhagic disease, a single water-soluble dose of vitamin K is given prophylactically at birth.

Vitamin K deficiency does not occur from inadequate intake. Malabsorption syndromes may cause vitamin K deficiency, as can certain medications, namely anticoagulants and antibiotics, that interfere with vitamin K metabolism or synthesis. Anticoagulants, such as coumadin, interfere with hepatic synthesis of vitamin K-dependent clotting factors. People who take anticoagulants do not need to avoid vitamin K, but they should try to maintain a consistent intake. Antibiotics kill the intestinal bacteria that synthesize vitamin K. Clinically significant vitamin K deficiency is defined as vitamin K responsive hypoprothrombinemia and is associated with an increase in prothrombin time.

Due to the lack of data to estimate an average requirement, an Adequate Intake, not an RDA, has been set. And because no adverse effects are associated with vitamin K intake from food or supplements, an upper limit has not been set.

Water-Soluble Vitamins

Table 5.3 highlights sources, functions, deficiency symptoms, and toxicity symptoms of each water-soluble vitamin. Recommended intakes, median intakes, and tolerable upper limit values appear in Table 5.2. As a group, water-soluble vitamins

- Are absorbed directly into the bloodstream.
- Move freely through the watery environment of blood and within cells.
- Are excreted in the urine when consumed in excess amounts; however, some tissues may hold limited amounts of certain water-soluble vitamins. For instance, adult men can store up to 3000 mg of vitamin C (most of which is contained within cells) at daily intakes of about 200 mg.
- Were historically believed to be nontoxic because the body can protect itself from large doses by increasing excretion. This belief has come under scrutiny since the discovery of neurologic abnormalities caused by high-dose vitamin B_6 supplements used for a prolonged period.
- Must be consumed daily because there is no reserve in storage.
- Are found in the watery portion of foods.

TABLE 5.3

SUMMARY OF WATER-SOLUBLE VITAMINS

Vitamin and Sources	Functions	Deficiency/Toxicity Signs and Symptoms
Thiamin (Vitamin B_1) • Whole grain and enriched breads and cereals, liver, nuts, wheat germ, pork, dried peas and beans	Coenzyme in energy metabolism Promotes normal appetite and nervous system functioning	*Deficiency* Beriberi Mental confusion, decrease in short-term memory Fatigue, apathy Peripheral paralysis Muscle weakness and wasting Painful calf muscles Anorexia, weight loss Edema Enlarged heart Sudden death from heart failure *Toxicity* No toxicity symptoms reported
Riboflavin (Vitamin B_2) • Milk and other dairy products; whole grain and enriched breads and cereals; eggs, meat, green leafy vegetables	Coenzyme in energy metabolism Aids in the conversion of tryptophan into niacin	*Deficiency* Dermatitis Cheilosis Glossitis Photophobia Reddening of the cornea *Toxicity* No toxicity symptoms reported
Niacin (Vitamin B_3) • All protein foods, whole grain and enriched breads and cereals	Coenzyme in energy metabolism Promotes normal nervous system functioning	*Deficiency* Pellagra: 4 (Ds) Dermatitis (bilateral and symmetrical) and glossitis Diarrhea Dementia, irritability, mental confusion → psychosis Death, if untreated *Toxicity* (from supplements/drugs) Flushing, liver damage, gastric ulcers, low blood pressure, diarrhea, nausea, vomiting
Vitamin B_6 Meats, fish, poultry, fruits, green leafy vegetables, whole grains, nuts, dried peas and beans	Coenzyme in amino acid and fatty acid metabolism Helps convert tryptophan to niacin	*Deficiency* Dermatitis, cheilosis, glossitis, abnormal brain wave pattern, convulsions, and anemia

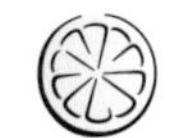

TABLE 5.3
(continued)

SUMMARY OF WATER-SOLUBLE VITAMINS

Vitamin and Sources	Functions	Deficiency/Toxicity Signs and Symptoms
	Helps produce insulin, hemoglobin, myelin sheaths and antibodies	*Toxicity* Depression, fatigue, irritability, headaches; sensory neuropathy characteristic
Folate • Leafy vegetables, dried peas and beans, seeds, liver, orange juice, some fruits; breads, cereals and other grains are fortified with folic acid	Coenzyme in DNA synthesis, therefore vital for new cell synthesis and the transmission of inherited characteristics	*Deficiency* Glossitis, diarrhea, macrocytic anemia, depression, mental confusion, fainting, fatigue *Toxicity* Too much can mask B_{12} deficiency
Vitamin B_{12} • Animal products: meat, fish, poultry, shellfish, milk, dairy products, eggs • Some fortified foods	Coenzyme in the synthesis of new cells Activates folate Maintains nerve cells Helps metabolize some fatty acids and amino acids	*Deficiency* GI changes: glossitis, anorexia, indigestion, recurring diarrhea or constipation, and weight loss Macrocytic anemia: pallor, dyspnea, weakness, fatigue, and palpitations Neurologic changes: paresthesia of the hands and feet, decreased sense of position, poor muscle coordination, poor memory, irritability, depression, paranoia, delirium, and hallucinations *Toxicity* No toxicity symptoms reported
Pantothenic Acid • Widespread in foods • Meat, poultry, fish, whole grain cereals, and dried peas and beans are among best sources.	Part of coenzyme A used in energy metabolism	*Deficiency* Rare; general failure of all body systems *Toxicity* No toxicity symptoms reported, although large doses may cause diarrhea
Biotin • Widespread in foods • Eggs, liver, milk, and dark green vegetables are among best choices • Synthesized by GI flora	Coenzyme in energy metabolism, fatty acid synthesis, amino acid metabolism, and glycogen formation	*Deficiency* Rare; anorexia, fatigue, depression, dry skin, heart abnormalities *Toxicity* No toxicity symptoms reported

(table continues on page 110)

TABLE 5.3
(continued)

SUMMARY OF WATER-SOLUBLE VITAMINS

Vitamin and Sources	Functions	Deficiency/Toxicity Signs and Symptoms
Vitamin C • Citrus fruits and juices, red and green peppers, broccoli, cauliflower, Brussels sprouts, cantaloupe, kiwifruit, mustard greens, strawberries, tomatoes	Collagen synthesis Antioxidant Promotes iron absorption Involved in the metabolism of certain amino acids Thyroxin synthesis Immune system functioning	*Deficiency* Bleeding gums, pinpoint hemorrhages under the skin Scurvy, characterized by Hemorrhaging Muscle degeneration Skin changes Delayed wound healing: reopening of old wounds Softening of the bones → malformations, pain, easy fractures Soft, loose teeth Anemia Increased susceptibility to infection Hysteria and depression *Toxicity* Diarrhea, abdominal cramps, nausea, headache, insomnia, fatigue, hot flashes, aggravation of gout symptoms

Thiamin

Thiamin (vitamin B_1) is a coenzyme in the metabolism of carbohydrates and branched chain amino acids. In addition to its role in energy metabolism, thiamin is important in nervous system functioning.

In the United States and other developed countries, the use of enriched breads and cereals has virtually eliminated the thiamin deficiency disease known as beriberi. Today thiamin deficiency is usually seen only in alcoholics with limited food consumption because chronic alcohol abuse impairs thiamin intake, absorption, and metabolism. Edema occurs in wet beriberi; muscle wasting in prominent in dry beriberi. Cardiac and renal complications can be fatal.

Because thiamin is not stored in the body, a daily intake is essential. No adverse effects have been noted from high intakes of thiamin from food or supplements, so an upper limit has not been set.

Riboflavin

Riboflavin (vitamin B_2) is an integral component of the coenzymes flavin adenine dinucleotide (FAD) and flavin mononucleotide (FMN) that function to release energy

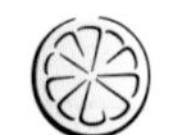

Homocysteine: an amino acid correlated with increased risk of heart disease.

Methionine: an essential amino acid.

from nutrients in all body cells. Flavin coenzymes are also involved in the formation of some vitamins and their coenzymes and in the conversion of homocysteine to methionine. Riboflavin is unique among water-soluble vitamins in that milk and dairy products contribute the most riboflavin to the diet.

Biochemical signs of an inadequate riboflavin status can appear after only a few days of a poor intake. The elderly and adolescents seem to be at greatest risk for riboflavin deficiency. Riboflavin deficiency interferes with iron handling and contributes to anemia when iron intake is low. Other deficiency symptoms include sore throat, cheilosis, stomatitis, glossitis, and dermatitis, many of which may be related to the effect riboflavin deficiency has on the metabolism of folate and vitamin B_6. Cancer, heart disease, and diabetes precipitate or exacerbate riboflavin deficiency.

Niacin

Niacin (vitamin B_3) exists as nicotinic acid and nicotinamide. The body converts nicotinic acid to nicotinamide, which is the major form of niacin in the blood. All protein foods provide niacin, as do whole-grain and enriched breads and fortified ready to eat cereals.

Niacin Equivalents (NE): the amount of niacin available to the body including that made from tryptophan.

A unique feature of niacin is that the body can make it from the amino acid tryptophan: approximately 60 mg of tryptophan is used to synthesize 1 mg of niacin. Because of this additional source of niacin, niacin requirements are stated in niacin equivalents (NEs). Median intake in the United Stakes generously exceeds the RDA.

Niacin is part of the coenzymes nicotinamide adenine dinucleotide (NAD) and nicotinamide adenine dinucleotide phosphate (NADP), which are involved in energy transfer reactions in the metabolism of glucose, fat, and alcohol in all body cells. Reduced NADP is used in the synthesis of fatty acids, cholesterol, and steroid hormones.

Pellagra, the disorder caused by severe niacin deficiency, is rare in the United States and usually is seen only in alcoholics. However, pellagra is widespread in areas that rely on corn as a staple, such as parts of Africa and Asia, because corn is low in niacin and tryptophan. Before grain products were enriched with niacin in the early 20th century, pellagra was also common in the southern United States.

Niacin deficiency may be treated with niacin, or tryptophan, or both. Because a deficiency of niacin rarely occurs alone, treatment is most effective when other B-complex vitamins are also given, especially thiamin and riboflavin.

Large doses of niacin in the form of nicotinic acid (1 g to 6 g/d) are used therapeutically to lower total cholesterol and LDL-cholesterol and raise high-density lipoprotein (HDL)–cholesterol. Flushing is a common side effect caused by vasodilation. Large doses may also cause liver damage and gout. Large doses of niacin should be used only with a doctor's supervision. The upper limit of 35 mg of NE does not apply for clinical applications using niacin as a drug.

Vitamin B_6

Vitamin B_6 and pyridoxine are group names for related compounds that include pyridoxine, pyridoxal, and pyridoxamine. All three forms can be converted to the pyridoxal phosphate, which is a coenzyme for more than 100 enzymes involved in amino acid metabolism. Vitamin B_6 helps to convert amino acids into other amino acids and tryptophan to niacin. It plays a role in the formation of heme for hemoglobin and in the synthesis of myelin sheaths and neurotransmitters. Vitamin B_6 helps to regulate blood glucose levels by assisting in the release of stored glucose from glycogen and is important in the maintenance of cellular immunity. Unlike other B vitamins, vitamin B_6 is stored extensively in muscle tissue.

Elevated blood levels of homocysteine seem to increase the risk for coronary heart disease, stroke, peripheral vascular disease, and venous thrombosis. Evidence suggests that blood concentrations of homocysteine are inversely related to blood concentrations of vitamin B_6, folate, and vitamin B_{12} and that vitamin intervention can lower homocysteine levels. Studies show that people with the highest vitamin B_6 intakes have a twofold decrease in MI (myocardial infarction) and CHD compared to people with the lowest intakes.

Deficiencies of vitamin B_6 are uncommon but are usually accompanied by deficiencies of other B vitamins. Secondary deficiencies are related to alcohol abuse (the metabolism of alcohol promotes the destruction and excretion of vitamin B_6) and to other drug therapies such as isoniazid, the antituberculosis drug that acts as a vitamin B_6 antagonist.

Large oral doses of vitamin B_6 are used experimentally for a variety of conditions such as carpal tunnel syndrome, painful neuropathies, seizures, asthma, and sickle cell disease, and malaise and depression in women who use oral contraceptives. Historically, vitamin B_6 was considered nontoxic like all the other water-soluble vitamins, and indeed, there are no known adverse effects from high intakes of vitamin B_6 from food. However, the notion of safety was dispelled when women taking 2000 mg of vitamin B_6 daily for 2 months to relieve PMS developed sensory neuropathy, a nerve disorder that began with the sensation of numb feet and progressed to the inability to ambulate. Fortunately, the damage was not permanent and symptoms improved gradually when the vitamin was discontinued.

Folate

Dietary Folate Equivalents (DFE): 1 DFE = 1 microgram of food folate = 0.6 micrograms of folic acid from fortified food or as a supplement consumed with food = 0.5 microgram of a supplement taken on an empty stomach.

Folate is the generic term for this B vitamin that includes folic acid found in vitamin supplements and fortified foods such as fortified ready-to-eat cereals, and natural folate in food such as green leafy vegetables, dried peas and beans, seeds, liver, and orange juice. Natural food folate is only half as available to the body as man-made folic acid is, so dietary folate equivalents (DFE) are used in establishing folate requirement.

As part of the coenzymes tetrahydrofolate (THF) and dihydrofolate (DHF), folate's major function is in the synthesis of DNA. With the aid of vitamin B_{12}, folate is vital for synthesis of new cells and transmission of inherited characteristics. Folate is also involved in the conversion of homocysteine to methionine; adequate folate prevents the deleterious accumulation of homocysteine, which increases the risk of heart disease and stroke.

Because folate is recycled through the intestinal tract (much like the enterohepatic circulation of bile), a healthy gastrointestinal tract is essential to maintain folate balance. When gastrointestinal integrity is impaired, as in malabsorption syndromes, fail-

ure to reabsorb folate quickly leads to folate deficiency. Gastrointestinal cells are particularly susceptible to folate deficiency because they are rapidly dividing cells that depend on folate for new cell synthesis. Without the formation of new cells, gastrointestinal function declines and widespread malabsorption of nutrients occurs.

Folate deficiency is prevalent in all parts of the world. In developing countries, folate deficiency commonly is caused by parasitic infections that alter gastrointestinal integrity. In the United States, alcoholics are at highest risk of folate deficiency because of alcohol's toxic effect on the gastrointestinal tract. Groups at risk because of poor intake include the elderly, fad dieters, and people of low socioeconomic status. Because new tissue growth increases folate requirements, infants, adolescents, and pregnant women may have difficulty consuming adequate amounts.

Studies show that adequate intake of folate before conception and during the first trimester of pregnancy can reduce the incidence of neural tube defects (e.g., spina bifida) by as much as 50%. This discovery has prompted the U.S. Public Health Service to recommend that all women of childbearing age who are capable of becoming pregnant consume 400 micrograms of synthetic folic acid from food and/or supplements in addition to folate from a varied diet. To increase folate intake, mandatory folic acid fortification of enriched bread and grain products began on January 1, 1998. However, this policy alone does not ensure adequate folate intake among women of childbearing age; supplements and wise food choices continue to be important.

The UL for folate is 1000 micrograms/day from fortified food or supplements, exclusive of food folate. Consistently high intakes of folate can mask vitamin B_{12} deficiency, which can cause permanent neurologic damage if left untreated. Large doses may interfere with anticonvulsant therapy and precipitate convulsions in patients with epilepsy controlled by phenytoin.

Vitamin B_{12}

Vitamin B_{12} (cobalamin) has several interesting features. First, vitamin B_{12} has an interdependent relationship with folate: each vitamin must have the other to be activated. Because it activates folate, vitamin B_{12} is involved in DNA synthesis and maturation of red blood cells. Like folate, vitamin B_{12} functions as a coenzyme to convert homocysteine to methionine. Unlike folate, vitamin B_{12} has important roles in maintaining the myelin sheath around nerves. For this reason, large doses of folate can alleviate the anemia caused by vitamin B_{12} deficiency (a function of both vitamins), but folate cannot halt the progressive neurologic impairments that only vitamin B_{12} can treat. Nervous system damage may be irreversible without early treatment with vitamin B_{12}.

Vitamin B_{12} also holds the distinction of being the only water-soluble vitamin that does not occur naturally in plants. Fermented soy products and algae may be enriched with vitamin B_{12} but it is in an inactive, unavailable form. Some ready-to-eat cereals are fortified with vitamin B_{12}. All animal foods contain vitamin B_{12}.

Another unique feature of vitamin B_{12} is that it requires an intrinsic factor, a glycoprotein secreted in the stomach, to be absorbed from the terminal ileum. But before it can bind with the intrinsic factor, vitamin B_{12} must first be separated from the small peptides to which it is bound in food sources. Separation is accomplished by pepsin and gastric acid.

Vitamin B_{12} deficiency symptoms may take 5 to 10 years or longer to develop, because the liver can store relatively large amounts of B_{12} and the body recycles B_{12} by reabsorbing it.

Dietary deficiencies of vitamin B_{12} are rare and are likely to occur only in strict vegans who consume no animal products and do not adequately supplement their diet. A more frequent cause of deficiency is the lack of intrinsic factor, which prevents absorption of vitamin B_{12} regardless of intake; this condition is known as pernicious anemia. People with pernicious anemia, which can occur secondary to gastric surgery or gastric cancer, require parenteral injections of vitamin B_{12}. Most commonly, B_{12} deficiency arises from inadequate gastric acid secretion, which prevents protein-bound vitamin B_{12} in foods from being freed. As many as 10% to 30% of adults older than 50 years of age may have this type of vitamin B_{12} deficiency as a result of atrophic gastritis or from gastric resection, use of medications that suppress gastric acid secretion, or gastric infection with *Helicobacter pylori*. Because people with protein-bound vitamin B_{12} deficiency are able to absorb synthetic (free) vitamin B_{12}, the National Academy of Sciences Institute of Medicine recommends that people in this age group obtain most of their requirement from fortified foods or supplements.

Other B Vitamins

Pantothenic acid is part of CoA, the coenzyme involved in the formation of acetyl-CoA and in the TCA cycle. Pantothenic acid participates in more than 100 different metabolic reactions. It is widespread in the diet. The best sources of pantothenic acid are meat, fish, poultry, whole-grain cereals, and dried peas and beans.

As a coenzyme, biotin is involved in the TCA cycle, gluconeogenesis, fatty acid synthesis, and chemical reactions that add or remove carbon dioxide from other compounds. Biotin is widely distributed in nature and significant amounts are synthesized by GI flora, but it is not known how much is available for absorption. It is assumed that the average American diet provides adequate amounts of both pantothenic acid and biotin.

Non-B Vitamins

Other substances, such as inositol, choline, and carnitine are sometimes inaccurately referred to as B vitamins because they are coenzymes. Only choline has been assigned an Adequate Intake value. Research is needed to determine if these substances are essential in the diet.

Other substances that are not essential nutrients but often are falsely promoted as B vitamins include para-aminobenzoic acid (PABA), bioflavonoids (vitamin P or hesperidin), ubiquinone, vitamin B_{15}, and vitamin B_{17}.

Vitamin C

Vitamin C (ascorbic acid), most notably found in citrus fruits and juices, may be the most famous vitamin (Fig. 5.2). Its long history dates back more than 250 years when it was determined that something in citrus fruits prevents scurvy, a disease that killed as many

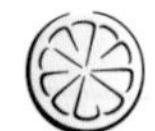

as two-thirds of sailors on long journeys. Years later, British sailors acquired the nickname "Limeys" because of Great Britain's policy to prevent scurvy by providing limes to all navy men. It wasn't until 1928 that the antiscurvy agent was identified as vitamin C. Since then, vitamin C has been touted as a cure for a variety of ills, including cancer, colds, and infertility.

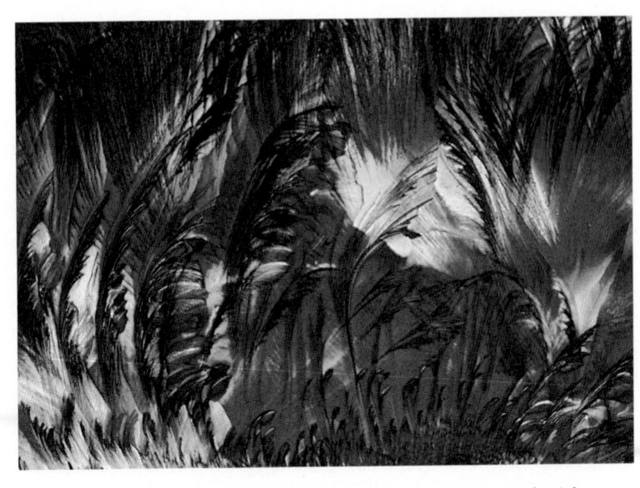

FIGURE 5.2 Photo of vitamin C. (Source: Florida State University.)

Vitamin C prevents scurvy by promoting the formation of collagen, the most abundant protein in fibrous tissues such as connective tissue, cartilage, bone matrix, tooth dentin, skin, and tendon. Without adequate vitamin C, the integrity of collagen is compromised; muscles degenerate, weakened bones break, wounds fail to heal, teeth are lost, and infection occurs. Hemorrhaging begins as pinpoints under the skin and progresses to massive internal bleeding and death. Even though scurvy is deadly, it can be cured within a matter of days with moderate doses of vitamin C.

Vitamin C is a water-soluble antioxidant that protects vitamin A, vitamin E, PUFA, and iron from destruction. As an antioxidant, vitamin C is being studied for its ability to prevent heart disease, certain cancers, cataracts, and asthma. It is involved in many metabolic reactions including the promotion of iron absorption, the formation of some neurotransmitters, the synthesis of thyroxine, the metabolism of some amino acids, and normal immune system functioning.

The newest RDA for vitamin C represents an increase from the previous recommendation. Cigarette smokers are advised to increase their intake by 35 mg/d because smoking increases oxidative stress and metabolic turnover of vitamin C. The need for vitamin C also increases in response to other stresses such as fever, chronic illness, infection, and wound healing as well as from chronic use of certain medications such as aspirin, barbiturates, and oral contraceptives.

Intakes higher than the UL may cause osmotic diarrhea and gastrointestinal disturbances. Because vitamin C facilitates the absorption of iron, excessive amounts can in theory cause iron overload. Large doses of vitamin C can interfere with the blood thinning affect of anticoagulants.

There is no clear and convincing evidence that large doses of vitamin C prevent colds, although some studies suggest that it may lessen the severity of cold symptoms because vitamin C reduces blood histamine levels. Its role in normal immune system functioning may also be involved.

VITAMINS IN HEALTH PROMOTION: VITAMIN SUPPLEMENTS

Headlines and research findings fuel strong consumer interest in supplements. Intrigued by the prospect of defying aging and avoiding disease without the effort of changing their eating and exercise behaviors, Americans swallow supplements with abandon. They rationalize that supplements make up for "bad" food choices. They are spurred on by the misplaced philosophy that "if a little is good, a lot is better." Of the more than $13.9 billion spent on supplements annually in the United States, vitamins account for approximately 40%. The most commonly used supplements are multivitamins, vitamin C, and the mineral calcium.

Although vitamin supplements are popular, are they necessary? Can vitamin supplements prevent chronic disease? Who needs vitamin supplements? Can they be used as a safeguard against less than optimal food choices? And what do you look for when buying a vitamin supplement?

Are They Necessary?

With few exceptions, healthy people who eat a variety of nutritious foods are able to obtain an adequate and balanced intake of vitamins, other essential nutrients, and healthy food components for which no recommendations have been made. Yet an estimated 40 to 47% of Americans use vitamin and mineral supplements at least occasionally. Supplement users are more likely to be Caucasian, female, and older; have higher personal incomes and education levels; live in the western United States; and have healthier diets (e.g., eat less fat, more fiber, and more fruit and vegetables). In other words, people who take vitamin supplements are probably not the people who need them. On the plus side, multivitamins have been shown to help people consume the recommended levels of folic acid and vitamin D as well as the minerals iron and calcium-nutrients that are often consumed in less than optimal amounts.

Can Vitamin Supplements Prevent Chronic Disease?

Without doubt, vitamin supplements can prevent *deficiency* diseases (e.g., scurvy, beriberi) that occur when vitamin intake is inadequate. But can certain vitamins in amounts greater than the RDA help to prevent *chronic* diseases? That is the area of current of vitamin research.

Phytochemicals: plant chemicals that, though not essential for life, are thought to promote health.

Convincing evidence shows that fruit and vegetables help to protect against certain cancers, birth defects, and cardiovascular disease. While the evidence is less compelling, fruit and vegetables may be protective against several other chronic diseases (Box 5.1). That does not specifically mean that the credit goes to vitamins. Other substances in fruit and vegetables, such as the content of fiber, minerals, phytochemicals, or low caloric density, may be at least partially responsible. Or it may be that a food synergy exists between the components of fruit and vegetables, causing the whole to be greater than the sum of

 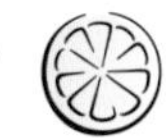

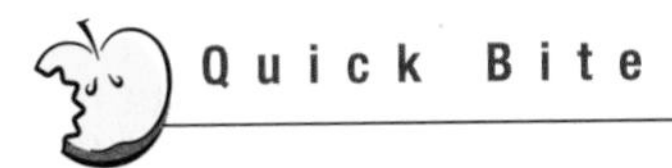

Facts about fruit and vegetable intake among Americans

When French fries and potato chips are excluded, Americans eat only about 3.6 servings of fruits and vegetables daily.

Nine out of 10 teenage girls do not eat five servings of fruit and vegetables daily.

Fruit and vegetable intake is declining. Romaine lettuce and bag lettuce are the only vegetables Americans are eating more of.

Obesity levels are lowest for people who eat the most fruit and vegetables.

their individual parts. With few exceptions (e.g., folate preventing birth defects), benefits are attributed to fruit and vegetables not from individual vitamins or vitamin supplements.

Clients who are tempted to use vitamin supplements to prevent chronic disease should be advised that

- **Proof is difficult to document.** Observational studies, such as those that detect an association between lower cancer rates and diets rich in fruits and vegetables, do not *prove* anything. To prove cause-and-effect (e.g., that vitamin C prevents cancer), all types of research must be considered—clinical, pathologic, animal, experimental, epidemiologic—and, when available, randomized, double-blind, placebo-controlled clinical intervention trials. There is no conclusive evidence yet to prove that supplements prevent chronic disease. In fact, several well-designed clinical trials have shown that the beneficial effects associated with high intakes of fruits and vegetables may not be replicated by the use of supplements of individual nutrients such as vitamin E, C, or beta-carotene.

BOX 5.1

THE EVIDENCE LINKING FRUIT AND VEGETABLE CONSUMPTION WITH DECREASED RISK OF DISEASE

Convincing Evidence

For many cancers
Cardiovascular disease
Birth defects

Convincing as Adjunct

Hypertension
Obesity

Highly Suggestive

COPD, lung function

Plausible

Longevity
Bone health
Cognition and aging
Neurodegenerative disorders

Suggestive

Cataracts

Produce for Better Health Foundation. (2002). The health benefits of fruits and vegetables. A scientific overview for health professionals. Available at www.5aday.org.

- **The responsible substances are not even known.** Perhaps the antioxidant vitamins in fruit and vegetables do help to prevent cancer, but maybe that is only true when they are consumed with other food components. But which ones? And how much of each substance is optimal? People eat food, not nutrients, and food provides a variety of nutrients and compounds, not single active ingredients.

Also, fruit and vegetables provide phytochemicals, biologically active compounds produced by plants to protect themselves against viruses, bacteria, and fungi. In foods, phytochemicals impart color, taste, aroma, and other characteristics. When eaten, they can have important physiologic effects; they serve as antioxidants, enhance immune response, alter estrogen metabolism, or detoxify carcinogens through enzyme systems. Table 5.4 outlines potential health benefits and dietary sources of selected phytochemicals.

At this time, researchers are not able to create a perfect pill to substitute for a varied diet rich in plants. We simply do not know all the components in plant foods, how they function, which ones are beneficial, which ones are potentially harmful, and the ideal combination and concentration of these chemicals. More than likely it is the total package and balance of nutrients, fiber, and phytochemicals that makes fruits and vegetables so healthy. Until science catches up to nature, the best advice is to eat a diet rich in plants, including fruit and vegetables. Variety is important because different plants supply different types and amounts of nutrients and phytochemicals.

- **Abnormally high intakes of one or more vitamins may adversely affect other vitamins.** For instance, high doses of vitamin E interfere with the function of vitamin K and excess folic acid can mask vitamin B_{12} deficiency. In contrast, when the vehicle is food, it is almost impossible to overdose on vitamins or to create a pseudo vitamin deficiency related to an imbalance of vitamins.
- **Potential long-term risks are unknown.** Controlled studies testing supplement use in humans have been of relatively short duration. They have not lasted long enough (e.g., years) to indicate if there are any risks from high doses of multiple or single vitamins taken for a prolonged period.

Who Needs Vitamin Supplements?

Leading health and nutrition authorities agree that the best way to get nutrients is through food, not supplements, with a few noted exceptions:

- Women capable of becoming pregnant are urged to obtain 400 micrograms of folic acid through supplements or fortified food in addition to natural folate obtained through a normal mixed diet. Notice the word "or." Women who consume folic acid fortified cereal do not need a supplement; in fact, they may be at risk for an excessive folic acid intake if they consume both. Although fortified cereals only provide 400 micrograms folic acid per serving, actual portion sizes eaten are usually much bigger. During pregnancy, the recommendation for folic acid jumps to 600 micrograms.
- Men and women over age 50 are urged to consume most of their RDA for vitamin B_{12} via fortified cereals or supplements because they may not adequately absorb adequate B_{12} from protein-bound food sources.

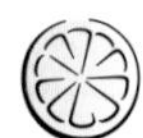

TABLE 5.4

POSSIBLE EFFECTS AND SOURCES OF SELECTED PHYTOCHEMICALS

Phytochemical Name or Class	Possible Effects	Sources
Isothiocyanates (including sulphoraphane)	Neutralize free radicals; inhibit enzymes that activate carcinogens; promote production of enzymes that detoxify carcinogens	Broccoli, broccoli sprouts, cabbage, cauliflower, horseradish, mustard greens
Lycopene	Potent antioxidant that may reduce risk of prostate cancer	Tomatoes, tomato products, red grapefruit, dried apricot, guava, watermelon
Allyl sulfides	Boosts levels of naturally occurring enzymes that may help to maintain healthy immune system	Garlic, onions, leeks, chives
Isoflavones (genistein and daidzein)	Antiestrogen activity, which may decrease risk of estrogen-dependent cancers; may inhibit formation of blood vessels that enable tumors to grow	Soybeans, soy flour, soy milk tofu, other legumes
Phenolic acids (including ellagic acid)	May block production of enzymes needed for cancer cells to replicate	Grapes, strawberries, raspberries, coffee beans, blueberries, apples, cherries, pears, prunes, oats, potatoes, soybeans
Limonene	Boosts levels of body enzymes that may destroy carcinogens	Oranges and lemons
Polyphenols (catechins)	May help to prevent DNA damage by neutralizing free radicals	Onion, apple, tea, red wine, grapes, grape juice, strawberries, green tea, wine
Lignans	Act as a phytoestrogen; may reduce risk of certain kinds of cancer	Flaxseed, whole grains
Phytic acid	May inhibit oxidative reactions in the colon that produce harmful free radicals	Whole wheat
Lutein	Acts as antioxidant; may reduce risk of heart disease, age-related eye diseases, and cancer	Peaches, orange juice, kale, spinach, broccoli, pumpkin, dark leafy greens, tomatoes, carrots

- The elderly are not likely to consume the new AI for vitamin D unless they drink liberal amounts of fortified milk.
- Vegans, who eat no animal products, need supplemental B_{12} and vitamin D if sunlight exposure is inadequate. Vitamin B_{12} is found naturally only in animal products and the only plant sources of vitamin D are some fortified margarines and some fortified cereals.

Career Connection

How can you tell if a client is getting enough vitamins through food? In a nutshell, you can't. First of all, an individual's actual nutrient requirements are almost never known: RDAs are proposed to meet the needs of 97 to 98% of all healthy people but not necessarily individuals. Secondly, day-to-day variation in intake makes it extremely difficult to accurately determine the long-term average intake of any particular nutrient and people tend to underreport their actual food intake. In addition, food composition data may be inaccurate (as in the case of vitamin E, which includes all types of E, not just the active form) or limited (e.g., biotin and pantothenic acid content). Thus is it not possible to state with complete certainty that an individual's intake meets his or her nutrient requirements. For practical purposes, it is more useful to talk about food than individual nutrients. The food groups of most concern are fruits and vegetables. To boost their intake, encourage clients to

- Eat at least five servings of fruits and vegetables every day. More is even better.
- Choose wholesome, nutrient-dense foods over refined or processed foods. For instance, fortified whole-grain cereal (e.g., Total) is more nutritious than refined cereal (e.g., puffed wheat), and orange juice is more nutritious than carbonated beverages.
- Concentrate on variety and color.
- Make an effort to preserve the vitamin content of foods during storage and preparation; avoid overcooking vegetables; microwave them instead of boiling.
- Start at least one meal each day with a fresh salad.
- Eat raw vegetables or fresh fruits for snacks.
- Add vegetables to other foods such as zucchini to spaghetti sauce, grated carrots to meat loaf, and spinach to lasagna.
- Double the normal portion size of vegetables.
- Buy a new fruit or vegetable when you go grocery shopping.
- Eat occasional meatless entrees such as pasta primavera, vegetable stir-fry, or black beans and rice.
- Order a vegetable when you eat out.
- Choose 100% fruit juice at breakfast and instead of drinks, cocktails, ades, and/or carbonated beverages during the day.
- Eat fruit for dessert.
- Make fruits and vegetables more visible. Leave a bowl of fruit on the center of your table. Keep fresh vegetables on the top shelf of the refrigerator in plain view.

On a hedge-your-bet basis, multivitamin supplements may be a good idea for others such as

- Dieters consuming less than 1200 calories. Even with optimal food choices, it may not be possible to consume adequate amounts of all nutrients on a low-calorie diet.
- Finicky eaters and people who eliminate one or more food groups from their typical diet. For instance, someone who cannot tolerate citrus juices because of gastric reflux may not consistently obtain adequate vitamin C without the use of a vitamin supplement.
- The elderly, who may have an inadequate food intake related to income restraints, impaired chewing and swallowing, social isolation, physical limitations that make shopping or cooking difficult, or a decreased sense of taste leading to poor appetite. In addition, their vitamin requirements may be elevated as a result of chronic disease or as a side effect of certain medications. And as already noted, the ability to synthesize vitamin D decreases with aging, as does the ability to absorb vitamin B_{12}. Studies show that low-dose multivitamin and mineral supplements may improve immune function in the elderly.
- Alcoholics, because alcohol alters vitamin intake, absorption, metabolism, and excretion. The nutrients most profoundly affected are thiamin, riboflavin, niacin, folic acid, and pantothenic acid.

Can They Be Used as a Safeguard Against Less Than Optimal Food Choices?

While there is little scientific evidence to suggest vitamin supplements can benefit the average person, there is also little evidence of harm from low-dose multivitamin or multivitamin and mineral supplements. Because vitamins work best together and in balanced proportions, a multivitamin is usually better than single vitamin supplements that tend to provide doses much greater than the RDA. Remember that pills are not a substitute for healthy food: "supplement" means "add to," not "replace."

What to Look for in a Vitamin Supplement

The FDA requires a standardized Supplement Facts label on all supplements. Like the Nutrition Facts label, the supplement label is intended to provide consumers with better information. Labels must divulge serving sizes, calories per serving (if any), and a complete ingredient list. Vitamins with established DVs must appear at the top of the panel. Ingredients that have not been proven to be important in health (e.g., inositol, garlic, bioflavonoids) must appear at the bottom of the panel and must be separated from the established nutrients by a solid line. The amount of each ingredient and the Percent Daily Value (%DV) must be listed. For ingredients that do not have a DV, an asterisk must be used to indicate that there is no official government recommendation for that substance.

Choose multivitamins with 100% DV. For most people, the best bet for an all-purpose, safeguard-type supplement is one that provides no more than 100% of the DV for the 12 vitamins and 8 minerals for which there are established DVs. Clients who opt for megavitamins should be aware that, with few exceptions, manufacturers are free to add or leave out whatever nutrients they choose. What they put in is often based on economics, not health. For instance, because biotin is expensive, only small amounts, if any, are found in supplements. Conversely most of the other B vitamins are cheap so they are often used abundantly.

Take note of serving size. The nutrient content on some brands is listed as a "serving" but two or three "servings" may be needed daily, adding to cost and inconvenience.

Not dangerous, but not necessary. The median U.S. intake for thiamin, riboflavin, niacin, and vitamin C meets or exceeds recommendations. Likewise, deficiencies of biotin and pantothenic acid almost never occur. Taking more in supplement form is usually not harmful but it does not offer any advantage. Ingredients such as bee pollen, silica, and yarrow flowers add to the price but not the nutritional value.

Potentially dangerous. Taking more than 100% of the DV for vitamins A, D, and B_6 is potentially harmful. Because studies of beta-carotene supplements have failed to show health benefits and some have shown increased health risks, it is best to get beta-carotene from fruits and vegetables, not supplements. At the very least, avoid taking more than 15,000 IU of beta-carotene.

Natural is not naturally better. Marketing tactics that promote vitamins as "natural" and "organic" are open to interpretation. In this situation, "natural" often means synthetic mixed with plant extracts. Sometimes synthetic is even better than natural. For instance, synthetic folic acid is much better absorbed than natural folate in foods. The exception is supplemental vitamin E: synthetic vitamin E, commonly labeled as dl-alpha tocopherol, has lower bioavailability than "natural" vitamin E labeled d-alpha-tocopherol.

Cost is not necessarily an indication of quality. Vitamin supplements do not necessarily follow the dictum, "You get what you pay for." Because large retail chains are high-volume customers, they can demand and get their own top-quality, private-label brand supplements from vitamin manufacturers. The cost of these supplements is usually significantly less than that of brand-name varieties, yet the quality and content are similar.

Look for USP on the label. The United States Pharmacopeia (USP) has established strict quality standards for vitamins and minerals to enable consumers to identify products whose quality can be trusted. The designation *USP* on the label means that the product passes tests for disintegration, dissolution, strength, and purity. An expiration date is also included; beyond this date, the ingredients may no longer meet USP standards of purity, strength, and/or quality. What the quality indicators do not ensure is that the supplement is safe or beneficial to health.

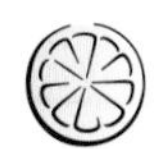

Beware of label claims. Because the FDA does not closely regulate the supplement industry, manufacturers' claims may be less than reliable and not defined.

- **"High potency,"** at least to the FDA, means that at least two-thirds of the product's nutrients are provided at 100 % of the DV. To most people, "high potency" means more than the DV.
- **"Advanced," "Complete," or "Maximum"** formulas are not defined; manufacturers can use those terms as desired.
- **"Mature" or "50+" formulas** usually have less iron and vitamin K. While seniors do need less iron, the need for vitamin K does not decrease with aging. In fact, vitamin K may help prevent hip fractures. However, people using anticoagulants should strive for a consistent vitamin K intake.
- **"Women's" formulas** have 18 mg of iron, which is appropriate for premenopausal women. Postmenopausal women need around 8 mg, which is the same amount of iron as men need.

How Do You Respond?

Is it better to take vitamin supplements with meals or between meals? In general, it is better to take supplements with meals, because food enhances the absorption of some vitamins.

Should I choose vitamin-fortified foods over those that are not fortified? For the most part, fortified foods are a good bet. Fortified milk and fortified cereals provide nutrients (vitamin D and iron respectively) that otherwise may not be consumed in adequate amounts by some people. On the other hand, a vitamin-fortified candy bar is still a candy bar. Be aware of slick marketing techniques that might lead you to believe that junk food with vitamins is healthy.

I am under a lot of emotional stress. Should I take stress vitamins? Although significant physical stress (e.g., thermal injury, trauma) increases the requirements for certain vitamins, mental stress does not. Misleading advertising is to blame for this widespread misconception.

▲ Focus on Critical Thinking

Respond to the following statements:

1. With vitamins, if a little is good, more is better.
2. Because there is little danger from taking a low dose multivitamin, people should be encouraged to do so as added protection against less than optimal food choices.
3. Most people do not consume adequate amounts of vitamins from food.

Key Concepts

- Vitamins do not provide energy (calories) but they are needed for metabolism of energy. Most vitamins function as coenzymes to activate enzymes.
- The body needs vitamins in small amounts (microgram or milligram quantities). Vitamins are essential in the diet because they cannot be made by the body or they are synthesized in inadequate amounts.
- Fortification and enrichment have virtually eliminated vitamin deficiencies in healthy Americans.
- It is assumed that if a variety of nutritious foods are consumed, the diet's vitamin content will be generally be adequate for most people.
- Vitamins are organic compounds that are soluble in either water or fat; their solubility determines how they are absorbed, transported through the blood, stored, and excreted.
- Vitamins A, D, E, and K are the fat-soluble vitamins. Because they are stored in liver and adipose tissue, they do not need to be consumed daily. Vitamins A and D are toxic when consumed in large quantities over a long period.
- The B-complex vitamins and vitamin C are water-soluble vitamins. Although some tissues are able to hold limited amounts of certain water-soluble vitamins, they are not generally stored in the body so a daily intake is necessary. Because they are not stored, they are considered nontoxic; however, adverse side effects can occur from taking megadoses of certain water-soluble vitamins over a prolonged period.
- Although diets rich in fruits and vegetables appear to be protective against chronic diseases such as heart disease, cancer, and hypertension, it is not known what components in them are responsible for the health benefits. Antioxidant vitamins in foods are suspected of being beneficial, but high-dose supplements have not been proven to prevent disease and may disrupt nutrient balances. Long-term safety has not been established; some reports indicate that single-nutrient supplements may actually increase, not decrease, health risks.
- It is recommended that women who are capable of becoming pregnant consume 400 micrograms of folic acid through supplements or fortified food daily. People over the age of 50 are urged to consume most of their B_{12} requirement from supplements or fortified food. Vegans need supplemental B_{12} and D, if exposure to sunshine is inadequate.
- Multivitamin supplements provide a limited safeguard when food choices are less than optimal. Other groups who may benefit from taking a daily multivitamin are the elderly, dieters, finicky eaters, and alcoholics.
- People who choose to take an all-purpose multivitamin should select one that provides 100% of the DV for vitamins with an established DV. The USP stamp ensures the quality, but not safety or benefits. High-cost supplements are not necessarily superior to lower-cost ones.

ANSWER KEY

1. **FALSE** In theory, healthy people should be able to obtain all the nutrients they need by choosing a varied diet of nutrient dense foods.

 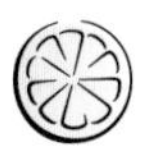

2. **FALSE** Vitamins are needed to release energy from carbohydrates, protein, and fat but are not a source of energy (calories).
3. **FALSE** Adverse side effects can occur from taking large doses of certain water-soluble vitamins over a long period of time. For instance, adverse effects can be seen from large doses of B_6 (neuropathy), vitamin C (GI upset and diarrhea), and niacin (flushing).
4. **FALSE** Median intake of vitamin C for both men and women exceeds the RDA. Other vitamins consistently eaten in excess of need include thiamin, riboflavin, and niacin.
5. **FALSE** Cost and quality are not necessarily related.
6. **FALSE** "Natural" vitamins are not naturally better.
7. **TRUE** Under optimal conditions, such as exposing unprotected skin to the sun in the southern United States for several minutes, the body can make all the vitamin D it needs providing that kidney and liver functions are normal. However, sunscreen, smog, dark skin, clothing, and dense cloud cover hinder vitamin D synthesis.
8. **FALSE** Natural folate in foods is only half as available to the body as man-made folic acid.
9. **FALSE** USP on a vitamin label means that the product passes tests that evaluate disintegration, dissolution, strength, and purity. It does not mean the product is safe. For instance, large doses of vitamin A are not safe but they may have USP on the label.
10. **TRUE** The percentage of Americans consuming five or more servings of fruit and vegetables daily is 23.1%, which represents a decrease in fruit and vegetable intake over the recent past.

WEBSITES

Produce for Better Health Foundation at **www.5aday.org**
Dietary Reference Intakes from the Institute of Medicine at **www.nap.edu**

REFERENCES

American Dietetic Association. (2001). Position of the American Dietetic Association: Food fortification and dietary supplements. *Journal of the American Dietetic Association, 101,* 115–125.

Barr, S., Murphy, S., & Poos, M. (2002). Interpreting and using the Dietary References Intakes in dietary assessment of individuals and groups. *Journal of the American Dietetic Association, 102,* 780–788.

Brigelium-Flohe, R., Keyy, F., Salonen, J., et al. (2002). The European perspective on vitamin E: Current knowledge and future research. *American Journal of Clinical Nutrition, 76,* 703–716.

Food and Nutrition Board, Institute of Medicine. (2001). *Dietary Reference Intakes for vitamin A, vitamin K, arsenic, boron, chromium, copper, iodine, iron, manganese, molybdenum, nickel, silicon, vanadium, and zinc.* Washington, DC: National Academy Press.

Food and Nutrition Board, Institute of Medicine. (2000). *Dietary Reference Intakes for vitamin C, vitamin E, selenium, and carotenoids.* Washington, DC: National Academy Press.

Food and Nutrition Board, Institute of Medicine. (1998). *Dietary Reference Intakes for thiamin, riboflavin, niacin, vitamin B_6, folate, vitamin B_{12}, pantothenic acid, biotin, and choline.* Washington, DC: National Academy Press.

Jacobs, D., & Steffen, L. (2003). Nutrients, foods, and dietary patterns as exposures in research: A framework for food synergy. *American Journal of Clinical Nutrition, 78*(Suppl.), 508S–513S.

Janssen, H., Samson, M., & Verhaar, H. (2002). Vitamin D deficiency, muscle function, and falls in elderly people. *American Journal of Clinical Nutrition, 75,* 611–615.

Liebman, B. (2003). Spin the bottle. How to pick a multivitamin. *Nutrition Action Health Letter, 30*(1), 1, 3–9.

Liebman, B. (2003). Soaking up the D's. *Nutrition Action Health Letter, 30*(10), 1, 3–6.

Mennen, L., Potier de Courcy, P., Guilland, J., et al. (2002). Homocysteine, cardiovascular disease risk factors, and habitual diet in the French supplementation with antioxidant vitamins and minerals study. *American Journal of Clinical Nutrition, 76,* 1279–1289.

Penniston, K., & Tanumihardjo, S. (2003). Vitamin A in dietary supplements and fortified foods: Too much of a good thing? *Journal of the American Dietetic Association, 103,* 1185–1187.

Powers, H. (2003). Riboflavin (vitamin B_2) and health. *American Journal of Clinical Nutrition, 77,* 1352–1360.

Produce for Better Health Foundation (2002). *The health benefits of fruits and vegetables. A scientific overview for health professionals.* Available at www.5aday.org. Accessed on 2/19/04.

Produce for Better Health Foundation. *Consumption statistics.* Available at www.5aday.org. Accessed on 2/20/04.

Troppmann, L., Gray-Donald, K., & Johns, T. (2002). Supplement use: Is there any nutritional benefit? *Journal of the American Dietetic Association,* 102, 818–825.

United States Department of Agriculture Beltsville Agricultural Research Center (BARC). *Frequently asked questions about phytonutrients.* Available at www.barc.usda.gov/bhnrc/pl/pl_fac.html. Accessed on 2/18/04.

For information on the new dietary guidelines 2005 and MyPyramid, visit **http://connection.lww.com/go/dudek**

6

Water and Minerals

TRUE	FALSE	
⬭	⬭	**1** Most people have an inadequate intake of fluid.
⬭	⬭	**2** Minerals consumed in excess of need are excreted in the urine.
⬭	⬭	**3** Sodium is the most plentiful mineral in the body.
⬭	⬭	**4** An increase in sodium intake is associated with an increase in blood pressure.
⬭	⬭	**5** Bottled water is superior to tap water.
⬭	⬭	**6** Foods high in sodium tend to be low in potassium and foods high in potassium tend to be low in sodium.
⬭	⬭	**7** Major minerals are more important for health than trace minerals.
⬭	⬭	**8** For most people, thirst is a reliable indicator of fluid needs.
⬭	⬭	**9** A deficiency of zinc can cause impaired sense of taste.
⬭	⬭	**10** A chronically low intake of calcium leads to hypocalcemia.

UPON COMPLETION OF THIS CHAPTER, YOU WILL BE ABLE TO

- Name sources of fluids.
- Discuss method of estimating fluid requirements.
- Explain mechanisms by which the body maintains mineral homeostasis.
- Describe general functions and sources of minerals.

WATER

Life as we know it does not exist without water. It is the largest single constituent of the human body, averaging 60% of total body weight. It is the medium in which all biochemical reactions take place. Although most people can survive 6 weeks or longer without food, death occurs in a matter of days without water.

Functions of Water

Water occupies essentially every space within and between body cells and is involved in virtually every body function. Water

- **Provides shape and structure to cells.** Approximately two-thirds of the body's water is located within cells (intracellular fluid). Muscle cells have a higher concentration of water (73%) than fat, which is only about 25% water. Men generally have more muscle mass than women have and, therefore, have a higher percentage of body water.
- **Regulates body temperature.** Because water absorbs heat slowly, the large amount of water contained in the body helps to maintain body temperature homeostasis despite fluctuations in environmental temperatures. Evaporation of water (sweat) from the skin cools the body.
- **Aids in the digestion and absorption of nutrients.** Approximately 7 to 9 L of water is secreted in the gastrointestinal tract daily to aid in digestion and absorption. Except for the approximately 100 mL of water excreted through the feces, all of the water contained in the gastrointestinal secretions (saliva, gastric secretions, bile, pancreatic secretions, and intestinal mucosal secretions) is reabsorbed in the ileum and colon.
- **Transports nutrients and oxygen to cells.** By moistening the air sacs in the lungs, water allows oxygen to dissolve and move into blood for distribution throughout the body. Approximately 92% of blood plasma is water.
- **Serves as a solvent for vitamins, minerals, glucose, and amino acids.** The solvating property of water is vital for health and survival.
- **Participates in metabolic reactions.** For instance, water is used in the synthesis of hormones and enzymes.
- **Eliminates waste products.** Water helps to excrete body wastes through urine, feces, and expirations.
- **Is a major component of mucus and other lubricating fluids.** As such, it reduces friction in joints where bones, ligaments, and tendons come in contact with each other and it cushions contacts between internal organs that slide over one another.

Water Output

Water is an essential nutrient because the body cannot produce as much water as it needs. On average, adults lose approximately 1450 to 2800 mL of water daily (Table 6.1).

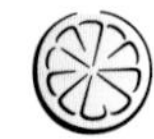

TABLE 6.1 SOURCES AND AVERAGE AMOUNTS OF DAILY WATER LOSS

Source of Water Loss	Average Amount Lost (mL/d)
Perspiration	450–900
Exhalations	350
Urine	500–1400
Feces	150
Total	1450–2800

Insensible Water Loss: immeasurable losses.

Sensible Water Loss: measurable losses.

Insensible water losses from the skin and expirations account for approximately half of the total water lost daily. Extreme environmental temperatures (very hot or very cold), high altitude, low humidity, and strenuous exercise increase insensible losses. Water evaporation from the skin is also increased by prolonged exposure to heated or recirculated air such as during long airplane flights. Sensible water losses from urine and feces make up the remaining water loss. Because the body needs to excrete a minimum of 500 mL of urine daily to rid itself of metabolic wastes, the minimum daily total fluid output is approximately 1500 mL. To maintain water balance, intake should approximate output.

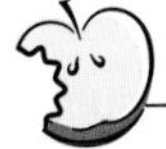

Quick Bite

Percentage of water in selected foods

	% water by weight
Lettuce	95
Watermelon	92
Broccoli	91
Milk	89
Carrot	87
Yogurt	85
Chicken	65
Whole wheat bread	38
Honey	17
Vegetable oil	0

Water Intake

An AI for total water, which includes drinking water, other beverages, and water in food, is based on the median total water intake from U.S. food consumption survey data. For men ages 19 to 30 the Adequate Intake (AI) is 3.7 L/day; for women of the same age, the AI is 2.7 L. Fluid (water and other beverages) accounts for approximately 81% of usual total water intake, with the remaining 19% coming from water in food. Similar to AIs set for other nutrients, daily intakes below the AI may not be harmful to healthy people because normal hydration is maintained over a wide range of intakes. Intakes higher than the AI are recommended for rigorous activity in hot climates.

Career Connection

Plain water is the best thirst-quenching fluid and is readily available and calorie free. Yet it is not everyone's beverage of choice. Of concern is the high intake of soft drinks, particularly among children and adolescents, which has increased dramatically in recent decades. A recent survey indicates the mean daily intake of soft drinks is 12 oz/day—approximately 150 calories of sugar water. The problem with the ever-growing use of soft drinks is that

- Soft drinks are 100% empty calories that may increase the risk of weight gain and obesity. Studies indicate that when extra calories are consumed in liquid form, the body does not compensate for those additional calories by eating less later on as it tends to do when extra carbohydrate calories are consumed in solid form. Liquid calories appear to lack satiety value and so are major contributors to obesity. In children, one serving of soft drink per day increases the risk of becoming overweight by 60% during the course of 1 year.
- Although the mean intake is 12 ounces/day, an actual serving can be much larger. For instance, a king-sized soft drink at Burger King is 35 ounces, slightly more than 1 quart and about 426 calories.
- Soft drinks that displace milk remove the primary source of calcium in the typical American diet, increasing the risk of osteoporosis. Low calcium intakes may also increase the risk of bone fractures among children and adolescents.
- High soft drink consumption is associated with lower total diet quality, not just because less milk is consumed, but also because intake of 100% fruit juice may be less. High soft drink consumers tend to have lower intakes of vitamin A, vitamin D, riboflavin, and phosphorus.

Encourage healthy beverage choices:

- Replace soft drinks with calorie-free versions such as diet soda or sparkling water.
- Use bottled water if the taste of tap water is objectionable. Artesian water, mineral water, purified water, spring water, and sparkling water are basically water. In contrast, soda water, tonic water, and club soda are carbonated soft drinks, not different varieties of water.
- Refrigeration usually improves the taste of tap water.
- Drink a glass of water before each meal, especially if weight control is a concern. Water can blunt appetite and help people to eat less. Weight management programs often urge participants to drink adequate water as a means to control appetite.
- Eat enough fruits and vegetables. Fruits and vegetables are generally high in water even though the water they provide is usually not counted when fluid intake is calculated. Their fiber, vitamins, minerals, phytochemicals, and satiety value are bonuses.

 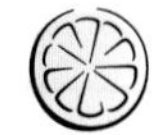

TABLE 6.2 **METHODS TO ESTIMATE FLUID NEEDS**

Based upon	Guidelines	Example of calculation (40 year old weighing 70 kg who consumes 2000 cal/day with 1300 mL urine output)
Calories consumed	1 mL water/calorie	2000 cal × 1 mL/cal = 2000 mL
Age and body weight in kilograms	40 mL/kg for active people aged 16–30 35 mL/kg for 20–55 year olds 30 mL/kg for 55–74 year olds 25 mL/kg for >75 year olds	35 mL × 70 kg = **2450 mL**
Weight	100 mL/kg body weight for the first 10 kg of weight 50 mL/kg body weight for the next 10 kg of weight 20 mL/kg body weight for each kg >20 kg	100 mL × 10 kg = 1000 mL + 50 mL × 10 kg = 500 mL + 20 mL × 50 kg = 1000 mL 70 kg 2500 mL
Fluid balance	Urine output (mL) + 500 mL/day	1300 mL + 500 mL = 1800 mL

In clinical situations, fluid needs can be estimated by a variety of methods (Table 6.2). However, actual water requirement is highly variable. Vomiting, diarrhea, and fever increase water losses. Certain other clinical conditions are characterized by high water losses, including thermal injuries, fistulas, uncontrolled diabetes, hemorrhage, and certain renal disorders. The use of drainage tubes contributes to increased water losses. Intake and output records are used to assess adequacy of intake.

KEYS TO UNDERSTANDING MINERALS

Although minerals account for only about 4% of the body's total weight, they are found in all body fluids and tissues. Major minerals are present in the body in amounts greater than 5 g (the equivalent of 1 teaspoon). Calcium, phosphorus, magnesium, sulfur, sodium, potassium, and chloride are major minerals. Iron, iodine, zinc, selenium, copper, manganese, fluoride, chromium, and molybdenum are classified as trace minerals or trace elements because they are present in the body in amounts less than 5 g, not because they are less important than major minerals. Both groups are essential for life. As many as 30 other, potentially harmful minerals are present in the body such as lead, gold, and mercury. Their presence appears to be related to environmental contamination.

General Chemistry

Inorganic: not containing carbon or concerning living things.

Unlike the energy nutrients and vitamins, minerals are inorganic elements that originate from the earth's crust, not from plants or animals. Minerals do not undergo digestion nor are they broken down or rearranged during metabolism. Although they combine with other elements to form salts (e.g., sodium chloride) or with organic compounds (e.g., iron in hemoglobin), they always retain their chemical identities.

Unlike vitamins, minerals are not destroyed by light, air, heat, or acids during food preparation. In fact when food is completely burned, minerals are the ash that remains. Minerals are lost only when foods are soaked in water.

General Functions

Minerals function to provide structure to body tissues and to regulate body processes such as fluid balance, acid–base balance, nerve cell transmission, muscle contraction, and vitamin, enzyme, and hormonal activities.

- **Structure.** Calcium, phosphorus, magnesium, and fluorine provide structure to bones and teeth. Soft tissues gain structural support from phosphorus, potassium, iron, and sulfur. Sulfur is also a fundamental constituent of skin, hair, and nails.
- **Fluid balance.** The volume of water in the body and its distribution among body compartments are determined largely by the concentrations of solutes in solution. Fluid balance is influenced by sodium, potassium, chloride, and all the major minerals (calcium, phosphorus, magnesium).
- **Acid–base balance.** This term refers to the maintenance of the body's concentration of hydrogen ions. Sodium hydroxide and sodium bicarbonate are part of the carbonic acid–bicarbonate system that regulates the pH of blood. Phosphorus is involved in buffer systems that regulate the pH of red blood cells and the kidney tubular fluids.
- **Nerve cell transmission and muscle contraction.** The exchange of sodium and potassium across nerve cell membranes causes the transmission of nerve impulses. Calcium stimulates muscles to contract. Sodium, potassium, and magnesium are involved in muscle relaxation. Mineral imbalances interfere with normal muscle functioning.
- **Vitamin, enzyme, and hormone activity.** Minerals help to regulate body processes through their role in activation of vitamins, enzymes, and hormones.

 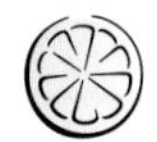

For instance, cobalt's sole function is as an essential component of vitamin B_{12}. Zinc is a constituent of many enzymes used in energy and nucleic acid metabolism, and manganese is part of an enzyme involved in fat synthesis. Iodine is needed for synthesis of the hormone thyroxine, and chromium is involved in insulin production.

Mineral Balance

The body has several mechanisms by which it maintains mineral balance, depending on the mineral involved such as

- **Releasing minerals from storage for redistribution.** Some minerals can be released from storage and redistributed as needed, which is what happens when calcium is released from bones to restore normal serum calcium levels.
- **Altering rate of absorption.** For example, normally only about 10% of the iron consumed is absorbed but the rate increases to 50% when the body is deficient in iron.
- **Altering rate of excretion.** Virtually all of the sodium consumed in the diet is absorbed; the only way the body can rid itself of excess sodium is to increase urinary sodium excretion. For most people, the higher the intake of sodium, the greater the amount of sodium excreted in the urine. Excess potassium is also excreted in the urine.

Mineral Toxicities

Minerals that are easily excreted, such as sodium and potassium, do not accumulate to toxic levels in the body under normal circumstances. Stored minerals can produce toxicity symptoms when intake is excessive, but excessive intake is not likely to occur from eating a balanced diet. Instead, mineral toxicity is related to excessive use of mineral supplements, environmental or industrial exposure, human errors in commercial food processing, or alterations in metabolism. For instance, more than a dozen Americans developed selenium toxicity after taking an improperly manufactured dietary supplement than contained 27.3 mg of selenium per tablet (500 times the Recommended Dietary Allowance [RDA] of 55 micrograms/day).

Mineral Interactions

Mineral balance is significantly influenced by hundreds of interactions that occur among minerals and between minerals and other dietary components. For instance, caffeine promotes calcium excretion, whereas vitamin D and lactose promote its absorption. Therefore, mineral status must be viewed as a function of the total diet, not only from the standpoint of the quantity consumed.

Sources of Minerals

Generally, unrefined or unprocessed foods have more minerals than refined foods. Trace mineral content varies with the content of soil from which the food originates. Within all food groups, processed foods are high in sodium and chloride. Drinking water contains varying amounts of calcium, magnesium, and other minerals; sodium is added to soften water. Fluoride may be a natural or added component of drinking water.

▶ MAJOR ELECTROLYTES

Sodium, chloride, and potassium are major minerals that are also major electrolytes in the body. Salient features for each electrolyte are presented in the following paragraphs. Table 6.3 details their sources, functions, recommended intakes, and signs and symptoms of deficiency and toxicity.

Sodium

By weight, sodium accounts for 39% of salt (sodium chloride); therefore, 1 teaspoon of salt (5g) provides approximately 2000 mg of sodium. Approximately 75% of the sodium consumed in the typical American diet comes from salt or sodium preservatives added to foods by food manufacturers. Only 10% of total sodium intake is from sodium that occurs naturally in foods such as sodium from milk and certain vegetables. Salt added during cooking or at the table accounts for the remaining sodium intake. Wide variations in sodium intake exist between cultures and between individuals within a culture related to the amount of processed foods consumed (Fig. 6.1).

As the major extracellular cation, sodium is largely responsible for regulating fluid balance. It also regulates cell permeability and the movement of fluid, electrolytes, glucose, insulin, and amino acids. Sodium is pivotal in acid–base balance, nerve transmission, and muscular irritability.

Although sodium plays vital roles, under normal conditions the amount of sodium actually needed is very small, maybe even less than less than 200 mg/day. However, American men consume approximately 3300 mg sodium/day, American women slightly less. In northern Japan, daily sodium intake is more than 10.3 g/day. Although almost 98% of all sodium consumed is absorbed, humans are able to maintain homeostasis over a wide range of intakes, largely through urinary excretion.

If sweating is not excessive, the amount of sodium in the urine closely mirrors the amount of sodium eaten. For instance, a salty meal causes a transitory increase in serum sodium, which triggers thirst. Drinking fluids dilutes the sodium in the blood to normal concentration, even though the volume of both sodium and fluid are increased. The increased volume stimulates the kidneys to excrete more sodium and fluid

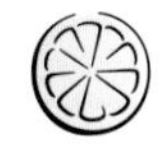

TABLE 6.3

SUMMARY OF MAJOR ELECTROLYTES

Electrolyte and Sources	Functions	Deficiency/Toxicity Signs and Symptoms
Sodium (Na) Adult AI: 19–50 yr: 1.5 g 50–70 yr: 1.3 g 71+ yr: 1.2 g Adult UL: 2.3 g • 1 tsp salt = 2400 mg Na • 75% of Na intake is from processed foods: canned soups, meats, vegetables; convenience and restaurant foods; pizza; processed meats	Fluid and electrolyte balance, acid–base balance, maintains muscle irritability, regulates cell membrane permeability and nerve impulse transmission	*Deficiency* Rare except with chronic diarrhea or vomiting and renal disorders; nausea, dizziness, muscle cramps, apathy *Toxicity* Hypertension, edema
Potassium (K) Adult AI: 4.7 g No UL • Fruits and vegetables, dried peas and beans, whole grains, milk, meats	Fluid and electrolyte balance, acid–base balance, nerve impulse transmission, catalyst for many metabolic reactions, involved in skeletal and cardiac muscle activity	*Deficiency* Muscular weakness, paralysis, anorexia, confusion (occurs with dehydration) *Toxicity (from supplements/drugs)* Muscular weakness, vomiting
Chloride (Cl) Adult AI: 19–50 yr: 2.3 g 50–70 yr: 2.0 g 71+ yr: 1.8 g Adult UL: 3.6 g • 1 tsp salt ≈ 3600 mg Cl • Same sources as sodium	Fluid and electrolyte balance, acid–base balance, component of hydrochloric acid in stomach	*Deficiency* Rare; may occur secondary to chronic diarrhea or vomiting and certain renal disorders: muscle cramps, anorexia, apathy *Toxicity* Normally harmless; can cause vomiting

together to restore normal blood volume. Conversely, low blood volume or low extracellular sodium stimulates the hormone aldosterone to increase sodium reabsorption by the kidneys. In people who have minimal sweat losses, sodium intake and sodium excretion are approximately equal.

Because there are insufficient data from dose–response trials, an Estimated Average Requirement (EAR) has not been established; therefore, there is no RDA for sodium. Instead, an Adequate Intake is set at 1.5 g/day for young adults to ensure that the total diet provides adequate amounts of other essential nutrients and to compensate for

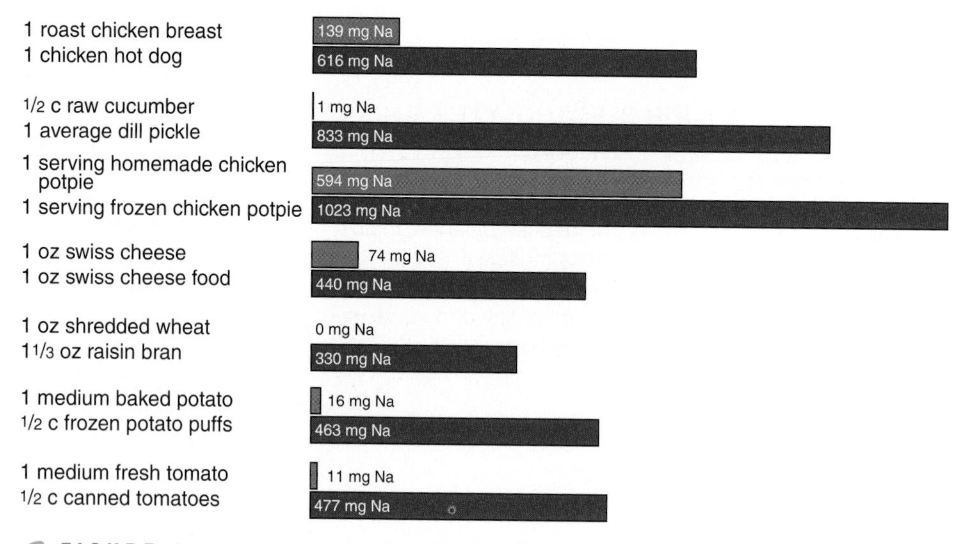

FIGURE 6.1 Effect of food processing on the sodium content of selected foods.

sodium lost in sweat in unacclimatized people exposed to high temperatures or who become physically active. For men and women ages 50 to 70 years old, the AI is 1.3 g and after age 70 AI decreases to 1.2 g. There are no benefits to consuming amounts greater than the AI, yet the typical American consumes approximately twice the recommended amount of sodium.

The major problem with a high sodium intake is elevated blood pressure, a risk factor for coronary heart disease and renal diseases. Generally, blood pressure increases as sodium intake increases. The dose-dependent rise in blood pressure is progressive and continuous and appears to occur throughout the continuum of sodium intake without an obvious threshold. However, certain groups are more "salt sensitive" and so have greater responses to changes in sodium intake, namely people with hypertension, diabetes, older people, and African Americans. Evidence suggests that salt sensitivity is blunted when potassium intake is high or a when a low-fat, high-mineral diet is followed. In normotensive people, lowering sodium intake can decrease the risk of developing hypertension. An UL for adults is set at 2.3 g/day, an amount less than the average American adult consumes.

Because the Daily Value (DV) for sodium used on food labels predates the latest AI and UL set for sodium, their values are inconsistent. The daily reference value for sodium used on the Nutrition Facts label is 2400 mg. Thus, although one would assume a food that supplies 50% of the DV for sodium in a serving has perhaps 650 mg of sodium (e.g., 50% of 1.3 g), it actually provides 1200 mg of sodium (50% of 2400 mg), which is almost the AI for the entire day. Until the Daily Value figure is updated, %DV is best used to compare the sodium content of similar products, not to estimate intake with the goal of consuming the AI. Descriptive terms on food labels do have legally defined meanings and can assist in food selection (Box 6.1).

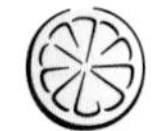

BOX 6.1 **DESCRIPTORS OF SODIUM CONTENT**

If the label says . . .	One serving contains . . .
Sodium free	<5 mg
Very low sodium	<35 mg
Low sodium	<140 mg
Reduced or less sodium	At least 25% less sodium compared with a standard serving size of the traditional food
Light in sodium	50% less sodium than the traditional food (restricted to >40 cal/serving or >3 g fat/serving)
Salt free	<5 mg
Unsalted or no added salt	No salt added during processing (this does not necessarily mean the food is sodium free)

Potassium

Most of the body's potassium is located in the cells as the major cation of the intracellular fluid. The remainder is in the extracellular fluid, where it works to maintain fluid balance, maintain acid–base balance, transmit nerve impulses, catalyze metabolic reactions, aid in carbohydrate metabolism and protein synthesis, and control skeletal muscle contractility.

An AI for potassium is set at 4.7 g/day for all adults. This level is believed to maintain lower blood pressure levels, lessen the adverse effects of high sodium intake on blood pressure, reduce the risk of kidney stones, and possibly reduce bone loss. However, the median intake of potassium in the United States is approximately 2.9 to 3.2 g/day in men and 2.1 to 2.3 g/day in women. Because African Americans have a relatively low potassium intake and a high prevalence of salt sensitivity and hypertension, a higher potassium intake may be even more beneficial for this population group.

In healthy people with normal kidney function, a high intake of potassium does not lead to an elevated serum potassium concentration because the hormone aldosterone promotes urinary potassium excretion to keep serum levels within normal range. Therefore, an UL has not been set. However, when potassium excretion is impaired, such as secondary to diabetes, chronic renal insufficiency, end stage renal disease, severe heart failure, and adrenal insufficiency, high potassium intakes can lead to hyperkalemia and life-threatening cardiac arrhythmias.

Moderate potassium deficiency, typically occurring without hypokalemia, is characterized by increased blood pressure, increased salt sensitivity, an increased risk of kidney stones, and increased bone turnover. An inadequate potassium intake may also increase the risk of cardiovascular disease, particularly stroke. Generally, sodium and potassium content are inversely related: processed foods are low in potassium and high in sodium; fresh, wholesome foods are high in potassium and lower in sodium.

Chloride

Chloride is the major anion in the extracellular fluid, where it helps to maintain fluid and electrolyte balance in conjunction with sodium. Chloride is an essential component of hydrochloric acid in the stomach and, therefore, plays a role in digestion and acid–base balance. Its concentration in most cells is low.

Because almost all of the chloride in the diet comes from salt (sodium chloride), the AI for chloride is set at a level equivalent (on a molar basis) to that of sodium. The AI for younger adults is 2.3 g/day, the equivalent to 3.8 g/day of salt or 1500 mg sodium. Sodium and chloride share dietary sources, conditions that cause them to become depleted in the body, and signs and symptoms of deficiency.

MAJOR MINERALS

The remaining major minerals are calcium, phosphorus, magnesium, and sulfur. They are summarized in Table 6.4; additional salient information appears below.

Calcium

Calcium is the most plentiful mineral in the body, making up about half of the body's total mineral content. Almost all of the body's calcium (99%) is found in bones and teeth, where it combines with phosphorus, magnesium, and other minerals to provide rigidity and structure. Bones serve as a large, dynamic reservoir of calcium that readily releases calcium when serum levels drop; this helps to maintain blood calcium levels within normal limits when calcium intake is inadequate.

The remaining 1% of calcium in the body is found in plasma and other body fluids, where it has important roles in blood clotting, nerve transmission, muscle contraction and relaxation, cell membrane permeability, and the activation of certain enzymes. Studies suggest that calcium plays a role in the prevention and treatment of hypertension and has a possible protective effect on the development of colon cancer. In addition, preliminary studies show that adequate calcium may play a role in maintaining healthy body weight or facilitating weight loss by promoting the breakdown of fat or by inhibiting fat cells from making fat.

Calcium balance—or, more accurately, calcium balance in the blood—is achieved through the action of vitamin D and hormones. When blood calcium levels fall, the parathyroid gland secretes parathormone (PTH), which promotes calcium reabsorption in the kidneys and stimulates the release of calcium from bones. Vitamin D has the same effects on the kidneys and bones and additionally increases the absorption of calcium from the gastrointestinal tract. Together, the actions of PTH and vitamin D restore low blood calcium levels to normal, even though bone calcium content may fall. A chronically low calcium intake compromises bone integrity without affecting blood calcium levels. When blood calcium levels are too high, the thyroid gland secretes calcitonin, which promotes

 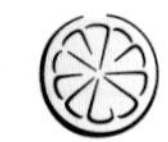

TABLE 6.4

SUMMARY OF MAJOR MINERALS

Mineral and Sources	Functions	Deficiency/Toxicity Signs and Symptoms
Calcium (Ca) *Adult AI* 19–50 yr: 1000 mg 51+ yr: 1200 mg Adult UL: 2.5 g/d • Milk and milk products, fortified orange juice, green leafy vegetables, small fish with bones, dried peas and beans	Bone and teeth formation and maintenance, blood clotting, nerve transmission, muscle contraction and relaxation, cell membrane permeability, blood pressure	*Deficiency* Children: impaired growth Adults: osteoporosis *Toxicity* Constipation, increased risk of renal stone formation, impaired absorption of iron and other minerals
Phosphorus (P) *Adult RDA* Men and women: 700 mg Adult UL: To age 70: 4 g/d 70+ yr: 3 g/d • All animal products (meat, poultry, eggs, milk), bread, ready-to-eat cereal	Bone and teeth formation and maintenance, acid–base balance, energy metabolism, cell membrane structure, regulation of hormone and coenzyme activity	*Deficiency* Unknown *Toxicity* Low blood calcium
Magnesium (Mg) *Adult RDA* Men: 19–30 yr: 400 mg 31+ yr: 420 mg Women: 19–30 yr: 310 mg 31+ yr: 320 mg Adult UL: 350 mg/d from supplements only (does not include intake from food and water) • Green leafy vegetables, nuts, dried peas and beans, whole grains, seafood, chocolate, cocoa	Bone formation, nerve transmission, smooth muscle relaxation, protein synthesis, CHO metabolism, enzyme activity	*Deficiency* Weakness, confusion; growth failure in children Severe deficiency: convulsions, hallucinations, tetany *Toxicity* No toxicity demonstrated from food Supplemental Mg can cause diarrhea, nausea, and cramping Excessive Mg from magnesium in Epsom salts causes diarrhea
Sulfur (S) No recommended intake or UL • All protein foods (meat, poultry, fish, eggs, milk, dried peas and beans, nuts)	Component of disulfide bridges in proteins; component of biotin, thiamin, and insulin	*Deficiency* Unknown *Toxicity* In animals, excessive intake of sulfur-containing amino acids impairs growth

the formation of new bone by taking excess calcium from the blood. A high calcium intake does not lead to hypercalcemia but rather maximizes bone density. Abnormal blood concentrations of calcium occur from alterations in the secretion of PTH.

Many factors influence calcium absorption, which averages about 30% of the total calcium consumed. The percentage of calcium absorbed increases in response to body need such as during pregnancy, lactation, growth, and recovery from bone fractures. Lactose, the carbohydrate in milk, and vitamin D promote calcium absorption. Calcium absorption is impaired by vitamin D deficiency, phytates, and oxalates. Fat malabsorption syndromes cause calcium to precipitate into insoluble calcium soaps, which are excreted in the feces.

An adequate calcium intake early in life helps to maximize bone density and strength and, therefore, offers protection against the inevitable net bone loss that occurs in all people after the age of about 35 years. Daily Adequate Intake (AI) recommendations are set at 1300 mg for adolescents up to 18 years of age, 1000 mg between the ages of 19 and 50 years, and 1200 mg thereafter. Three daily servings of milk, yogurt, or cheese as well as nondairy sources of calcium are needed to ensure an adequate calcium intake. Women older than 12 years of age in almost all racial and ethnic groups consistently fail to consume adequate calcium.

Career Connection

The National Academy of Science recommends American adults consume 1000 to 1200 mg of calcium daily. Food is the best source with milk and other dairy products considered "nearly perfect" sources because they contain vitamin D and lactose that promote calcium absorption. Low oxalate green vegetables, namely bok choy, broccoli, Chinese/Napa cabbage, collards, kale, okra, and turnip greens have significant calcium with high bioavailability, unlike the calcium in spinach, beet greens, and Swiss chard that is poorly absorbed due to the presence of oxalates. Significant amounts of calcium can be found in calcium fortified foods such as fruit juices, tomato juice, and ready-to-eat breakfast cereals.

Although various foods contribute calcium, it is not likely that the recommendation for calcium will be consistently met without an ample intake of milk. However, many adults shy away from milk due to lactose intolerance or because they perceive milk as an infant food. Still others, particularly women, avoid milk in an attempt to control calorie intake even though skim milk provides approximately 300 mg of calcium in a mere 80 calories. Yogurt is an excellent source of calcium, as are hard natural cheeses, but again, their calorie content is often seen as prohibitive. Hence many adults resort to calcium supplements to meet their daily need.

Calcium supplements are not created equally. The percent of elemental calcium found in a supplement varies with the type of compound used such as

- Calcium carbonate 40%
- Calcium phosphate (tribasic) 38%
- Calcium citrate 21%
- Calcium lactate 13%
- Calcium gluconate 9%

 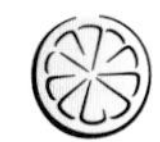

Career Connection (Continued)

The amount of elemental calcium available in a supplement can be calculated when the type of compound and the number of milligrams/tablet are known. For instance, a 500-mg tablet of calcium carbonate provides 200 mg of elemental calcium (500 mg × 40% = 200 mg elemental calcium). Thus 5 tablets/day are required to provide a total day's intake of calcium. Compare that to a 500-mg tablet of calcium gluconate, which provides only 45 mg of elemental calcium. (500 mg × 9% = 45 mg). More than 22 tablets of calcium gluconate are needed to meet the AI for calcium. It is clear why calcium gluconate and calcium lactate are generally not recommended as calcium supplements.

Other considerations for calcium supplements are as follows:

- TUMS is made of calcium carbonate; it is 40% elemental calcium and is generally the least expensive calcium supplement.
- Calcium carbonate supplements can cause constipation. Encourage an adequate fluid intake and a high-fiber diet as needed.
- Avoid calcium supplements made from bonemeal, oyster shell, or dolomite because some may contain heavy metals, particularly lead.
- Calcium citrate contains acids that promote calcium absorption, which is particularly beneficial in elderly people who normally produce less stomach acid than younger adults.
- Calcium citrate is less likely to cause constipation than calcium carbonate.
- Calcium from supplements is absorbed best in doses of 500 mg or less. Tablets should be spread out over the day.
- Calcium carbonate is better absorbed with food, especially with acidic foods such as citrus juice or fruit. Calcium citrate is better absorbed on an empty stomach.
- "Supplement" means to add to, not to replace. Encourage the intake of calcium rich foods.

Phosphorus

After calcium, the most abundant mineral in the body is phosphorus. Approximately 85% of the body's phosphorus is combined with calcium in bones and teeth. The rest is distributed in every body cell, where it performs various functions such as regulating acid–base balance (phosphoric acid and its salts), metabolizing energy (adenosine triphosphate), and providing structure to cell membranes (phospholipids). Phosphorus is an important component of RNA and DNA and is responsible for activating many enzymes and the B vitamins.

Normally about 55% of phosphorus in the adult diet is absorbed. As with calcium, phosphorus absorption is enhanced by vitamin D and regulated by PTH. The major route of phosphorus excretion is in the urine.

Because phosphorus is pervasive in the food supply, dietary deficiencies of phosphorus do not occur. Animal proteins, soft drinks, and food additives are major sources of phosphorus.

Magnesium

More than half of the body's magnesium content is deposited in bone with calcium and phosphorus; the rest is distributed in various soft tissues, muscles, and body fluids. Magnesium is a cofactor for more than 300 enzymes in the body, including those involved in energy metabolism, protein synthesis, and cell membrane transport.

Mean magnesium intake among American adults is approximately 80% of the Daily Value. A low magnesium intake is related to the increased use of refined grains over whole grain breads and cereals. Magnesium is a mineral lost in the refining process that is not added back through routine enrichment. However, food consumption data does not include the magnesium content of water, which is significant in water classified as "hard." Despite chronically low intakes, deficiency symptoms appear only in conjunction with certain diseases such as alcohol abuse, protein malnutrition, renal impairments, endocrine disorders, and prolonged vomiting or diarrhea.

Net magnesium absorption in a typical diet is approximately 50%. Phytates, oxalates, and fat inhibit magnesium absorption.

Magnesium supplements that have 350 mg or more are not recommended because although magnesium from food is beneficial, that much supplemental magnesium can cause diarrhea, nausea, and cramping.

Sulfur

Sulfur does not function independently as a nutrient but it is a component of biotin, thiamin, and the amino acids methionine and cysteine. The proteins in skin, hair, and nails are made more rigid by the presence of sulfur.

There is neither an RDA nor an AI for sulfur, and no deficiency symptoms are known. Although food and various sources of drinking water provide significant amounts of sulfur, the major source of inorganic sulfate for humans is body protein turnover of methionine and cysteine. The need for sulfur is met when the intake of sulfur amino acids is adequate. A sulfur deficiency is likely only when protein deficiency is severe.

TRACE MINERALS

Although their presence in the body is small, their impact on health is significant. Each trace mineral has its own range over which the body can maintain homeostasis (Fig. 6.2). People who consume an adequate diet derive no further benefit from supplementing their intake with minerals and may induce a deficiency by upsetting the delicate balance that exists between minerals. Even though too little of a trace mineral can be just as deadly as too much, routine supplementation is not recommended. Factors that complicate the study of trace minerals include

- The high variability of trace mineral content of foods. The mineral content of the soil from which a food originates largely influences trace mineral content. For instance, grains, vegetables, and meat raised in South Dakota, Wyoming, New

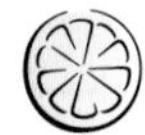

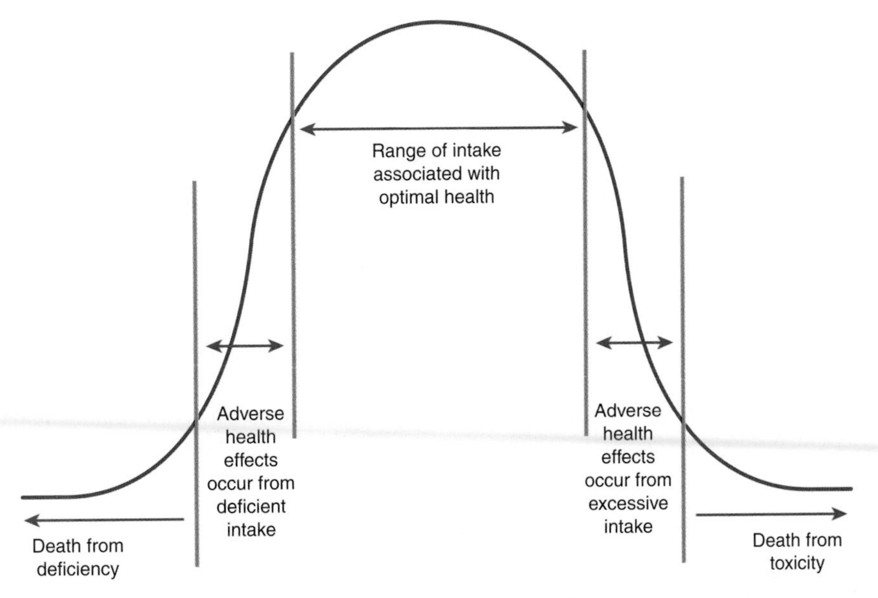

FIGURE 6.2 Health effects seen over a range of trace mineral intakes.

Mexico, and Utah are high in selenium, whereas foods grown in the southern states and from both coasts of the United States have much less selenium. Other factors that influence a food's trace mineral content are the quality of the water supply and food processing. Because of these factors, the trace mineral content listed in food composition tables may not represent the actual amount in a given sample.

- Food composition data are not available for all trace minerals. Food composition tables generally include data on the content of iron, zinc, manganese, selenium, and copper, but data on other trace minerals, such as iodine, chromium, and molybdenum, is not be readily available.
- Bioavailability varies within the context of the total diet. Even when trace element intake can be estimated, the amount available to the body may be significantly less because the absorption and metabolism of individual trace elements is strongly influenced by mineral interactions and other dietary factors. An excess of one trace mineral may induce a deficiency of another. For instance, a high intake of zinc impairs copper absorption. Conversely, a deficiency of one trace mineral may potentiate toxic effects of another, as when iron deficiency increases vulnerability to lead poisoning.
- Reliable and valid indicators of trace element status (e.g., measured serum levels, results of balance studies, enzyme activity determinations) are not available for all trace minerals, so assessment of trace element status is not always possible.

Table 6.5 summaries the sources, functions, recommended intakes, and signs and symptoms of deficiency and toxicity of trace minerals that have either a RDA or AI. Additional salient features are presented below.

TABLE 6.5

SUMMARY OF TRACE MINERALS

Mineral and Sources	Functions	Deficiency/Toxicity Signs and Symptoms
Iron (Fe) *Adult RDA* Men: 8 mg Women (19–50 yr): 18 mg (51+ yr): 8 mg Adult UL: 45 mg • Beef liver, red meats, fish, poultry, clams, tofu, dried peas & beans, fortified cereals, bread, dried fruit	Oxygen transport via hemoglobin and myoglobin; constituent of enzyme systems	*Deficiency* Impaired immune function, decreased work capacity, apathy, lethargy, fatigue, itchy skin, pale nailbeds and eye membranes, impaired wound healing, intolerance to cold temperatures *Toxicity* Increased risk of infections, apathy, fatigue, lethargy, joint disease, hair loss, organ damage, enlarged liver, amenorrhea, impotence Accidental poisoning in children causes death
Zinc (Zn) *Adult RDA* Men: 11 mg Women: 8 mg Adult UL: 40 mg • Oysters, red meat, poultry, dried peas and beans, certain seafood, nuts, whole grains, fortified breakfast cereals, dairy products	Tissue growth and wound healing, sexual maturation and reproduction; constituent of many enzymes in energy and nucleic acid metabolism; immune function; vitamin A transport, taste perception	*Deficiency* Growth retardation, hair loss, diarrhea, delayed sexual maturation and impotence, eye and skin lesions, anorexia, delayed wound healing, taste abnormality, mental lethargy *Toxicity* Anemia, elevated LDL, lowered HDL, diarrhea, vomiting, impaired calcium absorption, fever, renal failure, muscle pain, dizziness, reproductive failure
Iodine *Adult RDA* 150 µg Adult UL: 1100 µg • Iodized salt, seafood, bread, dairy products	Component of thyroid hormones that regulate growth, development, and metabolic rate	*Deficiency* Goiter, weight gain, lethargy During pregnancy may cause severe and irreversible mental and physical retardation (cretinism) *Toxicity* Enlarged thyroid gland, decreased thyroid activity
Selenium (Se) *Adult RDA* Men and women: 55 µg Adult UL: 400 µg/d • Seafood, liver, kidney, other meats. • Grains grown in selenium-rich soil, Brazil nuts, walnuts	Component of antioxidant enzymes, immune system functioning, thyroid gland activity	*Deficiency* Enlarged heart, poor heart function, impaired thyroid activity *Toxicity* Rare; nausea, vomiting, abdominal pain, diarrhea, hair and nail changes, nerve damage, fatigue

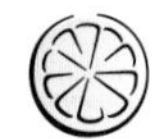

TABLE 6.5
(continued)

SUMMARY OF TRACE MINERALS

Mineral and Sources	Functions	Deficiency/Toxicity Signs and Symptoms
Copper (Cu) *Adult RDA:* 900 μg Adult UL: 10,000 μg • Organ meats, seafood, nuts, seeds, whole grains, drinking water	Used in the production of hemoglobin; component of several enzymes; used in energy metabolism	*Deficiency* Rare; anemia, bone abnormalities *Toxicity* Vomiting, diarrhea, liver damage
Manganese (Mn) *Adult AI* Men: 2.3 mg Women: 1.8 mg Adult UL: 11 mg • Widely distributed in foods. Best sources are whole grains, tea, pineapple, kale, strawberries	Component of enzymes involved in the metabolism of carbohydrates, protein, and fat, and in bone formation	*Deficiency* Rare *Toxicity* Rare; nervous system disorders
Fluoride (Fl) *Adult AI* Men: 4 mg Women: 3 mg Adult UL: 10 mg • Fluoridated water, water that naturally contains fluoride, tea, seafood	Formation and maintenance of tooth enamel, promotes resistance to dental decay, role in bone formation and integrity	*Deficiency* Susceptibility to dental decay, may increase risk of osteoporosis *Toxicity* Fluorosis (mottling of teeth), nausea, vomiting, diarrhea, chest pain, itching
Chromium (Cr) *Adult AI* Men: 19–50: 35 μg Women 51+: 30 μg Women 19–50: 25 μg Men 51+: 30 μg Adult UL: Undetermined • Meat, whole grains, nuts, cheese	Cofactor for insulin	*Deficiency* Insulin resistance, impaired glucose tolerance *Toxicity* Dietary toxicity unknown Occupational exposure to chromium dust damages skin and kidneys
Molybdenum (Mo) *Adult RDA:* 45 μg Adult UL: 2000 μg • Milk, legumes, bread, grains	Component of many enzymes; works with riboflavin to incorporate iron into hemoglobin	*Deficiency* Unknown *Toxicity* Occupational exposure to molybdenum dust causes gout-like symptoms

Iron

Approximately two-thirds of the body's 3 to 5 g of iron is contained in the heme portion of hemoglobin. Iron is also found in transferrin, the transport carrier of iron, and in enzyme systems that are active in energy metabolism. Ferritin, the storage form of iron, is located in the liver, bone marrow, and spleen.

Iron in foods exists in two forms: heme iron found in meat, fish, and poultry, and nonheme iron found in plants such as grains, vegetables, legumes, and nuts. The majority of iron in the diet is nonheme iron.

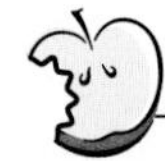

Quick Bite

Factors influencing nonheme iron absorption

Absorption enhancers (when consumed at the same meal)

- Vitamin C
- Meat, fish, and poultry

Absorption inhibitors

- Polyphenols found in coffee and tea (in the form of tannic acid), many grain products, and red wine
- Vegetable proteins found in soybeans, other dried peas and beans, and nuts
- Calcium
- Phytates found in dried peas and beans, rice, and grains
- Oxalic acid found in spinach, chard, berries, chocolate

Normally the overall rate of iron absorption, which includes both heme and nonheme iron, is only 10 to 15% of total intake. During times of need such as during growth, pregnancy, or iron deficiency, iron is absorbed more efficiently to boost the overall absorption rate to as high as 50%.

The bioavailability of heme and nonheme iron differs greatly. The rate of heme iron absorption is normally about 15% and is influenced only by need, not by dietary factors. In contrast, nonheme iron absorption is enhanced or inhibited by numerous dietary factors. Only 1% to 7% of nonheme iron is absorbed from plant foods when they are consumed as a single food. That rate increases when nonheme iron is consumed with an absorption enhancer. For instance, consuming 50 mg of vitamin C with a meal, which is the amount of vitamin C found in one small orange, can increase nonheme iron absorption three to six times above normal. Conversely, tea, an absorption inhibitor, can reduce iron absorption in a meal by 60%.

Based on average absorption rates and to compensate for daily (and monthly) iron losses, the RDA for iron is set at 8 mg for men and postmenopausal women and 18 mg for premenopausal women. Iron requirements increase during growth and in response to heavy or chronic blood loss related to menstruation, surgery, injury, gastrointestinal bleeding, or aspirin abuse. Iron recommendations for vegetarians are 1.8 times higher than nonvegetarians due to the lower bioavailability of iron from a vegetarian

 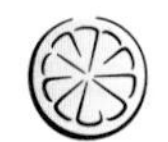

diet. Most adult men and postmenopausal women consume adequate amounts of iron. Women of childbearing age, pregnant women, and breastfeeding women generally do not consume the recommended amounts of iron.

Microcytic: small blood cells.

Hypochromic: pale red blood cells related to the decrease in hemoglobin pigment.

Pica: ingestion of nonfood substances such as dirt, clay, or laundry starch.

Iron deficiency anemia, a microcytic, hypochromic anemia, occurs when total iron stores become depleted, leading to a decrease in hemoglobin. The World Health Organization considers iron deficiency the most common nutritional disorder in the world, affecting more than 30% of the world's population. In the United States, about 10% of the population is iron deficient. Because the typical American diet provides only 6 to 7 mg of iron per 1000 calories, many menstruating women simply do not eat enough calories to satisfy their iron requirement. Other groups most likely to be deficient from an inadequate iron intake are older infants and toddlers, adolescent girls, and pregnant women. Some people with iron deficiency anemia practice pica which impairs iron absorption. Because symptoms of iron deficiency are similar to iron overload, namely apathy, lethargy, and fatigue, iron supplements should not be taken on the basis of symptoms alone.

Because very little iron is excreted from the body, the potential for toxicity is moderate to high. Although repeated blood transfusions, rare metabolic disorders, and megadoses of supplemental iron can cause iron overload, the most common cause is a genetic disorder known as hemochromatosis. In fact, hereditary hemochromatosis is the most common genetic disorder in the United States. The absorption of excessive amounts of iron leads to iron accumulation in body tissues, especially the liver, heart, brain, joints, and pancreas. Left untreated, excess iron can cause heart disease, cancer, cirrhosis, diabetes, and arthritis. Phlebotomies are used to reduce body iron. Given the prevalence of iron enrichment and iron fortification in the U.S. food supply, a low-iron diet is not recommended nor could it be realistically achieved.

Acute iron toxicity, caused by the overdose of medicinal iron, is the leading cause of accidental poisoning in small children. As few as 5 to 6 high-potency tablets can provide enough iron to kill a child weighing 22 pounds. In adults, high intakes of iron supplements can cause constipation, nausea, vomiting, and diarrhea, especially when the supplements are taken on an empty stomach.

Zinc

The small amount of zinc contained in the body (about 2 g) is found in almost all cells and is especially concentrated in the eyes, bones, muscles, and prostate gland. Zinc in tissues is not available to maintain serum levels when intake is inadequate, so a regular and sufficient intake is necessary.

Zinc is a component of DNA and RNA and is part of more than 100 enzymes involved in growth, metabolism, sexual maturation and reproduction, and the senses of taste and smell. Zinc plays important roles in immune system functioning and in wound healing. Most Americans consume adequate amounts of zinc.

There is no single laboratory test that adequately measures zinc status, so zinc deficiency is not readily diagnosed. Risk factors for zinc deficiency include poor calorie intake, alcoholism, and malabsorption syndromes such as celiac disease, Crohn's disease, and short bowel syndrome. Vegetarians are also at increased risk because zinc is only half as well absorbed from plants as it is from animal sources. Although overt zinc deficiency is not common in the United States, the effects of marginal intakes are poorly understood.

The effectiveness of zinc lozenges in reducing the severity or duration of the common cold is controversial. Although some studies indicate that zinc lozenges decrease the duration of common colds, others have found cold symptoms are no better with zinc lozenges than with a placebo. Research suggests that the effectiveness of zinc may be dependent upon how well zinc ions are delivered to the oral mucosa. Until more studies are done, it is not unreasonable or unsafe to use zinc lozenges to treat a cold. However, long-term use to prevent colds is not recommended because regular consumption of too much zinc can impair the immune system and lower the concentration of high-density lipoprotein ("good") cholesterol.

Supplemental zinc given to people who are deficient in zinc leads to an increase in the numbers of T-cell lymphocytes and enhances their ability to fight infection. Although zinc supplements are often given to promote healing of skin ulcers, they do not increase rates of wound healing when zinc levels are normal.

Iodine

Iodine is found in muscles, the thyroid gland, skin, the skeleton, endocrine tissues, and the bloodstream. It is an essential component of thyroxine (T_4) and triiodothyronine (T_3), the thyroid hormones responsible for regulating metabolic rate, body temperature, reproduction, growth, the synthesis of blood cells, and nerve and muscle function.

In the United States, approximately 50% of the population uses iodized salt, making it the biggest source of iodine in the American diet. The RDA for iodine is easily met with ½ teaspoon of iodized salt daily. Seafood is naturally high in iodine derived from ocean water. Food processing techniques incidentally add iodine to the food supply. For instance, milk is naturally low in iodine, but it has become a significant source of iodine because of the iodized salt licks given to cows and the use of iodine chemicals to sanitize and disinfect udders, milking machines, and milk tanks. Processed foods may also contain higher amounts of iodine due to the addition of iodized salt or additives containing iodine.

Goitrogens: thyroid antagonists found in cruciferous vegetables (e.g., cabbage, cauliflower, broccoli), soybeans, and sweet potatoes.

The RDA for iodine includes a built-in measure of safety for the unquantified effect of goitrogens on iodine requirements. The average American adult consumes more than the RDA for iodine, and it is recommended that no new sources of iodine be added to the U.S. food supply.

Selenium

Selenium is a component of a group of enzymes, called glutathione peroxidases, that function as antioxidants to disarm free radicals produced during normal oxygen metabolism. As such, its roles as an antioxidant in the prevention of heart disease and cancer are being investigated. Selenium is also essential for normal immune system functioning and thyroid gland activity.

 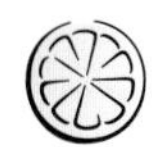

Although areas of the country with selenium-poor soil produce selenium-poor foods, mass transportation mitigates the effect on total selenium intake. Also because selenium is associated with protein, some meats and seafood provide selenium. In the United States, bread also supplies selenium. The average American adult consumes adequate amounts of selenium.

Selenium deficiency is rare in the United States. People who rely on total parenteral nutrition as their sole source of nutrition have developed selenium deficiency when not given supplemental selenium. Severe malabsorption syndromes can also lead to selenium deficiency. Selenium deficiency is associated with HIV/AIDS and is correlated to a high risk of death from this disease. Researchers speculate that selenium is important in HIV because of its role in immune system functioning and as an antioxidant. In addition, selenium may be used by the HIV virus to replicate, thus creating a deficiency in the host. Clinical trials are needed to evaluate the impact of selenium supplementation on HIV progression.

Copper

Copper is distributed in muscles, liver, brain, bones, kidneys, and blood. Copper is a component of several enzymes involved in hemoglobin synthesis, collagen formation, wound healing, and maintenance of nerve fibers. Copper also helps cells to use iron and plays a role in energy metabolism.

Americans typically consume adequate amounts of copper. Excess zinc intake has the potential to induce copper deficiency by impairing its absorption, but copper deficiency is rare. Supplements, not food, may cause copper toxicity, as do some genetic disorders.

Manganese

Mean manganese intake among American adults is well above the AI, and dietary deficiencies have not been noted. Manganese toxicity is a well-known occupational hazard for miners who inhale manganese dust over a prolonged period of time, leading to central nervous system abnormalities with symptoms similar to those of Parkinson's disease. There is some evidence to suggest that high manganese intake from drinking water, which may be more bioavailable than manganese from food, also produces neuromotor deficits similar to Parkinson's disease. The UL for adults is set at 11 mg/day, approximately four times the usual intake.

Fluoride

Cariogenic: cavity-promoting.

Fluoride promotes the mineralization of developing tooth enamel prior to tooth eruption and the remineralization of surface enamel in erupted teeth. It concentrates in plaque and saliva to inhibit the process by which cariogenic bacteria metabolize carbohydrates to produce acids that cause tooth decay. Fluoridation of municipal water in the second half of the 20th century is credited with a major decline in the prevalence and severity of dental caries in the U.S. population.

Fluoridation of municipal water is considered to be the most cost-effective, equitable, and cost-saving method of delivering fluoride to the community. It is endorsed by the National Institute of Dental Health, the American Dietetic Association, the American Medical Association, the National Cancer Institute, and the Centers for Disease Control and Prevention (CDC). Yet fluoridation often meets with some degree of public opposition. According to the CDC, almost 66% of Americans had access to optimally fluoridated water in 2000. National health goals are to increase fluoridation to 75% of the U.S. population served by municipal water systems.

Children under the age of 8 are susceptible to mottled tooth enamel if they ingest several times more fluoride than the recommended amount during the time of tooth enamel formation. The swallowing of fluoridated toothpaste is to blame.

Chromium

Chromium enhances the action of the hormone insulin to help regulate blood glucose levels. A deficiency of chromium is characterized by high blood glucose and impaired insulin response.

Even though chromium is widespread in foods, many foods provide less than 1 to 2 micrograms per serving. Because existing databases lack information on chromium, few food intake studies utilizing few laboratories are available to estimate usual intake. However, it appears that average intake is adequate. Unrefined foods are higher in chromium than processed foods.

Molybdenum

Molybdenum plays a role in red blood cell synthesis and is a component of several enzymes. Average American intake falls within the recommended range. Dietary deficiencies and toxicities are unknown.

Other Trace Elements

Although definitive evidence is lacking, future research may reveal that other trace elements are essential for human nutrition. However, evidence is difficult to obtain and quantifying human need is even more formidable. In addition, as with all trace minerals, the potential for toxicity exists. Consider that

- Nickel, silicon, vanadium, and boron have been demonstrated to have beneficial health effects in some animals and may someday be classified as essential for humans.
- Cobalt is an essential component of vitamin B_{12} but it is not an essential nutrient and does not have an RDA.
- It is possible that minute amounts of cadmium, lithium, tin, and even arsenic are also essential to human life.

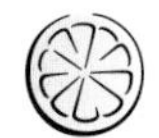

HEALTH PROMOTION: ARE WE DRINKING ENOUGH FLUID?

For healthy people, the universal, age-old advice has been to drink at least eight 8-ounce glasses of fluid daily ("8 × 8")—preferably in the form of water and discounting beverages containing alcohol or caffeine because of their diuretic effect. However, the validity of that recommendation has been questioned after a recent search failed to uncover scientific proof supporting this practice. Indeed, results of food surveys show that thousands of men and women habitually consume less than "8 × 8" without suffering any adverse effects, thanks to the precision and effectiveness of the body's osmoregulatory system that maintains fluid balance. The bottom line is that healthy adults leading a mostly sedentary lifestyle in a temperate climate—in other words, a large proportion of Americans—may not *need* "8 × 8" to maintain health. What *is* supported by scientific evidence is that eight glasses of fluid or more are recommended to treat or prevent some diseases (e.g., kidney stones, constipation) and for vigorous work and exercise, especially in hot climates.

In addition, several published studies show that caffeine is not the dehydrating culprit as is commonly believed. In fact, an analysis of the scientific literature dealing with moderate caffeine consumption (e.g., the equivalent of 1 to 4 cups of coffee/day) found:

- The body retains some fluid from caffeinated beverages.
- The mild diuresis seen with moderate caffeine consumption is similar to that of water. Strictly speaking, large amounts of water are a diuretic because they increase urine output.
- People who regularly consume caffeine develop a higher tolerance to its diuretic effect.
- There is no proof that consuming caffeinated beverages causes a fluid and electrolyte imbalance detrimental to health or interferes with the ability to perform physical activity.

The conclusion is that caffeinated beverages *can* count toward the day's total fluid intake, providing that caffeine consumption is not excessive.

For healthy adults, thirst is usually a reliable indicator of water need and fluid intake is assumed to be adequate when the color of urine produced is pale yellow. However, the sensation of thirst is blunted in the elderly, in children, and during hot weather or strenuous exercise. For these people and conditions, drinking fluids should not be delayed until the sensation of thirst occurs because by then fluid loss is significant. Because the body cannot store water, it should be consumed throughout the day.

How Do You Respond?

Is bottled water better than tap water? Both bottled water and tap water are safe. The advantages of bottled water are that it is usually chlorine free so the taste is more appealing to some people and it is lead-free, unlike tap water in some areas. Lead can accumulate in the body, damaging the brain, nervous system, kidneys, and red blood cells. Unborn babies, infants, and children are especially vulnerable to lead poisoning. However, tap water is treated with chlorine to reduce the risk of cholera, hepatitis, and other diseases and may be a source of minerals such as fluoride, calcium, iron, and magnesium. In the end, the decision to use bottled water instead of tap water is a personal choice usually based on taste. However, if nonfluoridated bottled water is used by children, a fluoride supplement is prudent to help strengthen and protect teeth from decay.

Does chlorine in drinking water cause cancer? When organic matter is present in water, chlorine reacts with it to form a byproduct called trihalomethane (THM). If THM forms, it is in such small quantities that it is not a cancer risk. The benefits of chlorine in preventing outbreaks of cholera, hepatitis, and other diseases far outweigh the negligible effects of THM.

What are chelated minerals? A chelated mineral is surrounded by an amino acid to protect it from other food components such as oxalates and phytates that can bind to the mineral and prevent it from being absorbed. Chelated minerals are probably not worth the added expense: chelated calcium is absorbed 5 to 10% better than ordinary calcium but costs about five times more.

▲ Focus on Critical Thinking

Respond to the following statements:

1. Supplemental vitamins are generally less likely to cause adverse effects than supplemental minerals.
2. Do you personally drink at least eight 8-ounce glasses of fluid daily?
3. Trace element toxicities are more dangerous than trace element deficiencies.

Key Concepts

- Because water is involved in almost every body function, is not stored, and is excreted daily, it is more vital to life than food.
- Under normal conditions, water intake equals water output to maintain water balance. In most healthy people, thirst is a reliable indicator of need.
- The body's need for water is influenced by many variables. A general guideline is to consume 1.0 mL of fluid per calorie consumed, with a minimum of 1500 mL/day.
- Minerals are inorganic substances that cannot be broken down and rearranged in the body.
- Mineral toxicities are not likely to occur from diet alone. They are most often related to excessive use of mineral supplements, environmental exposure, or alterations in metabolism.

 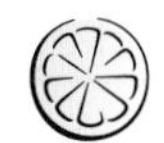

- Depending on the mineral involved, the body can maintain mineral balance by altering the rate of absorption, altering the rate of excretion, or releasing minerals from storage when needed.
- The absorption of many minerals is influenced by mineral-mineral interactions. Too much of one mineral may promote a deficiency of another mineral.
- Sodium, potassium, and chloride are electrolytes because they carry electrical charges when they are dissolved in solution.
- Macrominerals are needed in relatively large amounts and are found in the body in quantities greater than 5 g. Trace minerals are needed in very small amounts and are found in the body in amounts less than 5 g.
- As much as 75% of sodium consumed in the average American diet is from processed food. Americans are urged to reduce their intake of sodium because of its potential role in the development of hypertension.
- Many American adults consume less than optimal amounts of calcium, placing them at risk of osteoporosis and possibly hypertension. Milk and yogurt are the richest sources of calcium, and their vitamin D and lactose content promote its absorption.

ANSWER KEY

1. **FALSE** Although many healthy people do not consume the eight 8-ounce glasses of fluid recommended daily, the body is able to maintain homeostasis over a wide range of intakes.
2. **FALSE** Although the body rids itself of some excess minerals such as sodium and potassium through urinary excretion, homeostasis of other minerals is achieved by adjusting the rate of mineral absorption (e.g., iron, calcium).
3. **FALSE** Calcium is the most plentiful mineral in the body. For most Americans, sodium is the most abundant mineral in the diet.
4. **TRUE** An increase in sodium intake is associated with an increase in blood pressure. In addition, the dose-dependent rise in blood pressure is progressive, continuous, and appears to occur throughout the continuum of sodium intake without an obvious threshold.
5. **FALSE** Bottled water may taste better than tap water to some people but it usually lacks fluoride, the trace element that protects against dental decay.
6. **TRUE** Foods high in sodium tend to be low in potassium (e.g., processed foods like frozen entrees) and foods high in potassium tend to be low in sodium (e.g., fresh vegetables and whole grains).
7. **FALSE** The "major" and "trace" descriptions refer to the relative quantity of the mineral found in the body, not to their importance in maintaining health.
8. **TRUE** For most people, thirst is a reliable indicator of fluid needs. Exceptions are the elderly, children, and during hot weather or strenuous exercise.
9. **TRUE** Impaired sense of taste is a symptom of zinc deficiency.
10. **FALSE** A chronically low intake of calcium compromises the density and strength of bones but does not lead to hypocalcemia. Serum levels of calcium are maintained within normal range, regardless of calcium intake via the actions of hormones and vitamin D.

WEBSITES

Iron Overload Diseases Association at **www.ironoverload.org**
National Dairy Council at **www.nationaldairycouncil.org**
National Academy of Sciences, Institute of Medicine for Reference Dietary Intakes at **www.nap.edu**
Facts about dietary supplements (including mineral supplements) from the National Institutes of Health at **www.cc.nih.gov/ccc/supplements**

REFERENCES

American Dietetic Association. (2003). Position of the American Dietetic Association and Dietitians of Canada: Vegetarian diets. *Journal of the American Dietetic Association, 103,* 748–765.
Centers for Disease Control and Prevention. (2002). *Populations receiving optimally fluoridated public drinking water–United States, 2000.* Available at www.cdc.gov/mmwr/preview/mmwrhtml/mm5107a2.htm. Accessed on 2/25/04.
Chicago Dietetic Association, The South Suburban Dietetic Association, Dietitians of Canada. (2000). *Manual of clinical dietetics* (6th ed.). Chicago: The American Dietetic Association.
French, S., Lin, B., & Guthrie, J. (2003). National trends in soft drink consumption among children and adolescents age 6 to 17 years: Prevalence, amounts, and sources, 1977/1978 to 1994/1998. *Journal of the American Dietetic Association, 103,* 1326–1331.
International Food Information Council. (2002). *Caffeine and dehydration: Myth or fact?* Available at www.inif.org/foodinsight/2002. Accessed on 2/23/04.
Marcason, W. (2002). How much calcium is really in that supplement? *Journal of the American Dietetic Association, 102,* 1647.
National Academy of Sciences Institute of Medicine. (2004). *Dietary Reference Intakes for water, potassium, sodium, chloride, and sulfate.* Available at www.nap.edu. Accessed on 2/23/04.
National Academy of Sciences Institute of Medicine. (2001). *Dietary Reference Intakes for vitamin A, vitamin K, arsenic, boron, chromium, copper, iodine, iron, manganese, molybdenum, nickel, silicon, vanadium, and zinc.* Washington, DC: National Academy Press.
National Academy of Sciences Institute of Medicine. (2000). *Dietary Reference Intakes for vitamin C, vitamin E, selenium, and carotenoids.* Washington, DC: National Academy Press.
National Academy of Sciences Institute of Medicine. (1997). *Dietary Reference Intakes for calcium, phosphorus, magnesium, vitamin D, and fluoride.* Washington, DC: National Academy Press.
National Institutes of Health, Office of Dietary Supplements. (2002). *Facts about dietary supplements: Zinc.* Available at www.cc.nih.gov/ccc/supplements/zinc.html. Accessed on 2/25/04.
National Institutes of Health, Office of Dietary Supplements. (2002). *Facts about dietary supplements: Iron.* Available at www.cc.nih.gov/ccc/supplements/iron.html. Accessed on 2/25/04.
National Institutes of Health, Office of Dietary Supplements. (2001). *Facts about dietary supplements: Selenium.* Available at www.cc.nih.gov/ccc/supplements/selenium.html. Accessed on 2/25/04.
Rosenberg, I. (Ed.). (2003). Magnesium: Are you getting enough? *Tufts University Health & Nutrition Letter, 21*(6), 8.
Shanta-Retelny, V. (2004). Beverage calories: Are they going to waist? *Communicating Food for Health,* March, 21.
Valtin, H. (2002). *"Drink at least eight glasses of water a day"-Really? Is there scientific evidence for "8 × 8"?* Available at http://ajpregu.physiology.org/cgi. Accessed on 2/24/04.

For information on the new dietary guidelines 2005 and MyPyramid, visit **http://connection.lww.com/go/dudek**

7

Energy Metabolism

TRUE	FALSE	
		1 A food that is high in "energy" is high in calories.
		2 An excess of carbohydrates is more likely to cause weight gain than an excess of fat.
		3 When glucose from food or glycogen is not available to meet glucose need, the body converts fatty acids into glucose for energy.
		4 Starvation diets (e.g., fasting) may cause less loss of body fat than low-calorie diets.
		5 Ketones result from the incomplete breakdown of fatty acids.
		6 The majority of calories expended daily by most Americans are on basal needs.
		7 Building muscle speeds metabolic rate.
		8 To reap health benefits, you must participate in continuous activity for at least 30 minutes.
		9 The best exercise is one the individual sticks with.
		10 To lose weight, what matters is the amount of calories burned not whether those calories are from stored fat or stored glycogen.

UPON COMPLETION OF THIS CHAPTER, YOU WILL BE ABLE TO

- Discuss how the body breaks down glucose into energy.
- Discuss how the body breaks down amino acids into energy.
- Discuss how the body breaks down triglycerides into energy.
- Describe how the body handles excess intakes of carbohydrate, protein, and fat.
- Explain the body's use of fuels during a prolonged fast.
- List factors that influence basal metabolic rate.
- Name health benefits from regular physical activity.
- Discuss how physical activity recommendations differ when the goal is health benefits vs. weight management.

Energy is relatively abstract in that it cannot be defined by its size, shape, or mass. According to basic principles of thermodynamics, energy is neither created nor destroyed but changes from one form to another without being used up. In the body, energy is extracted from nutrients. Tiny amounts of energy are stored within cells as a source of immediate fuel. Much larger amounts of energy are available in glycogen and fat tissue to fuel activity of longer duration. The metabolism of energy is a dynamic process that constantly changes with the influx of nutrients, the availability of stored energy, and the demands of fueling activity.

This chapter addresses how the body breaks down nutrients for energy and how it stores energy to meet future needs. Energy metabolism during fasting and physical activity is presented. Total energy requirements and the topic of increasing physical activity for health promotion are discussed.

ENERGY METABOLISM

Calorie: unit by which energy is measured; the amount of heat needed to raise the temperature of 1 kg of water 1 degree Centigrade. Technically, calorie is actually kilocalorie or kcal.

From a nutritional standpoint, energy is synonymous with calories. The more energy a food has, the higher its caloric value. Carbohydrates and protein provide 4 calories/gm, fat has 9 cal/gm. Vitamins are needed for the metabolism of energy but they do not supply calories.

Energy metabolism encompasses the processes of anabolism and catabolism that occur continuously as the body uses energy to synthesize compounds or extracts energy from the breakdown of nutrients from food or body storage. For instance immediately after eating, nutrients are used for energy as needed and the remainder is reconfigured into compounds for storage. When food is not available to meet energy needs, those storage compounds break down to release energy to fuel the body. In people who eat three meals daily, the amount of time spent on synthesizing storage compounds is approximately the same as the time spent on breaking down stored nutrients.

Anabolism

Metabolism: the sum total of all physical and chemical changes that occur in living cells; it encompasses the two fundamental processes of anabolism and catabolism.

Anabolism is an energy-using process that occurs continuously in all people as cells or substances are replaced after normal wear and tear. Anabolism also reassembles nutrients into compounds for storage. As illustrated in Figure 7.1, each of the energy-yielding nutrients consumed in excess of need can ultimately be synthesized into body fat. Specifically,

- Glucose remaining after energy needs are met is converted to glycogen and stored in the liver and muscle if those stores are not saturated. However, glycogen storage is limited so any glucose left is converted to fatty acids and stored as body fat.
- Amino acids that are not needed for energy or to replace protein tissue are converted to fatty acids for storage as body fat. The body does not store protein although body tissues can give up protein when needed.
- Fatty acids that are not needed for energy recombine with glycerol to form triglycerides for storage as body fat. The body has a virtual limitless capacity to

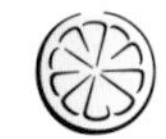

Anabolism: energy-using reactions that build.

Catabolism: energy-producing reactions that break down.

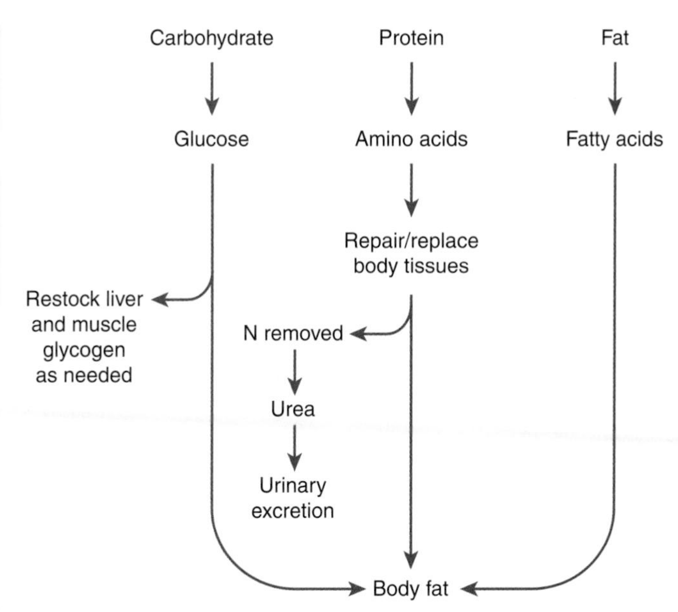

FIGURE 7.1 Fate of energy yielding nutrients when they are consumed in excess of need.

Tricarboxylic Acid (TCA) Cycle: also known as the Krebs' cycle, is a complex series of reactions during which acetyl coenzyme A (acetyl-CoA) is broken down to carbon dioxide and hydrogen atoms.

store excess nutrients in adipose. Figure 7.2 illustrates the average glycogen and body fat stores in an 80-kg (176-pound) person.

The rate of anabolism exceeds the rate of catabolism during times when the demand for new tissue is increased such as periods of growth, pregnancy, lactation, and the recovery phase following injury or illness. For healthy nonpregnant adults, the rate of anabolism equals the rate of catabolism.

Catabolism

Acetyl Coenzyme A (Acetyl-CoA): a two-carbon compound made of acetic acid formed from the break down of pyruvate with a molecule of CoA attached to it.

Catabolism is the breakdown of large molecules into smaller ones: glycogen is broken down into glucose, protein into amino acids, and triglycerides into glycerol and fatty acids. These four basic units can be further catabolized into smaller substances and ultimately into energy. This energy is trapped in adenosine triphosphate (ATP) and stored in every cell until needed. Whether from food or body storage, glucose, amino acids, glycerol, and fatty acids all eventually enter the tricarboxylic acid cycle and electron transport chain to yield energy as needed (Fig. 7.3).

Energy From Glucose

Glucose catabolism begins with the anaerobic process of glycosis which splits glucose (six carbon atom molecule) into pyruvate molecules (three carbon atoms each). Glycosis produces only about 10% of the total energy available from glucose; in other

Electron Transport Chain: also known as oxidative phosphorylation, the final pathway in the release of energy as hydrogen atoms from the Krebs' cycle are oxidized to generate ATP.

Anaerobic: not requiring oxygen.

Pyruvate: a three-carbon atom compound made from the breakdown of glucose, glycerol, and glucogenic amino acids.

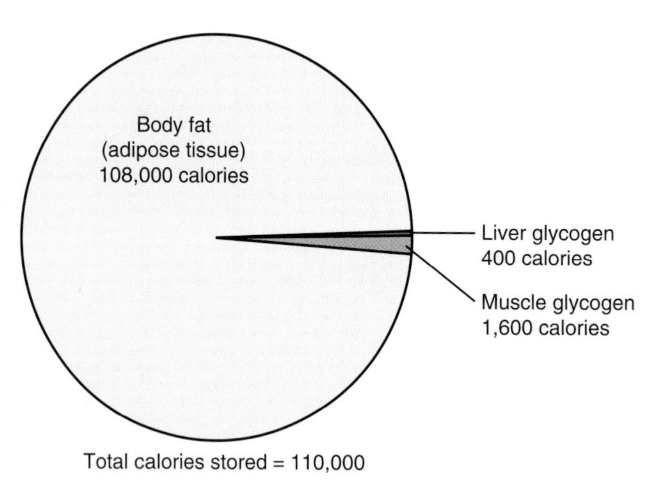

FIGURE 7.2 Average glycogen and body fat (adipose) storage in a person weighing 80 kg.

words, if more energy is needed, the process continues. Notice in Figure 7.3 that pyruvate can be reassembled into glucose; therefore, any compound that can be converted to pyruvate can be reassembled into glucose.

If the cell needs more energy and oxygen is available, catabolism continues as an additional carbon splits off from pyruvate forming the two-carbon compound known as acetyl-CoA. Notice that the reaction from the three-carbon molecule into a two-carbon molecule is irreversible, so compounds broken down into acetyl CoA (e.g., fatty acids) cannot be reassembled into glucose.

Acetyl CoA enters the TCA cycle, where it is degraded to carbon dioxide and hydrogen. Hydrogen atoms oxidize and energy is captured and stored in ATP molecules through a complex series of reactions known as the electron transport chain.

Energy From Protein

Glucogenic Amino Acids: amino acids that are broken down into the three-carbon compound pyruvate and are able to be synthesized into glucose.

Normally the body uses little protein for energy as long as intake and storage of carbohydrate and fat are adequate. However, amino acids are broken down for energy if carbohydrate and fat are insufficient for energy use or if protein is consumed in excessive amounts.

First, amino acids are stripped of their nitrogen through the process of deamination. The freed nitrogen can be used to synthesize nonessential amino acids or it may be converted to urea and excreted in the urine.

Deaminated amino acids enter the TCA cycle by one of three different paths. Approximately half are broken down into pyruvate, which means they are capable of being reassembled into glucose. They are classified as glucogenic. Other deaminated amino acids classified as ketogenic amino acids are converted into acetyl CoA; they cannot be reassembled into glucose. The remaining amino acids enter the TCA cycle directly without first being transformed into either pyruvate or acetyl CoA.

Energy From Fat

By weight, 95% of a typical triglyceride molecule is fatty acids and 5% is glycerol. Fatty acids and glycerol are catabolized differently in the body.

Through the process of beta-oxidation, fatty acids are split, two carbon atoms at a time, into fragments that combine with CoA to form acetyl CoA, which can then con-

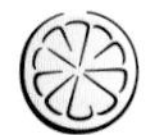

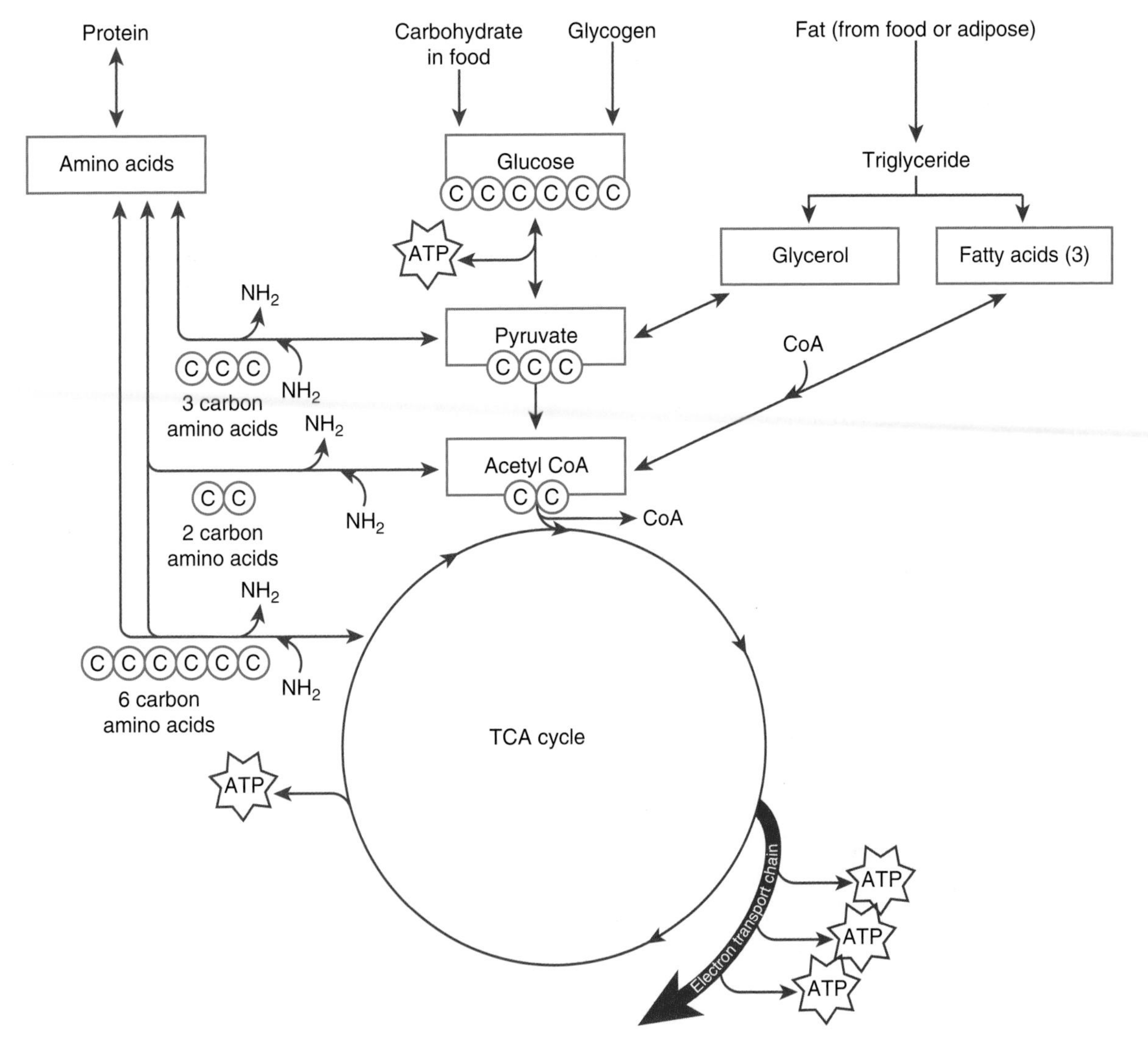

FIGURE 7.3 Summary of energy metabolism.

tinue through the TCA cycle and electron transport chain. Because fatty acids break down into two carbon molecules, not a three-carbon molecule, they cannot be reassembled to make glucose. Thus, 95% of a triglyceride molecule cannot be converted to glucose.

Glycerol, a three-carbon compound, is easily converted to pyruvate. From there, it can be oxidized through the TCA cycle and electron transport chain. During times of need, glycerol can be reassembled into glucose by way of pyruvate. Converting fat to glucose is extremely inefficient because it represents only 5% of the total triglyceride molecule.

THE BODY'S CHOICE OF FUELS

As previously stated, the type and source of energy nutrients actually used at any given time depend on the influx of nutrients, the availability of stored nutrients, and the demands of fueling physical activity. Fasting and exercise metabolism are discussed below.

Fasting

Ketogenic Amino Acids: amino acids that are broken down into the two-carbon compound acetyl CoA and cannot be synthesized into glucose but can be used to make fat if are not further catabolized to release energy.

Deaminated: an amino acid that has had it amino (NH_2) group removed.

Ketone Bodies: acidic compounds formed from the incomplete breakdown of fat when carbohydrate is not available.

Temporary routine fasting occurs during late morning, late afternoon, and most of the evening beginning about 4 hours after the previous meal. During this time the body's energy needs are met from stored nutrients. Liver glycogen and fatty acids from fat storage are released into the bloodstream, where body cells catabolize them to produce energy. A slight dip in blood glucose level signals hunger, which normally stimulates eating and body refueling.

If eating does not occur because of either voluntary or involuntary fasting, fat breakdown continues and liver glycogen becomes depleted. Most body cells can use fatty acids for energy. The exceptions are brain cells, nerve cells, and red blood cells, which normally rely exclusively on glucose for energy. When liver glycogen is depleted, the body's next best source of glucose is glucogenic amino acids. Unfortunately, whole body proteins must be sacrificed to free these glucogenic amino acids so that they may be synthesized into glucose. During the first few days of a fast, brain and nerve cells obtain about 90% of the glucose they need from the catabolism of body proteins, such as muscle and lean tissue, and the remaining 10% from glycerol in triglycerides. Breaking down body protein for energy is expensive, yet it is more efficient than using the small amount of glucose available from glycerol in stored triglycerides. If protein catabolism were to continue at this rate, death would occur within 3 weeks, regardless of the amount of stored fat a person might have.

Fortunately, the body adapts to starvation by attempting to conserve body protein. Some brain cells are able to switch to using ketone bodies, derivatives of fat, for energy. Ketone production increases gradually and after several weeks of fasting, ketones supply about two-thirds or more of the nervous system's energy requirements. However, many brain cells are unable to convert to ketone use, so some body protein catabolism continues to provide glucose, albeit at a much slower rate.

Another adaptive mechanism that occurs during prolonged fasting is a reduction in metabolic rate to slow the sacrifice of body fat and protein. The ultimate result of lowered metabolism is that *fat tissue* is conserved even though *weight loss* (due to protein loss) may be significant. In fact, because of the lowered metabolic rate, less body fat may be lost during fasting than during a low-calorie diet.

 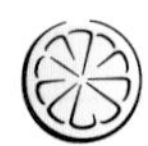

In long-term fasting, fatty acids supply about 90% of total energy requirements. If adequate fluids are consumed, a normal-weight person can survive up to 60 days before fat stores are exhausted. After that, protein catabolism quickly accelerates and death follows.

Fueling Physical Activity

The body's energy needs are always met with a mixture of fuels. At rest that mixture is about 35% glucose, about 60% fat, and about 2% to 5% amino acids. During activity, the mix of fuels used is constantly changing in response to the duration and intensity of the exercise. Other factors, such as the individual's fitness level and usual diet, also influence the proportion of nutrients used.

Energy for Exercise

The immediate fuel of muscle cells when activity begins is the energy trapped in ATP, which is in small supply in every cell. Because half or more of the energy released is lost as heat, exercise has an immediate warming effect. Muscle cells also use creatine phosphate, a high-energy compound, to augment the supply of ATP. Neither ATP nor creatine phosphate is dependent on the availability of oxygen. However, the supply of creatine phosphate is small, and another source of fuel is needed if the activity lasts longer than 10 to 20 seconds.

During the first 1 to 2 minutes of exercise, when oxygen has not yet arrived at the muscles, stored muscle glycogen is the primary fuel; it generates energy through anaerobic glycolysis. As exercise continues, glucose from liver glycogen is released and picked up by muscle cells for their use. After several minutes, the body shifts to aerobic metabolism as increased breathing increases the supply of oxygen. The body can quickly alternate between aerobic and anaerobic metabolism as the supply of oxygen changes.

For activities lasting longer than a few minutes, the mixture of fuels used depends on the intensity and duration of the exercise. In general

- **As the intensity of activity increases, the proportion of glucose used increases** because glucose is the only fuel that can be burned anaerobically via glycolysis.
- **As the duration of activity increases, the proportion of fat used increases.** At the onset of moderate exercise fueled aerobically, muscle glycogen serves as the primary source of energy. After 20 to 30 minutes, the proportion of fat used increases to 50% to 60% of the total in an attempt to conserve glycogen. (However, glycogen use continues and glycogen stores become depleted if the activity is intense enough and lasts long enough.) Likewise, a mixture of fat and glucose is the fuel source used in high-intensity endurance events such as marathons whereas glucose is used almost exclusively in high-intensity, short-duration activities.
- **Physically fit people have a higher aerobic capacity, allowing them to use more fat and spare more glycogen.** Fat can be used for energy only when adequate

oxygen is available. Regular aerobic exercise three times per week for at least 20 to 30 minutes improves heart and lung capacities, which increases oxygen delivery to muscle cells, allowing for more aerobic metabolism. It also stimulates muscle cells to produce more structures within the cell in which aerobic metabolism takes place (mitochondria), thereby increasing the rate of energy synthesis. Furthermore, trained muscles are able to store more glycogen and are better at conserving glycogen because they rely more on fat for energy.

When Exercise Leaves You Breathless

To extract all available energy, nutrients must undergo complete oxidation by way of the TCA cycle and the electron transport chain. Both pathways are aerobic, meaning that oxygen—obtained through deep, regular breathing—is required. However, sometimes oxygen is not available quickly enough or in large enough supply, as in the case of intense bursts of activity or prolonged exercise. Without sufficient oxygen, the body switches to anaerobic metabolism (glycolysis) to keep things moving when you can't "catch your breath."

During moderate aerobic exercise, a trained heart and circulatory system can adequately meet the muscles' demand for oxygen. However, when conditioning is less than optimal or when activity is intense or prolonged, the heart and lungs cannot supply adequate oxygen quickly enough to maintain aerobic metabolism. When this occurs, muscles switch from using a glucose/fat mix to using only glucose, the only fuel that can be metabolized anaerobically, albeit incompletely. Fat can be broken down for energy only when oxygen is present; in fact, more oxygen is needed to catabolize fat than glucose.

In anaerobic metabolism, glucose is broken down into pyruvate but pyruvate catabolism cannot continue without oxygen. Instead, pyruvate accumulates, which stimulates the heart and lungs to work harder. If there is a break in the action, the increase in breathing (and, therefore, oxygen) allows the body to switch back to aerobic metabolism and catabolize pyruvate through the TCA cycle (aerobically). Without adequate oxygen, the accumulated pyruvate is transformed into lactic acid, which accumulates until adequate oxygen becomes available.

The accumulation of lactic acid is deleterious: it is responsible for the burning-type pain in muscles and can quickly lead to muscle exhaustion if it is not carried away by the blood. To avoid problems with lactic acid accumulation, it is necessary to rest periodically, to breathe deeply, and most importantly to increase the level of fitness.

TOTAL ENERGY REQUIREMENTS

The total number of calories a person needs in a day is the sum of the number of calories spent for basal metabolism, physical activity, and the thermic effect of food. In practical terms, the thermic effect of food is an additional energy expense but is usually not factored in total calorie expenditure.

 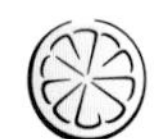

Basal Metabolism

Basal Metabolic Rate (BMR) or Basal Energy Expenditure (BEE): the minimum caloric requirement to sustain life in a resting individual.

Basal metabolism is the amount of calories required to fuel the involuntary activities of the body at rest after a 12-hour fast. These involuntary activities include maintaining body temperature and muscle tone, producing and releasing secretions, propelling the gastrointestinal tract, inflating the lungs, and beating the heart. In essence, it is the caloric cost of staying alive.

Basal metabolic rate (BMR) differs only slightly from resting energy expenditure (REE) in that REE does not adhere to the criterion of a 12-hour fast and, therefore, includes the energy spent on digesting, absorbing, and metabolizing food. In practice, BMR and REE are often used interchangeably.

A rule-of-thumb guideline for calculating BMR is to multiply healthy weight (in pounds) by 10 for women and 11 for men. For example, a 130-pound woman expends approximately 1300 cal/day on BMR:

$$130 \text{ lb} \times 10 \text{ cal/lb} = 1300 \text{ cal}$$

Another method is to use the Harris-Benedict equation, which is as follows:

$$\text{Males: } 66 + (13.7 \times W) + (5 \times H) - (6.8 \times A)$$

$$\text{Females: } 655 + (9.6 \times W) + (1.7 \times H) - (4.7 \times A)$$

Where W = actual weight in kg

H = height in cm

A = age in years

Example: the 130-pound (59-kg) woman mentioned above is 5 ft 4 in tall (162 cm) and is 21 years old.

$$\text{BMR} = 655 + (9.6 \times 59) + (1.7 \times 162) - (4.7 \times 21)$$

$$\text{BMR} = 1397$$

Although the results are similar, both methods are approximations. Unless physical activity is unusually high, BMR accounts for 60% to 70% of total energy requirements in most people. The less active a person is, the greater the proportion of calories used for BMR.

BMR is influenced by numerous factors, especially body composition. Lean tissue (muscle mass) contributes to a higher metabolic rate than fat tissue. Therefore, people with more muscle mass have higher metabolic rates than do people with proportionately more fat tissue. This explains why men, who have a greater proportion of muscle, have higher metabolic rates than women, who have a greater proportion of fat. Conversely, the loss of lean tissue that usually occurs with aging beginning sometime around age 30 is one reason why energy requirements decrease as people get older. However, the loss of lean tissue is not an inevitable consequence of aging; strength training exercises can maintain or restore muscle mass at any age.

Other factors that affect BMR include

- **Growth.** The formation of new tissue as seen in children and during pregnancy, increases BMR.
- **Hormones.** The thyroid gland secretes two active hormones that regulate BMR: tetraiodothyronine (thyroxine, or T_4) and triiodothyronine (T_3). When the body oversecretes thyroid hormones (hyperthyroidism), metabolism speeds up, often causing dramatic weight loss even though appetite is ravenous and food intake is high. BMR may increase by 15% to 25% in mild cases and up to 50% to 75% in severe cases. A rapid metabolic rate causes nervousness; decreased attention span; increased pulse rate, palpitations, and increased systolic blood pressure; intolerance to heat and profuse perspiration; and diarrhea or constipation. Drug therapy, radiation, or surgical removal of part or all of the thyroid gland is needed to treat hyperthyroidism.

When the body's production of thyroid hormones is inadequate (hypothyroidism), the rate of metabolism slows often by 15% to 30% or more. Significant weight gain occurs despite calorie restriction. Other symptoms of a slowed metabolism include fatigue, decreased body temperature, and pulse rate; physical and mental slowness; constipation; and an intolerance to cold. Hypothyroidism is responsible for only a small percentage of obesity.

- **Fever.** Metabolism increases 7% for each degree Fahrenheit above 98.6.
- **Height.** When considering two people of the same gender who weigh the same, the taller one has a higher metabolic rate than the shorter one because of a larger surface area.
- **Environmental temperature.** Very hot and very cold environmental temperatures increase the metabolic rate because the body expends more energy to regulate its own temperature.
- **Starvation, fasting, and malnutrition.** Part of the decline in BMR that occurs with these conditions is attributed to the loss of lean body tissue. Hormonal changes may contribute to the decrease in metabolic rate.
- **Weight loss from dieting.** With smaller body mass, less energy is required to fuel metabolism.
- **Stress.** Stress hormones raise the metabolic rate.
- **Certain drugs,** such as barbiturates, narcotics, and muscle relaxants, decrease the metabolic rate, as does sleep and paralysis.

Physical Activity

Over the last 50 years, calorie expenditure on physical activity has declined for most Americans as a result of the increase in mechanization and the proliferation of laborsaving devices. Physical activity, or voluntary muscular activity, accounts for 25% to 30% of total calories used, although this varies among individuals. The actual amount of energy expended on physical activity depends on the intensity and duration of the activity and the weight of the person performing the activity. The more intense and

 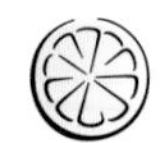

longer the activity, the greater the amount of calories burned. Heavier people, who have more weight to move, use more energy than lighter people to perform the same activity.

Although it is possible to get a fairly accurate estimate of total calories expended in a day by keeping a thorough record of all activity for a 24-hour period, it is a tedious process. An easier rule-of-thumb method for estimating daily calories expended on physical activity is to calculate the percent increase above BMR based on the intensity of usual activity. Multiply

- BMR × 1.2 if you are sedentary such as mainly sitting, driving, lying down, standing, reading, typing, or other low-intensity activities
- BMR × 1.3 if you are lightly active such as walking no more than 2 hours daily or participate in sports 1 to 3 days/week
- BMR × 1.4 if you are moderately active such as heavy housework, gardening, dancing, and very little sitting or participate in moderate exercise or sports 3 to 5 days/week
- BMR × 1.5 if you are highly active such as active physical sports 6 to 7 days/week or have a labor-intensive occupation (e.g., construction work, ditch digging)

For example, a 130-pound woman who is lightly active expends a total of 1690 calories/day:

1300 cal for BMR × 1.3 for light activity = 1690 total calories/day

Box 7.1 describes the steps to estimating your own calorie requirements.

BOX 7.1

ESTIMATING TOTAL CALORIE EXPENDITURE

1. Estimate basal metabolic rate

Multiply your healthy weight (in pounds) by 10 for women or 11 for men. If you are overweight, multiply by the average weight within your healthy weight range (see Chapter 14).

____ (weight in pounds) × ____ = ________ calories for BMR

2. Estimate total calories according to usual activity level

Choose the category that describes your usual activities.

Multiply BMR by	For this type of usual activity
1.2	Sedentary: mostly sitting, driving, sleeping, standing, reading, typing, other low-intensity activities
1.3	Light activity: light exercise such as walking not more than 2 h/d
1.4	Moderate activity: moderate exercise such as heavy housework, gardening, and very little sitting
1.5	High activity: active in physical sports or a labor-intensive occupation such as construction work

____ (calories for BMR) × ____ (calories for activity level) = ____ total daily calories expended

Thermic Effect of Food

Thermic Effect of Food: an estimation of the amount of energy required to digest, absorb, transport, metabolize, and store nutrients.

The thermic effect of food is the "cost" of processing food. In a normal mixed diet, it is estimated to be about 10% of the total calorie intake. For instance, people who consume 1800 cal/day use about 180 cal to process their food. The actual thermic effect of food varies with the composition of food eaten, the frequency of eating, and the size of meals consumed. Although it represents an actual and legitimate use of calories, the thermic effect of food in practice is usually disregarded when calorie requirements are estimated because it constitutes such a small amount of energy and is imprecisely estimated.

ENERGY IN HEALTH PROMOTION

Despite the proven benefits of regular exercise, most Americans are not getting enough. According to data from the 2000 National Health Interview Survey, 64% of men do not engage regularly in leisure-time physical activity. Among women, the figure jumps to 72%. It is estimated that physical inactivity together with unhealthy eating contributes to 400,000 preventable deaths in the United States annually. Only tobacco use is responsible for more preventable deaths in the United States.

The terms *activity, exercise, and fitness* are frequently used interchangeably but they have very different meanings. Physical activity is voluntary muscular activity that results in energy expenditure. Washing your face is a physical activity but it is not exercise. Exercise is a structured and repetitive physical activity done to improve or maintain one or more aspects of physical fitness. Running is both a physical activity and exercise. Physical fitness refers to a person's ability to perform physical activity. A person who is physically fit has a high level of capacity in each of three areas: cardiorespiratory endurance, muscular endurance and strength, and flexibility.

Benefits of Regular Physical Activity

Benefits of increasing activity are dose-dependent and occur along a continuum: a modest amount of activity is enough to reap health benefits while additional exercise promotes weight management and moves people toward achieving optimal physical fitness (Fig. 7.4). A greater increase in benefits occurs when sedentary people become moderately active than when moderately active people become vigorous exercisers.

Subjectively, regular physical activity provides pleasure, improves productivity, instills a sense of accomplishment, increases creativity, relieves stress, and makes people feel more energetic. Objectively, physical activity increases bone strength, improves serum cholesterol, lowers blood pressure, relieves stiffness related to osteoarthritis, stimulates metabolism, and reduces falls among the elderly. Improved sleep quality, improved immune system functioning, and reduced levels of body fat occur. These benefits translate to lowered risk of (or improvements in) cardiovascular disease, hyper-

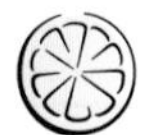

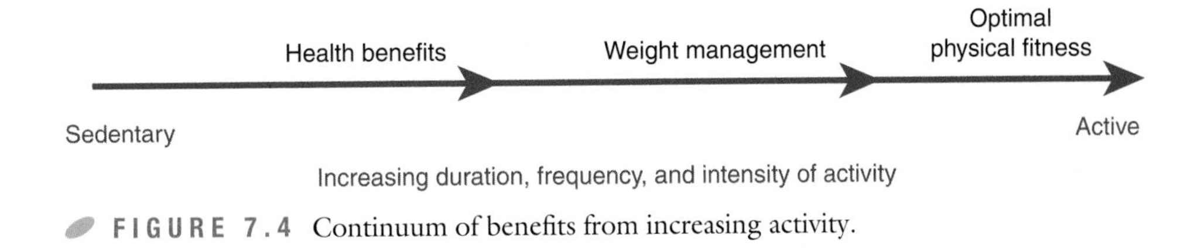

FIGURE 7.4 Continuum of benefits from increasing activity.

tension, type 2 diabetes, obesity, osteoporosis, depression, infection, and cancers of the colon and breast. Regular physical activity is credited with helping to reduce the number of hospitalizations, physician visits, and medications. Both quality and length of life are enhanced by increasing physical activity. Actual benefits derived vary with the type of exercise (Table 7.1).

How Much Aerobic Exercise Is Enough?

Aerobic Exercise: activity requiring oxygen; provides cardiovascular benefits because the cardiovascular system must work harder to deliver oxygen to the tissues.

Not too long ago, exercise philosophy was based on the idea of "no pain, no gain" and "go for the burn." Since the mid-1990s, health organizations ranging from the Centers for Disease Control and Prevention (CDC) and American College of Sports Medicine (ACSM) have softened their stance in view of evidence that moderate intensity activity provides most of the health benefits that come from exercising.

The total dose of exercise is the primary determinant of the benefits received. For health benefits, the ACSM recommends a minimum of 30 minutes of moderate intensity physical activity most days of the week. The activity need not be continuous to provide benefits; in other words, 30 minutes of walking can be accrued in three 10-minute walks.

TABLE 7.1 POTENTIAL BENEFITS AND MINIMUM FREQUENCY RECOMMENDED FOR VARIOUS TYPES OF EXERCISE

Type	Benefits	Minimum Frequency
Aerobic exercise (e.g., walking, jogging)	Cardiovascular fitness	3 ×/week
	Lowered blood pressure	3 ×/week
	Fat loss	Daily
	Improved insulin sensitivity	3 ×/week
Strength training	Increased bone density	3 ×/week
Stretching	Improved flexibility	3–4 ×/week, preferably daily

For health benefits *and* prevention of weight gain, the Institute of Medicine recommends 60 min/day of moderate intensity physical activity (e.g., walking/jogging at 4 to 5 mph) in addition to normal lifestyle activity. The increase in exercise duration promotes fat burning to help manage weight. For children, the recommendation is 60 minutes or more of daily physical activity and exercise. While ACSM applauds the Institute of Medicine's inclusion of physical activity in its report, they acknowledge that the amount of physical activity needed for "optimal benefits" is still unknown. Also unknown is the amount of activity needed to prevent weight gain, for which individual variation is considerable. For instance, some people never exercise and are able to maintain their weight throughout adulthood while others gain significant weight despite faithfully exercising. The danger with increasing the recommendation to 60 minutes/day is that most sedentary people may be discouraged from doing anything. Just as eating plans and nutrition therapy need to be individualized, so too do physical activity and exercise plans.

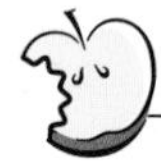

Quick Bite

Maximal heart rate is approximately 220 minus the individual's age. The target heart rate is obtained by multiplying maximum heart rate by the desired percent.

Example: For a 30 year old who wants to exercise at 75% of maximal heart rate

1. Subtract age from 220 to obtain maximum heart beats/minute.

   $220 - 30 = 190$ beats/min

2. Multiply maximal rate by 75% to obtain desired maximum heart beats/minute.

   $190 \times 75\% = 142.5$ beats/min

3. Divide by 6 to calculate maximum beats/10 second interval.

   142 divided by 6 $\approx$ 24 beats/10 seconds

Ergogenic Aid: products used to enhance physical performance.

For optimum physical fitness, the recommendation is to engage in moderate to high intensity aerobic exercise at 60 to 90% maximal heart rate three to five times/week, with each session lasting 20 to 60 minutes plus additional time for warm-up and cool-down. In other words, you have to work up a sweat. Table 7.2 summarizes selected supplements used as ergogenic aids by athletes.

Other Exercises

In addition to regular aerobic exercises, strength training and stretching exercises are recommended for a well-rounded exercise program. Specifically

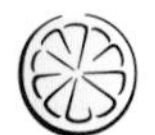

Career Connection

Carbohydrate-loading is an effective way to maximize glycogen storage for endurance events by simply adjusting carbohydrate intake and training schedule. The idea is to increase the already high carbohydrate sports diet even higher while tapering training. The combined effect of a greater influx of carbohydrates (food) while fewer carbohydrates are being used (less exercise) results in a significant increase in muscle glycogen available on the day of the endurance event. Specifically, clients are urged to eat 55 to 65% of total calories from carbohydrate with adequate protein. The last hard training session should be approximately 3 weeks from the day of the event with tapering starting at least 2 weeks before the event. Little exercise is recommended during the last 7 to 10 days before the event (other than some short, intense speed intervals) to allow maximum glycogen saturation. Carbohydrate loading is considered successful if the client gains 2 to 4 pounds, which is mostly water weight. Each ounce of stored glycogen is accompanied by about 3 ounces of water, which is available during exercise to reduce the risk of dehydration.

Sample Carbohydrate Loading Menu

Breakfast
¾ cup orange juice
½ cup oatmeal with 1 Tbsp brown sugar
1 cup skim milk
1 pumpernickel bagel
1 Tbsp jelly
1 banana

Lunch
¾ cup grape juice
2 slices wheat bread
3 oz lean roast beef
1 tsp mayonnaise
1 cup plain yogurt with 1 cup fresh blueberries

Snack
5 vanilla wafers
1 frozen fruit juice bar

Dinner
3 cups spaghetti
1 cup spaghetti sauce
3 oz lean meatballs
1 slices multigrain bread with 1 tsp margarine
1 cup watermelon
½ cup lowfat pudding

Snack
Fruit smoothie made with 1 cup vanilla yogurt, ¾ cup skim milk, 1 frozen banana, 1 cup sliced strawberries

Approximately 2800 cal; 68% carbohydrate (478 g), 19% protein (131 g), 13% fat (40 g)

TABLE 7.2

SUMMARY OF SELECTED ERGOGENIC AIDS USED BY ATHLETES

Ergogenic Aid	Proposed Benefit	Study Results
Androstenedione ("Andro")	Steroid hormone that increases testosterone levels	No documented benefit; potential side effects are major, including increased levels of estrogen and decreased HDL cholesterol Banned by International Olympic Committee, NCAA
Caffeine	Increases fat metabolism to spare muscle glycogen; CNS stimulant	Increases endurance times. Ergogenic dose is approximately 250–500 mg of caffeine, the amount in 3 cups of coffee
Creatine	Delays fatigue; improves performance during short-duration, high-intensity sports	Effective for short burst (e.g., weight lifting, sprinting); no positive effect on endurance, performance
HMB (beta-hydroxy beta-methylbutyrate	Improves nitrogen balance; speeds muscle repair	No benefits noted in humans
Protein	Essential amino acids help muscles to recover more quickly	Athletes do have increased protein needs, which may be 1.4–1.8 g/kg (normal RDA is 0.8 gm/kg). Intakes higher than this do not provide additional gains in muscle strength or mass
Glutamine	Improves nitrogen retention; prevents or reduces muscle breakdown	No effect on muscle recovery

- Perform strength training exercises 2 to 3 times per week with each session lasting at least 15 minutes. Use additional time for warm-up and cool-down. Strength training builds muscle, raising the metabolic rate and increasing the likelihood of weight loss and body fat loss. Changes in body composition—more muscle, less fat—are positive outcomes of strength training that are not reflected on the scale. Strength training also improves bone density to decrease the risk of osteoporosis and falls in the elderly.
- Do stretching exercises at least 3 to 4 times/week, preferably every day. Stretching uses few calories but increases range of motion, enabling the body to move more. Flexibility can improve by more than 100% in a week; it's the easiest area of fitness to improve.

The Bottom Line on Increasing Activity

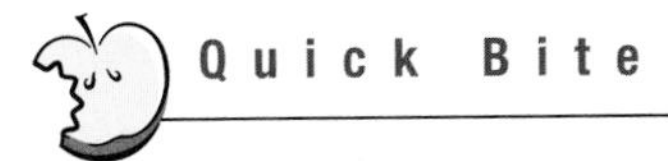

How to burn 150 calories (based on a 150-pound person)

Pedal a stationary bicycle for 20 minutes.
Practice fast dance steps for 24 minutes.
Work in the garden for 27 minutes.
Walk briskly (3.5 mph) for 33 minutes.
Clean the house for 38 minutes.

The bottom line is that almost all Americans can benefit from doing more, whether it is simply more physical activity, such as taking the stairs instead of the elevator, or adding regular (almost daily) exercise, such as power walking or jogging, to their normal routine. Both 20 minutes of vigorous activity 3 times/week and 30 minutes of more moderate activity 5 to 7 days/week ("moderate" activity is defined as activity that uses approximately 150 cal/day) provide about the same dose of activity—about 1000 calories a week of exercise for a 160-pound person. Both regimens will provide health benefits. For additional goals of weight management and physical fitness, more is needed, but exactly how much varies among individuals. Here are some suggestions for increasing activity:

- **Find something enjoyable.** The best chance of success comes from choosing activities that are enjoyable to the individual. The best activity or exercise is one that is done, not just contemplated.
- **Use the buddy system.** Committing to an exercise program or increased physical activity with a friend makes the activity less of a chore and helps to sustain motivation.
- **Spread activity over the entire day if desired.** This recommendation is particularly important for people who "don't have time to exercise." Many people find it easier to fit three 10-minute activity periods into a busy lifestyle than to find 30 uninterrupted minutes to dedicate to activity.
- **Start slowly and gradually increase activity.** For people who have been inactive, the recommendation is to start with only a few minutes of daily activity, such as walking, and gradually increase the frequency, duration, then intensity. For people who are already regularly exercising, increasing the frequency or intensity by 50% is a reasonable goal. Benefits are gained when exercise increases from 2 days/week to 3 or from 30 minutes/day to 45 minutes. People with existing health problems such as diabetes, heart disease, and hypertension should consult a physician before beginning a physical activity program, as should all men older than 40 and all women older than 50 years of age.
- **Move more.** Just moving more can make a cumulative difference in activity. Take the stairs instead of the elevator, park at the far end of the parking lot, walk around while talking on the portable phone, walk instead of driving short distances, play golf without a golf cart or caddy, fidget.
- **Keep an activity log.** Just as people tend to underestimate the amount of food they eat, people usually overestimate the amount of physical activity they perform. Documenting the type and duration of activity can help to track progress.

Career Connection

Many people use activity and exercise to manage their weight. Understanding the basic principle of weight management—that weight changes as the balance between calorie intake and calorie output changes—enables people to tailor their activities and exercises according to their calorie intake and weight goals. For greatest effectiveness, exercise is best combined with a controlled calorie intake.

Physical activity should be an integral component of weight management programs because it (1) modestly contributes to weight loss in overweight and obese adults, (2) reduces body fat, (3) improves cardiorespiratory fitness, and (4) promotes muscle development to help offset the metabolism-lowering effect of dieting and losing weight. In practice, exercise may have only a modest effect on weight if used alone. If the goal is to promote weight loss as well as reap health benefits, exercise should be more intense, of longer duration, and more frequent. Exercise is vital to maintain weight loss.

- **Aim to increase energy expenditure by 1000 to 2000 calories per week.** Encourage clients to start slowly and gradually build to at least 45 minutes of moderate-intensity exercise on at least 5 days a week, preferably daily. Most experts recommend first increasing the duration and frequency of the activity and then the intensity.
- **Don't expect pounds to melt away.** Note that the goal of increasing activity is to burn an extra 1000 to 2000 cal/week. Because 1 pound of body fat is the equivalent of 3500 cal, you need to incur a *daily* calorie deficit of 500 calories to lose 1 pound of weight in 1 week (3500 cal ÷ 7 days/week = 500 cal/day). A 2-pound weight loss occurs when the daily deficit is 1000 cal/*day*. Without a reduction of food intake to contribute to this needed calorie deficit, the 1000 to 2000 extra calories burned each week would amount to a weight loss of only about ⅓ to ½ pound, an amount too low to be reflected on the bathroom scale.

  Many people overestimate the effect that activity and exercise will have on their weight. They expect rapid and sustained weight loss and become discouraged when the scale fails to reflect their hard work. It is important to remember that, even before weight changes are evident, exercise produces positive health benefits such as improvements in blood pressure and blood cholesterol levels and lowered risks of heart disease, diabetes, and colon cancer. People who undertake activity and exercise programs with realistic expectations are more likely to remain committed.

- **Remember that what is important is burning calories, not the actual type of fuel used.** Low- and moderate-intensity exercises performed for longer than 20 minutes are fueled primarily by fat, and when people say they want to lose weight, what they really mean is that they want to lose fat. Therefore, low- and moderate-intensity exercises are desirable, particularly because they are easier on unconditioned or overweight bodies and can be performed for longer periods. But high-intensity exercise, even though fueled mostly by glucose, burns more calories per unit of time. The downside is that it usually requires higher motivation to sustain, and the risk of injury is greater. Ultimately what is important is the *amount* of fuel used, not the *type.*

How Do You Respond?

Does exercise make you hungrier? During and immediately after exercise, blood flow is drawn away from the gastrointestinal tract to the muscles to deliver fuel and oxygen. Because of this, the process of digestion slows and the sensation of hunger is absent. Long, strenuous exercise can cause low blood glucose but that is not the same as hunger. Hunger occurs when calories burned create a calorie deficit, but the increased energy expenditure allows for greater food intake without causing an increase in weight.

Do calories eaten at night promote weight gain? What determines whether or not calories are stored as fat is not when they are eaten but in what quantity. Food eaten in the evening does not provide more calories than it does during the day, but mindless snacking in the evening can accumulate an abundance of calories that can lead to weight gain over time.

When is the best time to exercise? The best time to exercise is what works for the individual. But if exercise time varies from day to day and a clear-cut best time does not seem apparent, circadian rhythms may help to sort out the best time to exercise. These rhythms, which dictate the daily cycles the body follows, influence body temperature, which seems to influence the quality of a workout. Exercise performed when body temperature is at its highest (usually late afternoon) is likely to be more productive than when body temperature is low (generally early morning). Studies show that exercise late in the day produces better performance and more power: muscles are warm and more flexible, perceived exertion is low, reaction time is quicker, strength is at is peak, and resting heart rate and blood pressure are low. To find your own circadian peak, experts recommend recording your temperature every couple of hours for 5 to 6 consecutive days. But if you are a morning exerciser and it works for you, there is no need to change your schedule. In fact, morning exercisers are more successful at making it a habit. And experts agree that exercise at any time is better than no exercise at all.

▲ Focus on Critical Thinking

Respond to the following statements:

1. Fasting is counterproductive to losing weight.
2. It is better to do less intense physical activity for longer periods of time than it is to do a high intensity exercise for a shorter duration.
3. Calculate your own total energy requirements using Box 7.1. Do you think it is an accurate estimate?

Key Concepts

- Energy metabolism refers to how energy from carbohydrates, proteins, and fats is extracted and used. It is a dynamic process that constantly changes with the influx of nutrients, the availability of stored energy, and the demands of fueling activity.

- Anabolism is an energy-using process that occurs continuously in all people as cells or substances are replaced after normal wear and tear. Anabolism also reassembles nutrients into compounds for storage. Regardless of the source, calories eaten in excess of need are converted to fatty acids and stored as body fat.
- Catabolism is the breakdown of large molecules into smaller ones. Energy is released and trapped in ATP when glucose, amino acids, and glycerol and fatty acids undergo oxidation via the TCA cycle and electron transport chain.
- Nutrients broken down into pyruvate, namely glucose, glycerol, and glucogenic amino acids, can be synthesized into glucose as needed by the body. Nutrients broken down into acetyl CoA, namely fatty acids and ketogenic amino acids, cannot be resynthesized into glucose and so cannot normally fuel glucose-requiring cells of the brain, nervous tissue, and red blood cells when glucose from food or glycogen is unavailable.
- Breaking down body protein to yield glucose is expensive because only about half of amino acids can actually be converted to glucose. Yet it is more efficient compared to the small amount of glucose available from glycerol in stored triglycerides (5% of the triglyceride molecule is glycerol).
- During prolonged fasting, the brain and nervous system adapt to the glucose shortage by using ketones produced by fat catabolism. However, body protein catabolism continues (although at a slower rate) because not all cells are able to adapt to ketone use. Another adaptive mechanism is that metabolism slows to preserve both protein tissue and fat tissue.
- Cells' immediate source of fuel is stored in ATP, which is supplemented with a small supply of creatine phosphate; neither requires oxygen to be burned. Glucose is the only fuel that can be burned without oxygen through the process of glycolysis, but glycolysis extracts only a small amount of the total available energy from glucose. Aerobic metabolism includes the TCA cycle and the electron transport chain; it yields the maximum amount of available energy.
- The body uses a mixture of fuels at rest and at work. In general as the duration of activity increases, the amount of fat burned increases in an attempt to conserve the body's supply of glycogen. As the intensity of activity increases, the amount of glucose burned increases because glucose is the only fuel that can be metabolized anaerobically. Breathlessness that occurs with vigorous exercise indicates anaerobic metabolism.
- Total daily calorie expenditure equals the amount of calories spent on voluntary activities (physical activity) and on involuntary activities (basal metabolism). For most Americans, basal metabolism represents 60% to 70% of total calories burned. The thermic effect of food is the cost of digesting, absorbing, and metabolizing food. At about 10% of total calories consumed, it is a small part of total energy requirements.
- The vast majority of Americans do not get the recommended amount of physical activity. The benefits of physical activity are dose-dependent and range from significant health benefits to weight management to optimal physical fitness.

 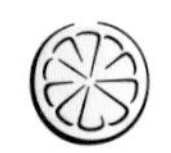

- In the short term, exercise leads to modest weight loss if calories are not also restricted. In the long term, exercise promotes weight loss by promoting fat loss and preventing loss of muscle, which contributes to metabolic rate.

ANSWER KEY

1. **TRUE** Calorie is a unit of measure pertaining to energy in foods. Thus a food that is high in "energy" is high in calories.
2. **FALSE** An excess of any calorie-yielding nutrient, whether carbohydrate, protein, or fat, is converted to fatty acids and stored as fat.
3. **FALSE** The body cannot convert fatty acids into glucose; only the glycerol portion of a triglyceride can be transformed into glucose. Because fatty acids can't become glucose, the body must break down muscle tissue to provide glucose to meet minimum needs when glucose is not available from diet or stored glycogen.
4. **TRUE** Starvation diets (e.g., fasting) may cause less loss of body fat than low-calorie diets because the body seeks to lower its metabolic rate to sustain life when food is not available. It does so by breaking down muscle. Hormonal changes also promote fat-sparing.
5. **TRUE** Ketones result from the incomplete breakdown of fatty acids when adequate glucose is available. Ketones inhibit appetite and increase the risk of acidosis.
6. **TRUE** Depending on the individual's activity level, basal metabolism accounts for 60 to 70% of total calories expended in a day.
7. **TRUE** Building muscle speeds metabolic rate because lean tissue is metabolically active.
8. **FALSE** Activity does not need to be sustained for any given duration to provide health benefits. Snippets of activity accumulated over the entire day can provide the same health benefits as one exercise session of the same total length of time.
9. **TRUE** The best exercise is one the individual sticks with. Exercise prescriptions are not one-size-fits-all.
10. **TRUE** The bottom line for losing weight is that calorie expenditure must exceed calorie consumption over time. It does not matter if the calories used are predominately from glucose (e.g., a high intensity activity) or fat (a lower intensity activity) as long as a calorie deficit is created. The benefit of intense exercise is that more calories are burned per unit of time so total time exercising can be less than when moderate intensity activity is chosen. The benefits of moderate intensity activity are that it is less physically demanding and is easier to perform for longer periods of time. Whether exercise is intense or moderate is a matter of individual preference.

WEBSITES

American College of Sports Medicine at **www.acsm.org**
American Council on Exercise at **www.acefitness.org**
Calculate your own BMR at **www.room42.com/nutrition/basal.shtml**
Exercise: A Guide from the National Institute on Aging at **www.nia.nih.gov/exercisebook/index.htm**
Improving Nutrition and Increasing Physical Activity at **www.cdc.gov/nccdphp/bb_nutrition/index.htm**

National Institute of Diabetes and Digestive and Kidney Diseases, Active at Any Size at **www.niddk.nih.gov/health/nutrit/pubs/physact.htm**
President's Council on Physical Fitness and Sports at **www.fitness.gov**

REFERENCES

Ahrendt, D. (2001). Ergogenic aids: Counseling the athlete. *American Family Physician, 63,* 913–922.
American Council on Exercise. (2001). Fit facts. The best time to exercise. Available at www.acefitness.org. Accessed on 3/6/04.
Centers for Disease Control and Prevention, Department of Health and Human Services. (2003). Physical activity and good nutrition: Essential elements to prevent chronic disease and obesity. Available at www.cdc.gov/nccdphp/dnpa. Accessed on 3/1/04.
Clark, N. (2003). *Sports nutrition guidebook* (3rd ed.). Champaign, IL: Human Kinetics.
Institute of Medicine. (2002). *Dietary Reference Intakes for energy, carbohydrate, fiber, fat, fatty acids, cholesterol, protein, and amino acids.* Washington, DC: The National Academies Press.
International Food Information Council Foundation. (2003). Calories count: Balancing the energy equation. *Food Insight,* March/April, 1, 6.
Liebman, B. (2002). Your exercise Rx. *Nutrition Action Health Letter, 29*(10), 1, 3–7.
McCaffree, J. (2003). Physical activity: How much is enough? *Journal of the American Dietetic Association, 103,* 153–154.
Mohr, C. (2004). Supplement update. *Sports, Cardiovascular, and Wellness Nutritionist's Pulse, 23*(2), 15–16.
Rosenberg, I. (Ed.) (2002). To work up a sweat, or not? *Tufts University Health & Nutrition Letter,* 20(10), 6.
United States Department of Health and Human Services. Office of the Assistant Secretary for Planning and Evaluation. (2002). *Physical activity fundamental to preventing disease.* Available at http://aspe.hhs.gov/health/reports/physicalactivity/. Accessed on 3/1/04.

For information on the new dietary guidelines 2005 and MyPyramid, visit **http://connection.lww.com/go/dudek**

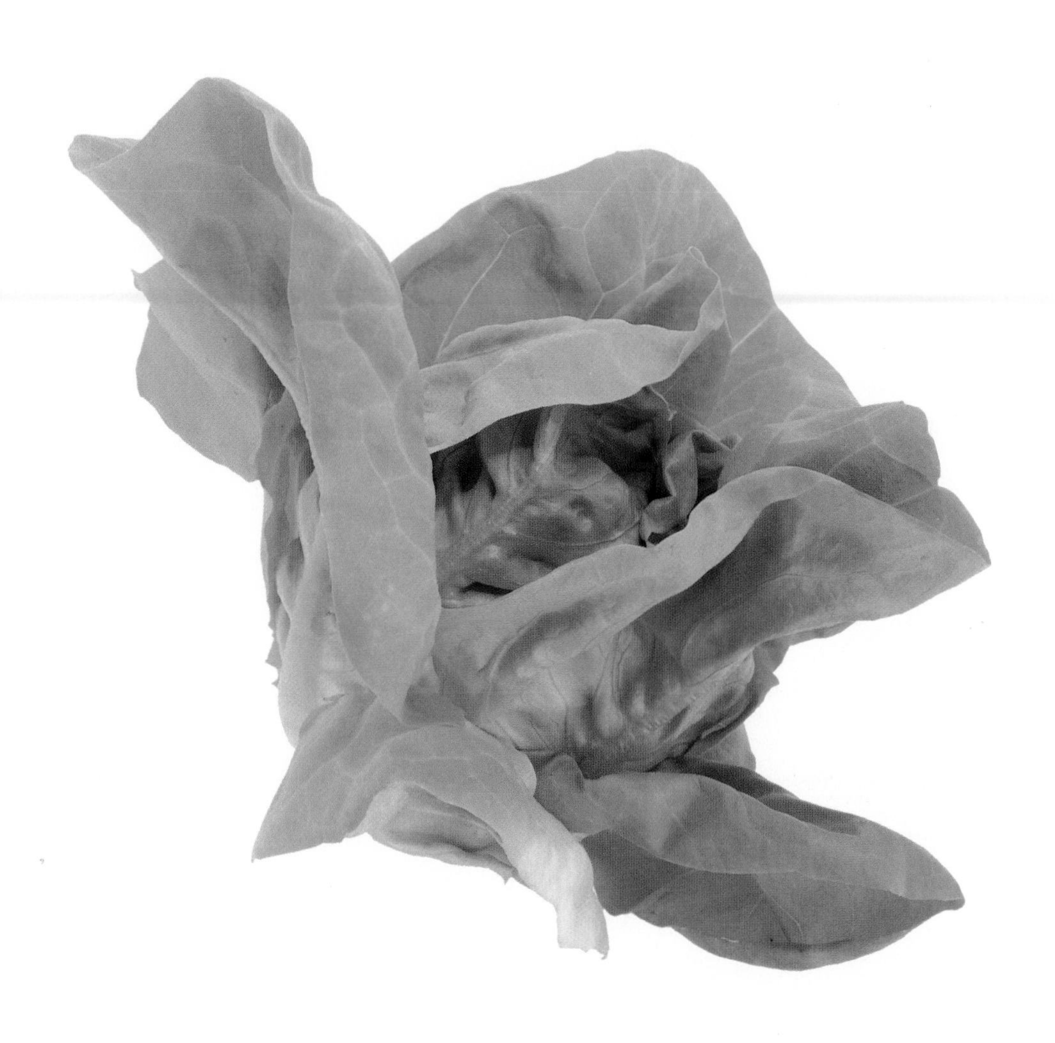

UNIT TWO

Nutrition in Health Promotion

8

Guidelines for Healthy Eating

TRUE	FALSE	
⬭	⬭	**1** The Recommended Dietary Allowances (RDAs) are intended for healthy people only.
⬭	⬭	**2** The Dietary Reference Intakes (DRIs) are useful to teach people how to choose a healthier diet.
⬭	⬭	**3** The Tolerable Upper Intake Level (UL) is the optimal level of nutrients that people should try to consume.
⬭	⬭	**4** The Dietary Guidelines for Americans are intended to promote wellness and decrease the risk of chronic disease in healthy Americans 2 years of age and older.
⬭	⬭	**5** MyPyramid is the graphic used to illustrate the Dietary Guidelines for Americans.
⬭	⬭	**6** A person's individual MyPyramid is based on gender, age, and activity patterns.
⬭	⬭	**7** MyPyramid specifies how many servings from each group a person should consume daily.
⬭	⬭	**8** All high carbohydrate foods are healthier than all high fat foods.
⬭	⬭	**9** MyPyramid recommends regular physical activity on most days of the week, with a suggested minimum of 30 minutes/day.
⬭	⬭	**10** Research suggests that 30 to 40% of all cancers could be prevented by changes in intake and activity.

UPON COMPLETION OF THIS CHAPTER, YOU WILL BE ABLE TO

- Describe how the old RDAs differ from the new Dietary Reference Intakes.
- List the three basic messages of the *Dietary Guidelines for Americans.*
- Describe the purpose of MyPyramid.
- Discuss how MyPyramid conveys the concepts of variety, moderation, proportionality, gradual improvement, personalization, and physical activity.
- Define the term "discretionary calories" and how they may be appropriated.
- Compare MyPyramid to the Healthy Eating Pyramid.
- Discuss similarities and differences between nutrition recommendations from the American Heart Association, the American Cancer Society, and the American Institute for Cancer Research.

HOW TO CHOOSE A "HEALTHY DIET"

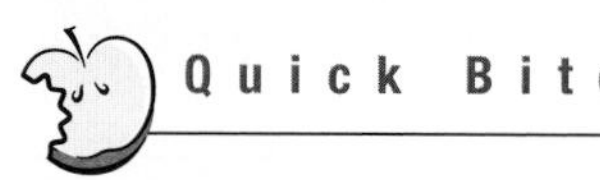

The 10 leading causes of death in the United States in 2001 (in descending order)

1. Heart disease
2. Cancer
3. Stroke
4. Chronic obstructive pulmonary disease
5. Accidents
6. Diabetes
7. Pneumonia/flu
8. Alzheimer's disease
9. Kidney disease
10. Suicide

Source: Anderson, R., & Smith, B. (2003). Deaths: Leading causes for 2001. *National Vital Statistics Reports,* 52(9), November 7, 2003. Available at www.cdc.gov

A healthy diet provides enough of all essential nutrients to avoid deficiencies but not excessive amounts that may increase the risk of nutrient toxicities or chronic disease such as heart disease, cancer, and hypertension. Today, nutrient deficiency diseases are rare in the United States except among the poor, elderly, alcoholics, fad dieters, and ironically hospitalized patients. Conversely, four of the 10 leading causes of death in the United States are associated with dietary excesses. Cardiovascular disease and cancer account for almost two-thirds of all deaths in the United States; diet, in addition to smoking and physical inactivity, is thought to play a major role in the development of these diseases. Likewise, diet plays a major role in stroke and type 2 diabetes. Researchers are investigating how nutrition—whether too much or too little of any particular nutrients—impacts the risk of Alzheimer's disease.

This chapter focuses on how to consume optimal levels of nutrients without consuming too much from professional and consumer perspectives. Tools covered include the Dietary Reference Intakes, Dietary Guidelines for Americans, MyPyramid, the Healthy Eating Pyramid, and diet recommendations from leading health agencies.

Primarily Professional

Previously, the Recommended Dietary Allowances in the United States and the Recommended Nutrient Intakes in Canada defined recommended levels of nutrients that were intended to protect people from inadequate diets and deficiency diseases. As the science of nutrition grew, it became clear that nutrient excesses contribute to chronic disease and that recommendations needed to expand their focus from simply preventing deficiencies to achieving optimal health and avoiding excesses. To that end, the old RDAs have been replaced with a new set of standards that fall under the umbrella of Dietary Reference Intakes.

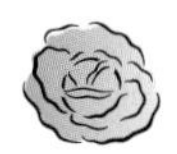

Dietary Reference Intakes

Dietary Reference Intakes: a set of four nutrient-based reference values used to plan and evaluate diets.

The monumental process of determining the amounts of nutrients and calories necessary for optimal health for both genders and across all life stages began in the early 1990s. Together, Canadian scientists and the Food and Nutrition Board of the Institute of Medicine embarked on a comprehensive, multiyear project to update and expand nutrient intake recommendations. The outcome has been a series of reports featuring a new set of references called Dietary Reference Intakes. The first report was issued in 1997 and covered five nutrients: calcium, phosphorus, magnesium, vitamin D, and fluoride. Since then, five additional reports have been released covering vitamins, minerals, the energy nutrients, cholesterol, fiber, electrolytes, and water. Two additional reports are slated for future release: one will feature bioactive compounds such as phytoestrogens and other phytochemicals and the other will cover the role of alcohol in health and disease.

Dietary Reference Intakes is a set of four separate reference values: updated RDAs, Estimated Average Requirement (EAR), Adequate Intake (AI), and the Tolerable Upper Intake Level (UL). Each of these reference values has a specific purpose and represents a different level of intake. Figure 8.1 is a representation of EAR, RDA, and UL points along a continuum. Additional references include Acceptable Macronutrient Distribution Ranges (AMDRs) and an Estimated Energy Requirement (EER).

Recommended Dietary Allowances

Recommended Dietary Allowances: the average daily dietary intake level sufficient to meet the nutrient requirement of 97 to 98% of healthy individuals in a particular life stage and gender group.

The RDAs continue to represent the recommended intake for healthy individuals by life stage and gender. This definition is similar to past descriptions of the RDAs but in the DRI framework, this is the only use of the RDA—as a goal for individuals. The recommendations are set high enough to account for daily variations in intake. They are

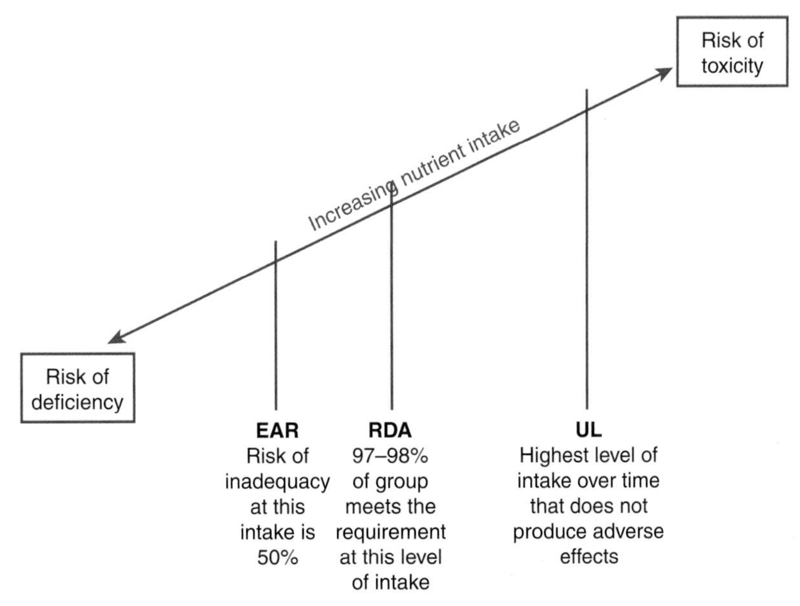

FIGURE 8.1 Representation of DRI along a continuum of intake.

based on specific criteria indicators for estimating requirements such as plasma and serum nutrient concentrations. When estimating the nutritional needs of people with health disorders, health professionals use the RDAs as a starting point and adjust them according to the individual's need.

Estimated Average Requirement (EAR)

The EAR is the amount of a nutrient that is estimated to meet the requirement of half of healthy people in a lifestyle or gender group. "Average" actually means *median*. By definition, the EAR exceeds the requirements of half of the group and falls below the requirements of the other half. The EAR is not based solely on the prevention of nutrient deficiencies but includes consideration for reducing the risk of chronic disease and takes into account the bioavailability of the nutrient, that is, how its absorption is impacted by other food components. EAR values are used to determine RDA values.

Estimated Average Requirement: the nutrient intake estimated to meet the requirement of half of the healthy individuals in a particular life stage and gender group.

Adequate Intake (AI)

An AI is set when an RDA cannot be determined due to lack of sufficient data on requirements. It is a recommended average daily intake level thought to meet or exceed the needs of virtually all members of a life stage/gender group. The primary purpose of the AI is as a goal for the nutrient intake of individuals. This is similar to the use of the RDA except that the RDA is expected to meet the needs of almost all healthy people, while in the case of an AI, it is not known what percentage of people are covered.

Adequate Intake: an intake level thought to meet or exceed the requirement of almost all members of a life stage/gender group. An AI is set when there are insufficient data to define a RDA.

Tolerable Upper Intake Level (UL)

The UL is the highest level of daily nutrient intake that is likely to pose no risk of adverse health effects to almost all individuals in the general population. The term "Tolerable Upper Intake Level" does not imply a possible beneficial effect in consuming that amount but rather indicates the level that can be physiologically tolerated with chronic daily use. It is not intended to be a recommended level of intake. There is no benefit in consuming amounts greater than the RDA or AI.

Tolerable Upper Intake Level: the highest average daily intake level of a nutrient likely to pose no danger to most individuals in the group.

Acceptable Macronutrient Distribution Ranges (AMDRs)

Acceptable Macronutrient Distribution Ranges are defined as a range of intakes for a particular energy source that is associated with reduced risk of chronic disease while

Acceptable Macronutrient Distribution Ranges: an intake range as a percentage of total calories for energy nutrients.

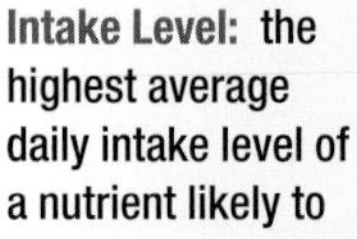

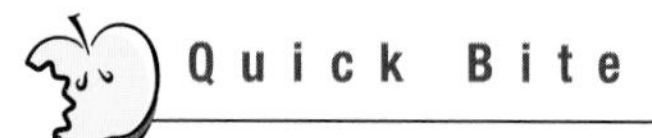

Quick Bite

The Acceptable Macronutrient Distribution Ranges for adults are

	% of total calories consumed
Carbohydrate	45–65%
Protein	10–35%
Fat	20–35%
Linoleic acid (n-6)	5–10%
Alpha-linolenic (n-3)	0.6–1.2%

Source: Dietary Reference Intakes for energy, carbohydrate, fiber, fat, fatty acids, cholesterol, protein, and amino acids (2002). This report may be accessed via www.nap.edu.

providing adequate intakes of essential nutrients. They are ranges expressed as a percentage of total calories consumed. Intakes above or below this range may increase the risk of chronic disease or deficiency, respectively.

A positive linear trend exists between coronary heart disease and the intake of saturated fat, trans fat, and cholesterol; even low intakes of each of these may increase risk. However, it is recognized that it is not possible to eliminate them from the diet and still obtain adequate amounts of essential nutrients. The recommendation is that they be consumed in as low an intake as possible while consuming a nutritionally adequate diet.

Estimated Energy Requirements: level of calorie intake estimated to maintain weight in normal weight individuals based on age, gender, height, weight, and activity.

Estimated Energy Requirements

Similar to the EAR, the EER is defined as the dietary energy intake predicted to maintain energy balance in healthy, normal weight individuals of a defined age, gender, weight, height, and level of physical activity consistent with good health. Exceeding the EER may produce weight gain.

How Are the DRIs Used?

For the most part, DRIs are used by scientists and nutritionists who work in research or academic settings and by dietitians who plan menus for specific populations such as elderly feeding programs, schools, prisons, hospitals, nursing homes, and military feeding programs. In the future, it is likely they will impact food labeling, the Dietary Guidelines for Americans, and MyPyramid. But because consumers eat food and not nutrients, they are not suited to teaching people how to make healthy choices.

Conveying the Concept of Healthy Diet to Consumers

The most prominent tools to assist Americans in making wise food choices are the Dietary Guidelines for Americans and MyPyramid. Numerous health agencies, including the American Heart Association, the American Cancer Society, and the American Institute of Cancer Research, have also issued dietary recommendations to help Americans choose diets aimed at reducing the risk of chronic diseases.

Dietary Guidelines for Americans

The Dietary Guidelines for Americans, published jointly every 5 years by the U.S. Department of Health and Human Services and the U.S. Department of Agriculture, provides science-based recommendations on diet and physical activity to promote health and decrease the risk of chronic diet-related diseases such as hypertension, diabetes, abnormal blood lipid levels, overweight, and obesity. The most recent edition, published in 2005, includes 9 major messages, 23 key recommendations, and 18 additional recommendations for specific population groups (Box 8.1). The Guidelines are intended to represent a pattern of eating for Americans over the age of 2 years and should ideally be implemented as a whole. The major themes are to eat fewer calories, be more physically active, and make wiser food choices.

BOX 8.1

DIETARY GUIDELINES FOR AMERICANS, 2005

Key Recommendations for the General Population

Adequate Nutrients Within Calorie Needs

- Consume a variety of nutrient-dense foods and beverages within and among the basic food groups while choosing foods that limit the intake of saturated and *trans* fats, cholesterol, added sugars, salt, and alcohol.
- Meet recommended intakes within energy needs by adopting a balanced eating pattern, such as the U.S. Department of Agriculture (USDA) MyPyramid or the Dietary Approaches to Stop Hypertension (DASH) Eating Plan.

Weight Management

- To maintain body weight in a healthy range, balance calories from foods and beverages with calories expended.
- To prevent gradual weight gain over time, make small decreases in food and beverage calories and increase physical activity.

Physical Activity

- Engage in regular physical activity and reduce sedentary activities to promote health, psychological well-being, and a healthy body weight.
  - To reduce the risk of chronic disease in adulthood: Engage in at least 30 minutes of moderate-intensity physical activity, above usual activity, at work or home on most days of the week.
  - For most people, greater health benefits can be obtained by engaging in physical activity of more vigorous intensity or longer duration.
  - To help manage body weight and prevent gradual, unhealthy body weight gain in adulthood: Engage in approximately 60 minutes of moderate- to vigorous-intensity activity on most days of the week while not exceeding caloric intake requirements.
  - To sustain weight loss in adulthood: Participate in at least 60 to 90 minutes of daily moderate-intensity physical activity while not exceeding caloric intake requirements. Some people may need to consult with a health care provider before participating in this level of activity.
- Achieve physical fitness by including cardiovascular conditioning, stretching exercises for flexibility, and resistance exercises or calisthenics for muscle strength and endurance.

Food Groups to Encourage

- Consume a sufficient amount of fruits and vegetables while staying within energy needs. Two cups of fruit and 2½ cups of vegetables per day are recommended for a reference 2,000-calorie intake, with higher or lower amounts depending on the calorie level.
- Choose a variety of fruits and vegetables each day. In particular, select from all five vegetable subgroups (dark green, orange, legumes, starchy vegetables, and other vegetables) several times a week.

BOX 8.1 (continued)

DIETARY GUIDELINES FOR AMERICANS, 2005

- Consume 3 or more ounce-equivalents of whole-grain products per day, with the rest of the recommended grains coming from enriched or whole-grain products. In general, at least half the grains should come from whole grains.
- Consume 3 cups per day of fat-free or low-fat milk or equivalent milk products.

Fats

- Consume less than 10% of calories from saturated fatty acids and less than 300 mg/day of cholesterol, and keep *trans* fatty acid consumption as low as possible.
- Keep total fat intake between 20 to 35% of calories, with most fats coming from sources of polyunsaturated and monounsaturated fatty acids, such as fish, nuts, and vegetable oils.
- When selecting and preparing meat, poultry, dry beans, and milk or milk products, make choices that are lean, low-fat, or fat-free.
- Limit intake of fats and oils high in saturated and/or *trans* fatty acids, and choose products low in such fats and oils.

Carbohydrates

- Choose fiber-rich fruits, vegetables, and whole grains often.
- Choose and prepare foods and beverages with little added sugars or caloric sweeteners, such as amounts suggested by the USDA MyPyramid and the DASH Eating Plan.
- Reduce the incidence of dental caries by practicing good oral hygiene and consuming sugar- and starch-containing foods and beverages less frequently.

Sodium and Potassium

- Consume less than 2,300 mg (approximately 1 teaspoon of salt) of sodium per day.
- Choose and prepare foods with little salt. At the same time, consume potassium-rich foods, such as fruits and vegetables.

Alcoholic Beverages

- Those who choose to drink alcoholic beverages should do so sensibly and in moderation—defined as the consumption of up to one drink per day for women and up to two drinks per day for men.
- Alcoholic beverages should not be consumed by some individuals, including those who cannot restrict their alcohol intake, women of childbearing age who may become pregnant, pregnant and lactating women, children and adolescents, individuals taking medications that can interact with alcohol, and those with specific medical conditions.
- Alcoholic beverages should be avoided by individuals engaging in activities that require attention, skill, or coordination, such as driving or operating machinery.

(box continues on page 186)

BOX 8.1 (continued)

DIETARY GUIDELINES FOR AMERICANS, 2005

Food Safety

- To avoid microbial foodborne illness:
  - Clean hands, food contact surfaces, and fruits and vegetables. Meat and poultry should not be washed or rinsed.
  - Separate raw, cooked, and ready-to-eat foods while shopping, preparing, or storing foods.
  - Cook foods to a safe temperature to kill microorganisms.
  - Chill (refrigerate) perishable food promptly and defrost foods properly.
  - Avoid raw (unpasteurized) milk or any products made from unpasteurized milk, raw or partially cooked eggs or foods containing raw eggs, raw or undercooked meat and poultry, unpasteurized juices, and raw sprouts.

Note: The *Dietary Guidelines for Americans 2005* contains additional recommendations for specific populations. The full document is available at www.healthierus.gov/dietaryguidelines.

(U.S. Department of Health and Human Services and U.S. Department of Agriculture.)

The Food Guide Pyramid

The Food Guide Pyramid, which debuted in 1992, was the original graphic used to illustrate the Dietary Guidelines for Americans. It was divided into five horizontal food groups with an apex representing "other" items high in fat and/or sugar. As a teaching tool to help people choose healthy diets, the Pyramid gained widespread recognition and became nearly ubiquitous on food labels, shopping bags, and nutritional brochures. However, over time the Pyramid was criticized for being obsolete and incompatible with the latest research findings. The epidemic of obesity was cited as proof that the Pyramid failed to teach Americans how to choose a healthy diet. Specific complaints were as follows:

- Quality distinctions were not made between items within each food group. For instance, white bread was equivalent to whole wheat bread.
- The range of servings given for each group was misinterpreted by some people to mean that it is appropriate for all people to choose any number of servings within each given range, when in effect the range was supposed to represent a range of different total calorie needs.
- There was confusion over serving sizes.
- The concepts of balance and moderation were vague. To many people, "moderation" loosely meant not "overdoing it" instead of an intended message such as "limit red meat to a 3-oz piece of lean meat one or two times per week."
- Weight and physical activity were not addressed.
- Visually, the apex intuitively represented the pinnacle, the highest level of achievement, the goal to strive for, when it was supposed to represent the smallest portion of the diet.

MyPyramid

As criticism mounted, experts speculated that the Food Guide Pyramid would undergo a major overhaul. In early 2005, MyPyramid was launched as the next generation of the food guidance system (Fig. 8.2). The new symbol has vertical groups and a three-dimensional shape that depicts physical activity on the side. MyPyramid actually represents 12 customized pyramids of the food intake patterns from the Dietary Guidelines for Americans, each one representing a different calorie level. Total calories provided in the pyramids range from 1000 to 3200 calories in increments of 200 calories (Table 8.1). Visitors to www.MyPyramid.gov enter their age, gender, and usual activity level to see the pyramid most appropriate for their estimated calorie needs.

Like its predecessor, MyPyramid is designed to convey the concepts of variety and moderation. Additional themes incorporated into MyPyramid include proportionality, gradual improvement, personalization, and physical activity. Basic messages appropriate for all Americans appear in colored boxes at the base of MyPyramid (see Fig. 8.2). Two additional boxes discuss the balance between food and physical activity and address the concepts of limiting fat, sugar, and salt. In place of the vague term "servings," daily amounts are specified in cups or ounces—a big improvement over the old Food Guide Pyramid.

Variety

The six different color sections in the pyramid are intended to illustrate that foods from all groups are needed each day for good health. The importance of variety is also demonstrated by the use of subgroups in the grain and vegetable groups. For instance, in addition to recommending a specific amount of vegetables per day, MyPyramid also suggests a weekly breakdown of types of vegetables to consume to ensure variety and nutritional adequacy.

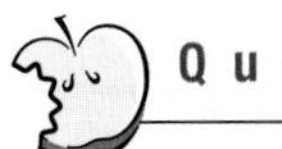

Quick Bite

For someone needing 2000 calories/day, the recommendation is to:

Consume 2½ cups of vegetables daily, with further guidance to eat:

- **3 cups/week of dark green vegetables**
- **2 cups/week of orange vegetables**
- **3 cups/week of legumes**
- **3 cups/week of starchy vegetables**
- **6½ cups/week of other vegetables**

Moderation

Moderation is depicted by the narrowing of each colored section from bottom to top, with the most nutrient-dense foods within each category representing the base of each section and the top of each section occupied by foods with added sugars and/or solid fats.

Proportionality

The varying widths on the bottom of each colored section represent the concept of proportionality, suggesting the proportion each group should contribute to overall in-

PHYSICAL ACTIVITY
30 min – most days
60 min – to prevent weight gain
60-90 min – to sustain weight loss
PEACHES
RAISINS
FAT-FREE MILK
Lowfat Yogurt
1% MILK
TUNA

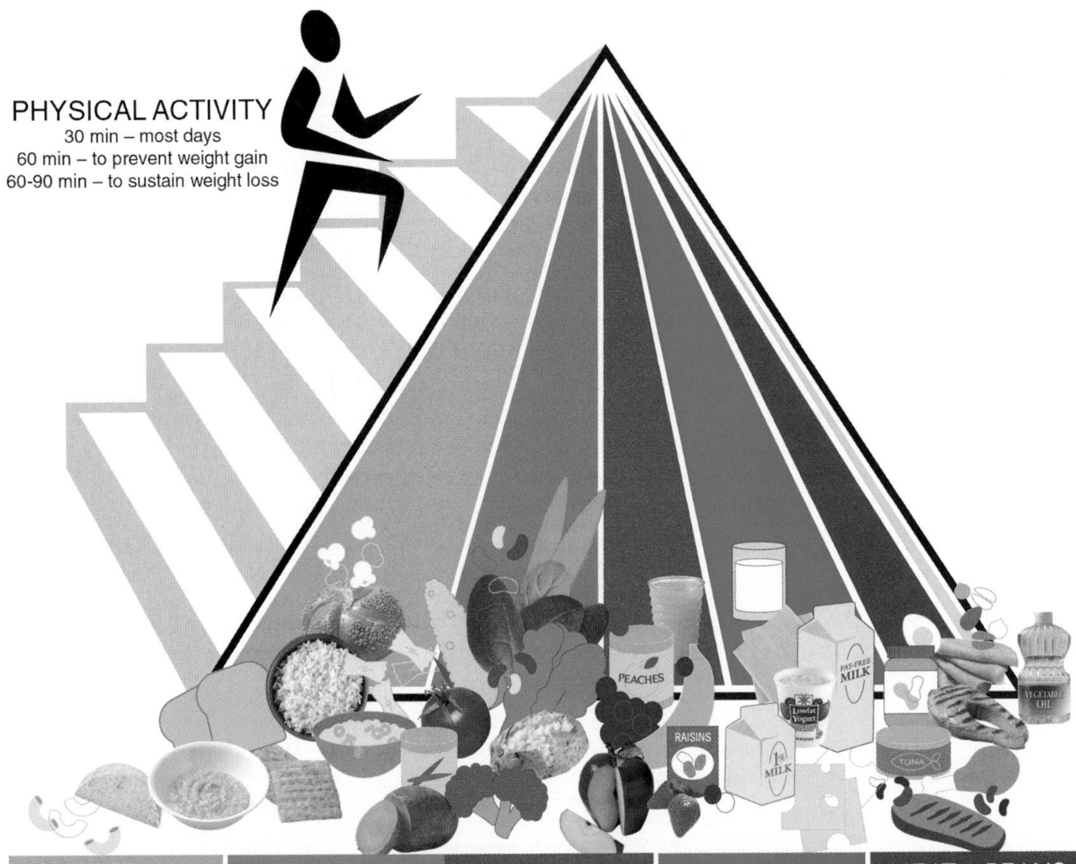

GRAINS Make half your grains whole	VEGETABLES Vary your veggies	FRUITS Focus on fruits	MILK Get your calcium-rich foods	MEAT & BEANS Go lean with protein
Eat at least 3 oz. of whole-grain cereals, breads, crackers, rice, or pasta every day 1 oz. is about 1 slice of bread, about 1 cup of breakfast cereal, or 1/2 cup of cooked rice, cereal, or pasta	Eat more dark-green veggies like broccoli, spinach, and other dark leafy greens Eat more orange vegetables like carrots and sweetpotatoes Eat more dry beans and peas like pinto beans, kidney beans, and lentils	Eat a variety of fruit Choose fresh, frozen, canned, or dried fruit Go easy on fruit juices	Go low-fat or fat-free when you choose milk, yogurt, and other milk products If you don't or can't consume milk, choose lactose-free products or other calcium sources such as fortified foods and beverages	Choose low-fat or lean meats and poultry Bake it, broil it, or grill it Vary your protein routine – choose more fish, beans, peas, nuts, and seeds
For a 2,000-calorie diet, you need the amounts below from each food group. To find the amounts that are right for you, go to MyPyramid.gov.				
Eat 6 oz. every day	Eat 2 1/2 cups every day	Eat 2 cups every day	Get 3 cups every day; for kids aged 2 to 8, it's 2	Eat 5 1/2 oz. every day

Find your balance between food and physical activity

- Be sure to stay within your daily calorie needs.
- Be physically active for at least 30 minutes most days of the week.
- About 60 minutes a day of physical activity may be needed to prevent weight gain.
- For sustaining weight loss, at least 60 to 90 minutes a day of physical activity may be required.
- Children and teenagers should be physically active for 60 minutes every day, or most days.

Know the limits on fats, sugars, and salt (sodium)

- Make most of your fat sources from fish, nuts, and vegetable oils.
- Limit solid fats like butter, margarine, shortening, and lard, as well as foods that contain these.
- Check the Nutrition Facts label to keep saturated fats, *trans* fats, and sodium low.
- Choose food and beverages low in added sugars. Added sugars contribute calories with few, if any, nutrients.

FIGURE 8.2 MyPyramid. (U.S. Department of Agriculture, Center for Nutrition Policy and Promotion, April 2005, CNPP-15.)

TABLE 8.1

FOOD INTAKE PATTERNS AT VARIOUS CALORIE LEVELS

Group	1000	1200	1400	1600	1800	2000	2200	2400	2600	2800	3000	3200
Grain	3 oz eq	4 oz eq	5 oz eq	5 oz eq	6 oz eq	6 oz eq	7 oz eq	8 oz eq	9 oz eq	10 oz eq	10 oz eq	10 oz eq
Vegetables	1 cup	1.5 cups	1.5 cups	2 cups	2.5 cups	2.5 cups	3 cups	3 cups	3.5 cups	3.5 cups	4 cups	4 cups
Fruits	1 cup	1 cup	1.5 cups	1.5 cups	1.5 cups	2 cups	2 cups	2 cups	2 cups	2.5 cups	2.5 cups	2.5 cups
Milk	2 cups	2 cups	2 cups	3 cups	3 cups	3 cups	3 cups	3 cups	3 cups	3 cups	3 cups	3 cups
Meat and Beans	2 oz eq	3 oz eq	4 oz eq	5 oz eq	5 oz eq	5.5 oz eq	6 oz eq	6.5 oz eq	6.5 oz eq	7 oz eq	7 oz eq	7 oz eq
Oils	3 tsp.	4 tsp.	4 tsp.	5 tsp.	5 tsp.	6 tsp.	6 tsp.	7 tsp.	8 tsp.	8 tsp.	10 tsp.	11 tsp.
Discretionary Calorie Allowance*	165	171	171	132	195	267	290	362	410	426	512	648

eq = equivalents

The following are considered 1 oz Grain equivalent:

1 slice of bread
1 cup of ready-to-eat cereal
½ cup cooked rice, pasta, or cooked cereal

1 oz Meat and Bean equivalent is:

1 oz lean meat, poultry, or fish
1 egg
1 tbsp peanut butter
½ cup cooked dry beans
½ oz nuts or seeds

*Discretionary Calorie Allowance is the remaining amount of calories in a food intake pattern after accounting for the calories needed for all food groups, using forms of foods that are fat-free or low-fat and with no added sugars.

take. Specifically, the widest segments represent the grain, vegetables, milk, and fruits groups; meat and beans and oils are depicted by smaller segments. The widths should be interpreted as a general guide, not exact proportions.

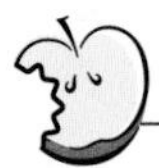

Quick Bite

A comparison between a standard *serving* and a usual *portion* for selected foods

	Standard serving	*Usual portion*
Bagel	½ small	1 large
Pasta	½ cup	2–3 cups
Rice	½ cup	1–2 cups
Orange juice	6 oz	12 oz
Banana	1 small	1 large
Canned tuna	⅓ of a 6 oz can	1 whole 6 oz can
Peanut butter	2 Tbsp	2–4 Tbsp
Chicken	2 oz drumstick	6 oz breast

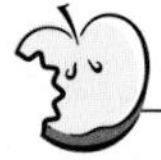

Quick Bite

Portion sizes in terms of common objects

3 oz of meat is approximately the size of a deck of cards.
2 tablespoons of peanut butter are approximately the size of a ping-pong ball.
1 ounce of cheese looks like four dice.
⅓ cup of nuts is a level handful for an adult.
½ cup cooked pasta, rice, or cereal looks like a scoop of ice cream.
1 medium-sized piece of fruit is the size of a baseball.
Eight cherry tomatoes are approximately ½ cup of vegetable as are seven packaged, peeled baby carrots.
15 grapes are approximately ½ cup of fruit.

Gradual Improvement

The slogan "Steps to a Healthier You" suggests gradual improvement that occurs step by step with small daily changes in food choices and physical activity.

Personalization

Personalization is illustrated by the individual on the steps of the pyramid, by the slogan "Steps to a Healthier You," and by the URL of "MyPyramid." Separate gender categories, seven age ranges, and three activity levels resulting in 12 different pyramids ensure personalization.

Physical Activity

For the first time, physical activity is incorporated into the food guidance system. Regular physical activity is recommended on most days of the week, ranging from

30 minutes/day for fitness and to lower the risk of chronic diseases to 60 to 90 minutes/day to sustain weight loss among people who have lost weight.

The MyPyramid website provides interactive features and a wealth of information for consumers, professionals, and kids. A sampling of the pages available includes:

- www.mypyramid.gov/downloads/MiniPoster.pdf. The basic messages of healthy eating and physical activity are discussed here.
- www.mypyramid.gov/professionals/food_tracking_wksht.html. From here, consumers can print a personalized mini-poster and worksheet they can use to track their own progress and set individual goals.
- www.mypyramid.gov/pyramid/index.html. Details about each food group, discretionary calories, and physical activity are found here.
- www.mypyramidtracker.gov. From this page, consumers can obtain a detailed assessment and analysis of their current eating and physical activity habits.

Career Connection

To customize the food guidance system for individual clients:

- **Identify one or two major messages of the Guidelines that target the client's primary health concerns. Because the nine messages are interrelated, other recommendations may be simultaneously met. Tackling all nine messages at once can lead to paralyzing information overload.**
- **Discuss the concept of discretionary calories, which gives the client flexibility to choose less-than-spectacular choices within food groups or to add "extras" for their taste and enjoyment factor. Emphasize that the allowance is small—only 150 to 300 calories, depending on the individual's total calorie requirements.**
- **Encourage clients to visit www.MyPyramid.gov to take advantage of the resources and interactive features.**

Other Tools

While the old Food Guide Pyramid was still in use, several other food guidance systems were created by researchers, universities, and health organizations to more accurately illustrate current research findings on diet and health. Two examples of other tools are the Alternative Health Eating Index (Table 8.2) and the Healthy Eating Pyramid (Fig. 8-3). Both tools feature specific dietary patterns and eating behaviors consistently associated with lower chronic disease risk based on epidemiological and clinical studies. After rigorously studying the diets of more than 100,000 men and women, researchers found that those whose diets most closely followed the AHEI guidelines and the Healthy Eating Pyramid lowered their risk of cardiovascular disease by 39% and 28%, respectively. Time will tell if MyPyramid is as effective at improving the health of Americans.

Healthy Eating Pyramid

The Healthy Eating Pyramid, created by nutrition researchers at the Harvard School of Public Health, offers sound advice on eating based on the latest scientific evidence

TABLE 8.2

ALTERNATE HEALTHY EATING INDEX: COMPONENTS, "IDEAL" INTAKES, AND RATIONALE

Component	"Ideal" Intake	Rationale
Vegetables	5 servings/day	Vegetable intake is associated with reduced risk of chronic disease; French fries were excluded because they have not been linked to lower disease risk.
Fruit	4 servings/day	Fruit intake is associated with decreased risk of CVD and cancer.
Nuts and soy protein	Combined average of 1 serving/day	Nuts and soy protein have been associated with lower rates of CVD; their relation to cancer is inconclusive.
Ratio of white meat to red meat	≥ 4:1 A maximum score was given to vegetarians and to people who eat red meat < 2 times/month	White meat is poultry or fish; white meat is associated with lower rates of CHD and cancer. Red meat is beef, pork, lamb, and processed meats; red meat, particularly processed meat, is associated with an increased risk of certain cancers.
Cereal fiber	15 g/day	Fiber from grains is associated with decreased risk of CHD and stroke; the relation with cancer is less clear.
Trans fat	≤ 0.5% of total calories	Trans fats raise LDL cholesterol, lower HDL, and are associated with increased risk of CHD.
P:S ratio (ratio of polyunsaturated fat to saturated fat)	≥ 1	A higher P:S is generally associated with lower risk of CHD, although n-3 and n-6 polyunsaturated fatty acids have different metabolic effects.
Duration of multivitamin use	≥ 5 years	Multivitamins contain folic acid, vitamin B_6, and other nutrients. Long-term folic acid is associated with lower risk of CHD and cancer.
Alcohol	Men: 1.5–2.5 drinks/day Women: .5–1.5 drinks/day	Moderate alcohol consumption is associated with substantially lower risk of CVD.

McCullough, M., Feskanich, D., Stampfer, M, et al. (2002). Diet quality and major chronic disease risk in men and women: moving toward improved dietary guidance. *American Journal of Clinical Nutrition, 76,* 1261–1271.

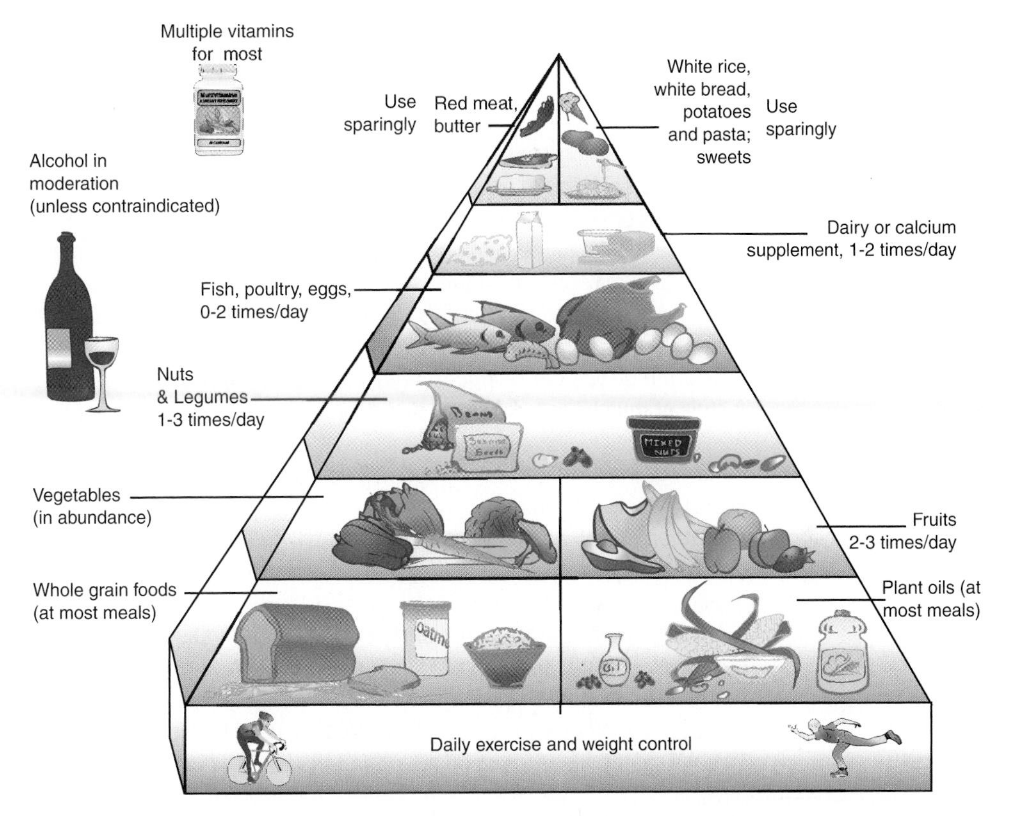

FIGURE 8.3 Healthy Eating Pyramid. (Reprinted with the permission of Simon & Schuster Adult Publishing Group from *Eat, drink and be healthy: The Harvard Medical School guide to healthy eating* by Walter C. Willett, M.D. Copyright © 2001 by President and Fellows of Harvard College.)

on the relationship between diet and disease. In fact, they believe that the risk of premature heart disease, type 2 diabetes, and colon cancers can be lowered by 70 to 90% with modest changes in diet and lifestyle as reflected in the Healthy Eating Pyramid (see Fig. 8.3). Notable features from the bottom up include the following:

- Daily exercise and weight control form the foundation of the pyramid. Both factors strongly influence health and what and how people eat.
- Whole grains are recommended daily; their fiber content helps to keep blood glucose levels from rising and falling too quickly. Better glycemic control may help to prevent the development of diabetes.
- Plant oils occupy the same level as whole grains. The average American consumes approximately 30% of total calories from fat, so placing fat near the bottom of the pyramid is realistic. A crucial point is that the recommendation specifies plant oils, not fat in general. Almost all plant oils are low in saturated fat and canola oil is a source of plant n-3 fatty acids.

Career Connection

To zero in on how well your client adheres to current concepts of healthy eating, ask specific questions about amounts and types of foods consumed such as

- ***How many servings of fruits and vegetables do you eat daily?*** Not only do fruits and vegetables provide an array of essential nutrients, fiber, and phytochemicals, but eating recommended amounts of plant foods helps to ensure a moderate fat intake. An optimum intake may be 8 to 10 total servings/day.
- ***What types of bread and cereals do you use?*** Without whole-grain bread and high-fiber cereals it may be difficult to achieve the recommended intake of fiber.
- ***How often do you eat red meat (beef, lamb, pork) and what is the usual portion size?*** A "rule of thumb" assumption is that people who eat red meat more than four times per week are least likely to be following a low-fat eating plan. Less frequent consumption is better; "use sparingly" may be optimal. Portion size should be approximately 3 oz or the size of a deck of cards.
- ***How often do you eat nuts and soy products?*** Both items may help to lower the risk of heart disease. The goal is that they are eaten once daily *in place of meat* as a source of protein.
- ***What kind of margarine or butter do you use?*** Soft, trans fat-free tub margarines are healthiest. Butter is high in saturated fat and contains cholesterol; hard stick margarine has heart-unhealthy trans-fatty acids.
- ***What type of oil do you use at home?*** Most oil used by the food industry as an ingredient in prepared foods is soy oil; therefore, the best oils to use at home are canola and olive.
- ***How frequently and how much alcohol do you drink?*** Although moderate alcohol consumption may help to protect against heart disease, higher intakes are associated with increased risks of cancer, liver diseases, and accidental death. From a nutritional standpoint, heavy alcohol consumption interferes with nutrient intake, metabolism, and excretion, and, therefore, is a risk factor for nutritional problems.
- ***Do you take a multivitamin, multimineral supplement?*** Certain nutrients in certain populations are best obtained through fortified foods or supplements, such as folic acid for women of childbearing age and vitamin B_{12} for people over 50. For general use, a multivitamin provides some insurance against day to day variations in nutrient intake.

Some additional revealing questions not tied to the Alternate Healthy Eating Index are

- ***How many hours of television do you watch daily?*** The longer the time spent watching television, the less time available to participate in physical activities. There is a correlation between television watching and obesity, especially among children who watch for longer than 2 hours daily.
- ***How much milk do you drink daily and what type do you consume?*** Two percent and whole milk provide unhealthy saturated fat. The DASH diet (see Chapter 18) recommends three servings of low-fat or fat-free milk and dairy products daily in contrast to the Healthy Eating Pyramid which recommends only one to two servings daily. People who do not consume ample amounts of milk and yogurt need a calcium supplement.

Career Connection (Continued)

- ***How often do you eat desserts and sweets?*** **Most desserts and sweets are empty calories—calories from fat and sugar with few nutrients.**
- ***What types of beverages do you consume?*** **Sugar-sweetened carbonated beverages are "liquid candy;" sweetened juices are basically no better. One 12 oz can of soda/day leads to a 15-pound weight gain in a year if it is not offset by a decrease in calories or an increase in physical activity.**
- ***How many meals per week do you eat away from home?*** **Generally, foods prepared outside the home are higher in fat, calories, and sodium and lower in fiber and nutrients than home-prepared meals. Restaurant portions usually exceed recommended portion sizes and selections of whole grains, fruits, and vegetables may be limited.**

- Vegetables are recommended in abundance and fruit two to three times daily. Diets rich in fruit and vegetables decrease the risk of heart disease, certain cancers, hypertension, cataracts, and macular degeneration.
- Nuts and legumes are recommended up to three times daily; they are excellent sources of protein, fiber, vitamins, and minerals. Nuts contain heart healthy fats.
- Fish, poultry, and eggs are recommended zero to two times daily as important sources of protein. Fish, especially fatty fish, is associated with a decreased risk of heart disease and arrhythmias. Skinless poultry is low in saturated fat and Harvard researchers state that eggs are not as damaging as once believed.
- Dairy or calcium supplement is recommended one to two times daily. Nonfat or low-fat versions are advised for people who like dairy products. For others, supplements are recommended to obtain adequate calcium.
- Red meat and butter occupy half the apex of the pyramid. They should be used sparingly because they are loaded with saturated fat.
- White rice, white bread, potatoes, pasta, and sweets are also at the apex of the pyramid. They are recommended sparingly based on the rationale that they cause rapid rises in blood glucose levels that can lead to diabetes, heart disease, and other chronic disorders.
- A daily multivitamin, multimineral supplement is recommended as insurance against less than perfect eating.
- Alcohol is advised in moderation unless contraindicated. Moderation is defined as one to two drinks/day for men and no more than one drink/day for women. Moderate alcohol consumption lowers the risk of heart disease.

Harvard researchers believe their Healthy Eating Pyramid reflects the best dietary advice available today. Yet some experts raise legitimate questions:

- Will putting plant fats at the bottom of the pyramid lead to an excess of calories? All fat—whether from plants or animals—is calorically dense. At 130 calories/tablespoon, the calories in oil add up quickly.
- Shouldn't "plant oils" be more precisely defined to mean oils with the best n-6 to n-3 fatty acid ratio such as canola oil and flaxseed? Americans already get plenty of n-6 but not nearly the recommended amount of n-3 fatty acids.

- Won't limiting dairy products to one to two times/day shortchange Americans from essential nutrients? Granted, calcium can be obtained from calcium supplements, but those supplements may or may not provide vitamin D and lack riboflavin, protein, potassium and other nutrients found in milk. The DASH diet, which has been found to lower blood pressure, recommends three daily servings of milk or lowfat dairy products (see Chapter 18).
- Are white bread, white rice, and pasta really the nutritional equivalent of sweets? Is it wise to condemn white rice when more than a billion people live on it and maintain superior health? The assumption that all refined carbohydrates are "bad" because they have a high glycemic index and all whole grain carbohydrates are "good" because they have a low glycemic index is oversimplified. For instance, all bread, whether whole grain or white, usually has a high glycemic index because the flour is finely ground. Pasta has a low glycemic index, whether made from whole wheat flour or white flour, but there are variations related to the shape: thin linguine has a higher glycemic index than thick linguine. A food's glycemic index is influenced by many variables, including how that food is processed, stored, ripened, cut, and cooked. There are reasons for limiting refined carbohydrates, such as the lack of fiber and lower amounts of nutrients and phytochemicals than whole grain carbohydrates, but glycemic index may not be one of them, at least in a practical sense. In their latest nutrition recommendations, even the American Diabetes Association discounts the usefulness of glycemic index in managing blood glucose levels (see Chapter 19).

No doubt the Healthy Eating Pyramid will require modification as our knowledge of diet and disease grows. For now, it may be the best tool available to help people improve their diets.

Food Guide Graphics in Other Countries

The Food Guide Pyramid is pervasive in the United States, appearing on food packages, grocery bags, and nutrition education materials. Yet because of cultural differences in communicating symbolism and other cultural norms, the pyramid shape is not necessarily superior or even appropriate for food guides in other countries. A circle or dinner plate with each section depicting relative proportion to the total diet is used by many countries, including the United Kingdom (Fig. 8.4), Germany, Australia, and Mexico. Korea and China use a pagoda shape and Canada uses a rainbow shape (Fig. 8.5). Japan does not have an official food guide illustration. Despite the differences in the shape of the graphics, the core recommendations are consistently similar: consume large amounts of grains, vegetables, and fruit and moderate amounts of milk, dairy products, and meat.

Recommendations From Health Agencies

Many health agencies publish guidelines or recommendations for healthy eating such as the American Heart Association, the American Cancer Society, and the American Institute of Cancer Research. Even though they are written from different health perspectives, the recommendations are remarkably similar (Box 8.2). Nutrition recommendations for the primary and secondary prevention of coronary heart disease are detailed in Chapter 18. Table 8.3 summarizes nutrition interventions that may decrease the risk of specific cancers.

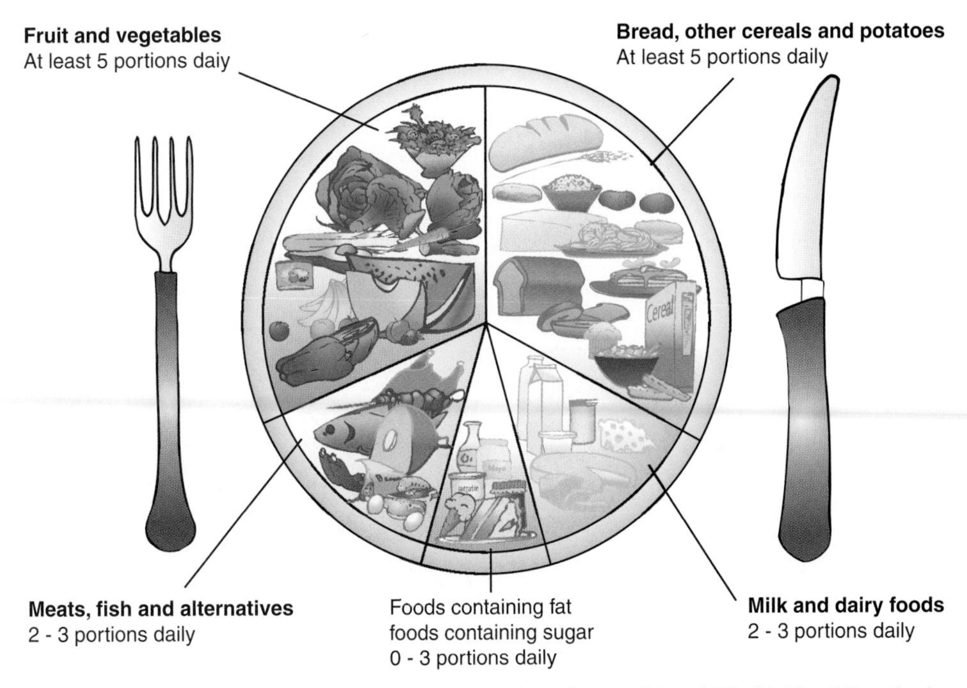

FIGURE 8.4 Great Britain's food guide: The Balance of Good Health Food Standards Agency (UK).

The New American Plate is a campaign by the American Institute of Cancer Research to teach Americans how to implement their diet guidelines using a dinner plate as a visual aid (Fig. 8.6). It is based on recommendations stemming from a comprehensive landmark report entitled *Food Nutrition and the Prevention of Cancer: A global perspective* that was based on more then 4500 research studies from around the world. The report estimates that 30 to 40% of all cancers could be prevented by changes in intake and activity. The guidelines are illustrated by a plate of food that is two-thirds or more covered with plants (fruit, vegetables, whole grains, and dried peas and beans) and one-third or less devoted to animal protein (fish, poultry, meat, low-fat dairy products). Additional recommendations regarding physical activity and weight management are discussed.

At Least Two-Thirds Plants

Plant foods contain a variety of antioxidant vitamins, minerals, phytochemicals, and fibers that are believed to be protective against cancer. Different plants have different types and combinations of protective substances. Because it is not known which substances have the greatest impact on cancer prevention, variety is important. The plant-based part of the plate should include

- Substantial portions of one or more fruits and vegetables. Research suggests that 20% of all cancers could be prevented if Americans ate at least five servings of fruits and vegetables daily. Dark green leafy vegetables and deep orange vegetables are recommended as are citrus fruits and other rich sources of vitamin C.

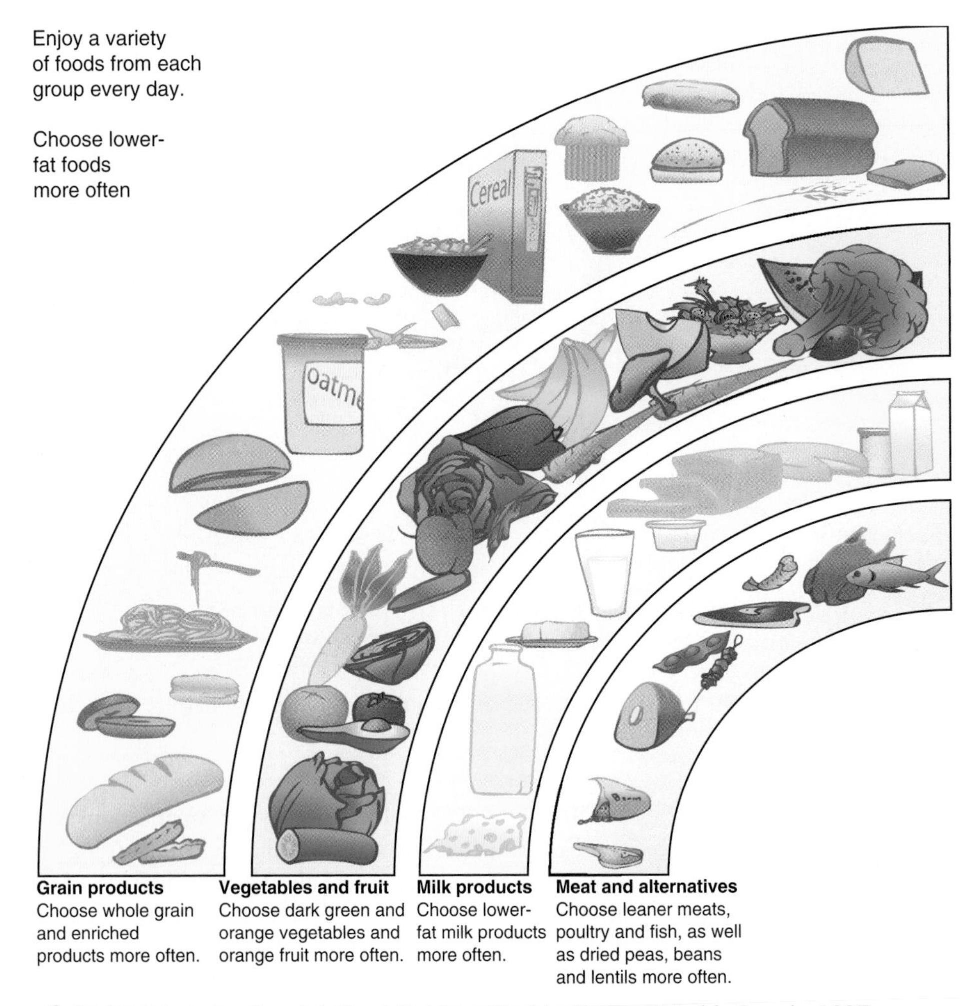

FIGURE 8.5 Canada's Food Guide to Healthy Eating. (Health Canada, 1997. Reproduced with the permission of the Minister of Public Works and Government Services Canada, 2004.)

According to the AICR, fruit juice does *not* count toward the goal of at least five servings of fruits and vegetables daily.

- Whole grain products daily and dried peas and beans. At least seven servings of these plant foods are recommended daily.
- Items that are not prepared with extra fat such as vegetables covered in cheese sauce, full fat salad dressing, regular sour cream, or butter and deep fried vegetables. Healthier alternatives to enhance the flavor of vegetables include herbs, spices, flavored vinegar, fresh lemon juice, salsa, marinara sauce, mustard, and light soy sauce. Baking, broiling, steaming, microwaving, and stir-fry are low fat methods of preparation.

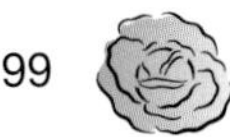

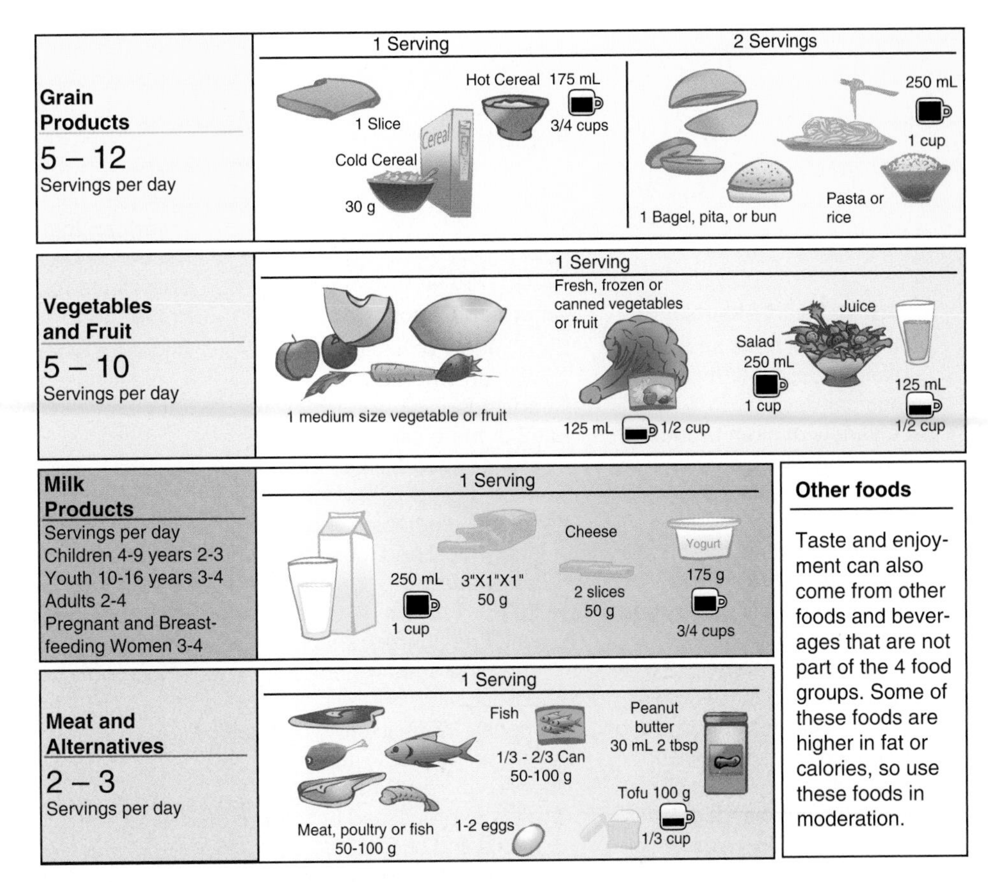

Different people need different amounts of food

The amount of food you need every day from the 4 food groups and other foods depend on your age, body size, activity level, whether you are male or female and if you are pregnant or breast-feeding. That's why the food guide gives a lower and higher number of servings for each food group. For example, young children can choose the lower number of servings, while male teenagers can go to the higher numbers. Most other people can choose servings somewhere in between.

FIGURE 8.5 (Continued)

One-Third or Less From Animal Protein

Because diets high in red meat may increase risk of colon and prostate cancers, consumers are urged to limit their intake of beef, pork, and lamb to no more than 3 oz cooked per day of only lean cuts. No specific limits are set for the intake of poultry, fish, and game other than keeping their place on the plate to less than one-third of the total space. Americans are urged to view meat not as the centerpiece of the meal but more like a side dish or condiment.

Physical Activity and Weight

Physical activity may reduce cancer risk by promoting weight management or avoiding obesity, which is linked to an increased risk for cancers of the colon, esophagus, gallbladder, pancreas, endometrium, kidney, and breast (in postmenopausal women).

BOX 8.2

SUMMARY OF NUTRITION AND LIFESTYLE GUIDELINES FROM THE AMERICAN HEART ASSOCIATION, THE AMERICAN CANCER SOCIETY, AND THE AMERICAN INSTITUTE FOR CANCER RESEARCH

American Heart Association

Eat a variety of fruits and vegetables. Choose 5 or more servings per day.

Eat a variety of grain products including whole grains. Choose 6 or more servings per day.

Include fat-free and low-fat milk products, fish, legumes (beans), skinless poultry and lean meats.

Choose fats and oils with 2 g or less saturated fat per tablespoon such as liquid and tub margarines, canola oil and olive oil.

Balance the number of calories you eat with the number you use each day.

Maintain a level of physical activity that keeps you fit and matches the number of calories you eat. Walk or do other activities for at least 30 minutes on most days.

Limit your intake of foods high in calories or low in nutrition including foods like soft drinks and candy that have a lot of sugars.

Limit foods high in saturated fat, trans fat and/or cholesterol such as full-fat milk products, fatty meats, tropical oils, partially hydrogenated vegetables oils and egg yolks.

American Cancer Society

Eat a variety of healthful foods with an emphasis on plant sources.

Eat 5 or more servings of a variety of vegetables and fruits each day.

- Include vegetables and fruits at every meal and for snacks.
- Eat a variety of vegetables and fruits.
- Limit French fries, snack chips, and other fried vegetables products.
- Choose 100% juice if you drink fruit or vegetable juices.

Choose whole grains in preference to processed (refined) grains and sugars.

- Choose whole grain rice, bread, pasta, and cereals.
- Limit consumption of refined carbohydrates including pastries, sweetened cereals, soft drinks, and sugars.

Limit consumption of red meats, especially those high in fat and processed.

- Choose fish, poultry, or beans as an alternative to beef, pork, and lamb.
- When you eat meat, select lean cuts and smaller portions.
- Prepare meat by baking, broiling, or poaching rather than by frying or charbroiling.

American Institute of Cancer Research Diet and Health Guidelines for Cancer Prevention

Choose a diet rich in a variety of plant-based foods.

Eat plenty of vegetables and fruits.

Maintain a healthy weight and be physically active.

Drink alcohol only in moderation, if at all.

Select foods low in fat and salt.

Prepare and store food safely.

And always remember . . . do not use tobacco in any form.

BOX 8.2
(continued)

SUMMARY OF NUTRITION AND LIFESTYLE GUIDELINES FROM THE AMERICAN HEART ASSOCIATION, THE AMERICAN CANCER SOCIETY, AND THE AMERICAN INSTITUTE FOR CANCER RESEARCH

American Heart Association	American Cancer Society	American Institute of Cancer Research Diet and Health Guidelines for Cancer Prevention
Instead choose foods low in saturated fat, trans fat and cholesterol from the first 4 points above. Eat less than 6 g of salt per day (2400 mg of sodium). Have no more than 1 alcoholic drink per day if you're a woman and no more than 2 if you're a man. One drink means is has no more than ½ oz pure alcohol. Examples of 1 drink are 12 oz of beer, 4 oz of wine, 1.5 oz of 80 proof spirits or 1 oz of 100-proof spirits.	Choose foods that help maintain a healthful weight. • When you eat away from home, choose food low in fat, calories, and sugar and avoid large portions. • Eat smaller portions of high-calorie foods. Be aware that "low fat" or "fat free" does not mean "low calorie" and that low-fat cakes, cookies, and similar foods are often high in calories. • Substitute vegetables, fruits, and other low-calorie foods for calorie-dense foods such as French fries, cheeseburgers, pizza, ice cream, doughnuts, and other sweets. Adopt a physically active lifestyle. Maintain a healthful weight throughout life. If you drink alcoholic beverages, limit consumption to no more than 2 drinks/day for men and 1 drink/day for women.	

TABLE 8.3 **DIETARY AND LIFESTYLE INTERVENTIONS THAT MAY REDUCE THE RISK OF CERTAIN CANCERS**

Bladder	Increase fluid intake. Increase intake of vegetables.
Breast	Limit alcohol intake to no more than 1 drink/day. Avoid obesity. Exercise vigorously at least 4 hours/week.
Colorectal	Increase physical activity. Increase fruit and vegetable intake. Limit red meat consumption. Avoid obesity. Avoid excessive alcohol.
Endometrial	Maintain healthy weight through diet and regular physical activity.
Kidney	Avoid becoming overweight.
Lung	Don't smoke. Eat at least 5 servings of fruits and vegetables daily.
Oral and esophageal	Avoid tobacco in any form. Limit alcohol intake. Avoid obesity. Eat at least 5 servings of fruits and vegetables daily.
Ovarian	Fruits and vegetables may lower risk.
Pancreatic	Avoid tobacco. Maintain healthy weight. Be physically active. Eat at least 5 servings of fruits and vegetables daily.
Prostate	Limit the intake of red meat and full fat (dairy products.) Eat at least 5 servings of fruits and vegetables daily. Studies suggest that diets high in certain vegetables, namely tomatoes and dried peas and beans, may lower prostate risk.
Stomach	Eat at least 5 servings of fruits and vegetables daily.

Career Connection

For clients who are ready to move toward a healthier lifestyle:

- Encourage the client to focus on only one behavior he/she wants to change and make a plan as to how to achieve that goal. For instance, if the client's goal is to eat more vegetables, potential actions may be to take mini carrots and low-fat dip to work for a mid-afternoon snack, eat a salad at dinner every night, double up on the normal vegetable portion at dinner, and eat a veggie burger for lunch every other day.
- Provide positive, proactive, and practical messages. In other words, emphasize what *can* be done, not what *shouldn't* be done.
- Tailor messages to meet the individual's needs within the cultural and social context.
- Emphasize food choices over time, not individual nutrients or individual foods.
- Encourage clients to obtain the nutrients they need from food, not supplements. Supplements are intended to add to, not to replace, food.
- Encourage more physical activity as a complement to healthy eating.

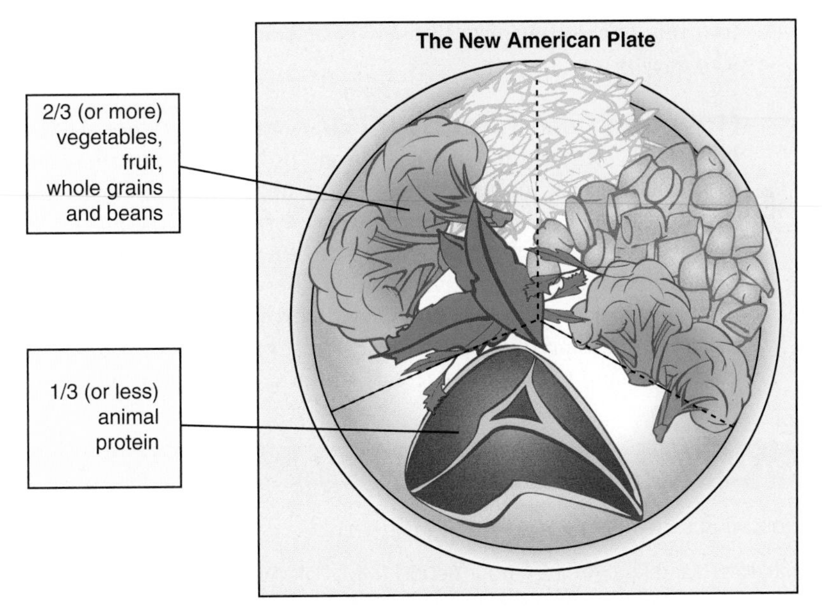

FIGURE 8.6 The New American Plate. Start reshaping your diet by looking at your plate. Is the greater proportion of your meal plant based? Are your portion sizes appropriate to your activity level? (Reprinted with permission from the American Institute for Cancer Research.)

Physical activity may also reduce risk by other mechanisms. For instance, it may reduce colon cancer risk by stimulating peristalsis, which decreases the amount of time potentially harmful substances are in the bowel. Physical activity may reduce the risk of breast cancer by influencing hormone levels. According to the AICR, 1 hour of brisk physical activity every day plus 1 hour per week of more vigorous exercise is needed to reduce the risk of cancer. However, any exercise is better than no exercise at all.

How Do You Respond?

Which foods are "good"? Which foods are "bad"? Instead of thinking as individual foods as "good" or "bad," consider how a food fits within the context of the total intake. For instance, broccoli is among the best plant foods available, yet if someone ate only broccoli all day long, it would not be "good" because it does not supply adequate amounts of all essential nutrients for health. Likewise, a chocolate candy kiss is certainly not "bad" if a person's intake consists of adequate amounts of healthful foods, calorie intake is appropriate for optimal weight, and the person engages in regular physical activity. What matters is how often a particular food is eaten, what size the portion is, *why* a particular food is eaten (e.g., by choice or from mindless eating), and overall calorie balance. If most of a person's intake is of healthful foods, small amounts of less-than-healthful choices can fit into the diet without wreaking great havoc as long as total calorie intake is appropriate. The keys to fitting in less-than-healthful foods are to eat them *infrequently, in small amounts, and by conscious decision.*

How can I eat healthy if I don't like whole wheat bread? Just as there are no "good" or "bad" foods, there is not one particular food you *must* eat in order to be healthy nor is there one particular food you *must never* eat to be healthy. Instead of whole wheat bread, consider whole wheat bagels or tortillas made with whole wheat flour for sandwiches and wraps. "Low-calorie" breads are another alternative; although they lack the phytochemicals, vitamins, and minerals of whole wheat bread, they do provide generous amounts of fiber added in place of some starch. Besides whole wheat bread, other sources of insoluble fiber include bran and whole grain cereals and dried peas and beans.

▲ Focus on Critical Thinking

Respond to the following statements:

1. Comparing someone's intake over a 24-hour period to MyPyramid recommendations is an accurate and reliable way of determining if a healthy diet is being consumed.
2. Scoring high in the Healthy Eating Index does not necessarily mean that a person's risk of chronic disease is lowered.
3. It would be easy for most Americans to change their perception of meat as the main entrée to meat as a side dish or condiment.

Key Concepts

- A healthy diet provides optimal amounts of all essential nutrients to prevent deficiency symptoms and not excessive amounts that may cause nutrient toxicities or increase the risk chronic diseases such as heart disease, cancer, and hypertension.
- Dietary Reference Intakes are a set of reference values: the new RDAs, Estimated Average Requirement, Adequate Intakes, and Tolerable Upper Limit. Individual nutrients do not have each of these reference values; a nutrient has either an EAR plus RDA or an AI. Upper limits are not established for all nutrients.
- The RDAs are amounts of essential nutrients considered adequate to meet the nutritional needs of 97 to 98% of healthy people in a gender/lifestage group. The AI are similar to the RDA but it is not known what percentage of people are meeting nutritional needs by consuming the AI.
- Tolerable Upper Limit is the highest intake of a nutrient over time that does not pose a risk. There is no benefit to consuming amounts between the RDA and UL of a nutrient.
- The DRIs are primarily for professional use because they deal with quantities of nutrients as opposed to amounts of food.
- The Dietary Guidelines for Americans are intended to help the public choose diets that are nutritionally adequate, promote health, and reduce the risk of chronic disease. They are revised every 5 years.
- The major messages conveyed by the Dietary Guidelines for Americans are to consume a variety of foods while staying within calorie needs; control calorie intake to manage body weight; be physically active every day; increase intake of fruits, vegetables, whole grains, and non-fat or low-fat milk and milk products; choose fats wisely; choose carbohydrates wisely; choose and prepare foods with little salt; if you drink alcohol, do so in moderation; and keep food safe to eat.
- MyPyramid is the newest generation of the graphic illustration of the Dietary Guidelines for Americans. To emphasize a personal approach to healthy eating and physical activity, MyPyramid is actually a series of pyramids providing different calorie levels for individualization based on a person's age, gender, and level of activity. MyPyramid is designed to convey the concepts of daily physical activity, moderation, personalization, proportionality, variety, and gradual improvement.
- A Healthy Eating Pyramid has been devised by researchers at Harvard University's School of Public Health. It is divided horizontally, with exercise and weight control serving as the foundation and whole grain foods and plant oils occupying the next tier. Nuts and legumes comprise their own group, as do fish, poultry and eggs. Dairy or a calcium supplement is recommended only 1 to 2 times/day; red meat and butter as well as white rice, white bread, potatoes, pasta, and sweets occupy the apex. Additional recommendations include alcohol in moderation (unless contraindicated) and a multivitamin for most people.
- An Adjusted Healthy Eating Index shows that adhering to the Healthy Eating Pyramid significantly reduces the risk of chronic disease.
- The pyramidal shape is not necessarily superior to other food guide graphics. Circles, a rainbow, a pagoda, and a plate are used as food graphics in other coun-

tries. Worldwide, food guides consistently recommend a high intake of grains, fruits, and vegetables.

- The American Heart Association, the American Cancer Society, and the American Institute for Cancer Research each recommend a plant-based diet to reduce the risk of chronic disease. The New American Plate, a nutrition campaign of the American Institute for Cancer Research, uses a plate to depict how a plant-based diet is achieved. It recommends two-thirds or more of the plate be devoted to plant foods and ⅓ or less feature animal protein.

ANSWER KEY

1. **TRUE** The RDAs are intended for healthy people only.
2. **FALSE** The DRIs are most often used by dietitians to plan and evaluate menus and by researchers studying nutrition. Because they focus on nutrients, not foods, they are of limited value in teaching people how to choose healthy diets.
3. **FALSE** The Tolerable Upper Intake Level is the highest intake of a nutrient that does not produce any adverse effects. There is no advantage in consuming amounts greater than the RDA.
4. **TRUE** The Dietary Guidelines for Americans are intended to promote wellness and decrease the risk of chronic disease in healthy Americans 2 years of age and older.
5. **TRUE** MyPyramid, like its predecessor, is the graphic designed to illustrate the Dietary Guidelines for Americans.
6. **TRUE** MyPyramid is actually a group of 12 different pyramids so that dietary advice can be personalized for a person's gender, age, and activity patterns.
7. **FALSE** Unlike its predecessor, MyPyramid specifies how many cups or ounces a person should consume from each group instead of using the vague term "servings."
8. **FALSE** There are differences in the nutritional value among different sources of carbohydrates and differences in the nutritional value of different fats. It is too simplistic to tell someone to eat a "high carbohydrate" or "moderate fat" diet without specifying the types of carbohydrates and fats that are recommended for optimal health.
9. **TRUE** MyPyramid recommends at least 30 minutes of physical activity on most days of the week. More than 30 minutes of activity may be needed to prevent weight gain or sustain weight loss.
10. **TRUE** Research suggests that 30 to 40% of all cancers could be prevented by changes in intake and activity. Eating at least five servings of fruits and vegetables daily may prevent at least 20% of all cancers.

WEBSITES

A comparison of international food guide pictorial representations is available at **www.eatright.org/images/journal/0402/commentary.pdf**
American Cancer Society at **www.cancer.org**
American Heart Association at **www.americanheart.org**
American Institute for Cancer Research at **www.aicr.org**
Analyze and compare your intake nutrients based on the RDAs for your gender and lifestage at **www.dietsite.com.**

An interactive Healthy Eating Index that enables the user to obtain a "score" for their diet quality based on five elements of the Dietary Guidelines and the five Food Guide Pyramid groups is available at **www.usda.gov/cnpp.**
Dietary Reference Intakes from the National Academy Press are found at **www.nap.edu**
Dietary Guidelines for Americans at **www.healthierus.gov/dietaryguidelines**
Healthy Eating Pyramid from Harvard School of Public Health at **www.hsph.harvard.edu**
MyPyramid: Steps to a Healthier You at **www.mypyramid.gov**

REFERENCES

American Cancer Society. (2002). *The complete guide—nutrition and physical activity.* Available at www.cancer.org. Accessed on 12/17/03.

American Dietetic Association. (2002). Position of the American Dietetic Association: Total diet approach to communicating food and nutrition information. *Journal of the American Dietetic Association, 102,* 100–108.

American Heart Association. *Dietary guidelines.* Available at www.americanheart.org. Accessed on 1/15/04.

American Institute for Cancer Research. (2002). *The new American plate. Meals for a healthy weight and a healthy life.* Available at www.aicr.org/brochures/napbook.htm. Accessed on 3/14/04.

Barr, S., Marphy, S., & Poos, M. (2002). Interpreting and using the Dietary References Intakes in dietary assessment of individuals and groups. *Journal of the American Dietetic Association, 102,* 780–788.

Cowley, G. (2003). A better way to eat. *Newsweek.* Jan 20, 46–54.

Harvard School of Public Health. (2002). *New alternative to U.S. Department of Agriculture Dietary Guidelines nearly twice as effective in reducing risk for major chronic disease.* Available at www.hsph.harvard.edu/press/releases/press11212202.html. Accessed on 3/10/04.

International Food Information Council. (2002). *Dietary Reference Intakes: An update.* Available at www.ific.org/publications/. Accessed on 3/8/04.

Liebman, B. (2004). Weighing the diet books. *Nutrition Action Health Letter, 31*(1), 1, 3–8.

McCullough, M., Feskanich, D., Stampfer, M., et al. (2002). Dietary quality and major chronic disease risk in men and women: Moving toward improved dietary guidance. *American Journal of Clinical Nutrition, 76,* 1261–1271.

Morton, C. (2003). Forum explores how and why to change eating patterns for better health. *Harvard Public Health NOW.* Available at www.hsph.harvard.edu/now/act3/formu.html Accessed on 3/10/04.

Nutrition Australia. (2003). *Dietary guidelines for adults in Australia.* Available at www.nutritionaustralia.org. Accessed on 3/8/04.

Painter, J., Rah, J.-H., & Lee, Y.-K. (2002). Comparison of international food guide pictorial representations. *Journal of the American Dietetic Association, 102,* 483–489.

United States Department of Agriculture. (2003). *Questions and answers about the food guide pyramid.* Available at www.usda.gov/news/releases/2003/09/qa0308.htm. Accessed on 3/10/04.

United States Department of Agriculture, Center for Nutrition Policy and Promotion. (2005). MyPyramid—Steps to a Healthier You Food Guidance System. Available at www.MyPyramid.gov.

United States Department of Health and Human Services, United States Department of Agriculture. (2005). *Dietary Guidelines for Americans* (7th ed.). Available at www.healthierus.gov/dietaryguidelines.

Willett, W. (2001). *Eat, drink, and be healthy.* New York: Simon & Schuster.

For information on the new dietary guidelines 2005 and MyPyramid, visit **http://connection.lww.com/go/dudek**

9

Consumer Issues

TRUE	FALSE	
⬭	⬭	**1** If a food misconception is harmless, it should be respected.
⬭	⬭	**2** The serving sizes listed on the Nutrition Facts label are based on amounts typically eaten.
⬭	⬭	**3** The % Daily Value listed on the Nutrition Facts label is based on a 2000-calorie diet.
⬭	⬭	**4** Structure/function claims that appear on food labels are accurate and reliable.
⬭	⬭	**5** Supplement manufacturers must prove that their products are safe and effective before they can be marketed.
⬭	⬭	**6** Supplement manufacturers must list potential side effects on the label.
⬭	⬭	**7** Organically grown foods are nutritionally superior to their conventionally raised counterparts.
⬭	⬭	**8** Bacteria cause the majority of foodborne illnesses.
⬭	⬭	**9** Genetically modified food is to be used with caution.
⬭	⬭	**10** Irradiated food contains small amounts of radioactive substances.

UPON COMPLETION OF THIS CHAPTER, YOU WILL BE ABLE TO

- Discuss why clients are often confused about nutrition messages.
- List six signs that may indicate a nutrition or health claim is not credible.
- Describe how to use food labels to make better food choices.
- Discuss how the regulation and marketing of dietary supplements differs from drugs.
- List three tips for supplement users.
- Name five ways to help retain the nutritional value of food.
- Name five functional foods.
- Describe how each functional food may improve health.
- Discuss what "organically grown" means.
- Describe four simple steps to keep food safe.
- Explain how food is genetically modified.
- Explain why some foods are irradiated.

It is a new age in nutrition. The proliferation of cyberspace information—and misinformation—gives millions of Americans ready access to nutritional concepts. Advances in food technology have brought us functional foods, bioengineering, and food irradiation as well as new questions about food safety and optimal nutrition. The ever-evolving science of nutrition has taken us from three square meals a day and a well-rounded diet to MyPyramid. A baby boomer's inspired quest for health and eternal youth has thrust nutrition into the spotlight not only as a means to prevent chronic health problems but also as a way to delay aging. This is an era that presents old and new challenges for health professionals.

This chapter explores how to identify and combat nutrition misinformation, with emphasis placed on how to read a food label. Dietary supplements are discussed. Consumer issues regarding food quality and safety are presented, namely organic foods, functional foods, foodborne illnesses, biotechnology, and irradiation.

INFORMATION AND MISINFORMATION

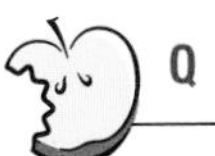

Quick Bite

Where Americans turn for nutrition information

Source	%
Television	48%
Magazines	47%
Newspapers	18%
Books	12%
Doctors	11%
Friends and family	11%
Dietitians and nutritionists	1%

Source: American Dietetic Association (2002). Position of the American Dietetic Association: Food and nutrition misinformation. *Journal of the American Dietetic Association, 102,* 260–266.

Americans have a big appetite for news on food and health, especially about the role particular foods may have in protecting health. Yet consumers are often confused by nutrition messages; what seems like fact today is often considered fiction tomorrow. It is said that the half-life of nutrition information is 3 years. In other words, 3 years from now, half of what we know about nutrition today will be out of date. For instance, between 1980 and 1995 the advice about dietary fat evolved from eat a low-fat diet to a low–saturated fat diet to a low–trans fat diet. Since then our fat phobia has given way to the current carbohydrate craze. In short, Americans recognize that nutrition is important but are confused about what to eat.

Judging Reliability

To protect yourself and your clients from misinformation, be cautious and skeptical about what you hear and read about nutrition. Resist jumping on the latest bandwagon until all the evidence is critically examined. Keep in mind that headlines sell but the bottom line, which is usually less sensational, may be buried deep in the article, the part least likely to be read. Ask yourself the age-old questions—who, what, when, where, and why—to test the validity and reliability of nutrition "news."

Who? Who is promoting the message? The name may or may not be important. A celebrity attracts more attention than an unknown spokesperson but may be equally unfit to summarize nutrition reports or provide nutrition advice. Investigate the validity of the author's or website's credentials. A "doctor" with a scientific breakthrough on how to combine foods to speed metabolism may be a doctor of education, theology, or economics. A supplement manufacturer whose website promotes the anti-aging effects of vitamin E is not the best authority on the subject. Look for ethical conflicts of interest. Anyone who stands to benefit economically by promoting a food, supplement, or diet is not likely to be an objective resource.

What? What is the message? Generally, if it sounds too good to be true, it usually is. Box 9.1 lists signs that may indicate that a health or nutrition claim may be fraudulent.

When? When was the study conducted, the results published, the web site updated? Even seemingly legitimate information can become quickly outdated. As previously stated, 3 years is a long time in the life of nutrition data.

Where? Where was the study conducted? Was the site a reputable research institution or an impressive-sounding but unknown facility? Internet addresses ending in .edu (educational institutions), .org (organizations), or .gov (government agencies) are more credible than those ending in .com (commercial), whose main objective may be to sell a product.

Why? Why was the article written—to further the reader's awareness and knowledge or to sell or promote a product? Freedom of speech guarantees Americans the right to express opinions about nutrition, but fraudulent claims cannot be used to advertise a product. Magazines and newsletters that blur the lines between articles and advertisements are misleading but legal. Question objectivity when the author or site has a financial interest in a supposed "breakthrough."

BOX 9.1

SIGNS THAT WHAT YOU READ OR HEAR MAY BE FRAUDULENT

- Claims of a quick-fix and effective cure-all for a wide variety of ills such as "Effective in the treatment of rheumatism, arthritis, infection, prostate problems, cancer, heart disease, and more"
- Promotions that use words like "scientific breakthrough," "miraculous cure," "exclusive formula," "secret formula," "ancient ingredient," "without risk," "all-natural"
- Statements that a product can treat or cure disease
- Undocumented case histories or personal testimonials from doctors that claim incredible results such as "After using this product for 10 days I have lost 25 pounds and I've never felt better. I don't know why I waited so long to try it."
- Statements that the product is available only from one source and only for a limited time
- Claims to be "scientifically proven" or "absolutely safe"
- Promises a no-risk money back guarantee
- Requires pre-payment

Source: Federal Trade Commission, Food and Drug Administration. (2001). "Miracle" health claims: Add a dose of skepticism. Available at: www.ftc.gov/bcp/conline/pubs/health/frdheal.htm. Accessed on 11/6/03.

Combating Nutrition Misinformation

Determining if information is valid and reliable may be easier than persuading a client that he or she has been a victim of hype. Many people assume that anything that appears in print form (e.g., in a book, magazine, or newspaper) is accurate. Not everyone recognizes the shortcomings of the world wide web. Smaller still is the number of people who acknowledge their susceptibility to nutrition fraud. Battling misinformation in a client convinced he or she has the facts requires objectivity, sensitivity, and consistency.

Career Connection

What can I do to combat misinformation?

- **Respect harmless food beliefs that do not financially exploit the client.**
- **Use reputable facts.**
- **Be brief in your explanation.**
- **Keep the message simple and positive.**
- **Don't over promise.**
- **Don't perpetuate the good food/bad food myth; instead, focus on the total diet.**
- **Provide written and verbal documentation about the true facts.**
- **Furnish a list of reputable nutrition resources (see websites for reliable nutrition information at the end of this chapter).**

Objectivity. First of all, the motto is "Do no harm." If clients' beliefs are unsupported but harmless, you may risk alienating them for no reason by waging a war to convince them they're misinformed. For instance, a male client who believes that using wheat germ will increase his libido nevertheless gets risk-free benefits from the fiber, vitamin E, and other nutrients in the wheat germ he consumes. Even though wheat germ does not objectively enhance sexual performance, the placebo effect may accomplish the same result.

Sensitivity. Be sensitive to the client's perspective including lifestyle, preferences, and culture. Determine how much of an emotional investment the client has in believing the misinformation. Casual or judgmental dismissal of misinformation can cause clients to become defensive and distrustful, as can being an alarmist and proclaiming imminent danger. With either scenario, clients may conclude that you are not as up-to-date as they are about nutrition and they may reject you as a credible reference.

Consistency. Client confusion is decreased when nutrition messages are consistent from all members of the health care team. Collaborate with dietetics professionals to stay up to date with current nutrition issues and sound nutrition advice.

One way to combat misinformation is to empower clients with knowledge and skill to make better decisions for themselves such as how to read a food label.

How to Read a Food Label

Reading labels can provide a wealth of information about individual foods and can enable clients to make healthier food choices. Information provided on a label includes Nutrition Facts and an ingredient list; nutrition descriptions, health claims, and structure/function claims may also be found.

Nutrition Facts

The aptly named Nutrition Facts label gives consumers "facts" they need to know to make informed decisions as they shop for food. Figure 9.1 lists facts about the Nutrition Facts label.

Daily Value: a reference created by the FDA for labeling purposes. Actually a group name for two distinct, behind-the-scenes sets of reference values: Daily Reference Values (DRVs) and Reference Daily Intakes (RDIs).

Daily Reference Values (DRV): are established for nutrients and food components that have important health implications, but no RDA. For some nutrients, they are amounts that should not be exceeded; for others, they are amounts to strive toward. For nutrient intakes that are based on the percentage of calories consumed, 2000 calories is the standard used.

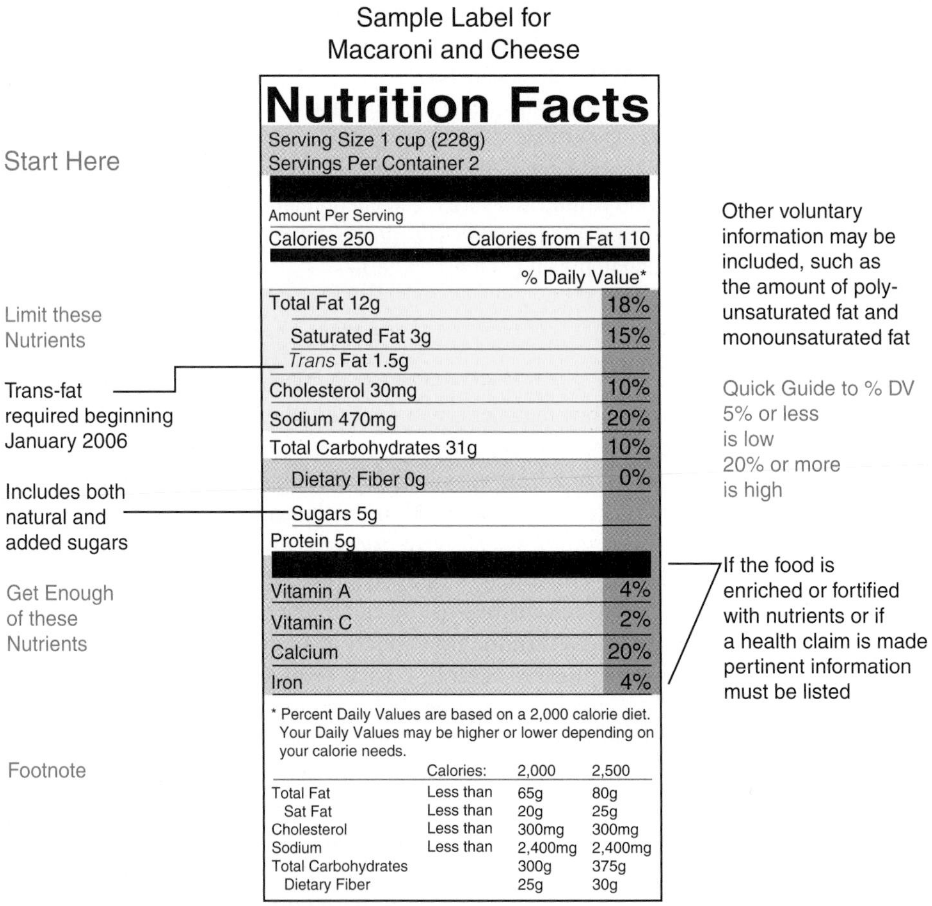

Sample Label for Macaroni and Cheese

Start Here

Nutrition Facts

Serving Size 1 cup (228g)
Servings Per Container 2

Amount Per Serving
Calories 250 Calories from Fat 110

	% Daily Value*
Total Fat 12g	18%
Saturated Fat 3g	15%
Trans Fat 1.5g	
Cholesterol 30mg	10%
Sodium 470mg	20%
Total Carbohydrates 31g	10%
Dietary Fiber 0g	0%
Sugars 5g	
Protein 5g	
Vitamin A	4%
Vitamin C	2%
Calcium	20%
Iron	4%

* Percent Daily Values are based on a 2,000 calorie diet. Your Daily Values may be higher or lower depending on your calorie needs.

	Calories:	2,000	2,500
Total Fat	Less than	65g	80g
Sat Fat	Less than	20g	25g
Cholesterol	Less than	300mg	300mg
Sodium	Less than	2,400mg	2,400mg
Total Carbohydrates		300g	375g
Dietary Fiber		25g	30g

Limit these Nutrients

Trans-fat required beginning January 2006

Includes both natural and added sugars

Get Enough of these Nutrients

Footnote

Other voluntary information may be included, such as the amount of polyunsaturated fat and monounsaturated fat

Quick Guide to % DV
5% or less is low
20% or more is high

If the food is enriched or fortified with nutrients or if a health claim is made pertinent information must be listed

FIGURE 9.1 Nutrition facts label. (Source: Food and Drug Administration.)

Reference Daily Intakes (RDI): represent amounts of nutrients people should strive to consume.

Percent Daily Value (%DV): the percent of how much of a particular nutrient or fiber a person should consume based on a 2000-calorie diet.

Tips to help clients understand the label are as follows:

Portion Size Is Everything. All information that appears on the Nutrition Facts label is specific for the size portion listed, so if the actual portion size eaten differs from that listed, all the "facts" are incorrect. Serving sizes must be listed in common household measurements (e.g., cups) and metric units (e.g., grams). Because different varieties of a food differ in weight, there may be slight differences in the serving size among different manufacturers. For instance, the serving size of Barbara's Bakery Puffins cereal is ¾ cup, 30g; Kellogg's Special K is 1 cup, 31 g; Kellogg's Rice Krispies is 1¼ cup, 33 g. Keep in mind that the actual calorie and nutritional values of a food are dependent on the size of the serving. Most Americans eat double the stated portion size of cereal.

The %DV May Underestimate or Overestimate the Contribution to an Individual's Diet. For nutrients whose amounts are based on a percent of total calories (e.g., carbohydrates, fiber, fat, saturated fat), the %DV is calculated on the basis of a 2000-calorie diet. For people who need less than 2000 calories daily, such as most women and elderly men, the %DV listed on the label actually underestimates the contribution a serving makes to the total needed daily. For instance, the Daily Reference Value upon which %DV for fat is calculated is 65 g, which is 30% of total calories in a 2000-calorie diet. (This number and others appear on the bottom of the Nutrition Facts label as a handy reference). Yet for someone who needs only 1600 calories daily, 30% or less of total calories from fat translates to approximately 53 g (1600 cal × .30 = 480 cal divided by 9 cal/g = 53 g). Therefore, a food that supplies 100% of the DV for fat (e.g., some frozen entrees) contains 65 g that actually provide 123% of the fat recommended for someone consuming 1600 calories daily. Conversely for young active men who need more than 2000 calories per day, the %DV overestimates actual contribution.

A more practical use for %DV than totaling the day's percentages and aiming for 100% is to use the percentages as a way to judge the quality of a food based on the nutrients listed. Generally for any nutrient, a %DV of 5 or less means the nutrient is low in that food. That is a positive attribute for saturated fat, cholesterol, or sodium but not generally desirable for calcium or fiber. Likewise, a %DV of 20 or higher means that nutrient is high in a serving of that food, which again is judged "good" or "bad" depending on the nutrient.

A wrinkle in the usefulness of the Nutrition Facts label is that the Daily Reference Values used to calculate the %DV are not all based on current recommendations. Surprisingly, the %DV for vitamin A, vitamin D, calcium, iron, vitamin E, folate, and zinc are based on the 1968 Recommended Dietary Allowances. Similarly the Daily Reference Value used for sodium is 2400 mg even though the new Adequate Intake set for sodium intake in adults is 1500 mg. Therefore %DV is of limited validity based on current nutrient recommendations.

Percent of Calories From Fat Is Not Listed on the Label. Many people are aware of the 30%-or-less suggestion for fat intake. Many people mistakenly think that the %DV for fat on the label is the percentage of calories from fat in a serving, not the percentage of total daily recommended fat intake provided in a serving. For example, the %DV for a serving of corn oil is 22% even though 100% of the calories in the oil come from fat (e.g., 1 tbsp of oil has 120 calories with 120 calories from fat).

Ingredient List

Ingredients are listed in descending order *by weight*. The further down the list an item appears, the less of that ingredient is in the product. This information enables the reader to discern the relative contribution an ingredient has in a product, but not the proportion. For instance, a cereal that lists its first four ingredients as yellow corn meal, corn bran, unsulphured molasses, and oat flour has more corn meal in than anything else, but how much more is unknown.

Buyer beware that products stating they contain certain ingredients *do* have those ingredients but they may not be present in large enough amounts to be nutritionally significant. For instance, analysis of a frozen vegetable and chicken pot pie found only 10 peas, 1⁄20 of a raw carrot, and 1⁄6 of a potato.

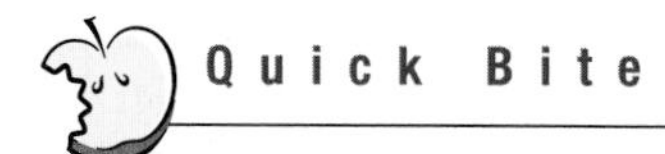

Sweeteners that basically mean "sugar"

- Brown sugar
- Cane sugar
- Confectioner's sugar
- Corn sweeteners
- Corn syrup
- Crystallized cane sugar
- Dextrin
- Evaporated cane juice
- Fruit juice concentrate
- High fructose corn syrup (HFCS)
- Honey
- Invert sugar
- Malt
- Maple syrup
- Molasses
- Raw sugar
- Turbinado sugar

It is also important to note that some ingredients have basically the same nutritional value yet go by different names and so are listed separately. For instance, many different forms of sugar may be listed individually; this makes the total concentration more difficult to determine than if all forms had appeared under the group name of sugar.

Nutrition Descriptions

Nutrient descriptions, such as "Low," "Free," and "High," are legally defined and so are reliable and valid. Any term used to describe the nutrient content of a food is uniform on all products on which the term appears. For example, "good source of fiber" means a serving of the product provides 10% to 19% of the DV for fiber (approximately 2.5 g to 4.5 g) regardless of whether the product is canned beans or dry cereal. Box 9.2 defines the terms used in nutrient claims.

Health Claims

Health claims are also reliable. The U.S. Food and Drug Administration (FDA) has approved certain health claims about the relationship between specific nutrients or foods and the risk of a disease or health related conditions that meet significant

BOX 9.2

DEFINITIONS OF TERMS USED IN NUTRIENT CLAIMS

Free means the product contains virtually none of that nutrient. "Free" can refer to calories, sugar, sodium, salt, fat, saturated fat, and cholesterol.

Low means there is a small enough amount of a nutrient that the product can be used frequently without concern about exceeding dietary recommendations. Low sodium, low calorie, low fat, low saturated fat, and low cholesterol are all defined as to the amount allowed per serving. For instance, to be labeled low cholesterol a product must have no more than 20 mg cholesterol/serving.

Very low refers to sodium only. The product cannot have more than 35 mg sodium/serving.

Reduced or less means the product has at least a 25% reduction in a nutrient compared to the regular product.

Light or lite means the product has 1/3 fewer calories than a comparable product or 50% of the fat found in a comparable product.

Good source means the product provides 10% to 19% of the Daily Value for a nutrient.

High, rich in, or excellent source means the product has at least 20% of the Daily Value for a nutrient.

More means the product has at least 10% more of a desirable nutrient than does a comparable product.

Lean refers to meat or poultry products with less than 10 g fat, less than 4 g saturated fat, and less than 95 mg cholesterol per standardized serving and per 100 g.

Extra lean refers to meat or poultry products with less than 5 g fat, less than 2 g saturated fat, and less than 95 mg cholesterol per standardized serving and per 100 g.

scientific agreement (SSA). All products that have health claims must (1) not exceed specific levels for total fat, saturated fat, cholesterol, and sodium and (2) contain at least 10% of the Daily Value (before supplementation) for any one or all of the following: protein, dietary fiber, vitamin A, vitamin C, calcium, and iron. Additional health claim criteria are specific for the claim made. For instance, the claim regarding calcium and osteoporosis is only allowed on foods that have at least 20% DV for calcium. Box 9.3 lists health claims approved by the FDA.

Relatively new is FDA approval for certain *qualified* health claims about diet and disease relationships when the science supporting the claim does not meet SSA standards yet may have value helping consumers to choose healthier foods or supplements. All current allowed qualified claims pertain to supplements with the exception of two: nuts and heart disease and walnuts and heart disease (Box 9.4). Qualified health claims must be accompanied by a disclaimer that the evidence supporting the claims may be limited and inconclusive.

Structure/Function Claims

Structure/function claims offer the possibility that a food may improve or support body function, which is a fine distinction from the approved health claims that relate

BOX 9.3

HEALTH CLAIMS BASED ON SIGNIFICANT SCIENTIFIC AGREEMENT APPROVED FOR USE BY THE FDA IF THEY MEET THE PROPER SPECIFICATIONS:

- Calcium and osteoporosis
- Dietary fat and cancer
- Saturated fat and cholesterol and risk of coronary heart disease
- Noncarcinogenic carbohydrate sweeteners and dental caries
- Fiber-containing grain products, fruits, and vegetables and cancer
- Folic acid and neural tube defects
- Fruits and vegetables and cancer
- Fruits, vegetables, and grain products that contain fiber, particularly soluble fiber, and risk of coronary heart disease
- Sodium and hypertension
- Soluble fiber from certain foods and risk of coronary heart disease
- Soy protein and risk of coronary heart disease
- Plant sterol/stanol esters and risk of coronary heart disease.

a food or nutrient to a disease. For instance, an example of disease claim needing approval is "suppresses appetite to treat obesity" whereas a function claim that does not need approval is "suppresses appetite to aid weight loss." These structure claims had previously been used primarily by supplement manufacturers with the disclaimer that "These statements have not been evaluated by the FDA. This product is not intended to diagnose, treat, cure or prevent any disease." Structure/function claims are now appearing on food labels and do not require a disclaimer. Unlike health claims that can only appear on foods that meet other nutritional criteria (e.g., they cannot be high in fat, cholesterol, sodium), structure/function claims can appear on "junk" foods. Structure/function claims do not require FDA approval so there may be no evidence to support the claim. See Box 9.5 for structure/function claims that do not need prior approval.

BOX 9.4

ALLOWED QUALIFIED HEALTH CLAIMS PERTAINING TO FOOD: REQUIRED STATEMENTS

"Scientific evidence suggests but does not prove that eating 1.5 ounces per day of most nuts {such as name of specific nut} as part of a diet low in saturated fat and cholesterol may reduce the risk of heart disease."

"Supportive but not conclusive research shows that eating 1.5 ounces per day of walnuts as part of a diet low in saturated fat and cholesterol may reduce the risk of heart disease" or "Scientific evidence suggests but does not prove that eating 1.5 ounces per day of most nuts such as walnuts, as part of a diet low in saturated fat and cholesterol may reduce the risk of heart disease."

BOX 9.5 **STRUCTURE/FUNCTION CLAIMS THAT DO NOT NEED APPROVAL**

Improves memory
Improves strength
Improves digestion
Boosts stamina
For common symptoms of PMS
For hot flashes
Helps you relax
Helps enhance muscle tone or size
Relieves stress
Helps promote urinary tract health
Maintains intestinal flora
For hair loss associated with aging
Prevents wrinkles
For relief of muscle pain after exercise
To treat of prevent nocturnal leg muscle cramps
Helps maintain normal cholesterol levels
Provides relief of occasional constipation
Supports the immune system

Putting Knowledge Into Practice

Armed with *what* the label means, consumers can use that knowledge to make informed decisions while shopping. Although two different brands of a reduced fat dressing have similar fat content, the taste, texture, and price may vary considerably. It is worth the initial investment in time to compare labels and try different brands. Questions for consumers to ask in choosing a product include

What is my reason for reading labels? Is it to choose higher fiber or lower fat? Is it to avoid certain ingredients because of a food allergy? Zero in on what's most important.

Will this food help to achieve my goal? If the primary objective is to eat more fiber, comparing the fiber content of various breakfast cereals is useful but comparing the fiber content of various cheeses is not.

How often do I eat this food? The label may indicate that a serving of canned soup provides 30% of DV for sodium, but if the client buys it to be used as a "standby" item, the sodium content may not be of much importance. Keep in mind that it is the total day's intake that matters, not necessarily individual foods.

How does it compare to similar items on the shelf? Are there other brands with a better nutrition profile? The differences among similar items of different brands can be significant. For instance, the sodium content of individual frozen pizzas may range from 550 mg to 2290 mg per serving.

Is it a nutrient-dense item or a nutritional liability? Does it matter that a fruit drink provides 100% DV for vitamin C given that it is basically colored sugar water with no other nutritional value?

DIETARY SUPPLEMENTS

Herbs: plants or parts of plants used to alleviate health problems or promote wellness.

The term dietary supplement is a group name for products that contain one or more dietary ingredients including vitamins, minerals, herbs or other botanicals, amino acids, and other substances. They are intended to *add to* (supplement) the diets of some people, not to replace a healthy diet. Supplements are to be taken by mouth as a capsule, tablet, or liquid. Labeling laws require the front label to state that the product is a dietary supplement. Figure 9.2 depicts a supplement label.

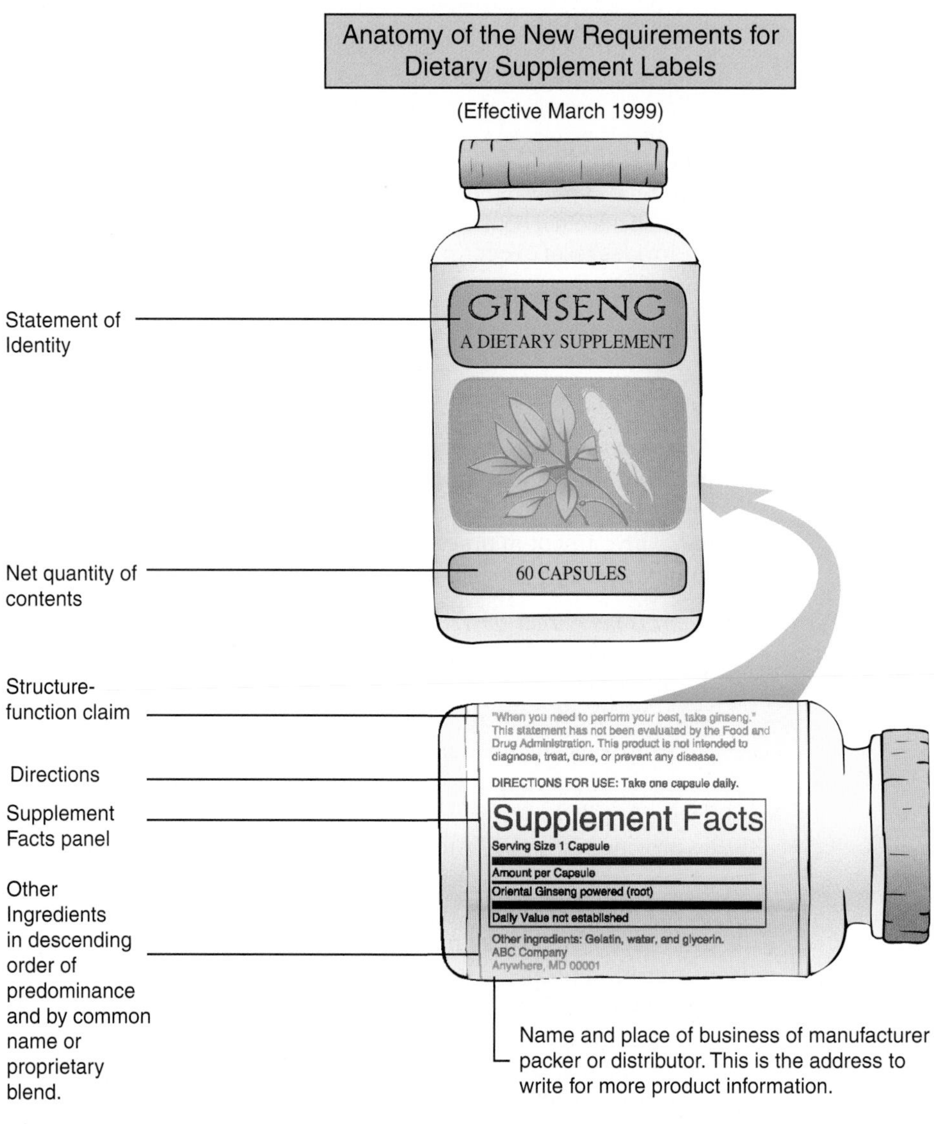

FIGURE 9.2 Supplement label. (Source: Food and Drug Administration.)

Career Connection

Ask about supplement use to identify potential drug-supplement interactions. Because clients usually take dietary supplements on the advice of friends, neighbors, advertisements, etc, and not on the advice of a physician, they may not realize there could be potential interactions with their regular medications, interactions among supplements, or pharmacologic effects such as the anticoagulant properties of gingko and vitamin E. Although some people may be reluctant to discuss supplement use with health care providers for fear of disdain, others may simply dismiss supplements as irrelevant to medical care because they are "natural" and self-prescribed. In a nonjudgmental manner, ask specific questions as to what kind of supplement they are using, the dosage, and frequency.

The U.S. Food and Drug Administration estimates there are more than 29,000 supplements on the market with more added daily. Supplements are widely popular among the American public: in 2001, sales reached an estimated $17.74 billion with an estimated 7 out of 10 adults taking some type of supplement. The top 10 selling herbal supplements in the United States are outlined in Table 9.1. People using supplements do so for a variety of reasons such as

- Distrust of traditional medicine
- Inadequate medical insurance coverage
- Traditional use of herbs based on ethnic or cultural background
- Pursuit of well-being
- Interest in homeopathic remedies and "natural" products

Whereas the functions and requirements of vitamins and minerals are fairly well understood, scientific research is lacking for many herbal products. Unfortunately, many people mistakenly believe "natural" is synonymous with "safe"; they assume that herbs must be harmless because they come from flowers, leaves, and seeds. In truth, herbs are not guaranteed to be safe or effective.

How Supplements Differ From Drugs

In their medicinal sense, herbs are technically unapproved drugs. In fact, approximately 30% of drugs used today originated from plants (e.g., Taxol, aspirin, digoxin). In the United States, dietary supplements are regulated by the FDA as *foods,* which mean they do not have to meet the same standards as drugs and over-the-counter medications. Herbs differ greatly from conventional drugs in how they are marketed and regulated.

Supplement Manufacturers Do Not Have to Prove Safety or Effectiveness Before Introducing a Product on the Market

Before a drug can be marketed, the FDA must authorize its use based on the results of clinical studies performed to determine safety, effectiveness, possible interactions

TABLE 9.1

TOP 10 SELLING HERBAL SUPPLEMENTS IN THE UNITED STATES

Supplement	Forms Available	Uses	Potential Side Effects	People Who Should NOT Use	Potential Herb–Drug Interactions
Black cohosh	Capsules, liquid, tablets	Relief of menopausal symptoms, PMS, dysmenorrhea	GI upset, headaches	Women with a history of breast cancer (an animal study showed black cohosh promoted cancer metastasis)	None known
Cranberry	Capsules, powder, tablets	Prevention and treatment of urinary tract infections	Prolonged or high use of concentrated tablets may increase risk of kidney stones	People at high risk for kidney stones	Antidepressants and prescription painkillers
Echinacea	Capsules, liquid, tablets	To prevent or treat colds and the flu	Minor GI upset, increased urination, allergic reactions (especially in people allergic to plants of the sunflower family)	People with autoimmune diseases such as multiple sclerosis, lupus. Not recommended to be used >8 successive weeks	None known
Garlic	Capsules, liquid, powder, tablets	To lower cholesterol +/or triglyceride levels; may be useful in the treatment of bacterial and fungal infections, digestive ailments, and hypertension	Large quantities may cause heartburn, flatulence, and GI distress	People about to have surgery, due to increased bleeding	Anticoagulants, nonsteroidal anti-inflammatories

TABLE 9.1
(continued)

TOP 10 SELLING HERBAL SUPPLEMENTS IN THE UNITED STATES

Supplement	Forms Available	Uses	Potential Side Effects	People Who Should NOT Use	Potential Herb–Drug Interactions
Ginkgo biloba	Capsules, gel caps, liquid, tablets	To improve memory, to treat peripheral vascular disease	Mild headache, GI upset	People scheduled for surgery or those with bleeding disorders. Diabetics	Anticoagulants, aspirin, vit E or garlic supplements, trazodone, antidiabetics, thiazide, diuretics
Ginseng	Capsules, gel caps, tablets, tea	To improve mental alertness or increase energy. As an aphrodisiac or stress reliever	Generally not associated with adverse side effects	People with untreated hypertension. Women with a history of breast cancer	MAO inhibitors, digitalis, insulin, oral hypoglycemics, coumadin, ticlopidine
Saw palmetto	Capsules, liquid, soft gels	To prevent or relieve symptoms of enlarged prostate	Mild GI upset	People scheduled to have surgery and those with bleeding disorders	Anticoagulants, aspirin, supplements of vit E or ginkgo
Soy isoflavones	Capsules, powder, tablets	To lessen symptoms of menopause such as hot flashes	None known	Women with a history of or at high risk for breast cancer. People with altered thyroid function	None known
St. John's wort	Capsules, liquid, teas	To treat depression, anxiety, seasonal affective disorder, sleep disorders	Dry mouth, dizziness, GI symptoms, increased sensitivity to sunlight, fatigue	People sensitive to sunlight or taking UV treatment. People with bipolar disorder	Ritalin, ephedrine, caffeine, protease inhibitors, digitalis, statins, warfarin, chemotherapy drugs, oral contraceptives, tricyclic antidepressants, olanzapine,

(table continues on page 222)

TABLE 9.1
(continued)

TOP 10 SELLING HERBAL SUPPLEMENTS IN THE UNITED STATES

Supplement	Forms Available	Uses	Potential Side Effects	People Who Should NOT Use	Potential Herb–Drug Interactions
					clozapine, theophylline, antirejection drugs
Valerian	Capsules, tablets	To relieve insomnia and other sleep disorders	Headache, dizziness, pruritus, GI upset	People about to drive or use heavy equipment	May increase the effects of barbiturates, Valium, and Halcion.

New Dietary Ingredient: supplement ingredient not marketed in the United States before October 15, 1994.

with other substances, and appropriate doses. In contrast, the regulations regarding dietary supplements are lax. Supplement ingredients sold in the United States before October 15, 1994 are assumed to be safe and so do not require FDA review for safety before they are marketed. Dietary supplement manufacturers that want to market a new dietary ingredient must submit information to the FDA that supports their conclusion that *reasonable* evidence exists that the product is safe for human consumption. Manufacturers do not have to *prove* to the FDA that dietary supplements are safe or effective; however, they are not supposed to market unsafe or ineffective products.

Once a product is marketed, the responsibility lies with the FDA to prove danger rather than with the manufacturer to prove safety. When the FDA determines a supplement is unsafe, it issues a consumer advisory discouraging its use but does not prohibit companies from continuing to sell the product. Many consumers mistakenly think that if a product is allowed to be sold, it must be safe. In truth, there are numerous active ingredients contained in products on the market that the FDA has warned against using (Table 9.2).

Dietary Supplements Are Not Yet Regulated for Quality

In March 2003, the FDA published a proposed rule intended to establish standards to ensure that supplements are not contaminated and are labeled accurately to reflect both active and other ingredients. This proposal seeks to require the use of new industry-wide standards in the manufacturing, packing, and holding of dietary supplements, thereby reducing the risk of contamination with harmful or undesirable substances such as pesticides, heavy metals, or other impurities. For the first time, identity, purity, quality, strength, and composition of dietary supplements

TABLE 9.2 **ACTIVE INGREDIENTS FOUND IN DIETARY SUPPLEMENTS LINKED TO HEALTH PROBLEMS**

The FDA Warns Against Using	Potential Problems
Aristolochic acid (including products with the words "Bragantia," "Asarum," or "Aristolochia")	Kidney damage; kidney failure; certain types of cancer, mostly in the urinary tract
Chaparral	Rapid liver disease that may be irreversible
Comfrey	Chronic liver disease; possible carcinogen
Kava	Liver damage, irreversible liver failure
LipoKinetix	Liver damage or liver failure
PC SPES and SPES	Found to contain undeclared prescription drugs
Tiractricol	Potent thyroid hormone marketed as a weight loss supplement; can cause CVA and MI
Usnic acid	Liver toxin

would be required to be accurately reflected on the label. Until this proposed rule is finalized, dietary supplements must comply with food Good Manufacturing Practice (GMP) regulations that are primarily concerned with safety and sanitation, not quality.

Dietary Supplements Are Not Standardized

Dietary supplements are not required to be standardized in the United States. In fact, there is no legal definition of standardization as it applies to supplements; therefore,

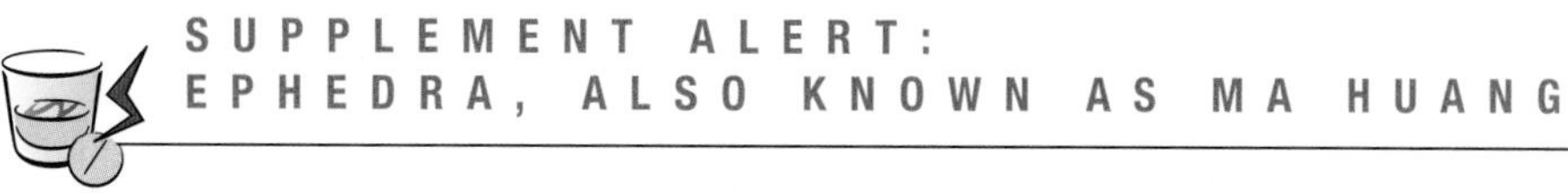

In an unprecedented move, the FDA banned the sale of ephedra-containing supplements in 2004, the culmination of a 7-year process that began when the FDA required a warning label on ephedra stating it is hazardous and should not be used for more than 7 days. Ephedra products are marketed as aid for weight control and to enhance athletic performance and energy. Yet after gathering and reviewing an extraordinary amount of data, the FDA concluded there is little evidence to support its effectiveness except for short-term weight loss, and that it presents an unreasonable risk of illness or injury and should not be consumed. It elevates blood pressure and stresses the circulatory system and is conclusively linked to heart attack and stroke. Despite the ban, it is likely that people who want to use ephedra will be able to purchase it via the internet or from other countries.

Standardization: a manufacturing process that ensures product consistency from batch to batch.

the concentration of active compounds in different batches of supposedly identical plant material can be highly variable. The difference in concentration may be related to different plant varieties, differences in harvesting techniques, the environmental conditions under which the plants were grown (e.g., fertility of the soil, amount of moisture), or how they were processed (e.g., temperature and length of time used to dry plant materials). Be aware that some manufacturers incorrectly use the term standardization to mean consistent manufacturing process, which is not the same thing as ensuring potency or quality.

Dietary Supplement Dosages Are Not Standardized

Recommended dosages vary among manufacturers. Because there is no premarket testing to determine optimum dosage or maximum safe dosage, it's anyone's guess as to what dose is appropriate. Also, recommended amounts of herbs to use when making tea are usually imprecise (e.g., "a heaping teaspoon"). When making tea, steeping times are also important, especially when the active ingredients are not highly water soluble.

Claims on Packaging for Dietary Supplements Do Not Require FDA Approval

Although dietary supplements cannot claim to be used for the diagnosis, treatment, cure, or prevention of disease, they can be labeled with statements explaining their purported effect on the structure or function of the human body (e.g., "alleviates fatigue") or their role in promoting well-being (e.g., "improves mood"). Although these statements do not require FDA approval, the manufacturer must provide the FDA with the text of the claim within 30 days of introducing a product on the market. Labels that make specific claims must include the following disclaimer: "This statement has not been evaluated by the FDA. This product is not intended to diagnose, treat, cure, or prevent any disease."

Warnings Are Not Required

Despite popular belief to the contrary, supplements are not required to carry warning labels about potential side effects, dangers, or supplement–drug interactions. Nor are there advisories about who should not use the product.

Dietary Supplements Are Self-Prescribed

In the United States, the use of herbs is self-prescribed. A major concern with self-medicating is that consumers may misdiagnose their condition or forsake effective conventional medical care to treat themselves "naturally." Another problem with self-medicating is that patients may not inform their physicians about their use of herbs, so that side effects and herb-drug interactions go undiagnosed and unreported.

 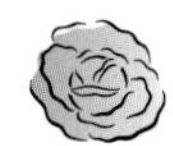

Advice for Supplement Users

Ask critical questions.

- What claims are made about the product? Are they valid?
- Can any dosage of the supplement cause harm?
- Does the company that manufactures the supplement use Good Manufacturing Practices?
- Are the active ingredients known and if so, how do they function in the body?
- How much active ingredient does the supplement contain? What other ingredients are in the supplement?
- What is the potential risk:benefit ratio?
- What scientific evidence supports the use of this product?
- What potential side effects may develop from using this product?
- How much and how often should this product be used? How long can it be taken safely?
- Are there known or suspected interactions with prescription medications?

Check with the FDA website for consumer advisories on supplements not to use. Go to www.cfsan.fda.fda.gov/~dms. Don't assume that because a product is available, it is safe.

Discuss supplement use with the physician. Physicians need to be aware of supplement use so they can monitor for side effects and supplement–drug interactions. People who take medications for high blood pressure, heart disease, or Parkinson's disease should consult their physicians before using supplements.

Beware of people who give unqualified advice. "Herbalist," "herb doctor," and "master herbalist" are unregulated job titles that anyone can use. Also beware of a product that claims to be "magical," a "new discovery," or "miraculous."

Take measures to prevent and manage adverse side effects and supplement–drug interactions. Stick to single supplement products and start with a small dose. Side effects and interactions are less likely to occur and easier to pinpoint when single supplements are used at low doses. Be alert to adverse side effects such as allergy, stomach upset, skin rash, or headache. Take supplements at different times from prescribed medications to help reduce the potential for supplement-drug interactions. Supplements taken with drugs have the potential to reduce the drug's effectiveness.

Supplements should be discontinued immediately if adverse side effects or supplement–drug interactions occur. Notify the physician so that a report can be filed with FDA MedWatch at 1-800-FDA-1088 or www.fda.gov/medwatch/report.hcp.ht. Consumers can file their own reports at the same telephone number or through www.fda.gov/medwatch/report/consumer/consumer.htm.

Avoid herbs and other botanical supplements during pregnancy and lactation and in children younger than 6 years of age. Herbs, like drugs, have the potential to cross the placenta to some degree, exposing the fetus to potential teratogenic effects. Herbs may also enter breast milk, resulting in adverse effects in the nursing infant.

The distribution of herbs in children's body tissue may be different than in adults because of differences in relative body composition.

Learn to read dietary supplement labels. Buy products that have the "USP" notation on the label. This indicates that the manufacturer follows standards established by the U.S. Pharmacopoeia for disintegration, dissolution, purity, strength, and expiration. See Fig. 9.2 depicts a supplement label and information required by the FDA.

FOOD QUALITY CONCERNS

Planning an adequate diet relates not only to nutritional adequacy but also to food quality considerations. For instance, proper storage and preparation are vital to ensure that the food's vitamin and mineral contents are retained. Incorporating functional foods or nutraceuticals into the diet may help to enhance health and prevent disease. Organically grown foods offer the allure of healthier products—but are they?

Retaining the Nutrient Content of Food

Even when it is carefully planned, an eating plan affords no guarantees that it will provide optimal amounts of all nutrients especially if the food eaten has been improperly stored or overly processed. Generally, food begins to lose its nutrients the moment that harvesting or processing begins; the more that is done to a food before it is eaten, the greater the nutrient loss. Heat, light, air, soaking in water, mechanical injury, dry storage, and acidic or alkaline food processing ingredients can all hasten nutrient losses. Vitamins, minerals, and fiber are particularly vulnerable to the effects of food processing. Tips to minimize nutrient losses are featured in Box 9.6.

Functional Foods and Nutraceuticals

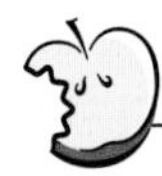

Quick Bite

A 2002 telephone survey on consumer attitudes revealed that

68% of Americans believe they have a "great amount" of control over their own health

71% of consumers believe that food and nutrition play "a great role" in maintaining or improving overall health

94% of Americans believe that some foods have health benefits than go beyond basic nutrition

85% of Americans are "very interested" or "somewhat interested" in learning more about functional foods

Source: International Food Information Council. (2002). The consumer view on functional foods: Yesterday and today. *Food Insight*, May/June, 5, 8.

Functional Foods: commonly (not legally) defined as foods that provide health benefits beyond basic nutrition. Often used as an all-inclusive generic term that includes nutraceuticals.

BOX 9.6

TIPS FOR RETAINING THE NUTRIENT VALUE OF FOODS

- Don't buy produce that is damaged or wilted or that has been improperly stored. Produce picked when fully ripe is higher in nutrients than produce picked when green.
- Refrigerate fruits and vegetables immediately to slow enzyme activity and retain nutrients. Keep produce in the refrigerator crisper or in moisture-proof bags.
- Wash, don't soak, produce to avoid leaching nutrients.
- Avoid peeling and paring vegetables before cooking because a valuable layer of nutrients is stored directly beneath the skin. If necessary, scrape or pare as thin a layer as possible.
- Avoid cutting produce into small pieces: The more surface area exposed, the greater the nutrient loss.
- Prepare vegetables as close to serving time as possible to avoid excessive exposure to light and air. Don't thaw frozen vegetables before cooking.
- Eat some fruits and vegetables raw.
- Cook produce in as little water as possible to avoid leaching vitamins. Stir-fry, steam, microwave, or pressure-cook vegetables to retain nutrients. If water is used in cooking, save and use it as stock for soups, gravies, or sauces.
- Shorten cooking time as much as possible. Cook vegetables to the tender crunchy, rather than to the mushy, stage of doneness; cover the pan to retain heat; and preheat the pan or water before adding foods to speed heating time.
- Cook only as many vegetables as are needed at a time because reheating causes considerable loss of vitamins.

Nutraceuticals: generally defined as foods that have been altered to provide medicinal benefits beyond basic nutrition. For instance, Benecol Spread (margarine-type product) has plant sterols added to help reduce serum cholesterol levels.

Functional foods are one of the fastest growing segments of the food industry. Although, broadly speaking, all foods may be considered "functional" in that they function at least to provide pleasure even if they do not impart nutritional benefits, the term functional foods applies to foods with components that appear to enhance health or prevent disease. Functional foods may be natural (Table 9.3) or manufactured.

Manufactured functional foods have one or more functional ingredients added such as vitamins, minerals, or herbs. New functional foods with unique combinations of ingredients are being introduced in the marketplace faster than science can provide information on their safety. Like supplements, once functional foods are marketed, adverse effects are brought to light only if consumers alert the FDA to suspected problems. Unlike natural functional foods, the use of manufactured foods raises several questions:

How much of a functional ingredient is contained in the product? Although infrequent consumption of a product containing gingko may have little impact on health, a high intake may result in unwanted and unregulated decreased platelet aggregation. Even too much of a known good thing, such as iron, can be detrimental.

TABLE 9.3

NATURAL FUNCTIONAL FOODS

Food	Active Ingredient	Effective Level	Potential Health Benefits
Garlic	Sulfur compounds	1 clove/day	May help to reduce blood pressure and blood cholesterol
Fatty fish	Omega-3 fatty acids	6 oz/week	May decrease risk of cardiovascular disease
Purple grape juice	Polyphenolic compounds	8–16 oz/day	May help to support normal heart function
Broccoli	Sulforaphane	Regular consumption	May decrease risk of cancer
Green and black teas	Catechins	3–5 cups/day	May decrease risk of cardiovascular disease and certain cancers; may boost immune system functioning
Yogurt and fermented dairy products	Probiotics	Not specified	Improve gastrointestinal health, aid in lowering cholesterol, and decrease risk for cancer
Oats and oat-containing foods	Soluble fiber (beta glucan)	3 g beta glucan/day (about 1.5 svgs oats/d)	Lowers cholesterol
Soy foods	Soy protein	25 g/day	Lowers cholesterol
Tomatoes and tomato products	Lycopene	Regular consumption	Reduces risk of certain cancers
Fruits and vegetables	Phytochemicals	5–9 servings/day	May decrease risk of cancer and may lower blood pressure

Is there a potential interaction with prescription medication? Consumers may not realize that potential herb–drug interactions exist not only from using some dietary supplements but also from consuming foods that contain those same ingredients.

Will the product do what it claims it will? With the exception of functional foods that carry one of the approved health claims (see Box 9.3), there is no regulation of the levels of functional ingredients required to support a structure/function claims. Dozens of products, particularly beverages, contain a variety of herbs with little or no evidence to support their efficacy. Even when scientific evidence supports the use of a functional ingredient, the quantity in the product may be too small to make an impact on health.

Are there potential dangers? For instance, it is known that groups of people who eat a diet rich in fruits and vegetables, especially those high in beta-carotene, have a decreased risk of certain cancers such as lung cancer. However, a clinical trial giving beta-carotene supplements to smokers to see if it could protect against lung

cancer had to be aborted when it became apparent that the participants receiving beta-carotene actually had higher rates of lung cancer than the controls. Conclusions from studies using whole foods may not extrapolate to individual food components.

As scientific evidence mounts in the role of specific nutrients or food substances in preventing chronic diseases such as heart disease, cancer, diabetes, hypertension, and osteoporosis, it is likely that more foods will be considered functional and that the supply of manufactured functional foods and nutraceuticals will expand exponentially. It is the position of the American Dietetic Association that functional foods, including nutraceuticals, have a potentially beneficial effect on health when consumed as part of a varied diet on a regular basis. Studies show that the intake of functional foods increases in response to an increased awareness about their potential health benefits. Functional foods should be viewed as an option in the continuum of good nutrition, not as a "magic bullet" to cure all dietary ills.

Organically Grown Foods

Organic: in a chemical sense, organic means carbon-containing. Generally, organic refers to living organisms; as such, all foods are technically organic.

During the 1990s, organic farming was one of the fastest growing segments of United States agriculture. Once found only in health food stores, organically grown foods are now mainstream in American grocery stores. The U.S. Department of Agriculture (USDA) estimates the retail sales of organic food is approximately $6 billion, a small but growing segment of the food market.

Organic farming uses "natural" products to fertilize crops such as manure, compost, and other organic wastes. Chemicals that occur naturally in the environment, such as sulfur, nicotine, and copper, may be used as pesticides. Insects that do not harm a particular crop may be used to control other insects known to cause crop damage. In addition, the National Organic Program of the USDA has an approved list of biological, botanical, or synthetic substances that can be used as pesticides. Crop rotation, tillage, and cover crops are used to manage soil. Food irradiation, sewage sludge, and bioengineered plants cannot be used.

Organically Grown or Organically Produced: foods produced with little or no synthetic fertilizers or pesticides (e.g., plants) and no antibiotics or hormones (e.g., livestock).

Regulations are also in place for raising organically grown livestock. Organically produced feed must be used for a specified period of time toward the end of gestation; animals may be given vitamin and mineral supplements but the use of growth hormones and antibiotics is prohibited; and animals treated with medication cannot be sold as organic.

The National Organic Program ensures that the production, processing, and certification of organically grown foods adhere to a comprehensive standard. Only foods that meet federal standards can be labeled with "100% organic," "organic," or "made with organic ingredients." Foods that contain at least 70% organic ingredients may bear the "USDA Organic" seal. Products containing less than 70% organic ingredients can only mention organic on the ingredient list for the specific organically produced ingredients.

Are organically produced foods superior to their conventionally raised counterparts? Studies show no significant difference in taste when foods are produced organically, nor is there evidence to suggest they are more nutritious or safer. And they look comparable to other foods. The biggest difference is cost: organically produced foods are more expensive because of higher production costs, greater losses, and smaller yields. Aside from price, there is no compelling intellectual reason to promote or discourage the use of organically produced foods.

FOOD SAFETY CONCERNS

Food safety concerns include preventing foodborne illnesses that can occur from improperly handled or stored food. Other current issues of food safety include biotechnology and irradiation.

Foodborne Illness

Foodborne Illness: an illness transmitted to humans via food.

In the United States, as many as 76 million illnesses, 325,000 hospitalizations, and 5000 deaths per year are attributed to consumption of contaminated food or water. The microorganisms that cause foodborne illness are found widely in nature. They are transmitted to people from within the food (e.g., meat and fish), on the food (e.g., eggshell or vegetables), from unsafe water, or from human or animal feces. Bacteria are responsible for more than 90% of all food borne illnesses. To spread, bacteria simply need food, moisture, a favorable temperature, and time to multiply. The remainder of cases are blamed on viruses, parasites, food toxins, and unknown causes. Although foodborne illness can be caused by any food, foods containing animal proteins are the most frequent vehicles. Table 9.4 outlines common foodborne illnesses caused by bacteria. Table 9.5 features foodborne illnesses caused by viruses.

The most common symptoms of foodborne illness may be mistaken for the flu: diarrhea, nausea, vomiting, fever, abdominal pain, and headaches. Most cases are self-limiting and run their course within a few days. Symptoms that warrant medical attention include bloody diarrhea (possible *E. coli* 0157:H7 infection), a stiff neck with severe headache and fever (possible meningitis related to *Listeria*), excessive diarrhea or vomiting (possible life-threatening dehydration), and any symptoms that persist for more than 3 days. Infants, pregnant women, the elderly, and people with compromised immune systems (people with acquired immunodeficiency syndrome [AIDS] or cancer, organ transplant recipients, people taking corticosteroids) are particularly vulnerable to the effects of foodborne illness.

The major cause of foodborne illnesses is unsanitary food handling. To reduce the risk of contamination, proper personal hygiene and handwashing must be practiced by all food handlers. Steps must be taken to prevent cross-contact between raw and cooked foods and through food handlers. Because heat kills most bacteria, thorough cooking of meat and fish is vital, as is pasteurization of all milk products. Adequate refrigeration inhibits the growth of bacteria. Figure 9.3 depicts the four simple steps to keep food safe promoted by the Fight BAC! (as in bacteria) Campaign of the

(*text continues on page 234*)

TABLE 9.4

COMMON FOODBORNE ILLNESSES IN THE U.S. CAUSED BY BACTERIA

Bacteria (illness)	Common Food Vehicles	Onset	Symptoms	Other
Escherichia coli (*E. coli* 0157-H7; hemorrhagic colitis hemolytic uremic syndrome)	Undercooked beef, especially ground beef; raw milk; unpasteurized fruit juice and cider; alfalfa sprouts; plant foods fertilized with raw manure or irrigated with contaminated water	2–5 days	Severe abdominal cramps and diarrhea Hemorrhagic colitis may lead to hemolytic-uremic syndrome (severe anemia and renal failure)	
Listeria monocytogenes (listeriosis)	Raw milk, deli-type salads, processed meats, soft cheese, undercooked poultry, ice cream, raw vegetables, raw and cooked poultry	3 days to 3 weeks	Sudden fever, chills, headache, backache, occasional abdominal pain, and diarrhea Septicemia and meningitis may lead to death May cause spontaneous abortion or stillbirth during pregnancy	This bacterium thrives in cold temperatures and appears to be able to survive short-term pasteurization Mortality from listeric meningitis may be as high as 70%
Salmonella species (salmonellosis)	Raw and undercooked eggs, poultry, meats, milk and dairy products, raw sprouts (alfalfa, bean), fish, shrimp, sauces and salad dressings, dried gelatin, peanut butter	6–48 hours	Nausea, vomiting, cramps, fever, diarrhea, headache Arthritic symptoms may occur 3–4 weeks after onset of acute infection	Can be fatal Incidence is increasing in US

(table continues on page 232)

TABLE 9.4
(continued)

COMMON FOODBORNE ILLNESSES IN THE U.S. CAUSED BY BACTERIA

Bacteria (illness)	Common Food Vehicles	Onset	Symptoms	Other
Shigella species (shigellosis)	Salads (potato, tuna, shrimp, macaroni, chicken) raw vegetables, milk and dairy products, poultry	12–50 hours	Severe diarrhea that may be bloody, abdominal pain, fever, vomiting	Fecally contaminated water and unsanitary food handling are most common causes of contamination
Staphylococcus aureus (staphylococcal food poisoning)	Custard- or cream-filled baked goods, sandwich fillings; meat and meat products; poultry and egg products; salad such as egg, tuna, chicken, potato, and macaroni; milk and dairy products	rapid	Severe nausea, vomiting, abdominal cramps, prostration	Of healthy people, 40%–50% are carriers. Most frequently found in the nose, throat, on skin, and in infected boils, pimples, cuts, and burns
Vibrio vulnificus (gastroenteritis; may lead to primary septicemia in people with chronic disease, especially liver disease)	Raw or undercooked shellfish, especially oysters	within 16 hours	Fever, chills, skin lesions, nausea, vomiting, diarrhea, hypotension, shock May lead to septicemia	Infection rarely occurs in healthy people; those at risk include people with compromised immune systems, achlorhydria, and chronic liver disease Mortality rate about 50% in immunocompromised people including those with liver disease

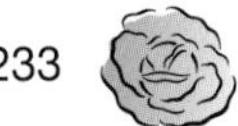

TABLE 9.4
(continued)

COMMON FOODBORNE ILLNESSES IN THE U.S. CAUSED BY BACTERIA

Bacteria (illness)	Common Food Vehicles	Onset	Symptoms	Other
Bacillus cereus (bacillus)	Meat products, soups, vegetables, puddings, sauces, milk and milk products	6–15 hours	Abdominal pain, watery diarrhea, nausea	Symptoms last for 24h in most cases
Campylobacter jejuni (campylobacter enteritis)	Untreated water, raw milk, undercooked poultry and meats, unchlorinated water	2–5 days	Diarrhea, muscle pain, fever, nausea, headache, abdominal pain	Leading cause of diarrhea in the United States: rarely life threatening symptoms. Symptoms may last 7–10 days
Clostridium botulinum (botulism)	Underheated, low-acid home canned foods (corn, peppers, green beans, mushrooms, tuna), vacuum-packed meats, sausage, fish, honey (in infants only)	Usually 18–36 hours after ingesting toxin, but onset may range from 4 hours to 8 days	Nausea, vomiting, diarrhea, fatigue, headache, dry mouth, double vision, difficulty speaking and swallowing, muscle paralysis	Fatal in 3–10 days if not treated
Clostridium perfringens (perfringens food poisoning)	Meat, poultry, stuffing, and gravy held or stored at inappropriate temperature	8–22 hours	Intense abdominal cramps	The "cafeteria germ," associated with steam table foods not kept hot enough Illness usually over within 24-hours One of most common foodborne illnesses in US

TABLE 9.5

MOST COMMON FOODBORNE VIRAL ILLNESSES IN THE UNITED STATES

Virus (Illness)	Common Food Vehicles	Onset	Symptoms	Other
Hepatitis A virus (hepatitis)	Food contaminated by infected food handlers, water, shellfish, and salads are the most common vehicles	10–50 days (average is 28–30 days)	Fever, malaise, nausea, vomiting, muscle pain, jaundice	Illness usually subsides after a few weeks; but may last for months
Norwalk virus (food poisoning; viral gastroenteritis)	Untreated water, shellfish, raw or undercooked clams, and oysters	24–48 hours	Nausea, vomiting, diarrhea, abdominal pain, headache, low-grade fever	Severe illness is rare

Partnership for Food Safety Education. See the Partnership for Food Safety Education website for additional food safety tips.

"Mad Cow Disease" (Bovine Spongiform Encephalopathy/BSE)

Mad cow disease is the common name for bovine spongiform encephalopathy (BSE), a slowly progressive, degenerative, fatal disease affecting the central nervous system of adult cattle. Although the exact cause is unknown, BSE is believed to be caused by prions, an infectious form of a type of protein. BSE was first reported in 1986 in the United Kingdom and is believed to have originated when scrapie-infected sheep meat and bone meal were fed to cattle (scrapie is the sheep version of BSE). Evidence suggests the disease proliferated when BSE-contaminated cattle protein was fed to calves. Unlike bacteria, prions are resistant to heat and so are not destroyed by cooking. Eating BSE-infected beef products is believed to cause a variant form of Creutzfeldt-Jacob disease (vCJD), which is the human version of BSE.

Although the FDA and other federal agencies have had regulatory measures in place since 1989 to prevent BSE from entering the United States' food supply, the first case of BSE in the United States was identified in December 2003. Fortunately, the animal's organs infected with prions never entered the food supply and the rest of the meat from that cow was successfully recalled from the marketplace. Since then, the USDA has enacted additional rules to enhance safeguards against BSE. Research is ongoing to better understand prion transmission and the diseases it causes.

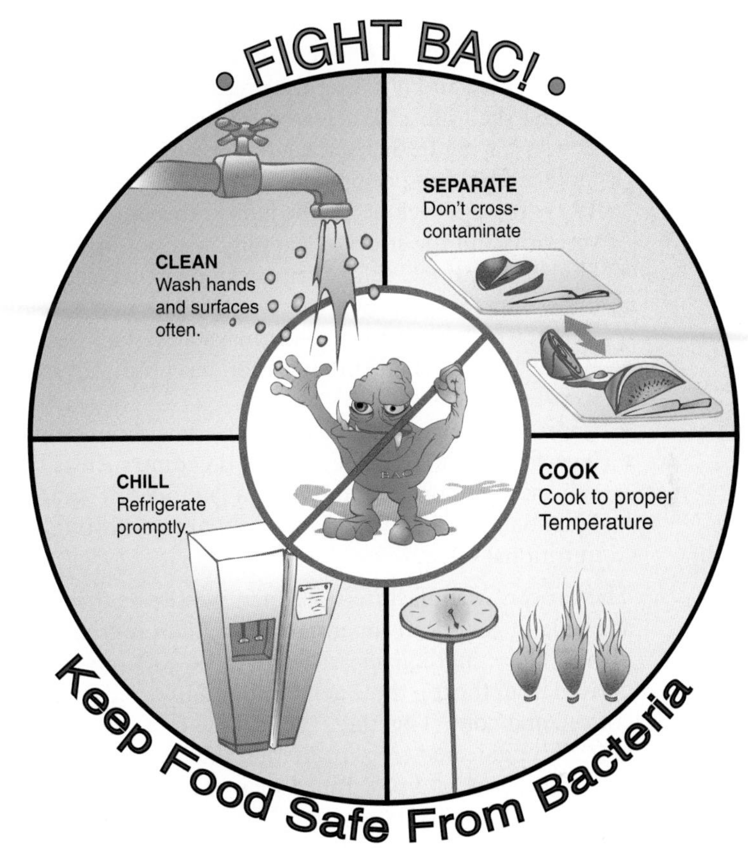

FIGURE 9.3 FightBAC! infographic. (Source: Partnership for Food Safety Education.)

Food Biotechnology

Food Biotechnology: a process that involves taking a gene with a desirable trait from one plant and inserting it into another with the goal of changing one or more of its characteristics. Also called genetically engineered food.

Many consumers believe that food biotechnology is a Pandora's box and inherently dangerous. Some religious leaders question the morality of changing nature. Concerns about food safety and adverse health effects are common. Can the proteins produced by these new genes cause allergies? Can genetically engineered foods be toxic with long-term use? Do genetically engineered foods have anti-nutrient effects? Will the ultimate outcome be a mutant plant or animal that cannot be controlled? Will any genetically engineered products have a negative impact on the environment?

Food biotechnology is used for a variety of reasons such as

- Healthier crops and greater yields. Some plants are genetically modified to increase their resistance to plant viruses and other diseases; this means they can be raised using fewer pesticides to help reduce production costs and environmental residues. One example is squash that has been made resistant to a common plant virus.

- Greater resistance to severe weather, which reduces crop losses and increases year-round availability of fresh crops. Tomatoes have been engineered to be resistant to both cold and hot temperatures.
- Longer shelf-life and increased freshness. Plants can be made to ripen more slowly, staying fresher longer—a big plus for transportation. The first genetically modified food to be approved by the FDA was Calgene's FlavrSavr tomato in 1994. It was developed to be left on the vine until fully ripened and flavorful and yet withstand the stress of shipping without bruising.
- Higher nutritional value. Plants can be genetically modified to contain more vitamins, minerals, or protein, or less fat. A potato is being developed that is higher in starch, which, compared to normal starch potatoes, absorbs less oil during frying.
- Better flavor. Genetic modification has produced sweeter melons and sweeter strawberries.
- Improved characteristics such as celery without strings.
- New food varieties through cross breeding such as broccoflower (a blend of broccoli and cauliflower) and tangelos (a tangerine–grapefruit hybrid).
- Potential benefits to alleviate world hunger through stronger crops with enhanced nutritional value.

The Grocery Manufacturers of America estimate that 70% to 75% of all processed foods available in American supermarkets contain ingredients from genetically engineered plants. Those ingredients are likely to be soybean oil, cottonseed oil, and corn syrup derived from the top three genetically engineered crops in the United States: soybeans, cotton, and corn. Together, those three crops dominate the 100 million acres of genetically engineered crops planted in the United States in 2003. Bread, cereals, frozen pizza, hot dogs, and soft drinks are some of the many products made with genetically engineered ingredients.

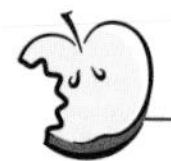

Quick Bite

Some genetically engineered foods determined to be safe according to the FDA

Canola oil
Corn
Cottonseed oil
Papaya
Potatoes
Soybeans
Squash
Sugar beets
Sweet corn
Tomatoes

Based on independent reports released by the National Academy of Science, the Organization for Economic Cooperation and Development, and the Subcommittee on Basic Research of the U.S. House of Representatives Committee on Science, food biotechnology is safe. The FDA asserts that genetically engineered foods do not pose a health or safety risk and, therefore, do not require mandatory labeling unless the food contains new allergens, has a modified nutritional profile, or represents a new plant. However, the USDA, FDA, and EPA (U.S. Environmental Protection Agency) actively monitor the development and testing of genetically engineered foods. Despite the relative consensus among the scientific community that it is safe, biotechnology

has not been used long enough to know if long-term complications may develop. People who do not want to consume genetically engineered foods can avoid these products by using organically produced foods.

Food Irradiation

Food Irradiation: treatment of food with approved levels of ionizing radiation for a prescribed period of time and a controlled dose to destroy bacteria and parasites that would otherwise cause foodborne illness.

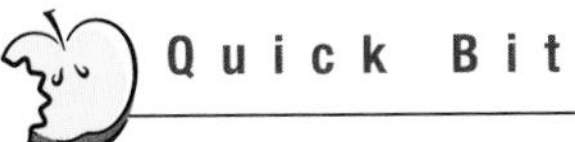

Quick Bite

Foods allowed to be irradiated in the United States include

- Wheat flour to control mold
- White potatoes to inhibit sprouting
- Pork to kill trichina parasites
- Fruits and vegetables to control insects
- Herbs and spices for sterilization
- Poultry to reduce bacterial pathogens
- Meat to reduce bacterial pathogens

To many consumers, the term irradiated food conjures up visions of radioactive fallout. In truth, irradiation used on approved foods does not produce radioactive food but does enhance food safety by reducing or eliminating pathogens, controlling insects, or killing parasites.

Irradiation does not use heat and so is sometimes referred to as "cold pasteurization." Bacteria, mold, fungi, and insects are destroyed as the food moves through a radiant energy field. A small amount of new compounds are formed that are similar to the changes seen in food as it is cooked, pasteurized, frozen, or otherwise prepared. Except for a slight decrease in thiamin, the nutrient content is essentially unchanged. Because irradiation kills any living cells that may be contained in the food, such as in seeds or potatoes, shelf life may be prolonged. For instance, irradiated potatoes do not sprout during storage. However, irradiation does not hide spoilage or eliminate the need for safe food handling; irradiated food can still become contaminated through cross-contamination.

Irradiation is the most extensively studied food processing technique available in the world and is used by 37 countries on more than 40 foods. In well-controlled animal and human studies, no adverse health effects have been identified from irradiation. In the United States, the FDA, the USDA, the U.S. Department of Defense, the U.S. Army, and NASA are among the agencies that either approve or establish guidelines for food irradiation. Federal law requires irradiated food to be labeled with the international symbol (the radura, Fig. 9.4) and state "Treated with irradiation" or "Treated by irradiation." Research on irradiation as a part of an overall system of ensuring food safety is ongoing.

FIGURE 9.4 Radura: international symbol for irradiation.

How Do You Respond?

Are all food labels required to have a Nutrition Facts label? Almost all processed foods require mandatory labeling. Only plain coffee and tea; some spices, flavorings, and other foods that contain no significant amounts of nutrients; ready-to-eat food prepared primarily on site such as deli and bakery items; restaurant food; bulk food that is not resold; and food that is produced by small businesses are exempt. Manufacturers of foods in small packages are not required to list nutrition information on their labels unless they make a nutrition claim. Nutrition information is voluntary (point-of-purchase) for many raw foods including frequently eaten raw fruits, vegetables, fish, and major cuts of meat and poultry.

Is "sugars" on the Nutrition Facts label just added sugar?
Sugars on the label refer to both added and natural sugars, which is why plain milk lists 12 g of sugar—all of it naturally occurring lactose.

▲ Focus on Critical Thinking

Respond to the following statements:

1. It is appropriate that structure/function claims be allowed on food labels without RDA regulation because they are not claiming that the product can diagnose, cure, treat, or prevent any disease.
2. Dietary supplements are safe because they are natural.
3. Food biotechnology is absolutely safe for short- and long-term use.
4. Food irradiation is absolutely safe for short- and long-term use.

Key Concepts

- The field of nutrition is rapidly changing and growing. New challenges in nutrition stem from advances in food technology, the explosion of information available on the world wide web, and the aging baby-boom generation's quest for quality of life.
- To judge the validity and reliability of nutrition "news," ask who, what, when, where, and why. Mental alarms should ring when claims sound too good to be true, when foods are listed as "good" or "bad," when the recommendations promise a quick fix, and when the recommendations are intended to help to sell a product.
- Nutrition misinformation is everywhere and can be difficult to refute in a client who is convinced that what he or she knows is accurate. Use objectivity, sensitivity, and consistency.
- The Nutrition Facts label is intended to provide consumers with reliable and useful information to help avoid nutritional excesses such as fat, saturated fat, cholesterol, and sodium.
- The Percent Daily Value listed on food labels for fat, saturated fat, carbohydrate, and dietary fiber is based on a 2000-calorie diet. The %DV for these nutrients underestimates the contribution in diets containing fewer than 2000 calories.
- Health Claims on food labels are legally defined such as "calcium may help prevent osteoporosis" and "low sodium may help prevent high blood pressure." In contrast,

structure/function claims, such as "improves mood," "relieves stress," and "for hot flashes," can be used without FDA approval and do not have to carry a disclaimer.
- Clients can use their knowledge of label reading to make better food choices.
- A dietary supplement is a product (other than tobacco) intended to supplement the diet and that contains one or more of the following: vitamins; minerals; herbs or other botanicals; amino acids; or any combination of these ingredients.
- Dietary supplements are regulated by the FDA like food; proof of their safety and effectiveness is not required before marketing. When a dietary supplement is deemed to be unsafe by the FDA, consumer advisories are issued and the manufacturer is requested, not ordered, to stop selling the product. As such, harmful supplements may remain on the market.
- People choosing to use supplements should first check with the FDA for consumer advisories and consult with their physicians. Many supplements can render certain drugs ineffective or potentiate the effectiveness of drugs.
- Pregnant and lactating women and children under the age of 6 should not use dietary supplements.
- To help to retain their nutrient value, plants should be purchased fresh, stored properly, and cooked for a minimum amount of time in a minimum amount of water.
- Functional foods contain substances that appear to enhance health beyond their basic nutritional value. Incorporating more natural functional foods into the diet is prudent; the use of manufactured functional foods may pose risks.
- Organically grown foods are comparable to conventionally grown foods in taste and nutritional value. Because of production costs, higher losses, and lower yields, they are more expensive than other foods.
- The majority of foodborne illnesses are caused by bacteria. Other causes include viruses, parasites, and molds. Chemical (e.g., agricultural chemicals) and physical (e.g., glass, bone, metal) hazards may also cause foodborne illness.
- The foods most commonly contaminated with bacterial are animal proteins—meat, fish, poultry, eggs, milk, and foods containing these items. Improper food handling, such as inadequate cooking and poor personal hygiene, is the major cause of foodborne illness.
- Food biotechnology uses genetic modification to improve the characteristics of a food. Biotechnology has brought us plant foods that are more resistant to disease, stay fresher longer, have higher nutritional value, or are more resistant to severe weather. The FDA considers biotechnology safe.
- Irradiation is used to reduce or eliminate pathogens that can cause foodborne illness. The food remains uncooked and completely free of any radiation residues. Strict regulations and ongoing research protect consumers from potential risks regarding irradiation.

ANSWER KEY

1. **TRUE** If a person's misconception about food is harmless, it is important to respect that belief.
2. **TRUE** The serving sizes used on the Nutrition Facts label are based on amounts typically eaten. However, they may not represent what an *individual* consumes.

3. **TRUE** The %DVs for fat, saturated fat, carbohydrate, and fiber listed on the Nutrition Facts label are based on a 2000-calorie diet. The values are not accurate percentages for anyone who eats more or less than 2000 calories/day. The %DV for other nutrients, such as cholesterol and sodium, are based on Daily Reference Values that are constant for all people over the age of 4 regardless of total calorie intake.
4. **FALSE** Structure/function claims are not regulated by the FDA; their use does not require prior approval nor is a disclaimer necessary.
5. **FALSE** Supplement manufacturers do not have to prove safety or effectiveness before marketing a product, although they are not supposed to sell dangerous or ineffective products.
6. **FALSE** Warning labels about potential side effects or supplement-drug interactions are not required. Nor is a statement regarding who should *not* use the product such as pregnant and lactating women, children under 6 years of age, people with certain chronic illnesses, etc.
7. **FALSE** Organically grown foods are similar to their conventionally grown counterparts in taste and nutritional value.
8. **TRUE** Bacteria are responsible for more than 90% of all foodborne illnesses.
9. **FALSE** Genetically modified foods are not labeled as such unless the food contains new allergens, modified nutritional profiles, or represents a new plant.
10. **FALSE** Irradiated food is completely free of radiation residues.

WEBSITES FOR RELIABLE NUTRITION INFORMATION

American Cancer Society at **www.cancer.org**
American Diabetes Association at **www.diabetes.org**
American Dietetic Association at **www.eatright.org**
Cancer Net, National Cancer Institute, National Institutes of Health at **www.nci.nih.gov**
Case Western Reserve consumer health information at **www.netwellness.org**
Center for Science in the Public Interest at **www.cspinet.org**
Government site for nutrition at **www.nutrition.gov**
Health On the Net Foundation at **www.hon.ch**
International Food Information Council at **www.ific.org**
Mayo Clinic at **www.mayohealth.org**
National Council Against Health Fraud, Inc. at **www.ncahf.org**
National Heart, Lung, and Blood Institute, National Institutes of Health at **www.nhlbi.nih.gov**
Office of Disease Prevention and Health Promotion, U.S. Department of Health and Human Services at **www.odphp.osophs.dhhs.gov**
PubMed, National Library of Medicine at **www.ncbi.nlm.nih.gov/Pubmed/**
Tufts Nutrition Navigator at **www.navigator.tufts.edu**
U.S. Department of Agriculture Food and Nutrition Information Center at **www.nal.usda.gov/fnic**
U.S. Department of Health and Human Services Healthfinder at **www.healthfinder.gov**
U.S. Food and Drug Administration Center for Safety and Applied Nutrition at **www.cfsan.fda.gov**
World Health Organization at **www.who.int**

WEBSITES FOR SUPPLEMENT INFORMATION

ConsumerLab (free subscription) at **www.consumerlab.com/indexasp**
Food and Nutrition Information Center Dietary Supplements Resource list at **www.nal.usda.gov/fnic/pubs/bibs/gen/dietsupp.html.**

Office of Dietary Supplements (ODS) of the National Institutes of Health at **http://dietarysupplements.info.nih.gov.**

SupplementWatch, Inc. (free subscription) at **www.supplementwatch.com/**

The International Bibliographic Information on Dietary Supplements (IBIDS) NIH-Office of Dietary Supplements at **http://ods.od.nih.gov**

U.S. Food and Drug Administration Center for Food Safety and Applied Nutrition at **www.cfsan.fda.gov.** Check out "Tips for the Savvy Supplement User: Making informed decisions and evaluating information.

US Pharmacopeia at **www.usp-dsvp.org/home-cons.html.**

WEBSITES FOR FOOD SAFETY

International Food Information Council at **www.ific.org**

Partnership for Food Safety Education at **www.fightbac.org**

U.S. Food and Drug Administration at **www.fda.gov**

REFERENCES

American Dietetic Association. (2003). Position of the American Dietetic Association: Food and water safety. *Journal of the American Dietetic Association,* 103, 1203–1218.

American Dietetic Association. (2002). Key trends affecting the dietetics profession and the American Dietetic Association. *Journal of the American Dietetic Association, 102,* S1821–1839.

American Dietetic Association. (2002). Position of the American Dietetic Association: Food and nutrition misinformation. *Journal of the American Dietetic Association, 102*(2), 260–266.

Bren, L. (2003). Genetic engineering: The future of foods? FDA Consumer magazine, November-December issue. Available at www.fda.gov/fdac/features/2003/603_food.html. Accessed on 11/22/03.

Brown, A. (2004). *Understanding food* (2nd ed.). Belmont, CA: Wadsworth/Thomson Learning.

Federal Trade Commission, Food and Drug Administration. (2001). "Miracle" health claims: Add a dose of skepticism. Available at: www.ftc.gov/bcp/conline/pubs/health/frdheal.htm. Accessed on 11/6/03.

Food and Drug Administration. (2004). Commonly asked questions about BSE in products prgulated by FDA's Center for Food Safety and Applied Nutrition (CFSAN). Available at www.cfsan.fda.gov/~comm/bsefaq.html. Accessed on 2/28/04.

Food and Drug Administration. (2003). Consumer Alert: FDA plans regulation prohibiting sale of ephedra-containing dietary supplements and advises consumers to stop using these products. Available at www.fda.gov/oc/initiatives/ephedra/december2003/advisory.html. Accessed on 1/2/04.

Hasler, C., Moag-Stahlberg, A., Webb, D., & Hudnall, M. (2001). How to evaluate the safety, efficacy, and quality of functional foods and their ingredients. *Journal of American Dietetic Association, 101,* 733–736.

International Food Information Council Foundation. (2002). Food for Thought IV. Reporting of diet, nutrition and food safety. Executive Summary. Available at: www.ific.org/research/fftivres.cfm?renderforprint=1.htm. Accessed on 11/6/03.

International Food Information Council Foundation. (2002). Emerging microbiological food safety issues . . . and solutions. *Food Insight,* March/April, 2–4.

International Food Information Council Foundation. (2002). Anatomy of a nutrition trend. *Food Insight,* March/April, 1, 3–4, 7.

International Food Information Council Foundation. (2002). Functional foods: Attitudinal research (2002). Available at www.ific.org/research/funcfoodsres02.cfm. Accessed on 11/11/03.

International Food Information Council Foundation. (2002). The consumer view on functional foods: Yesterday and today. *Food Insight*, May/June, 3, 8.

International Food Information Council Foundation. (2003). Questions and answers about food irradiation. Available at www.ific.org/publications/qa/irradiationqa.cfm. Accessed on 11/11/03.

Liebman, B. (2003). Claims crazy. Which can you believe? *Nutrition Action Health Letter, 30*(5), 1, 3–5.

Marcason, W. (2003). What are some resources that can help my clients sort through the conflicting information on dietary supplements? *Journal of the American Dietetic Association*, 103, 712–713.

Pelletier, S., Kundrat, S., & Hasler, C. (2002). Effects of an education program on intent to consume functional foods. *Journal of the American Dietetic Association, 102*, 1297–1300.

Schardt, D. (2003). Are your supplements safe? *Nutrition Action Health Letter, 30*(9), 1, 3–7.

Schardt, D. (2002). Food poisoning's long shadow. *Nutrition Action Health Letter, 29*(4), 1, 3–5.

U.S. Food & Drug Administration, Center for Food Safety & Applied Nutrition. (2002). Dietary supplements. Tips for the savvy supplement user: Making informed decisions and evaluating information. Available at: www.cfsan.fda.gov/~dms/ds-savvy.html. Accessed on 11/6/03.

For information on the new dietary guidelines 2005 and MyPyramid, visit
http://connection.lww.com/go/dudek

10

Cultural, Ethnic, and Religious Influences on Food and Nutrition

TRUE	FALSE	
◯	◯	**1** Culture defines what normal food behaviors are.
◯	◯	**2** Race and ethnicity are synonymous with culture.
◯	◯	**3** Core foods tend to be complex carbohydrates, such as cereal grains, starchy tubers, and starchy vegetables.
◯	◯	**4** Ethnocentrism is the belief that one's own culture is superior to all others.
◯	◯	**5** The hot-cold theory of health and diet refers to the temperature of the food eaten.
◯	◯	**6** First-generation Americans tend to adhere more closely to their cultural food patterns than subsequent generations.
◯	◯	**7** For many ethnic groups who move to the United States, breakfast and lunch are more likely than dinner to be composed of new "American" foods.
◯	◯	**8** People who eat out or get take-out food many times a week tend to eat more calories, fat, and sodium than people who eat out less often.
◯	◯	**9** Dietary acculturation produces unhealthy changes in eating.
◯	◯	**10** Like restaurant food, the portion sizes listed on convenience meals are much larger than they should be.

UPON COMPLETION OF THIS CHAPTER, YOU WILL BE ABLE TO

- Describe how culture influences food choices.
- Name the general ways in which people's food choices change as they become acculturated to a new area.
- List questions appropriate for cross-cultural assessment of food intake.
- Discuss trends in American culture with nutritional implications.
- Describe strategies for ordering food out healthily.

The nutritional requirements among people of similar age and gender are essentially the same throughout the world, yet an infinite variety of food and food combinations can satisfy those requirements. How a person chooses to satisfy nutritional requirements is influenced by many variables, including culture, socioeconomic status, and personal factors. Religion, even more than nationality or culture, also impacts food choices.

By the year 2050, it is estimated that only half of Americans will be Caucasian. The nutritional implication of this shift in cultural predominance is that cultural sensitivity will become increasingly important to nursing care. The key to cross-cultural assessment and counseling is an understanding of the client's cultural values and their impact on health and food choices. From this awareness, nutrition information can be tailored to the client's needs, desires, and lifestyle. Nutrition information that is technically correct but culturally inappropriate does not produce behavior change.

This chapter addresses the impact of culture on food choices. Traditional food practices of major cultural subgroups in the United States are presented, as are religious food practices. Trends in American culture with nutritional implications are discussed.

THE SIGNIFICANCE OF CULTURE

Culture: encompasses the total way of life of a particular population or community at a given time.

Every culture has an inherent value system that dictates behavior by defining what is normal and teaching that those norms are right. Culture is learned, is not instinctive, and is passed from generation to generation. Because culture's influence on its members is unconscious, members may not be aware of the unwritten rules governing their behavior. Culture resists change but is not static. For instance, food habits are basically stable and predictable but, paradoxically, they undergo constant and continuous change in response to changes in lifestyle, attitudes, technology, and environment.

What Culture Defines

Each culture has its own socially standardized foodway; however, within any culture individuals or groups of individuals behave differently based on age, gender, and socioeconomic status. Race, ethnicity, and geographic region are often inaccurately assumed to be synonymous with culture. This misconception leads to stereotypic grouping such as assuming that all Jews adhere to orthodox food laws or that all Southerners eat sausage, biscuits, and gravy. Subgroups within a culture display a unique range of cultural characteristics that affect food intake and nutritional status.

What Is Edible

Culture determines what is edible and what is inedible. To be labeled a food, an item must be readily available, safe, and nutritious enough to support reproduction. However, cultures do not define as edible all sources of nutrients that meet those cri-

teria. For instance in the United States, horse meat, insects, and dog meat are not considered food even though they meet food criteria. Culture overrides flavor in determining what is offensive or unacceptable. For example, you may like a food (e.g., rattlesnake) until you know what it is; this reflects disliking the *idea* of the food rather than the actual food itself. An unconscious food selection decision process appears in Figure 10.1.

The Role of Certain Foods in the Diet

Foodway: an all-encompassing term that refers to all aspects of food including what is edible, the role of certain foods in the diet, how food is prepared, the use of foods, the number and timing of daily meals, how food is eaten, and health beliefs related to food.

Edible: foods that are part of an individual's diet.

Inedible: foods that are usually poisonous or taboo.

Core Foods: the important and consistently eaten foods that form the foundation of the diet; they are the dietary staples.

Every culture has a ranking for its foods that is influenced by cost and availability. Major food categories include core foods, secondary foods, and occasional foods.

Core Foods

Core foods provide a significant source of calories and are considered an indispensable part of the meal. Core foods are cereal grains (rice, wheat, millet, corn), starchy

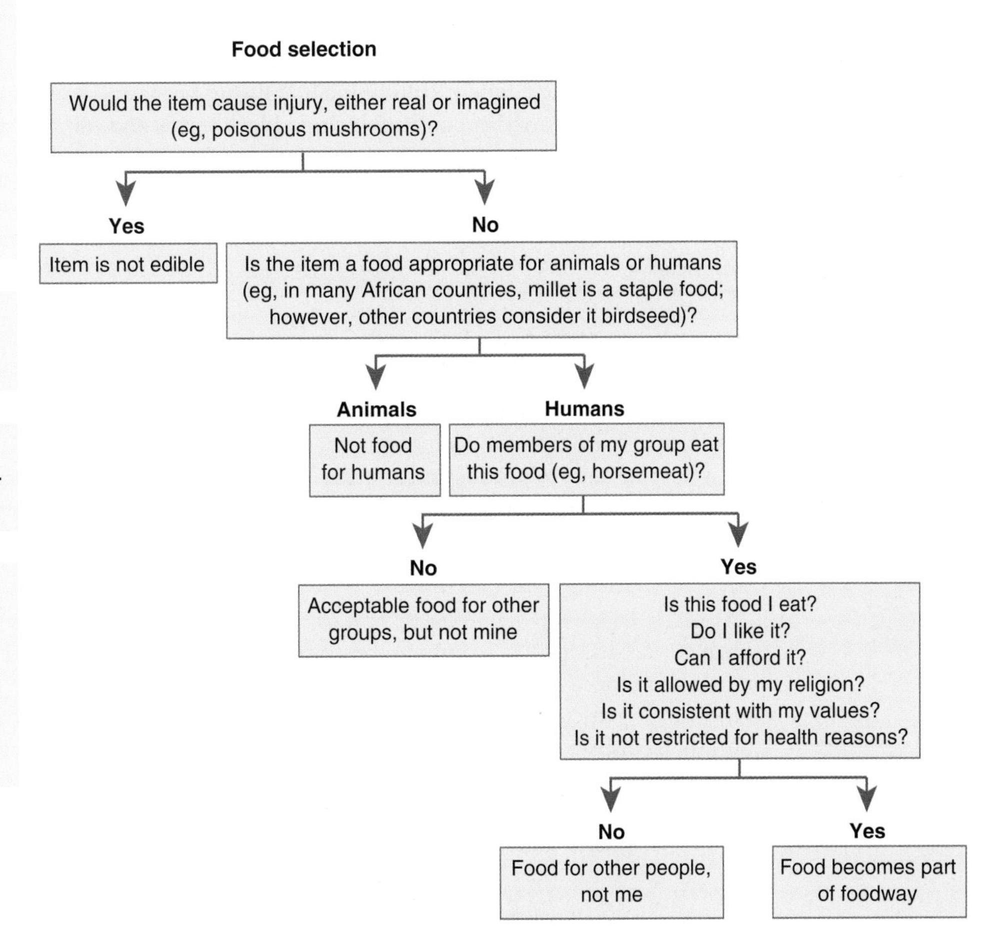

FIGURE 10.1 Food selection decision making.

Career Connection

Recognize that your "normal" may not be normal for others. Just as laboratory normal standards are not appropriate for all ages, races, and individuals, accepted "normal" eating plans may not be normal for all clients. Not everyone eats meat and not everyone drinks milk, yet neither scenario inevitably means a deficient intake. Eating styles that deviate from the typical American intake should not be automatically deemed inadequate or in need of repair. Keep an open mind.

tubers (potatoes, yams, taro, cassava), and starchy vegetables (plantain or green bananas).

Secondary Foods: foods that are widespread in the diet but not eaten consistently.

Secondary Foods

Vegetables, legumes, nuts, fish, eggs, and meats are secondary foods used in various combinations and with various seasonings to give flavor and ethnic identity to meals. Secondary foods used by a culture vary with availability. For instance, the types of legumes used in the Chinese culture include mung beans and soybeans, whereas those used in the Latin American culture include black beans and pinto beans.

Occasional or Peripheral Foods: foods that are infrequently consumed.

Occasional or Peripheral Foods

Occasional foods may be foods that are (1) reserved for special occasions, (2) not readily available, or (3) not generally well tolerated, as is the case with milk among Asian Americans.

Food Preparation

Traditional methods of preparation vary between and within cultural groups. For instance, vegetables often are stir-fried in Asian cultures but boiled in Hispanic cultures. Traditional seasonings also vary among cultures and may be the distinguishing feature between one culture's foods and another's. The choice of seasonings varies among geographic regions and between seasons, based on availability. For instance, fresh hot peppers are widely used in the tropics because they are plentiful.

Use of Foods

Each culture has food customs and bestows symbolism on certain foods. Custom determines what foods are served as meals versus snacks and what foods are considered feminine versus masculine. Symbolically, food can be used to express love, to reward or punish, to display piety, to express moral sentiments, to demonstrate belongingness to a group, or to proclaim the separateness of a group. On a personal level, food may be used inappropriately to relieve anxiety, reduce stress, ease loneliness, or to substitute for sex. Culture also determines which foods are used in celebration and which provide comfort.

Celebrations

All cultures use food during celebrations. Special foods may be reserved for or associated with certain celebrations such as birthdays, national holidays, religious holidays,

or family get-togethers. Celebration foods in the United States include birthday cake, Christmas cookies, Halloween candy, and Thanksgiving turkey. Families within a culture may establish their own food traditions for celebrations.

Comfort Foods

Comfort foods vary among cultures and individuals. In the United States, a child who falls might be offered cookies and milk for comfort; warm milk at bedtime is used to soothe and relax. During illness, people may resort to comfort foods. People who move from other cultures may retain their own cultural comfort foods as a link with the past.

Number and Timing of Meals

All cultures eat at least once a day. Typically, Americans have three meals daily; Mexicans might have four or five meals daily. In some places in Africa, one meal per day is standard.

When meals are eaten is also dictated by culture. Dinner takes place between 7 and 9 p.m. in Kenya and at approximately 6 p.m. in Australia. A Lebanese custom is to arrive anytime when invited for dinner, even as early as 9 or 10 a.m.

How Food Is Eaten

In China, food is usually eaten with chopsticks. In England, almost all foods are eaten with a knife and fork, even sandwiches. In the United States, bad manners in eating may be associated with animal behavior, as in "He eats like a pig," "She chews like a cow," or "Don't wolf down your food."

Health Beliefs Related to Food

Food may be thought to promote wellness, to cure disease, or to have medicinal properties. For instance, hot oregano tea seasoned with salt is used to treat an upset stomach in Vietnamese culture. In some Hispanic cultures, raw chopped onions with honey are believed to be good for a cold and other respiratory infections. In Caribbean cultures, chayote and papaya are used to treat high blood pressure.

Asian cultures believe that health and illness are related to the balance between yin and yang forces in the body. Yin represents female, cold, and darkness; yang represents male, hot, and light. Digested foods turn into air that is either yin or yang. Diseases caused by yin forces are treated with yang foods, and diseases caused by yang forces are treated with yin foods. For instance, pregnancy is considered a yang or "hot" condition, so women following traditional practices during pregnancy eat yin foods such as most fruits and vegetables, seaweed, cold drinks, juices, and rice water. Yang foods include chicken, meat, pig's feet, meat broth, nuts, fried food, coffee, and spices. The hot–cold theory of foods and illness also exists in Puerto Rico and Mexico. Although the theories are similar, the food designations are not universal within or across cultures.

Cultures often have varying views on what body types are attractive. Some cultures have a greater tolerance for heavier body weights than others.

Cultural Values

Ethnocentrism: the belief that one's own culture is superior to another or that the cultural practices of another are inappropriate or "wrong."

Underlying a culture's behavior patterns are cultural values that identify what is desirable and what is undesirable. Ethnocentric describes a person who believes that his or her own values and beliefs are superior to all other cultures. Replacing ethnocentrism with sensitivity to another's cultural values fosters more effective communication and can help to determine culturally appropriate interventions. A contrast between selected American cultural values and values of more traditional cultures follows.

Personal Control Versus Fate

Whereas many Americans have a sense of personal control over their future, members of other traditional cultures may accept what happens to them as fate. When illness is perceived as an affliction for sins, spiritual atonement and forgiveness are the ways to cure, not medical interventions. The idea of preventative health care may be unknown in cultures dominated by fate.

Individualism Versus Group Welfare

Individualism is the belief that the interests of the individual have preference over the interests of the group. Individual will and personality are valued. In contrast, group welfare values the group over the individual. Food intake decisions may not be made by the individual but rather by the consensus of the group or family.

Clock-Focused Versus Event-Focused Orientation

Americans tend to be ruled by time and schedules. "Being on time" and "not wasting time" are valued. Time-related misunderstandings can occur when fast-paced American culture encounters traditional cultures that are dominated by events or human interactions. This difference is particularly important when determining when and how to convey nutrition information.

Acculturation

Acculturation: the process that occurs as people who move to a different cultural area adopt the beliefs, values, attitudes, and behaviors of the dominant culture; not limited to immigrants but affects

Acculturation is influenced by many factors. Several studies show that the longer the residence in the host country, high education and income, employment outside the home, having young children, and fluency in the host language promote acculturation. Usually, first-generation Americans adhere more closely to cultural food patterns than subsequent generations do, and they may cling to traditional foods to preserve their ethnic identity. Subsequent generations may follow cultural patterns only on holidays and at family gatherings, or they may give up ethnic foods but retain traditional methods of preparation. Children tend to adopt new ways quickly as they learn from other children at school. People seeking higher education tend to have greater exposure to new ideas than those who remain more closely tied to their native cultural group.

anyone (to varying degrees) who moves from one community to another.

There are three types of interrelated changes in food choices that occur as part of acculturation: new foods are added to the diet, traditional foods are made in new ways, and some traditional foods are rejected. In addition, as part of dietary acculturation in the United States, individuals begin to adopt growing food trends in American culture such as changes in food purchasing and preparation methods and fewer meals eaten at home. Dietary changes through acculturation may have a positive or negative impact on health.

New Foods

Status, economics, information, taste, and exposure are some of the reasons why new foods are added to the diet. For instance, eating "American" food may symbolize status and make people feel more connected to their new culture. Frequently, new foods are added because they are relatively inexpensive and widely available.

Food Substitutions

Traditional foods may be replaced by new foods. This often occurs because traditional foods are difficult to find, are too expensive, or have lengthy preparation times. For many ethnic groups who move to the United States, breakfast and lunch are most likely to be composed of convenient American foods, whereas traditional foods are retained for the major dinner meal, which has greater emotional significance.

Rejection of Traditional Foods

Dietary Acculturation: the process that occurs as members of a minority group adopt the eating patterns and food choices of the host country.

To become more like their peers, children and adolescents are more likely than older adults to reject traditional foods. Traditional foods may also be rejected because of an increased awareness of the role of nutrition in the development of chronic diseases. For instance, one reason why Indians who have resided in the United States for a relatively long period tend to eat significantly less ghee (clarified butter served with rice or spread on Indian breads) may be that they are trying to decrease their intake of saturated fat.

TRADITIONAL DIETS OF SELECTED CULTURAL SUBGROUPS IN THE UNITED STATES

Subgroups: a unique cultural group that coexists within a dominant culture.

The major cultural subgroups in the United States are Hispanic American, African American, and Asian American. Within each of these subgroups are smaller subgroups. For instance, the term "Asian Americans" encompasses a diverse population originating from at least 17 Asian and 8 Pacific countries. Although generalizations can be made about traditional eating practices, actual food choices vary greatly among nations, regions, and individuals within a cultural subgroup.

African Americans

The majority of African Americans can trace their ancestors to West Africa, although some have immigrated from the Caribbean, Central America, and East African countries. Because most are many generations away from their original homeland, much of their native heritage has been assimilated, lost, or modified. For many, the biggest influence on their cultural identity is the lifestyle of their parents or grandparents who lived in the southern United States.

"Soul food" describes traditional southern African American food choices. It is a mixture of foods and cooking techniques brought from Africa, using foods available in the southern United States. Traditional soul foods tend to be high in fat, cholesterol, and sodium and low in protective nutrients such as potassium (fruits and vegetables), fiber (whole grains, vegetables), and calcium (milk, cheese, and yogurt). Although soul food has become a symbol of African American identity and African heritage, food choices of African American families may not differ from the conventional American diet. In such cases, soul food may be reserved for special occasions and holidays.

Traditional Food Practices

A MyPyramid featuring foods commonly eaten by African Americans in the southern United States appears in Figure 10.2. Comparisons show that African Americans may choose fried chicken, barbecued ribs, corn bread, sweet potato pie, collard greens, and fruit-flavored drinks and juices as favorite foods more often than whites. Compared to whites, African American households often purchase less cereal and bakery products, dairy products, sugar, and other sweets. However, food preferences do not vary greatly between blacks and whites in similar socioeconomic groups living in the same region of the United States.

A traditional soul food diet is high in protein and fat. Pork is the primary protein source and includes chitterlings, ham hocks, sausages, and variety cuts. Chicken is the second most popular meat. Frying and cooking with added fat, such as lard, bacon, shortening, and fatback or salt pork, are common. Many foods are served with gravy and sauces.

Milk and dairy products are not routinely consumed, so calcium intake is low. The incidence of lactose intolerance is estimated at 60% to 95% of the population.

The intake of fresh fruits and vegetables is generally low. Green leafy vegetables ("greens") are popular in all regions; other fruits and vegetables are consumed according to availability, although preference is generally low. Vegetables often are preferred cooked instead of raw. Bean dishes, such as those made with black-eyed peas, kidney beans, peanuts, pinto beans, and red beans, are popular.

Dietary Acculturation

Regional acculturation may result in

- Greater consumption of milk, at least among blacks living in urban areas.
- Popularity of luncheon and packaged meats; pork remains the preferred source of protein.
- Substitution of commercially made breads for homemade biscuits.

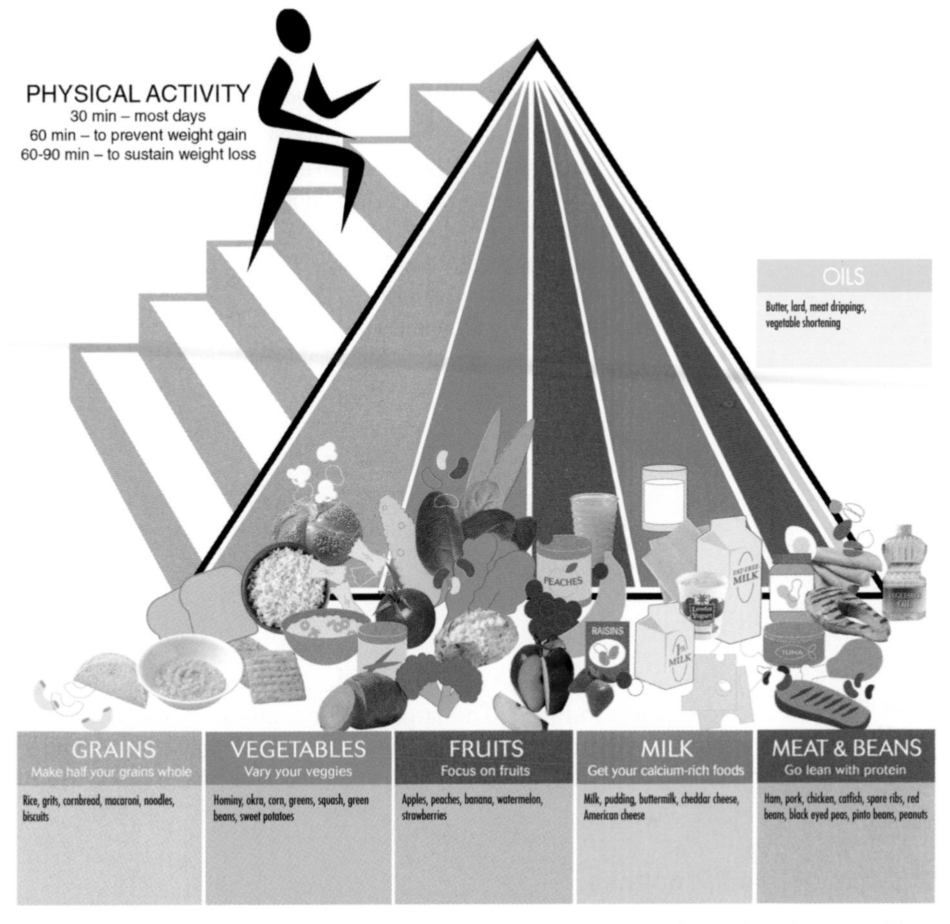

FIGURE 10.2 MyPyramid featuring traditional southern African-American "soul" foods.

- Fruit and vegetable intake remaining low; varies with availability. Greens remain popular in all regions.

Diet and Health

Obesity is prevalent among African Americans. Based on U.S. Centers for Disease Control (CDC) statistics for 1999–2000, the prevalence of obesity (BMI $\geq$ 30) among adult black American men is 28.8 %; among black women the prevalence is 50.8%. For the designation of overweight (BMI $\geq$ 25) the numbers climb to 60.0% and 78%, respectively. Studies suggest that African American women are less inclined to value thinness and may equate fatness with prosperity (Kittler & Sucher, 2001).

The prevalence of other chronic, diet-related diseases, namely diabetes, hypertension, and heart disease, is higher among African Americans than in whites. For instance, the incidence of Type 2 diabetes is 3 to 4 times higher among African Americans than

Career Connection

To encourage African American clients to modify traditional diet

- Focus on how food is prepared. Suggest removing the fat and skin from meat; limiting the amount of fats added to foods; using small amounts of canola or olive oil, or vegetable oil sprays in place of shortening or bacon drippings when frying; using turkey ham or smoke flavoring instead of bacon to season foods; and flavoring with herbs in place of sodium.
- Suggest eating less meat.
- Use sugar-free sweetened drinks in place of sweetened varieties.
- Encourage more fresh vegetables and fruit.
- Involve family in planning; offer immediate solutions and specific advice.

the American population as a whole. The incidence of hypertension is almost double that of whites, and it tends to occur at an earlier age, be more severe, and be more likely to cause death from renal failure, stroke, and heart attack.

Mexican Americans

Latino: refers to people originally from Mexico, the Caribbean, and Central and South America.

Latinos living in America are a diverse group differing in native language, customs, history, and foodways. The largest Latino group in the United States originates from Mexico. The majority of Mexican Americans live in California and Texas; 80% of Mexican immigrants settle in United States cities such as Los Angeles, San Antonio, and Chicago.

Traditional Food Practices

The traditional Mexican diet, influenced by Spanish and Native American cultures, is basically vegetarian with an emphasis on corn, corn products, beans, rice, and breads. It is rich in complex carbohydrates and is composed of mostly unprocessed foods. Tortillas and beans may be eaten at every meal. Foods eaten vary with income, education, urbanization, geographic region, and family customs.

Pork, goat, and poultry are common meats often served ground or chopped and mixed with vegetables and cereals. Stuffed foods are common such as enchiladas, bur-

Career Connection

Don't try to impose the American cultural value of slimness on other cultures.

A more effective approach to preaching the virtues of slimness is to encourage healthier food choices and increasing activity without mention of weight or size. To some people, "healthy eating" is synonymous with eating large quantities of food; use terminology that won't be misunderstood such as "more nutritious food choices."

Arroz Con Leche: rice with milk.

Flan: sweetened egg custard topped with carmelized sugar.

Atole: hot beverage of milk (or water) and sugar thickened with cornstarch.

Café Con Leche: coffee with milk.

ritos, tacos, and tamales. Cooking techniques may rely heavily on frying and stewing using oil or lard. Food tends to be heavily spiced; chilies are a mainstay.

Although unknown before Spanish colonization, milk, cheese, and other dairy foods are now widely consumed in Mexico. Milk is used in products such as arroz con leche, flan, atole and café con leche.

Semitropical and tropical fruits are popular where available. Vegetables often are consumed as ingredients in soups, rice, pasta, meat and tortilla-based items. Salads and vegetables as side dishes are less common. The use of sugar is not extensive. Figure 10.3 features a Latin American food pyramid.

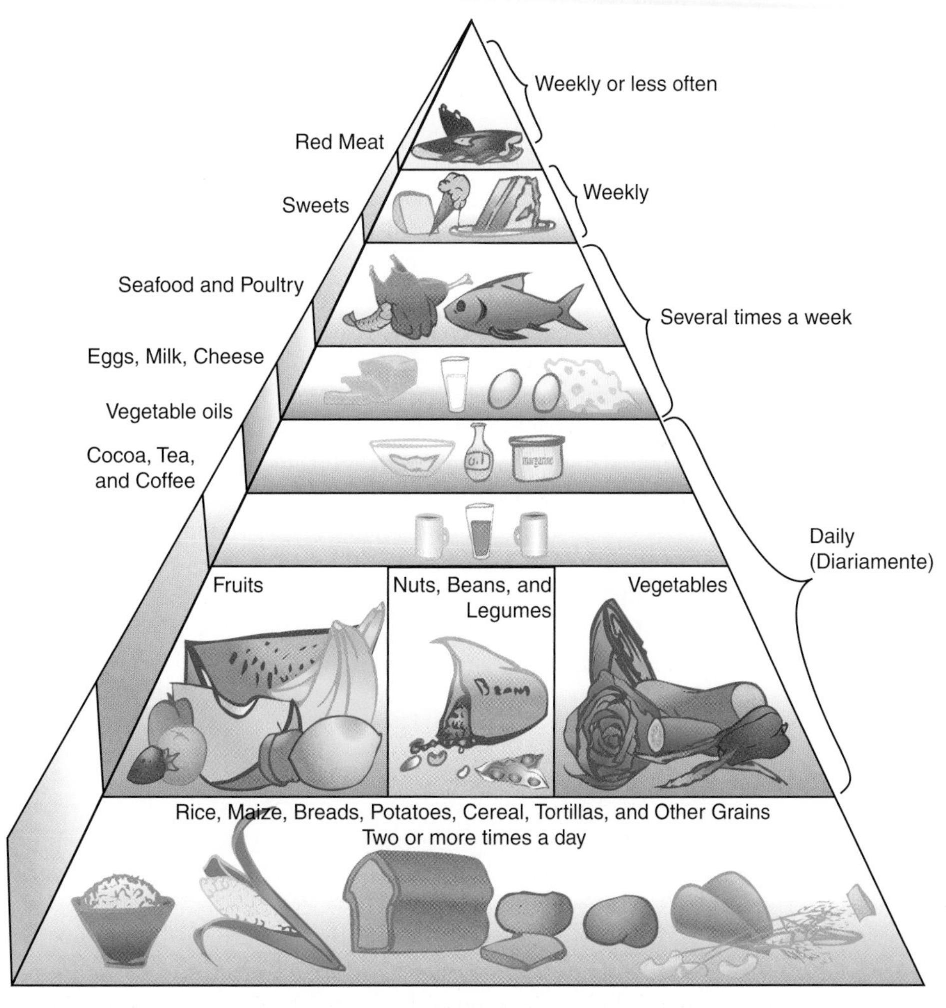

FIGURE 10.3 Latin American Food Pyramid. (Developed by the Nutrition Education for New Americans project of the Department of Anthropology and Geography at Georgia State University, Atlanta, Georgia.)

Dietary Acculturation

Acculturation tends to cause a decrease in total protein intake and an increase in fat intake among Mexican Americans. Although the traditional Mexican diet has good sources of vitamins A and C, thiamin, niacin, B_6, folate, phosphorus, zinc, and fiber, the intake of these nutrients by Mexican Americans has reported to be low because traditional sources of these nutrients are not available. Acculturation may cause the following changes:

- Milk intake increases related to its use with a new food such as ready-to-eat breakfast cereal.
- Meat remains popular, but the intake of traditional meat-vegetable preparations declines drastically. Protein intake may decline in second-generation Mexican Americans.
- Bean consumption falls.
- Rice remains a core food but may be prepared differently; consumption of rice prepared with vegetables, a major source of vegetables in the Mexican diet, decreases and the intake of plain boiled rice increases.
- Pasta consumption also falls; like rice, it is traditionally prepared with vegetables.
- Flour tortillas are used more often than corn; use of white bread increases.
- Fruit and vegetable intakes increase.
- Use of spices depends on availability.
- Severe decline in fruit-based beverages is concurrent with increased use of highly sweetened drinks (fruit drink, Kool-Aid, soft drinks).
- Introduction of cooked vegetables and salads leads to an increase in fat intake from butter and salad dressings.
- Use of lard and Mexican cream declines significantly; cooking oil use increases.
- Sugar intake increases.
- Traditional pattern of four to five meals daily is often retained, but the types of foods eaten at each meal tend to change. The largest meal may shift from the afternoon to the evening.

Diet and Health

Central Obesity: obesity characterized by the deposition of excess weight around the abdomen and waist, not the hips and thighs.

Mexican Americans have a high prevalence of obesity, particularly central obesity that raises the risk of diabetes and heart disease. Approximately 34.4% of Mexican Americans have a BMI $\geq$ 30. The prevalence of overweight (BMI $\geq$ 25) is at 73.4%.

The rate of type 2 diabetes among Mexican Americans is estimated to be 2 to 5 times higher than among the white population. The intake of traditional foods appears to be inversely related to the risk of diabetes: as intake of traditional food decreases, the risk of diabetes rises.

Career Connection

To encourage Mexican American clients to modify traditional diet

- Urge clients to retain the traditional high intake of complex carbohydrates, fruits, and vegetables.
- Recommend using less fat during cooking and substituting canola oil or olive oil for lard, bacon, and margarine.
- Target messages to emphasize the good of the entire family rather than individual benefits: Mexican-Americans encourage interdependence rather than independence in families.
- Focus not just on the potential health benefits of improving nutrition but also on potential savings in time and money, the maintenance of traditional food choices, and flavor.
- Be open and use a friendly conversational tone; treat older people with formality. Avoid prolonged eye contact.
- Involve family.
- Verbal and written messages in Spanish are important.

Asian Americans

The term "Asian Americans" encompasses a diverse population originating from at least 25 countries, including China, Japan, Hong King, South Korea, India, Thailand, Vietnam, Cambodia, Indonesia, Malaysia, the Philippines, and other Pacific Rim areas. Two dietary commonalities exist between these diverse cultures: (1) emphasis on rice and vegetables with relatively little meat, and (2) cooking techniques that include meticulous attention to preparing ingredients before cooking.

Traditional Food Practices

The traditional Asian diet is a plant-based diet and is, therefore, high in complex carbohydrates, fiber, and many nutrients. Rice is the primary staple and is eaten with every meal. Common foods consumed include noodles, flat breads, potatoes, fruits, vegetables (including sea vegetables), nuts, seeds, beans, soyfoods, vegetable and nut oils, herbs and spices, tea, wine, and beer. An Asian food pyramid appears in Figure 10.4.

Fat intake generally is low. Meat is considered more of a condiment than the focus of a meal. Poultry and eggs often are used in small amounts; red meat is used sparingly. The use of fish and seafood depends on availability. For instance, people who live in the interior of China or India consume little or no seafood, whereas people who live in seacoast and island areas (e.g., Japan, Vietnam) consume large amounts.

With the exception of India, milk and dairy products often are absent from traditional Asian diets; lactose intolerance affects 75% of Asians. Available sources of calcium include tofu, small fish (bones are eaten), and soups made with bones that have been partially dissolved by vinegar in making stock.

Sodium intake is generally assumed to be high because of traditional food preservation methods (salting and drying) and condiments (e.g., soy sauce).

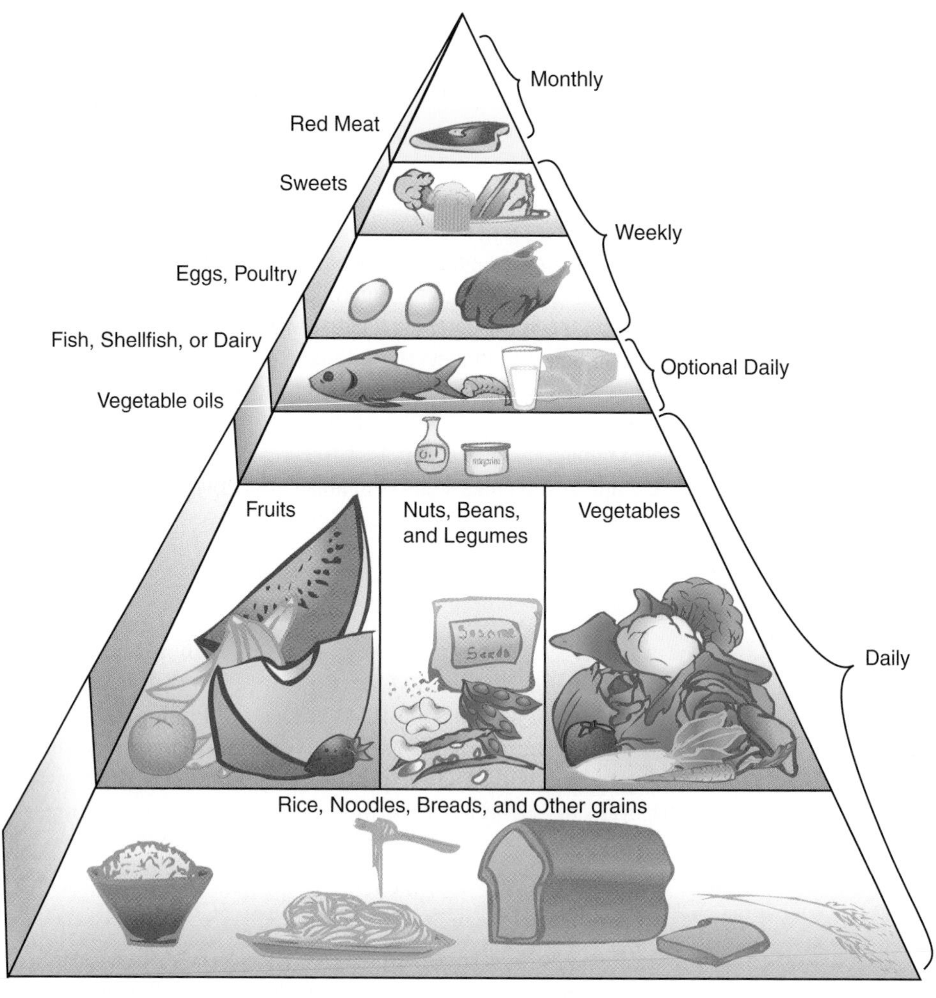

FIGURE 10.4 Asian-American Food Pyramid. (Developed by the Nutrition Education for New Americans project of the Department of Anthropology and Geography at Georgia State University, Atlanta, Georgia.)

Dietary Acculturation

With acculturation, intakes of fat, protein, sugar, and cholesterol increase and the intake of complex carbohydrates decreases. Specifically, the following changes in intake may be seen:

- Intakes of bread and cereals increase, although rice remains the primary staple.
- Intakes of raw vegetables and salads increase; traditional fruits and vegetables are replaced by more commonly available ones.
- Intakes of meats and ethnic dishes (e.g., Mexican, Italian) increase.
- Consumption of soft drinks, candy, and American desserts increases sugar intake.

Career Connection

To encourage Asian American clients to modify traditional diet

- Urge retention of a plant-based diet with meat used sparingly.
- Promote the healthier choices among American foods such as whole grain breads, low fat desserts, and limiting intake of soft drinks.
- Asian Americans consuming a traditional diet are not likely to achieve a low sodium intake due to the difficulty eliminating high-salt items. A more appropriate alternative to a low-sodium diet may simply be to consume less sodium.
- Use a quiet conversational approach with pauses. Avoid interruptions. Asking questions may be seen as a sign of disrespect.
- Use fleeting eye contact and be cautious about touching.
- Honor traditional beliefs. Some Chinese Americans may follow yin/yang customs without realizing the basis of their food choices.
- Determine if herbal supplements are used, and if so, which ones. It is believed that many Chinese Americans self-diagnose and self-treat at home before seeking medical attention.

Diet and Health

Moderation is valued; therefore, overeating and obesity are rare. Other positive factors related to diet include a lower incidence of heart disease, bowel cancer, and breast cancer. However, cancer risk increases with the length of stay in the United States and is the leading cause of death among Chinese Americans.

PROMOTING HEALTHY FOOD CHOICES

Promoting healthy food choices encompasses (1) identifying healthy traditional food practices that are retained and encouraging their use, (2) supporting healthy new food practices, and (3) discouraging the adoption of less healthy American dietary practices. Assessing the client's level of acculturation and offering culturally sensitive counseling are vital.

Assessing Acculturation

Think of dietary acculturation as a continuum of food choices that range from completely traditional on one end to completely American (if there is such a diet) on the other. It is essential to know where the client is on that continuum before interventions can be made to improve intake.

Some questions to consider are

- What is the country or region of origin and how long has the client been in the United States?

Career Connection

Points to keep in mind regarding acculturation

- Generally with acculturation, the intake of sweets and fats increases, neither of which has a positive effect on health.
- Because dietary acculturation is most likely to change food choices for breakfast and lunch rather than dinner, focus on promoting healthy "American" food choices for those meals.
- It is essential to determine how often a food is consumed in order to determine the potential impact of that food. For instance, lard is unimportant in the context of the total diet if it is used in cooking only on special occasions.

- What traditional foods does the client eat daily? Weekly? How often does the client currently eat traditional foods? What traditional foods does the client no longer eat? Why? Are there similar foods available? Does the client substitute new foods for traditional foods?
- What were the client's favorite cultural foods? Does the client still eat those foods? Are they still the client's favorite foods? If not, why not? Are similar foods available? Does the client substitute new foods for favorite foods?
- What new foods has the client tried? Which new foods did the client like? Which new foods did the client dislike? Does the client eat new foods regularly?
- What are the client's health beliefs related to food? Does the client use herbs or other dietary supplements?
- Who is responsible for procuring, storing, and preparing food? Does the client shop at grocery stores or ethnic specialty markets? Are refrigeration and cooking facilities adequate?
- Is the client intent on becoming "Americanized" or on trying to retain his or her ethnic identity?

Culturally Sensitive Nutrition Counseling

After gaining a sense of where the client is in terms of dietary acculturation, the health care professional can start to identify the client's needs. What positive aspects of the traditional diet has the client retained? What health-enhancing new foods has the client adopted? Has the diet been negatively impacted by the adoption of less-than-healthy new foods?

In counseling clients from other cultures about nutrition, it is important to remember that eating is a very personal matter. Be respectful and understanding of other cultures without being judgmental, especially regarding foods that you may personally find distasteful, such as turtle eggs or lizards. No one likes to have her or his food choices criticized. Clients may tell you what you want to hear to avoid the risk of being chastised. Other considerations include the following:

- Determine the client's level of fluency before beginning counseling. Obtain an interpreter if needed. Speak directly to the client even if an interpreter is used.
- Ask how the client wishes to be addressed.
- Avoid body language that may be misinterpreted.
- Determine reading ability before giving out written material.
- Reinforce positive eating habits. Promote change only in harmful practices.
- Remember that knowledge does not necessarily lead to behavior change.

TRADITIONAL FOOD PRACTICES OF SELECTED RELIGIOUS GROUPS

Religion tends to have a greater impact on food habits than nationality or culture does (e.g., Orthodox Jews follow kosher dietary laws regardless of their national origin). However, religious food practices vary significantly even among denominations of the same faith. National variations also exist. How closely an individual follows dietary laws is based on his or her degree of orthodoxy. An overview of religious food practices follows.

Christianity

The three primary branches of Christianity are Roman Catholicism, Eastern Orthodox Christianity, and Protestantism. Dietary practices vary from none to explicit.

Roman Catholics do not eat meat on Ash Wednesday or on Fridays of Lent. Food and beverages are avoided for 1 hour before communion is taken. Devout Catholics observe several fast days during the year.

Lacto-ovo Vegetarians: people who include milk products and eggs in their diets but no other sources of animal protein.

Eastern Orthodox Christians observe numerous feast and fast days throughout the year. The only denominations in the Protestant faith with dietary laws are the Mormons (Church of Jesus Christ of Latter-Day Saints) and Seventh-Day Adventists. Mormons do not use coffee, tea, alcohol, or tobacco. Followers are encouraged to limit meats and consume mostly grains. Some Mormons fast one day a month. Most Seventh-Day Adventists are lacto-ovo vegetarians; those who do eat meat avoid pork. Overeating is avoided, and coffee, tea, and alcohol are prohibited. An interval of 5 to 6 hours between meals is recommended with no snacking between meals. Water is consumed before and after meals. Strong seasonings, such as pepper and mustard, are avoided.

Judaism

In the United States there are three main Jewish denominations: Orthodox, Conservative, and Reform. Hasidic Jews are a sect within the Orthodox. These groups differ in their interpretation of the precepts of Judaism. Orthodox Jews believe that the laws are the direct commandments of God so they adhere strictly to dietary laws.

Reform Jews follow the moral law but may selectively follow other laws; for instance, they may not follow any religious dietary laws. Conservative Jews fall between the other two groups in their beliefs and adherence to the laws. They may follow the Jewish dietary laws at home but take a more liberal attitude on social occasions. Because Jews have diverse backgrounds and nationalities, their food practices vary widely.

Kosher: a word commonly used to identify Jewish dietary laws that define "clean" foods, "unclean" foods, how food animals must be slaughtered, how foods must be prepared, and when foods may be consumed (e.g., the timing between eating milk products and meat products).

Pareve: dairy-free.

Orthodox Jews eat only kosher meat and poultry that has been slaughtered according to ritual, soaked in water, salted, and washed. All crustaceans, shellfish, and fishlike mammals, such as catfish, shark, frog, crab, shrimp, lobster, scallops, oysters, and clams, are forbidden, as are all pork products. Milk and dairy products are used widely but cannot be consumed at the same meal with meat or poultry. Dairy products are not allowed within 1 to 6 hours after eating meat or poultry, depending on the individual's ethnic tradition. Meat and poultry cannot be eaten for 30 minutes after dairy products have been consumed. Margarine labeled *pareve,* nondairy creamers, and oils may be used with meats. Fruits, vegetables, plain grains, pastas, plain legumes, and eggs are considered kosher and can be eaten with either dairy or meat products. Separate utensils must be used for preparing and serving meat and dairy products.

Food preparation is prohibited on the Sabbath. Religious holidays are celebrated with certain foods. For example, only unleavened bread is eaten during Passover, and a 24-hour fast is observed on Yom Kippur. Because dietary laws are rigid, Orthodox Jews rarely eat outside the home except at homes or restaurants with kosher kitchens.

Islam

Halal: Islamic dietary laws.

Haram: foods that are prohibited.

Muslims eat as a matter of faith and for good health. Overindulgence is discouraged. Islamic dietary laws are called *halal,* which is also the term used to describe all permitted foods. *Haram* are prohibited foods such as pork in any form and birds of prey. Meats must be properly slaughtered. Alcohol is prohibited, and devout Muslims avoid stimulants such as coffee and tea. Muslims are required to fast during the entire month of Ramadan and on certain other days during the year.

Hinduism

Ahimsa: nonviolence as applied to foods.

Generally, Hindus avoid all foods that are believed to inhibit physical and spiritual development. Eating meat is not explicitly prohibited, but many Hindus are vegetarian because they adhere to the concept of ahimsa. Those who eat meat do not eat beef because cows are considered sacred. Pork is often avoided. Other food prohibitions vary by region and may include snails, crabs, fowl, cranes, ducks, boars, fish with ugly forms, and the heads of snakes. Devout Hindus may avoid alcohol. Those seeking spiritual unity may avoid garlic and onions.

The concept of purity influences Hindu food practices. Products from cows (e.g., milk, yogurt, ghee-clarified butter) are considered pure. Pure foods can improve the purity of unpure foods when they are prepared together. Some foods, such as beef or alcohol, are innately polluted and can never be made pure. Numerous feast and fast days are observed.

Jainism, a branch of Hinduism, also promotes the nonviolent doctrine of ahimsa. Devout Jains are complete vegetarians and may avoid blood-colored foods (e.g., tomatoes) and root vegetables (because harvesting them may cause the death of insects).

Sikhism

Sikhs participate in many Hindu practices. They abstain from beef, and alcohol is prohibited. Pork is allowed.

Buddhism

Buddhist dietary practices vary widely depending on the sect and country. Most Buddhists subscribe to the concept of ahimsa, so many are lacto-ovo vegetarians. Some eat fish; some avoid only beef. Feast days vary regionally. Buddhist monks avoid eating solid food after the noon hour.

CHANGES IN AMERICAN SOCIETY

The increase in ethnic diversity in the United States has impacted our own foodway as ethnic foods become mainstream. Not so long ago, foods such as yogurt and green tea were considered exotic. Today, ethnic restaurants and ethnic foods sections in grocery stores are commonplace and popular; salsa sales have outpaced ketchup sales for more than a decade. In fact, it is difficult to ascertain which foods are truly American foods and which are an adaptation from other cultures. Swiss steak, Russian dressing, and chili con carne are American inventions. Cross-cultural food creations include Tex-Mex wontons and tofu lasagna.

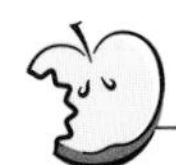

Quick Bite

What Americans eat

- **67% have hot or cold cereal for breakfast; 55% have toast, cereal or bagels; 31% have eggs.**
- **70% have a sandwich for lunch; 33% eat fast food for lunch.**
- **When dinner is take-out, the top three choices are pizza, Chinese, and fast food.**
- **Almost 66% of Americans snack in the evening usually while watching TV.**

The American foodway also evolves in response to societal changes. Our modern lifestyle presents many challenges that impact food choices: the traditional family structure has declined; more women than ever are in the workforce; time is in short supply. These and other societal or personal factors contribute to the increased reliance on convenience foods and eating out.

Increased Reliance on Convenience Foods

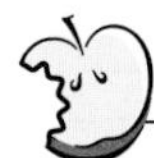

Quick Bite

Example of convenience items with a positive impact on nutrition

Fresh fruits and vegetables from the salad bar
Washed spinach
Presliced mushrooms
Bagged salad mixes
Frozen vegetables
Fresh sushi
Whole grain rolls from the bakery section
Prepared hummus
Fully cooked roasted chickens
Lean deli meats

Convenience Foods: broadly defined as any product that saves time in food preparation, ranging from bagged fresh salad mixes to frozen packaged complete meals.

For many, the pace of our American lifestyle is fast-forward. Time is at a premium. Our workdays—and sometimes workweeks—are longer. More women are in the workforce and the number of single-parent families is on the rise. The outcome: domestic chores, such as cooking, may be shared by family members or given up entirely. So we experience the universal popularity of products designed to save us time shopping, preparing meals, and cleaning up. According to *Food Technology* magazine, next to taste, what Americans value most in new foods is convenience in the form of ready-to-eat, heat-and-eat, and packaged grab-and-go items. In fact, taste and convenience outrank nutrition and health as important qualities in food selection.

Americans want simple recipes with few ingredients that can be prepared in a minimum amount of time. On average, Americans spend 31 minutes a day preparing weeknight dinners, down from 49 minutes just 10 years ago. That trend is likely to continue as convenience becomes a virtual necessity.

Convenience products exist on a continuum ranging from convenient ingredients to a quick "homemade" meal to a complete, ready-to-heat meal. Generally, the more convenient the meal is, the greater the impact all around on time, budget, and nutritional value. When time is short, frozen complete or nearly complete meals or boxed "helper" type entrees earn their designation as "convenient." They cost more than "from scratch" items and lack that "homemade" taste but are less expensive than take-out and are easy and quick to prepare. And variety abounds, from typical American fare such as meatloaf and pot roast to vegetarian, Mexican, Chinese, Southwestern, and Italian cuisines (Fig. 10.5). On the downside, these products are high in sodium and relatively low in fiber, and the 1- to 2-cup portion sizes listed on the label may leave many people hungry. Yet they are here to stay. With a little planning and effort, they can be part of a healthy diet. See Box 10.1 for tips on balancing convenience with nutrition.

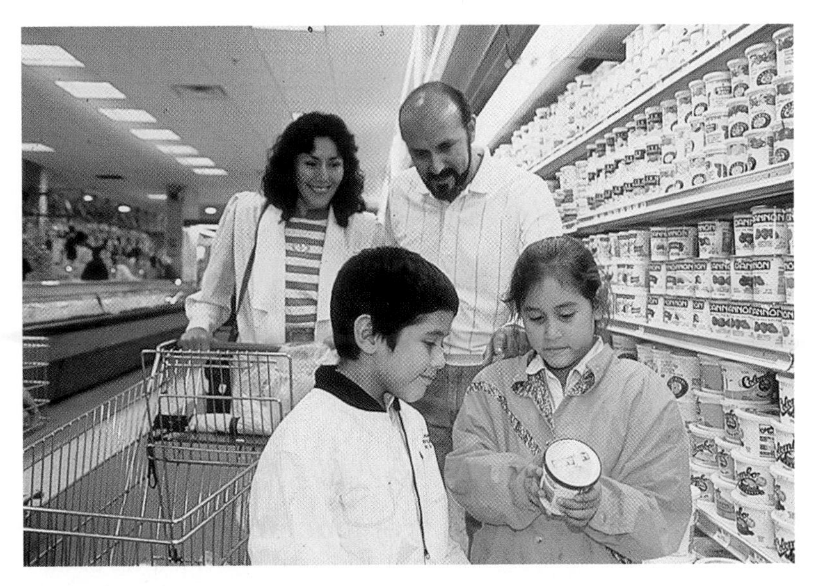

FIGURE 10.5 Parents and children can choose foods that are culturally appealing and nutritionally beneficial by learning to read food labels. (Copyright: Jeff Greenberg/Science Source/Photo Researchers.)

BOX 10.1

TIPS FOR BALANCING CONVENIENCE WITH NUTRITION

Read the label to comparison shop. Calories, fat, saturated fat, and sodium can vary greatly among different brands of similar items. A rule of thumb guideline is to limit sodium to less than 800 mg and fat to no more than 10 to 13 g in a meal that provides 300 to 400 calories.

Look for "healthy" on the label. The government allows "healthy" on the label of meals or entrees that limit sodium to 140 mg/100 g of food. And "healthy" foods must also provide 3 g or less of total fat or 1 g of saturated fat per 100 g of food. They are a better choice than the products not labeled with "healthy," yet may still lack adequate fiber.

Add additional ingredients to "stretch" the meal. For instance, adding a bag of frozen vegetables, a can of tomatoes, or a can of garbanzo or black beans provides nutrients and increases volume.

Add healthy side dishes. A convenience "meal" that provides 300 to 400 calories may leave many people hungry. Adding quick and easy side dishes, such as bagged salad mixes, raw vegetables, whole grain rolls, an instant cup of soup, or piece of fresh fruit, can greatly increase nutritional and satiety values.

Adjust the seasoning when possible. Some frozen meal solutions contain a separate seasoning packet; using half satisfies taste while cutting sodium.

Fewer Meals Prepared at Home

Eating out is a growing American cultural trend. It is estimated that on any typical day, half of American adults eat at least one meal outside the home. In an average month, 78% of American households order carry-out or delivered food. Meals ordered out tend to be higher in calories, fat, and sodium than home-cooked meals partly because portion sizes are bigger. Conversely, the fiber and calcium content of restaurant meals is usually less. Because eating out has evolved from a special treat to an everyday occurrence, planning and menu savvy are needed to ensure that eating out is consistent with, not contradictory to, eating healthy. Tips for eating healthy while eating out appear in Box 10.2. "Best bet" choices from various ethnic restaurants are listed in Box 10.3.

How Do You Respond?

What are "regional food practices"? Regional food practices are certain behaviors associated with specific areas of the country. Advances in food technology and transportation have diluted regional food practices by vastly increasing the variety and availability of foods across the country. The following "regional" foods are available anywhere:

- New England: Boston baked beans, clam chowder, lobster, and clam cakes
- Pennsylvania Dutch Country: shoofly pie, scrapple, and German-style sausage
- The South: grits, fried chicken, hot biscuits, greens, sweet potatoes, and corn bread
- Louisiana: French and Creole-style cooking
- Texas: chili con carne
- The Southwest: Mexican foods such as tortillas, tamales, enchiladas, and refried beans
- The Far West: citrus fruit, fresh produce, salads, and Asian-style cooking
- The Midwest: dairy products and beef

Will eating at Subway really help me lose weight? Subway can help to promote weight loss if the Subway meal provides fewer calories that what is typically eaten. In other words, if it helps you lose weight, it is because fewer calories were consumed but not because there is anything magical about a Subway sandwich that causes body fat to melt. Many Subway sandwiches are low in fat and calories and contain some fresh vegetables; however, processed meats tend to be high in sodium and if white rolls are chosen, the meal is low in fiber. There is no reason not to eat Subway subs—especially the low-fat 6-inch subs—but neither is there a compelling reason to buy them if someone does not like them.

(*text continues on page 268*)

BOX 10.2

TIPS FOR EATING HEALTHY WHILE EATING OUT

Plan ahead. Choose the restaurant carefully so you know there are reasonable choices available. Call ahead to inquire about menu selections. This is an especially important strategy when the location is not a matter of choice but rather a requirement such as for business luncheons or conferences. It may be possible to make a special request ahead of time.

Don't arrive starving. People become much less discriminating in their food choices when they are hungry. Having a small, high-fiber snack an hour or so before going out to dinner, such as whole wheat crackers with peanut butter or a piece of fresh fruit with milk, can take the edge off hunger without bankrupting healthy eating.

Balance the rest of the day. When eating out *is* an occasion, such as for a birthday or anniversary celebration, make healthier choices the rest of the day to compensate for a planned indulgence.

Practice portion control. Restaurant portions tend to be much bigger than the "standard" serving sizes used in MyPyramid or the Nutrition Facts label. And research shows that the more food people are served, the more they eat. Consider that a king-size steak may be 15 oz or more, which is enough for five meals of a standard 3-oz serving of meat. Order the smallest size meat available, cut away an estimated 3-oz portion (e.g., the size of a deck of cards) then put the remainder in a doggy bag *before eating;* if you wait until the end of the meal, there may not be any left. When ordering burgers, order regular size, not biggie size or super size. Ordering a la carte can help with portion control. Other strategies include requesting a half-portion; ordering two (carefully chosen) appetizers in place of an entrée; or ordering an appetizer and splitting a whole meal with a companion.

Know the terminology. A fat-free ingredient can turn into a high-fat disaster depending on the method of preparation such as eggplant made into eggplant parmigiana. "Fatty" words to watch out for include buttered, battered, breaded, deep fried, au gratin, creamy, crispy, alfredo, bisque, hollandaise, parmigiana, béarnaise, en croute, escalloped, French-fried, pan fried, rich, sautéed, with gravy, with mayonnaise, with cheese. Less fatty terms are baked, braised, broiled, cooked in its own juice, grilled, lightly sautéed, poached, roasted, steamed.

Beware of hidden fats. Even when less fatty terms are used to describe a menu choice, the item may be high in fat if is made from ingredients that are naturally high in fat. For instance, a hamburger may be "grilled" but if it is made from ground chuck instead of ground sirloin, it will be high in fat although additional fat may not have been added during preparation. Sources of hidden fat include meat products, nuts, and dairy products.

Make special requests. Most restaurants are eager to accommodate special requests. Order sauces and gravies "on the side" to control portions; ask that lower fat items be substituted for high fat items (e.g., a baked potato instead of French fries); request an alternate cooking method (e.g., broiled instead of fried).

BOX 10.3

BEST BET CHOICES FROM FAST FOOD AND ETHNIC RESTAURANTS

Fast Foods

English muffins or bagels with spreads on the side
Baked potato—plain or with reduced-fat or fat-free dressings or salsa
Regular, small, or junior sized hamburgers
Use ketchup, mustard, relish, BBQ sauce, and fresh vegetables as toppings
Grilled chicken sandwiches without "special sauce"
Veggie burger
Small roast beef on roll
Fruit 'n yogurt parfait
Lean, 6-inch subs
Side salads with reduced-fat or fat-free dressings
Salads with grilled chicken
Order specialty coffees with skim milk

Salad Bars

Dark, leafy greens
Plain raw vegetables
Chickpeas, kidney beans, peas
Hard cooked egg
Fresh fruit
Lean ham, turkey
Reduced-fat or fat-free dressings

Pizza

Thin crust
Vegetables: onion, spinach, tomatoes, broccoli, mushrooms, peppers
Lean meats: Canadian bacon, ham, grilled chicken, shrimp, crab meat
Order a ½-the-cheese pizza.
Eat salad with it.

Buffet

Survey the buffet before beginning.
Use a small plate.
Pile food no thicker than a deck of cards.
Practice the "plate method:" one-quarter meat, three-quarters plants.

Mexican

Sauces: salsa, mole, picante, enchilada, pico de gallo
Black bean soup, gazpacho
Soft, non-fried tortillas as in bean burritos or enchiladas
Soft-shell chicken or veggie tacos
Order a la carte or split an entrée
Ask for sour cream and guacamole on the side
Fajitas: chicken, seafood, vegetable, beef
Flan (usually a small portion)

Chinese

Hot-and-sour soup, wonton soup

BOX 10.3 (continued)

BEST BET CHOICES FROM FAST FOOD AND ETHNIC RESTAURANTS

Chicken chow mein
Chicken or beef chop suey
Szechuan dishes
Shrimp with garlic sauce
Stir-fried and teriyaki dishes
Noodles: lo mein, chow fun, Singapore noodle
Steamed rice instead of fried
Tofu
Steamed dumplings and other dim sum instead of egg rolls
Fortune cookies
Use chopsticks

Italian

Minestrone
Breadsticks, bruschetta, Italian bread
Sauces: red clam, marinara, wine, cacciatore, fra diavlo, marsala
Shrimp, veal, chicken without breading

Indian

Raw vegetables salads, Mulligatawny soup (lentil soup)
Tandoori meats
Condiments: fruits and vegetable chutneys, raita (cucumber and yogurt sauce)
Lentil and chickpea curries
Chicken and vegetables
Chicken rice pilaf
Basmati rice
Naan (bread baked in tandoori oven)
Dal

Japanese

Boiled green soybeans, miso soup, bean soups
Sushi—cooked varieties include imitation crab, cooked shrimp, scrambled egg
Most combinations of grilled meats or seafood
Teriyaki chicken
Steamed rice, rice noodles
Green tea

Greek

Lentil soup
Chicken, lamb, pork souvlaki salad or sandwich
Shish kebabs
Pita bread
Make a meal of appetizers: baba ghanoush (smoked eggplant), hummus (mashed chickpeas), dolma (stuffed grape leaves), tabooli (cracked wheat salad). Olive oil is often poured on the baba ghanoush, hummus, and other foods so ask for it on the side.

▲ Focus on Critical Thinking

Respond to the following statements:

1. Acculturation proceeds in a predictable sequence and timeframe for all new immigrants.
2. Ethnic foods tend to be healthier than typical American fare.
3. It is possible to eat out daily and still eating healthy.

Key Concepts

- Although culture defines what is edible; how food is handled, prepared, and consumed; what foods are appropriate for particular groups within the culture; the meaning of food and eating; attitudes toward body size; and the relationship between food and health, food habits vary considerably among individuals and families within a cultural group.
- Core foods are an indispensable part of the diet and consist of grains or starchy vegetables. Secondary foods are nutrient rich and add variety and ethnic identity to meals. Occasional or peripheral foods are used infrequently.
- It is important to understand a client's cultural values so that appropriate assessment data can be gathered and culturally sensitive interventions can be devised.
- As people move from one cultural area to another, they change their food habits to some degree. New foods are added to the diet or substituted for traditional foods and some traditional foods are rejected. Availability and cost influence food choices.
- Generalizations can be made about traditional eating practices of subcultures within the United States. However, an individual's food choices deviate from these based on personal preferences, socioeconomic status, and degree of acculturation.
- Cultural sensitivity is increasingly important to nursing care. The key to cross-cultural assessment and counseling is an understanding of the client's cultural values and their impact on health and food choices. From this awareness, nutrition information can be tailored to the client's needs, desires, and lifestyle.
- Religion tends to have a greater impact on food habits than nationality or culture.
- The "American" diet undergoes change as people from different cultures introduce their traditional foods to the mainstream culture.
- Americans are cooking less and eating out more, which tends to result in greater intakes of fat, cholesterol, and sodium. Clients need to learn how to use convenience products to prepare healthy meals at home and how to eat a healthy diet while eating out.

ANSWER KEY

1. **TRUE** Each culture has its own socially standardized food behaviors that dictate what is edible, the role of certain foods in the diet, how food is prepared, the use of

foods, the number and timing of daily meals, how food is eaten, and health beliefs related to food.

2. **FALSE** Race, ethnicity, and geographic region are often inaccurately assumed to be synonymous with culture. This misconception leads to stereotypical grouping.
3. **TRUE** Core foods tend to be complex carbohydrates, such as cereal grains, starchy tubers, and starchy vegetables. These core foods are the indispensable foundation of the diet and provide significant calories.
4. **TRUE** Ethnocentrism is the belief that one's own values and behaviors are "right," "normal," and "superior" compared to those of all other cultures, which are "wrong," "odd," or "inferior."
5. **FALSE** The hot–cold theory of health and diet refers to the Asian culture's belief that health and illness are related to the balance between yin and yang forces in the body. Yin represents female, cold, and darkness; yang represents male, hot, and light.
6. **TRUE** Usually, first-generation Americans adhere more closely to cultural food patterns to preserve their ethnic identity, compared with subsequent generations.
7. **TRUE** For many ethnic groups who move to the United States, breakfast and lunch are most likely to be composed of convenient American foods while traditional foods are retained for the major dinner meal, which has greater emotional significance.
8. **TRUE** People who eat at restaurants or buy take-out food tend to eat more calories, fat, and sodium than people who eat home-prepared meals.
9. **FALSE** Dietary acculturation can lead to positive or negative changes in food choices. For instance, Mexican Americans dramatically reduce their intake of lard and Mexican cream through the process of acculturation, which is a positive change. However, substituting sweetened drinks (e.g., Kool Aid, soft drinks) for the traditional beverage made from fruit has a negative impact on nutritional intake.
10. **FALSE** Although restaurant portions tend to be much larger than the standard serving size, the same is not true for convenience foods. The portion sizes listed on the label of convenience meals tend to be much smaller than what Americans typically consume in a meal.

WEBSITES FOR CULTURAL/ETHNIC FOOD GUIDE PYRAMIDS

The Department of Anthropology and Geography at Georgia State University for materials developed by the Nutrition Education for New Americans project at **www.multiculturalhealth.org**

Oldways Preservation & Exchange Trust at **www.oldwayspt.org**

WEBSITES FOR ETHNIC MEDICINE INFORMATION INCLUDING INFORMATION ON NUTRITION

Harborview Medical Center, University of Washington at **www.ethnomed.org**

www.EatEthnic.com

www.nal.usda.gov/fnic

WEBSITE FOR INFORMATION ON FAST FOOD AND EATING OUT

Center for Science in the Public Interest at **www.cspinet.org**

WEBSITE FOR NUTRITION FACTS OF 10 POPULAR FAST FOOD RESTAURANT CHAINS

www.fatcalories.com

REFERENCES

American Dietetic Association. (2002). Key trends affecting the dietetics profession and the American Dietetic Association. *Journal of the American Dietetic Association, 102,* S1821–S1839.

American Obesity Association. AOA Fact Sheet: Obesity in minority populations. Available at www.obesity.org/subs/fastfacts/Obesity_Minority_Pop.shtml. Accessed on 11/14/03.

Gentry, M. (Ed.). (2003). Selecting a frozen meal. *American Institute for Cancer Research Newsletter on Diet, Nutrition and Cancer Prevention, 79,* 12.

Hales, D. (2003). What (and who) is really cooking at your house. *Parade,* November 16, 2003. New York: Parade Publications.

Holzmeister, L. (2001). *Complete guide to convenience food counts.* Alexandria, VA: The American Diabetes Association.

Jones, D., & Darling, M. (1996). Ethnic foodways in Minnesota. Handbook of food and wellness across cultures. Available at www.agricola.umn.edu/foodways. Accessed 11/14/03.

Kittler, R., & Sucher, K. 2001. *Food and culture* (3rd ed.). Belmont, CA: Wadsworth/Thomson Learning.

Ohio State University Extension Fact Sheet, Family and Consumer Sciences. Cultural diversity: Eating in America, African-American. Available at http://ohioline.osu.edu/hyg-fact/5000/5250.html. Accessed on 11/14/03.

Ohio State University Extension Fact Sheet, Family and Consumer Sciences. Cultural diversity: Eating in America, Asian. Available at http://ohioline.osu.edu/hyg-fact/5000/5253.html. Accessed on 11/18/03.

Ohio State University Extension Fact Sheet, Family and Consumer Sciences. Cultural diversity: Eating in America, Mexican-American. Available at http://ohioline.osu.edu/hyg-fact/5000/5255.html. Accessed on 11/14/03.

Penn State Nutrition Center. (2001). *Pyramid packet.* University Park, PA: Pennsylvania State University.

Romero-Gwynn, E., & Gwynn, D. (1997). *Dietary patterns and acculturation among Latinos of Mexican descent,* Julian Samora Research Report #23. East Lansing, MI: The Julian Samora Research Institute, Michigan State University.

Satia-Abouta, J., Patterson, R., Neuhouser, M., & Elder, J. (2002). Dietary acculturation: Applications to research and dietetics. *Journal of the American Dietetic Association, 102,* 1105–1118.

For information on the new dietary guidelines 2005 and MyPyramid, visit
http://connection.lww.com/go/dudek

11

Healthy Eating for Healthy Babies

TRUE	FALSE	
⬭	⬭	**1** Adequate weight gain during pregnancy ensures delivery of a normal-weight baby.
⬭	⬭	**2** Obese women should not gain weight during pregnancy.
⬭	⬭	**3** An important source of folic acid is ready-to-eat breakfast cereals.
⬭	⬭	**4** Weight gain in excess of the recommended ranges is likely to lead to an increase in maternal fat stores and so increase the risk of postpartum weight retention.
⬭	⬭	**5** To get enough calcium during pregnancy, women need to consume the equivalent of six cups of milk daily.
⬭	⬭	**6** Pregnant and lactating women are advised to eliminate fish and seafood from their diets due to mercury contamination.
⬭	⬭	**7** Lactation increases calorie requirements more than pregnancy does.
⬭	⬭	**8** The vitamin content of breast milk is affected by the mother's vitamin intake.
⬭	⬭	**9** Thirst is a good indicator for the need for fluid in most lactating women.
⬭	⬭	**10** American women with human immunodeficiency virus (HIV) infection should be advised not to breast-feed.

UPON COMPLETION OF THIS CHAPTER, YOU WILL BE ABLE TO

- Discuss the recommended pattern and rate of weight gain during pregnancy for underweight, normal-weight, and obese women.
- Describe the number of servings recommended from each MyPyramid food group during pregnancy.
- Discuss other nutritional considerations during pregnancy such as meal frequency, fluid intake, the use of caffeine, and how to avoid foodborne illness.
- List nutritional interventions during pregnancy for nausea, constipation, heartburn, pica, and diabetes.
- Describe criteria for assessing nutritional needs during pregnancy.
- List benefits of breast-feeding.
- Discuss variables that affect the composition of breast milk.
- Describe the number of servings recommended from each MyPyramid food group during lactation.
- Describe criteria for assessing nutritional needs during lactation.
- List ways to promote breast-feeding.

Maternal diet and nutritional status have a direct impact on the course of pregnancy and its outcome. For instance, inadequate folate status prior to conception increases the risk of neural tube defects. Weight gain during pregnancy influences newborn size, which is an important indicator of infant survival and childhood morbidity and may influence the development of type 2 diabetes, hypertension, cardiovascular disease, and other disorders later in life. At no other time is the welfare of one so dependent on another.

This chapter discusses the role of nutrition prior to conception in optimizing pregnancy outcome. The impact of pregnancy-induced physiologic changes on nutritional requirements and intake is discussed. Guidance on food selection and supplements is offered. Problems and complications of pregnancy with nutritional implications are discussed. The advantages of breast-feeding and nutritional needs to support lactation are explained.

PREGNANCY

Nutrition Before Conception

Folic Acid: synthetic form of folate found in multivitamins, fortified breakfast cereals, and enriched grain products.

Both mother and infant have the potential to benefit when optimal maternal nutritional status is achieved prior to conception. For the mother, optimum nutrition, particularly regarding weight, has the potential to provide short- and long-term health benefits. For the infant, optimal nutritional status can reduce the risk of birth defects and chronic disease later in life. Folate intake and maternal weight are of particular concern for the general population; for women who have PKU, a low phenylalanine diet is necessary prior to conception.

Folic Acid

Folate: natural form of the B vitamin involved in the synthesis of DNA; only one-half as available to the body as manmade folic acid.

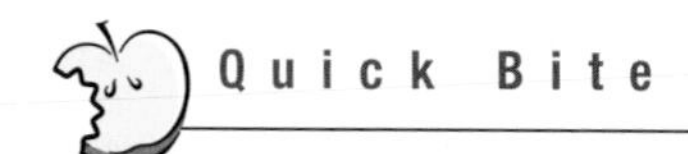

Sources of natural folate

	*Micrograms folate/cup (except where noted *)*
Cooked black-eyed peas, lentils	358
Cooked black, navy, or pinto beans; chickpeas	255–295
Okra (cooked from frozen)	269
Asparagus (cooked from frozen)	243
Spinach (cooked from frozen)	205
Orange juice (prepared from concentrate)	109
Broccoli (cooked from frozen)	104
Peas (cooked from frozen)	94
*Liver (3 oz braised)	280

Dietary Folate Equivalents (DFE): 1 DFE = 1 microgram food folate = 0.6 micrograms of folic acid from fortified food or as a supplement consumed with food = 0.5 microgram of a supplement taken on an empty stomach.

Women who consume adequate amounts of folic acid before conception and during pregnancy reduce their risk of having a baby with a neural tube defect (e.g., spina bifida, anencephaly), which develops 18 to 30 days after conception—often before the mother knows she is pregnant. Because more than 40% of pregnancies in the United States are unplanned, the March of Dimes recommends that all women who are capable of becoming pregnant consume a multivitamin containing 400 μg of synthetic folic acid daily from foods or supplements in addition to eating foods rich in natural folate. To ensure adequate blood levels of folate at the time of neural tube closure, supplementation should begin at least 1 month prior to conception.

Women age 19 and older should not exceed 1000 micrograms of synthetic folic acid per day because a high folic acid intake can mask a vitamin B_{12} deficiency. The exception is women who have previously delivered an infant with a neural tube defect. In those cases, up to 4 mg of folate equivalents daily may be recommended.

Career Connection

All women who are capable of becoming pregnant should consume 400 micrograms of folic acid daily through fortified foods and/or supplements . . . but who is getting enough through food and who needs a supplement? To decrease the risk of neural tube defects, the U.S. and Canada made folic acid fortification mandatory for grain products in 1998; thus white bread, rolls, pasta, and crackers are important sources. Even before that, many ready-to-eat breakfast cereals were fortified with varying amounts of folic acid. In fact, a study on the folic acid content of fortified cereals revealed that 14 of 27 cereals studied had *more than 150% more* folic acid in them than was listed on the label and the rest of the cereals had between 98% and 140%. The recommended amount of folic acid could easily be exceeded with fortified cereal. A potential danger from a high folic acid intake is that vitamin B_{12} deficiency in vegans could be masked.

On the other hand, women who do not eat fortified cereal may not get enough synthetic folic acid through foods, especially if they are restricting carbohydrates, a dietary strategy advocated by many fad diets. Consider this: prime "dieters"—women aged 15 to 35 years old—are also women of prime childbearing age. A dieting woman, eating suboptimal amounts of folic acid, could place her unborn infant at risk of a neural tube defect even before she realizes she is pregnant. To ensure an adequate but not excessive intake of folic acid, it is important to determine who is not routinely consuming adequate folic acid through fortified foods—ideally, at least 1 month prior to conception.

- Does the client eat folic acid fortified cereal regularly? How much, how often?
- How many servings from the grain group does the client consume daily? Does the client limit carbohydrates?
- Does the client take a multivitamin?
- Is the client a vegan, who may be at risk of vitamin B_{12} deficiency?

Maternal Weight

Healthy Weight Prior to Conception: BMI of 19.8–26.0.

Attaining healthy weight prior to pregnancy makes conception easier, improves pregnancy outcomes, and may facilitate breastfeeding. Health risks are higher for women weighing less than or more than healthy weight. For instance, women who are underweight before pregnancy tend to have smaller babies compared with heavier women with the same gestational weight gain. It appears that underweight women may reduce their risk of adverse pregnancy outcome by attaining a higher prepregnancy weight, by gaining extra weight during pregnancy, or both.

Conversely, obesity during pregnancy is associated with higher morbidity in both the mother and infant. Women who are obese at conception have a higher risk of hypertension, gestational diabetes, induced labor, and caesarean sections. Infants born to obese mothers are at increased risk of macrosomia, low Apgar scores, shoulder dystocia, and childhood obesity. Also, obesity during pregnancy is associated with an increased risk of neural tube defects regardless of folate intake. Finally, women who are overweight or obese tend to have more difficulty initiating breastfeeding than women of healthy weight do.

Maternal Phenylketonuria

Phenylketonuria (PKU): an inborn error of phenylalanine (an essential amino acid) metabolism that results in retardation and physical handicaps in newborns if it is not treated with a low-phenylalanine diet beginning shortly after birth.

The cornerstone of treatment for PKU is to limit (but not eliminate) phenylalanine intake. Mental retardation can be prevented in infants born with PKU if their diet consists primarily of a special low-phenylalanine formula instituted within 7 to 10 days after birth. Small amounts of breast milk or regular formula are used to provide just enough phenylalanine to support protein synthesis but not so much as to elevate blood levels. Later, certain vegetables, fruits, some grain products, and other low-phenylalanine foods are added to the diet. High-protein foods such as milk, cheese, eggs, and meat are never allowed, nor are products sweetened with aspartame (Nutrasweet).

Until the 1980s, a low-phenylalanine diet was generally discontinued around age 6 based on the premise that high levels of phenylalanine were not damaging once brain growth was completed. However, high levels of phenylalanine in children and adolescents can cause a decrease in IQ, learning disabilities, and behavioral problems. Current practice is to continue the diet throughout life, although some relaxation of the restrictions may be allowed with aging.

It is possible that women with PKU who discontinued the diet early in life may not remember they have PKU. Women who have PKU and who consume a normal diet before and during pregnancy have very high blood levels of phenylalanine, which are devastating to the developing fetus. As many as 90% of babies born to PKU mothers who do not control their blood level of phenylalanine have mental retardation, and many also have microcephaly, heart defects, and LBW. Most of these infants do not inherit PKU and cannot benefit from a low-phenylalanine diet after birth.

To prevent mental retardation and other problems associated with maternal PKU, a rigid low-phenylalanine diet is necessary at least 3 months before conception and throughout the duration of the pregnancy. With a low-phenylalanine diet, blood levels of phenylalanine are controlled to very low levels, eliminating risks to the develop-

ing fetus. Maternal PKU may present a bigger problem for an adolescent girl with an unexpected pregnancy, who may hide the pregnancy until late in gestation.

Clients who have a history of PKU should be advised that

- Complete understanding and strict adherence to the diet are vital.
- Protein foods are high in phenylalanine and must be eliminated: meat, fish, poultry, eggs, dairy products, and nuts.
- Diet drinks and foods sweetened with aspartame (Nutrasweet) are strictly forbidden.
- The special PKU formula is expensive and often offensive to adult palates but it must be consumed in adequate amounts to support fetal growth and to prevent maternal tissue breakdown that would have results similar to those caused by cheating on the diet.
- An adequate calorie intake is necessary for normal protein metabolism.
- Close monitoring of blood phenylalanine levels is essential.

Physiologic Changes Related to Pregnancy

Pregnancy produces physiologic changes that affect all the mother's body systems. Alterations in metabolism, gastrointestinal function, blood volume, and weight account for some changes that influence nutrient requirements and use of nutrients in the body.

Altered Metabolism

The basal metabolic rate increases by the fourth month of gestation and rises to 15% to 20% above normal by term. This increase reflects the increased oxygen demands of the fetus and maternal tissues. Calorie requirements increase proportionately.

In addition to the increased metabolic rate, the metabolism of nutrients is altered. Because the fetus' primary fuel for meeting energy requirements is glucose, fat becomes the major source of maternal fuel, making glucose available for the fetus. A decrease in insulin efficiency occurs during the latter part of pregnancy, which may be a compensatory mechanism to increase glucose availability for the fetus. Some women develop gestational diabetes, a type of diabetes that resolves itself after delivery.

Gastrointestinal Changes

Nausea and vomiting are common in the first trimester and may be related to hypoglycemia, decreased gastric motility, relaxation of the cardiac sphincter, or anxiety. Increases in appetite and thirst are also common.

Increased progesterone production has the effect of relaxing smooth muscle cells. This action helps the uterus expand to accommodate the growing fetus and also slows gastrointestinal motility. An advantage of slowed motility is that nutrient absorption increases. The disadvantages are an increased risk of esophageal reflux, heartburn, and constipation. As pregnancy progresses, the displacement of the stomach and intestines caused by the enlarging uterus contributes to heartburn and constipation.

Blood Volume Changes

Total body water increases throughout pregnancy and accounts for a large percentage of weight gain at term. The increase in blood volume exceeds the increase in red blood cell production, resulting in hemodilution or a physiologic anemia of pregnancy. Minor edema may be considered normal if it is not accompanied by hypertension and proteinuria.

Weight Gain

Weight gain during pregnancy results from the growth of the fetus, placenta, and maternal blood volume and tissues. Many women fail to understand that the increase in maternal fat tissue is a physiologic mechanism designed to prepare women for the energy demands of labor and lactation. Typical weight gain distribution in normal pregnancy is detailed in Box 11.1.

How Much Weight Should Be Gained?

The current recommended weight gain ranges during pregnancy are based on prepregnancy BMI (Table 11.1). Underweight women are urged to gain slightly more weight than normal weight women; obese women should gain less but at least 15 pounds and not more than 25 pounds. Women pregnant with twins or triplets need to gain somewhat more weight than that recommended for single births but not double or triple the amounts, respectively.

Low-Birth Weight (LBW): a baby weighing less than 2500 g or 5.5 pounds.

For any given prepregnancy weight, weight gain within these recommended ranges is associated with better pregnancy outcomes for both mother and infant. Conversely, weight gain outside of these ranges—whether below or above—increases risk to the infant and sometimes to the mother. For instance, inadequate weight gain during pregnancy, especially among underweight women, increases the risk of giving birth to a low-birth-weight (LBW) infant. LBW babies tend to be malnourished, especially if born full-term, and they have a high incidence of postnatal complications and mortality. In fact, birth weight may be the most important predictor not only of mortality but also of subsequent development. However, adequate

BOX 11.1 **WEIGHT GAIN DISTRIBUTION IN NORMAL PREGNANCY (POUNDS)**

Birth weight of baby	7.5
Placenta	1.5
Increase in maternal blood volume	4
Increase in maternal fluid volume	4
Increase in uterus	2
Increase in breast tissue	2
Amniotic fluid	2
Maternal fat tissue	7
	30

TABLE 11.1 RECOMMENDED WEIGHT GAIN RANGES BASED ON MATERNAL PREPREGNANCY BMI

Prepregnancy BMI	Category	Gestational Weight Gain (lb)
<19.8	Underweight	28–40
19.8–26.0	Normal weight	25–35
>26.0–29.0	Overweight	15–25
>29.0	Obese	≥15
Other:		
Twin pregnancy		34–45
Triplet pregnancy		50

weight gain during pregnancy cannot alone ensure the delivery of a normal-birth-weight infant.

Conversely, very high weight gain during pregnancy increases the risk of the infant being large-for-gestational age, which increases the risk of fetopelvic disproportion and is associated with excess body fat during childhood. Even more than fetal growth, weight gain in excess of the recommended ranges is likely to result in an increase in maternal fat stores, increasing the risk of postpartum weight retention.

The goal of gaining enough weight to prevent LBW, but not so much that it results in a high birth weight infant and excess postpartum weight retention, is especially difficult in teenagers. Teenagers who are still growing appear especially prone to excess weight gain during pregnancy and higher weight retention after pregnancy. However, birth weight tends to decline in multiparous teenagers; therefore, recommendations to limit weight gain should be approached cautiously.

Pattern of Weight Gain

The American College of Obstetricians and Gynecologists recommend a 2- to 4-pound weight gain during the first trimester. Thereafter, the recommended weight gain for normal-weight women is approximately 1 pound/week. Underweight women should gain slightly more than 1 pound/week, overweight women should gain about 0.66 pounds/week, and women pregnant with twins should be encouraged to gain at least 1 pound/week. The rate of weight gain for severely obese women should be determined on an individualized basis. However, weight reduction should never be undertaken during pregnancy. Although slightly higher or lower rates of weight gain can be considered normal, obvious or persistent deviations warrant further investigation.

Nutrient Requirements During Pregnancy

The requirements for most nutrients increase during pregnancy (Table 11.2). However, not all nutrient needs increase proportionately. For instance, the need for iron

Career Connection

Only one-third of pregnant American women gain weight within the recommended ranges. Women with high BMI are much more likely than normal BMI women to gain weight in excess of the recommended range and women with low BMI are significantly more likely to gain below the recommended weight gain range. Negative attitudes about gaining the recommended amount of weight are common even among well educated, relatively affluent women. Surprisingly, many women report getting no advice from health care workers on how much weight to gain during pregnancy. Although it is vital to discuss appropriate gestational weight gain early and often during prenatal care, nutrition counseling is not likely to be successful unless the woman's attitudes about her pregnancy and psychological well-being are considered. Probe for negative attitudes and restrictive behaviors that indicate the client may be at risk for inadequate weight gain. Does the client

- Worry about getting fat during pregnancy?
- Believe she must be very careful to avoid getting fat while pregnant?
- Feel embarrassed when she gets weighed?
- Dislike maternity clothes?
- Feel embarrassed about her size while pregnant?
- Try to limit weight gain one month if she gained too much weight the previous month?
- Avoid eating before going to the doctor?
- Have a partner who has a negative attitude about weight gain during pregnancy?

increases by 50% during pregnancy, yet the requirement for vitamin B_{12} increases by only about 10%. For all reference standards, the following points are notable:

- Actual requirements during pregnancy vary among individuals and are influenced by previous nutritional status and health history including chronic illnesses, multiple pregnancies, and closely spaced pregnancies.
- The requirement for one nutrient may be altered by the intake of another. For instance, women who do not meet their calorie requirements need higher amounts of protein.
- Nutrient needs are not constant throughout the course of pregnancy. Nutrient needs generally change little during the first trimester (folic acid is an exception) and are at their highest during the last trimester.
- Reference standards are usually meaningless to the general public. MyPyramid (see later discussion) can be used to teach women how to make food choices that will provide the balanced intake they need.

Calories

Calorie needs increase to support the growth of fetal and maternal tissues including the increase in maternal fat tissue deposited in preparation for lactation after delivery. Adequate intake of carbohydrate calories ensures that protein is "spared" and available for synthesis of new tissue instead of burned for energy.

TABLE 11.2 **NUTRITIONAL NEEDS FOR WOMEN (19–30 YEARS OLD) DURING PREGNANCY AND LACTATION**

Nutrient	Nonpregnant Women	Pregnancy	Lactation
Calories*		1st tri: +0 2nd tri: +300 3rd tri: +300	+500 1st 6 mo +400 2nd 6 mo
Protein (g)	**46**	**71**	**71**
Vit A (μg)	**700**	**770**	**1300**
Vit C (mg)	**75**	**85**	**120**
Vit D (μg)	5.0*	5.0*	5.0*
Vit E (mg)	**15**	**15**	**19**
Vit K (μg)*	90*	90*	90*
Thiamin (mg)	**1.1**	**1.4**	**1.4**
Riboflavin (mg)	**1.1**	**1.4**	**1.6**
Niacin (mg)	**14**	**18**	**17**
Vit B_6 (mg)	**1.3**	**1.9**	**2.0**
Folate (μg)	**400**	**600**	**500**
Vit B_{12} (μg)	**1.3**	**1.9**	**2.0**
Pantothenic acid (mg)	5*	6*	7*
Biotin (μg)	30*	30*	35*
Choline (mg)	425*	450*	550*
Calcium (mg)	1000*	1000*	1000*
Iron (mg)	**18**	**27**	**9**
Magnesium (mg)	**310**	**350**	**310**
Selenium (μg)	**55**	**60**	**70**
Zinc (mg)	**8**	**11**	**12**

tri, trimester; Vit, Vitamin.
Recommended Dietary Allowances are in **bold;** Adequate Intakes (AIs) in ordinary type followed by an asterisk (*).

The increased need for calories is surprisingly small—maybe even less than a mere 300 extra calories per day, which is approximately 15% of a woman's normal calorie requirement. Also, the increased need for calories does not occur until the beginning of the second trimester. Because calorie needs increase relatively little compared with the increased requirements for other nutrients (e.g., iron, folic acid), nutrient density is important.

Protein

Protein needs increase to support fetal growth and development, the formation of the placenta and amniotic fluid, the growth of maternal tissues, and the expanded blood volume. The RDA for protein for all age groups during pregnancy is 1.1 g/kg/day, or a daily increase of 25 g above normal. Women who fail to consume adequate protein may be at increased risk for development of anemia, poor uterine muscle tone, abortion, decreased resistance to infection, and shorter, lighter infants with low Apgar scores. However, most Americans, including vegetarians, consume more protein than they need, so most women do not need to adjust their usual protein intake. (See Box 11.2 for a sample lacto-ovovegetarian menu.) Eating more protein than is necessary offers no benefits and is potentially harmful.

B Vitamins

The requirement for folate increases 50% during pregnancy; it is a major player in the synthesis of DNA and, therefore, vital for the synthesis of new cells and transmission of inherited characteristics. Because vitamin B_{12} has an interdependent relationship with folate, the need for vitamin B_{12} also increases. The requirements for thiamin, riboflavin, and niacin increase in proportion to the increase in calories but are easily consumed within the context of a normal diet. The increased requirement for vitamin B_6 is approximately proportional to the increase in protein because it is involved in protein metabolism.

Calcium

The Dietary Reference Intakes (DRI) for women 19 to 50 years of age—whether pregnant or not—is 1000 mg. The reason why the DRI for calcium does not increase during pregnancy is that the body compensates for the increased need by more than doubling the rate of calcium absorption. If calcium intake was adequate before pregnancy, the amount consumed does not need to increase. However, 1300 mg/day of calcium is recommended for pregnant adolescents aged 14–18, and intakes higher than this may be beneficial. Women who do not consume enough calcium through foods require supplements of calcium with vitamin D.

Iron

Despite the increased rate of iron absorption and iron "saving" that occurs with the cessation of menstruation, the DRI for iron increases by 50% during pregnancy. An estimated 27 mg/day of iron is needed to support the increase in maternal blood vol-

BOX 11.2 **SAMPLE LACTO-OVOVEGETARIAN MENU FOR PREGNANT WOMEN**

Breakfast

Orange juice
Peanut butter and banana on wheat toast
1% milk

Snack

Fresh pear

Lunch

Baked corn tortillas with cheese
Black bean salad
Strawberries with yogurt
1% milk

Snack

Graham crackers
1% milk

Dinner

Veggie burger with lettuce and tomato on whole wheat bun
Baked sweet potato
Spinach salad
Apple crisp

Snack

Bran muffin
1% milk

ume and to provide iron for fetal liver storage, which will sustain the infant for the first 4 to 6 months of life.

Food Guidance During Pregnancy

MyPyramid is a tool that can be used to help pregnant women make healthy food choices. Because an individual's pyramid is specific for their gender, age, and activity pattern, there is not a separate pyramid appropriate for all pregnant women. In fact, there are 12 "individual" pyramids available that represent calorie levels from 1000 to 3200, each at 200-calorie increments. A pregnant woman simply has to determine her normal calorie requirements and move one or two channels higher (e.g., 200–400 calories more than she normally needs) to estimate the amount of food from each group she needs during pregnancy. For instance, a moderately active 30-year-old woman needs approximately 2000 calories; that amount increases to about 2300 calories during pregnancy, the midpoint between the 2200-calorie pyramid and the 2400-calorie pyramid. Table 11.3 shows food intake patterns at various calorie levels.

TABLE 11.3

FOOD INTAKE PATTERNS AT VARIOUS CALORIE LEVELS

Group	2000	2200	2400	2600	2800
Grains	6 oz equivalents	7 oz equivalents	8 oz equivalents	9 oz equivalents	10 oz equivalents
Vegetables	2.5 cups	3 cups	3 cups	3.5 cups	3.5 cups
Fruits	2 cups	2 cups	2 cups	2 cups	2.5 cups
Milk	3 cups	3 cups	3 cups	3 cups	3 cups
Meat and Beans	5.5 oz equivalents	6 oz equivalents	6.5 oz equivalents	6.5 oz equivalents	7 oz equivalents
Oils	6 tsp.	6 tsp.	7 tsp.	8 tsp.	8 tsp.
Discretionary Calories*	267	290	362	410	426

The following are considered 1 oz grain equivalent:
- 1 slice bread
- 1 cup of ready-to-eat cereal
- ½ cup cooked rice, pasta, or cooked cereal

1 oz meat and beans equivalent:
- 1 ounce of lean meat, poultry, or fish
- 1 egg
- 1 tbsp peanut butter
- ¼ cup cooked dry beans
- ½ ounce nuts or seeds

*Discretionary Calorie Allowance is the remaining amount of calories in a food intake pattern after accounting for the calories needed for all food groups, using forms of foods that are fat-free or low-fat and with no added sugars.

When using MyPyramid as a teaching tool, emphasize the important underlying concepts of variety, balance, and moderation to help ensure an adequate, but not excessive, intake all essential nutrients. Additional considerations for food selection during pregnancy include nutrient density; meal frequency; fluid consumption; salt intake; use of caffeine, alcohol, and artificial sweeteners; and avoiding foodborne illness.

Nutrient Density

Nutrient Density: relatively high in nutrients for the amount of calories provided.

Because the need for additional calories during pregnancy is proportionately much smaller than the increased need for many nutrients, making wise food decisions is vital to getting adequate amounts of nutrients without overeating calories. Generally, foods that are nutrient dense are those that are "wholesome"—whole grain breads and cereals; fresh fruits and vegetables that provide an array of color; dried peas and beans; low-fat or fat-free dairy products; lean meats; and nuts. "Extras" with low nutrient density, such as sweets and fats, are used sparingly.

Meal Frequency

Fasting, especially after midgestation, can result in hypoglycemia, hyperketonemia, acetonuria, and other signs of metabolic acidosis within 24 hours. Although ketonuria and acetonuria may occur normally in pregnancy (e.g., after overnight fasting) and probably do not threaten the fetus, the more serious condition of ketoacidosis, which results from severe calorie restriction, can pose a risk for the developing fetus. Therefore, women are advised to avoid periods of hunger by eating three meals and two or three nutritious snacks each day. Small, frequent meals may also help to alleviate nausea in the first trimester and heartburn during the second half of the pregnancy.

Fluid Consumption

Pregnant women need eight to ten 8-ounce glasses of fluid daily, preferably in the form of water, fruit juice, or milk. Empty-calorie drinks like carbonated beverages and fruitades are basically sugar water with few or no nutrients.

Salt Intake

Sodium needs increase during pregnancy to maintain normal sodium levels in the expanded blood volume and tissues. Restriction of sodium intake may adversely affect both mother and fetus. A moderate intake of iodized salt is recommended.

The Use of Caffeine

The question of whether or not caffeine use is safe during pregnancy is controversial. While some studies suggest moderate caffeine intake poses a risk to the fetus, other studies do not.

Caffeine easily crosses the placenta and can affect fetal heart rate and movement. Some evidence suggests that high intakes of caffeine (>500 mg/d) may impair fertility. Studies are conflicting as to whether or not caffeine increases the risk of sudden infant death syndrome. Although no human studies show an association between caffeine consumption and birth defects, high doses of caffeine produce birth defects in

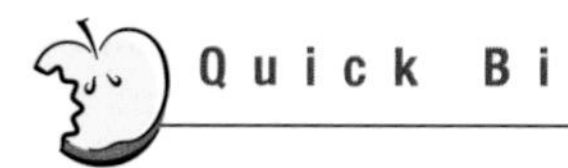

Caffeine content of selected beverages and foods

	Average caffeine content (mg)
8 oz coffee	
brewed, drip method	184
brewed, percolator	128
instant	104
decaffeinated	30
8 oz tea	
brewed, major U.S. brands	64
brewed, imported brands	96
instant	48
12 oz cola	36
12 oz hot cocoa	6.4
8 oz chocolate milk	5
1 oz milk chocolate	6
1 oz chocolate-flavored syrup	4

mice. Moderate use of coffee and caffeine (<300 mg/d) does not appear to pose any risk. Higher intakes should be avoided.

Avoid Alcohol

Fetal Alcohol Syndrome (FAS): a condition characterized by varying degrees of physical and mental growth failure and birth defects caused by maternal intake of alcohol.

Chronic or heavy alcohol consumption during pregnancy increases the risk of mental retardation, learning disabilities, and major birth defects such as those seen in fetal alcohol syndrome. Unlike other small-for-gestational-age infants, infants with FAS do not experience normal "catch-up" growth. Alcohol can cause damage by dehydrating fetal cells, leaving them dead or functionless, or by causing secondary nutrient deficiencies related to poor intake, decreased absorption, altered metabolism, or increased excretion.

Not all alcoholic mothers deliver FAS infants, yet even alcoholics who abstain during pregnancy have a higher incidence of LBW infants than women who do not have a history of alcoholism. Because alcohol is a potent teratogen and a "safe" level of consumption is not known, women are advised to completely avoid alcohol during pregnancy. Although an occasional drink may not cause damage, abstinence is recommended.

The Use of Artificial Sweeteners

The use of artificial sweeteners during pregnancy has been studied extensively. Even though there is no evidence that it is harmful to the fetus, women should consider carefully the use of saccharin during pregnancy because it crosses the placenta and remains in fetal tissues owing to slow fetal clearance. Except for women with PKU, aspartame (e.g., Nutrasweet, Equal) is safe during pregnancy at levels within the U.S. Food and Drug Administration (FDA) Acceptable Daily Intake (ADI) guidelines of 50 mg/kg body weight/day (the equivalent of 124 cans of diet soda for a person weighing 130 pounds). The use of acesulfame-K (e.g., Sunette, Sweet One) also appears to be safe for use during pregnancy when consumed within FDA guidelines of not more than 15 mg/kg body weight (the equivalent of about 20 diet sods or 10 sweetener packets).

Avoiding Foodborne Illness

Foodborne risks are more dangerous for pregnant women than for other adults. During pregnancy, listeriosis, caused by the bacterium *Listeria monocytogenes*, can cause meningitis and sepsis in the mother and infection in the fetus that results in premature delivery, miscarriage, or stillbirth. Pregnant women are 20 times more likely to get listeriosis than other healthy adults and also more likely to become dangerously ill from it. To reduce the risk of listeriosis, pregnant women should *not* consume

- Unpasteurized milk or products made with unpasteurized milk
- Raw or undercooked meat, poultry, eggs, fish, or shellfish
- Refrigerated pâtés or meat spreads
- Certain soft cheeses such as feta, Brie, bleu, and Camembert
- Leftover foods and ready-to-eat foods, including hot dogs and deli meats, unless heated until steaming hot

Pregnant women should also avoid raw vegetable sprouts and unpasteurized juices because of the risk of salmonella and *E. coli*.

The FDA has issued advisories regarding fish and shellfish consumption during pregnancy due to the risk of methylmercury contamination. Mercury occurs naturally in the environment, including waterways. Bacteria in the water convert mercury to methylmercury, which can be toxic, particularly to developing brains in fetuses and young children. Mercury poisoning in a fetus can result in learning delays in walking or talking to more severe problems such as cerebral palsy, seizures, and mental retardation. To reduce the risk of methylmercury poisoning, it is recommended that pregnant women, lactating women, and women who may become pregnant:

- Not eat shark, swordfish, king mackerel, and tilefish
- Limit the intake of other fish (including tuna fish) and shellfish to 12 oz/week
- Not eat the same type of fish and shellfish more than one time per week
- Check with the local health department or Environmental Protection Agency to determine which fish from local waters are safe to eat. If no advisories exist, up to 6 oz/week of local fish can be consumed but no other fish should be consumed that week.

Supplements

Use of vitamin and mineral supplements or herbal supplements during pregnancy should be carefully considered.

Vitamin and Mineral Supplements

Improved nutrient absorption and utilization and an increase in food intake means that most women who are at low nutritional risk can meet their nutrient needs throughout

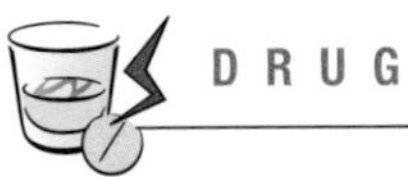

Iron Supplements

Use: Prevention and treatment of iron deficiency anemia

Possible adverse side effects: May cause diarrhea, constipation, dark-colored stools, and gastrointestinal upset. Although better absorbed when taken between meals, iron supplements are less irritating to the gastrointestinal tract when taken with food.

Actions: Observe for diarrhea and constipation. If constipation is not alleviated with a high-fiber diet, consider reducing the dosage or frequency. If supplements are irritating to the gastrointestinal tract when taken between meals, advise the client to take them with food. Advise the client that a change in stool color is to be expected.

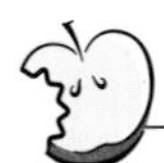

Quick Bite

Vegetarian sources of vitamin B_{12} (naturally found only in animal foods)

	Micrograms B_{12}
Fortified cereals, 1 oz	0.6–6.0
Milk, 1 cup	0.8–1.0
Egg, 1 large	0.5
Nutritional yeast, miniflakes, 1 Tbsp	1.5
Fortified soymilk or other nondairy milks, 1 cup	0.8–3.2
Fortified veggie "meats," 1 oz	0.5–1.2

pregnancy from food alone, with the exception of iron. The Centers for Disease Control and Prevention (CDC) recommend a routine low-dose iron supplement of 30 mg/day for all pregnant women, beginning at the first prenatal visit. Even though conclusive evidence supporting universal iron supplementation is lacking, the CDC defends its position because many women have difficulty maintaining iron stores during pregnancy and because there are no risks associated with prenatal iron supplementation. Also, iron supplementation may improve the mother's iron status during both pregnancy and postpartum, which may be especially beneficial for closely spaced pregnancies.

A multivitamin and mineral supplement is recommended for pregnant women in high-risk categories such as heavy smokers, drug or alcohol abusers, and those carrying two or more fetuses. A multivitamin and mineral supplement is also recommended for pregnant women who have iron deficiency anemia and those who are unlikely to consume an adequate diet despite nutritional advice or nutrition counseling. Other indications for supplements are as follows:

- Complete vegans who are pregnant or lactating should take supplements of vitamin B_{12} if a reliable dietary source is not consumed (RDA during pregnancy is

2.6 micrograms). All other nutrient needs can be met through a well planned lacto-ovo vegetarian or vegan diet, with the exceptions noted below.
- To prevent neural tube defects, all women of childbearing age should consume 400 micrograms/day of synthetic folic acid via fortified foods and/or vitamin supplements in addition to consuming natural folate in a mixed diet. As previously stated, supplementation should begin at least 1 month prior to conception to ensure adequate blood levels of folate.
- Women who do not receive adequate exposure to sunlight may need a vitamin D supplement. The Adequate Intake for vitamin D is 5 micrograms, the same as for nonpregnant women. The amount of vitamin D in prenatal supplements is 10 micrograms, an amount that is not excessive.
- Women who do not consume adequate calcium (e.g., the equivalent of about three 8-ounce glasses of milk daily) need calcium supplements. For maximum absorption, calcium supplements should be taken in doses of 500 mg or less and not at the same time as iron supplements.
- Women who take more than 30 mg of iron to treat iron deficiency anemia should take 15 mg of zinc and 2 mg of copper, the amount found in many prenatal vitamin and mineral supplements, because iron interferes with absorption and utilization of these trace elements.

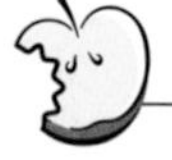
Quick Bite

Preformed vitamin A content of various types of liver

	IU Vitamin A
3 oz braised:	
beef liver	30,327
chicken liver	13,919
lamb liver	21,203
veal liver	22,851

There are instances in which vitamin or mineral supplements are dangerous. For example, accumulating data show that excessive consumption of preformed vitamin A (retinol) poses a teratogenic risk to the developing fetus. In the early weeks of pregnancy, excess preformed vitamin A from over-the-counter supplements or from the drug isotretinoin results in a variety of birth defects such as cleft lip or palate, hydrocephalus, or heart defects. Women of childbearing age should limit their intake of preformed vitamin A to 100% of the RDA. Women should check their supplements to make sure they are not taking too much vitamin A from retinol, and they should minimize their intake of liver and cereals fortified with preformed vitamin A (but not beta-carotene, the vegetable precursor of vitamin A).

Herbal Supplements

Because little is known about the safety and efficacy of herbal supplements during pregnancy, it is generally recommended that they not be used during pregnancy and lactation. Herbal products are technically unapproved drugs; most drugs cross the placental barrier to some degree, exposing the fetus to potentially teratogenic effects. Unlike approved drugs, little animal or human testing has been done to determine if herbs can cause birth defects or potentially harm mothers and infants. Even the use of herbal teas

should be limited: the American Academy of Pediatrics recommends that pregnant women use only filtered bag varieties of herbal tea and that consumption not exceed two 8 oz cups/day.

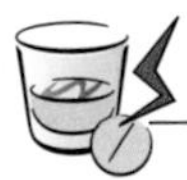

SUPPLEMENT ALERT

The following herbal supplements should be avoided because they stimulate uterine contractions and may increase the risk of miscarriage or premature labor:

Blue cohosh
Juniper
Pennyroyal or rosemary
Sage
Thuja
Raspberry tea

Nutritional Interventions for Specific Complaints and Health Conditions

Nausea and Vomiting

Nausea and vomiting, common during the first trimester, may be related to hypoglycemia, decreased gastric motility, relaxation of the cardiac sphincter, or anxiety. Interventions that can help to lessen nausea include eating small, frequent meals every 2 to 3 hours. Carbohydrates may be especially helpful because they leave the stomach quickly and readily raise blood glucose levels. Women should also be advised to

- Eat carbohydrate foods such as dry crackers, melba toast, dry cereal, or hard candy before getting out of bed in the morning
- Avoid drinking liquids with meals
- Avoid coffee, tea, and spicy foods
- Limit high-fat foods because they delay gastric emptying time
- Eliminate individual intolerances

Constipation

Constipation during pregnancy may be caused by relaxation of gastrointestinal muscle tone and motility related to increased progesterone levels, or it may result from pressure of the fetus on the intestines. Other contributing factors may include a decrease in physical activity and an inadequate intake of fluid and fiber. Constipation is also a common side effect of the consumption of iron supplements. If iron supplementation is contributing to constipation, the dosage or frequency should be reduced if possible.

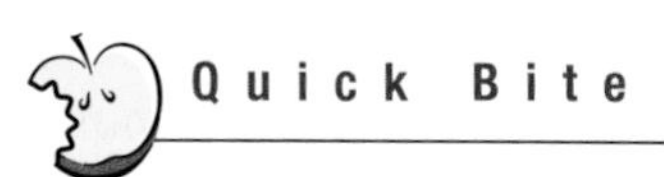

Fiber content of selected ready-to-eat cereals

	g fiber/1 cup serving
Fiber One	28.5
All-Bran with extra fiber	26.6
Kashi	12
Raisin Bran	8
Raisin Nut Bran	5.1
Shredded Wheat	5
Wheat Chex	4.1
Life	2.8
Wheaties	2.0
Cheerios	2
Total	1
Rice Chex	0.6
Corn Chex	0.5

Encourage the client to

- Increase fiber intake especially intake of whole-grain breads and cereals. Look for breads that provide at least 2 gm fiber per slice, and cereals with at least 5 g fiber per serving.
- Drink at least eight 8-ounce glasses of liquid daily.
- Try hot water with lemon or prune juice upon waking to help stimulate peristalsis.
- Participate in regular exercise.

Heartburn

A decrease in gastric motility, relaxation of the cardiac sphincter, and pressure of the uterus on the stomach are contributing factors to heartburn. Encourage the client to

- Eat small, frequent meals and eliminate liquids immediately before and after meals to avoid gastric distention
- Avoid coffee, high-fat foods, and spices
- Eliminate individual intolerances
- Avoid lying down or bending over after eating

Inadequate Weight Gain

Inadequate weight gain may occur secondary to a poor appetite related to nausea, vomiting, heartburn, or smoking, or from an inadequate intake related to lack of knowledge or fear of gaining weight. Women who mistakenly believe that the fetus is a perfect parasite and will be adequately nourished regardless of maternal intake may also experience inadequate weight gain. If an inadequate food budget is responsible for the inadequate intake, refer the client to social services. Determine if the client is eligible for the Women, Infants and Children (WIC) subsidy program (discussed later).

Although a short-term goal is to promote weight gain, the timing and the source of the weight gain are equally important. On a long-term basis, an improvement in overall eating habits benefits both the health of the family and any subsequent pregnancies.

Encourage the client to continue good eating practices and recommend specific ways to improve other habits. Depending on the cause, make appropriate dietary

modifications to improve appetite. Advise the client to quit smoking, not only to improve appetite but because smoking is detrimental to both maternal and infant health.

Counsel the client on the recommended rate and quantity of weight gain associated with optimal maternal and infant health and successful breast-feeding. Explain how the weight gain is distributed among the fetus, placenta, and maternal tissues. Encourage the client to ask questions and verbalize feelings. Advise the client that extra weight gained during pregnancy is quickly lost during lactation or through dieting *after* pregnancy. Set mutually agreeable weight gain goals.

Advise the client that

- If her diet is inadequate in calories, it probably is also inadequate in other nutrients.
- Although the fetus can use maternal nutrient stores if the mother's diet is inadequate, many nutrients are not stored by the body and require a daily dietary intake.
- An inadequate intake can adversely affect maternal health (e.g., poor iron intake leading to anemia) and infant health (e.g., LBW, anemia, other postnatal complications).

Excessive Weight Gain

Women who experience excessive weight gain related to overeating may do so because they lack knowledge concerning recommended weight gain, or they may believe that a pregnant woman must "eat for two." Other factors contributing to excessive weight gain are stress and a decrease in physical activity.

Although it is prudent to prevent excessive weight gain, weight reduction diets should *never* be undertaken during pregnancy because of the risk of ketonemia and its potential damage to the fetus. Likewise, counting calories should not take priority over the nutritional values of foods; a calorie-restrictive approach could result in a nutrient-poor diet. Again, one long-term objective of diet counseling is to improve eating habits for family health and any subsequent pregnancies. Recommend specific ways to limit the rate of weight gain without compromising nutrient intake such as to

- Substitute skim or low-fat milk for whole milk
- Bake, broil, or steam foods instead of frying
- Eliminate empty calories such as carbonated beverages, candy, rich desserts, and traditional snack foods
- Limit portion sizes to those recommended by MyPyramid
- Use fats and oils sparingly

Pica

Pica: a psychobehavioral disorder characterized by the ingestion of nonfood substances such as dirt, clay, starch, and ice.

Pica increases the risk of nutritional inadequacies because it may displace the intake of nutritious foods or interfere with nutrient absorption. Other potential complications vary with the items ingested and include lead poisoning, fecal impaction, parasitic infections, toxemia, prematurity, perinatal mortality, LBW, and anemia in the infant.

Iron deficiency was commonly considered to be a risk factor for pica, but studies suggest it is more likely a consequence. Pica can be a strongly rooted social tradition and is more prevalent among African-Americans and rural residents. Other suggested risk factors include low socioeconomic status, inadequate nutritional status, and a childhood or family history of pica.

Pica is surrounded by misconceptions about pregnancy and childbirth. Some women who practice pica claim that it "helps" babies, cures swollen legs, relieves nausea and vomiting, ensures beautiful children, helps infants "slide out" more easily, and prevents birthmarks. Pica may also be used to relieve tension or hunger, and some women claim they are merely satisfying cravings for clay or starch.

It is important to determine not only what is ingested but also why. *Remain nonjudgmental* but stress the importance of an adequate diet, the use of iron supplements during pregnancy, and the potential dangers of pica. Offer economical ways to obtain an adequate diet, and refer the client to social services or the WIC program if appropriate. Encourage women who experience constipation to consume a high-fiber, high-fluid diet. Women who experience diarrhea and vomiting may have a parasitic infection or lead poisoning.

Diabetes Mellitus

Diabetes mellitus, characterized by abnormal glucose tolerance, requires dietary management regardless of whether it was present before conception (preexisting diabetes) or developed during gestation (gestational diabetes) as a result of the metabolic changes of pregnancy. Preexisting diabetes increases the risk of congenital abnormalities, miscarriage, and neonatal death. Gestational diabetes appears in the latter half (after 24 weeks) of about 7% of all pregnancies. Gestational diabetes increases the risk of macrosomia and can make delivery difficult, increasing the risk of infant shoulder dislocation and cesarean delivery. Long-term, children born to diabetic mothers are at increased risk for hypertension and high BMI in childhood.

Women with preexisting diabetes should achieve glycemic control prior to conception. All women should be screened for gestational diabetes between 24 and 28 weeks of pregnancy. Check for ketonuria regularly. Diabetic management during pregnancy includes nutrition therapy and possibly multiple daily doses of insulin. Advise the client that

- Pregnant diabetics require the same nutrients and weight gain as nondiabetic pregnant women.
- She is not on a "diet." Weight loss and fasting should never be undertaken during pregnancy.
- Adequate food intake prevents ketone formation and promotes proper weight gain. The individualized meal plan should be high in complex carbohydrates and fiber and limited in fat and sugar.
- Three meals plus three snacks daily, preferably with foods of low glycemic index, may promote better glycemic control.
- Close monitoring (i.e., daily urine ketone testing for gestational diabetics, blood monitoring for established diabetics) and periodic evaluations are necessary throughout the course of pregnancy to meet nutritional needs and to control blood glucose levels.
- Although symptoms of gestational diabetes disappear after delivery, women who have had gestational diabetes, especially those who continue to have impaired glu-

cose tolerance in the postpartum period, are at high risk for type 2 diabetes later in life. Risk reduction strategies should be promoted.

Pregnancy-Induced Hypertension

Preeclampsia: a toxemia of pregnancy characterized by hypertension accompanied by proteinuria, edema, or both.

Eclampsia: a toxemia of pregnancy that develops with the occurrence of one or more convulsions resulting from preeclampsia.

Pregnancy-induced hypertension (PIH) is a hypertensive syndrome that occurs in approximately 8% to 10% of all pregnancies. More severe cases, preeclampsia and eclampsia, are associated with increased risks of preterm delivery, intrauterine growth restriction, neonatal death, and maternal morbidity and mortality. Risk factors include a history of chronic hypertension or preeclampsia in a prior pregnancy, nulliparity, very young or very old, obesity, change of partners, and genetic factors. A sudden weight gain (>2 pounds/week after the 20th week of gestation) may indicate preeclampsia.

No specific therapy has been proven effective in preventing or delaying preeclampsia and improving pregnancy outcomes. Some studies show that calcium supplements lower blood pressure and the risk of preeclampsia but have no significant impact on reducing maternal and infant morbidity and mortality. Likewise, supplements of vitamins C and E may reduce the risk of preeclampsia but do not improve gestational age or birth weight. Other dietary interventions, such as sodium restriction, magnesium supplements, zinc supplements, and the use of fatty fish oils, have not been proven effective.

Assessment of Nutritional Needs During Pregnancy

Initial evaluation of historical data, physical findings, and laboratory data should be performed to identify clients who are at risk for poor nutritional status during pregnancy (Box 11.3) and also to establish baseline data. Ongoing evaluation, performed regularly throughout the course of pregnancy, provides continuing surveillance and helps to identify clients in need of nutrition counseling or community assistance.

Historical Data

- Does the client have a medical condition that may benefit from nutrition therapy such as diabetes, hypertension, lactose intolerance, or PKU? Does the client have any gastrointestinal side effects of pregnancy such as nausea, vomiting, constipation, and heartburn? If so, assess onset, frequency, causative factors, severity, interventions attempted, and the results of these interventions.
- Is the client's usual 24-hour intake adequate for pregnancy? Pay particular attention to the total quantity of food consumed; the number of servings consumed from each of the major food groups and from the Fats, Oils, and Sweets group; and the amount of fluid consumed. Assess folic acid intake.
- Has the client made dietary changes in response to pregnancy or diet-related complications of pregnancy? What foods does the client avoid? What foods does the client prefer? Does the client use alcohol, tobacco, caffeine, or drugs? How frequently does the client eat?

BOX 11.3

RISK FACTORS FOR POOR NUTRITIONAL STATUS DURING PREGNANCY

Historical Data

Prepartum weight <85% or >120% of ideal weight
Use of a therapeutic diet for a chronic disease
Use of alcohol, tobacco, or drugs
Food faddism, unbalanced diet, pica
Teens and women older than 40 years of age
Poor obstetric history (LBW, stillbirth, abortion, fetal anomalies), high parity, multipara
Repetitive pregnancies at short intervals
Low socioeconomic status
Chronic preexisting medical problems such as hypertension, diabetes, heart disease, pulmonary disease, renal disease, maternal PKU
Untimely prenatal care

Physical Findings

Inadequate weight gain: <10 lb during the first 20 weeks of pregnancy; <2 lb/mo after the first trimester
Excessive weight gain: >2 lb/wk

Laboratory Data

Low or deficient hemoglobin and hematocrit

- What cultural, religious, and ethnic influences affect the client's food choices? Does the client practice pica? If so, what items are consumed and how does their consumption affect nutrition?
- Does the client have food allergies or intolerances (especially lactose intolerance)?
- Before pregnancy was the client underweight, normal weight, or overweight? Is her weight gain adequate and appropriate for the length of gestation?
- What is the client's attitude about weight gain? Is she fearful of becoming "fat"?
- Does the client take a vitamin and mineral supplement? Is it being used appropriately? Does the client use dietary supplements? What over-the-counter or prescribed medications does the client take? Does the client use herbal supplements?
- Has the client ever been pregnant before now? If so, how long ago was the pregnancy and what was the outcome? Is the client carrying more than one fetus?
- What is the client's knowledge of nutrition and is she able and willing to implement dietary changes? Is the client's food budget adequate? Women who are at nutritional risk because of inadequate nutrition and inadequate income may be eligible for the WIC program. WIC is a supplemental food program for pregnant women, postpartum women (up to 1 year if breast-feeding or up to 6 months if bottle-feeding), infants, and children up to 5 years of age. WIC provides nutrition counseling and vouchers for specified foods of high nutritional quality.
- Does the client plan to breast-feed?

Physical Findings

- Measure the client's present height and weight.
- Assess the client's blood pressure.
- Assess for severe dependent edema.
- Assess for abnormal findings of the skin, mucous membranes, gums, teeth, tongue, eyes, and hair. Although these findings (e.g., bleeding gums) may be related to normal physiologic changes of pregnancy, they may indicate potential nutritional problems that warrant further investigation.

Laboratory Data

Obtain the client's hemoglobin and hematocrit values to detect abnormal findings. Note that many laboratory values change during pregnancy because of normal adjustments in maternal physiology. For this reason, results of laboratory tests performed during pregnancy cannot be validly compared with nonpregnancy standards.

Nutrition Counseling During Pregnancy

Nutrition counseling is an essential component of prenatal care. For optimal impact on maternal and infant health, nutrition counseling ideally should begin before conception. However, before counseling can begin, it is necessary to identify the client's emotional needs by talking with her to learn about her attitudes, beliefs, and fears.

The most effective approach to nutrition counseling begins by determining the client's usual intake and food preferences and aversions to identify potential nutritional problems. Individualized nutrition counseling, initiated during the first prenatal visit and continued throughout the course of pregnancy, should stress the maintenance of good dietary habits and recommend realistic ways to improve intake. A variety of teaching materials are available. Select those appropriate for the client's level of understanding.

Because the risk of low gestational weight gain is higher among unmarried women, adolescents, African-American and Hispanic women, cigarette smokers, and women with low levels of education, these women should receive additional nutrition counseling to ensure an adequate weight gain during pregnancy.

Instruct the client and family:

About the importance of adequate nutrition and weight gain for maternal and infant health. Describe the optimal rate of weight gain. Explain that weight gain during pregnancy is not synonymous with "getting fat" and that weight reduction should never be undertaken during pregnancy, even by overweight women. Overweight women who require less weight gain than normal should be instructed on how to choose a nutrient-dense diet for a controlled amount of high-quality weight gain.

How to achieve nutritional adequacy by using MyPyramid. Stress the principles of variety, proportionality, and moderation. Nutrient-dense foods should provide the majority of the additional calories needed. Counsel the client regarding meal frequency, fluid requirements, and the use of salt, alcohol, caffeine, and artificial sweeteners.

To take supplements only as prescribed by the physician. Discourage the use of supplements that are not prescribed by the physician and stress the importance of taking only the prescribed dosage because megadoses of some vitamins and minerals can cause fetal malformations.

To avoid alcohol, tobacco, and drugs during pregnancy. These substances pose actual or potential adverse health effects to both mother and baby.

To use coffee, caffeine, and artificial sweeteners in moderation, if so desired. These items are not necessarily contraindicated during pregnancy but intake should be prudent.

That cravings during pregnancy do not appear to have a physiologic basis. Cravings are likely to be influenced by culture, geography, social traditions, the availability of foods, and previous experience. Satisfying cravings for foods is relatively harmless so long as the overall impact on nutrient intake is not negative. (For example, an occasional dill pickle is okay, but eating an entire jar of them is not.) Cravings for nonfood items should be investigated. Dispel myths about diet during pregnancy (Box 11.4).

About how to modify her diet to alleviate or avoid nutrition-related problems and complications of pregnancy as appropriate.

BOX 11.4

COMMON MYTHS ABOUT NUTRITION DURING PREGNANCY

You can eat anything you want because you're eating for two.
You can eat double portions because you're eating for two.
You should eat whatever you're craving; your body must need it.
If you take prenatal vitamins, you don't have to worry about what you eat.
You must take vitamins to have a healthy baby.
The baby gets what he or she needs first, and the rest goes to the mother.
If you breast-feed, you can lose all the weight you gain in pregnancy.
Obese women don't need to gain weight during pregnancy.
It doesn't matter what you eat because the baby will take what it needs from your body.
As long as you take vitamins, it's all right to skip meals.
When you are pregnant, you will crave pickles and ice cream.
Gaining lots of weight makes a healthy baby.
You lose a tooth with every baby if you don't drink milk.
Beets build red blood.
Food cravings during pregnancy determine your child's likes and dislikes later in life.
Give in to your cravings or you will mark the baby.
Do not eat fish and milk at the same meal.
Do not eat egg yolks because they will rot the uterus.
If you crave sweets, the baby will be a girl; if you crave pickles, the baby will be a boy.

 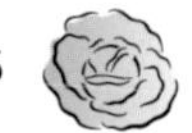

To avoid all medications unless approved by the physician.

That once labor begins, no foods or liquids should be consumed. This is to prevent aspiration if anesthesia must be used.

Adolescent Pregnancy

Each year approximately half a million American teenagers give birth. Compared with infants born to adults, those born to adolescent mothers are more likely to be preterm, to have LBW, to require intensive care, to have physical problems, or to die at birth or just after the newborn period. Pregnancy-induced hypertension, anemia, and sexually transmitted disease are the most common problems seen in pregnant adolescents younger than 16 years of age.

Gynecologic Age: age at conception minus age at menarche.

Pregnant adolescents are at increased risk for complications because of psychosocial and economic factors. Adolescents with a gynecologic age of less than 4 years are at high nutritional risk because the nutritional needs of the developing fetus are superimposed on the mother's own needs for growth. Those with gynecologic age of less than 2 years have the highest risk for pregnancy complications. Compared with adult women, pregnant adolescents

- Are more likely to be physically, emotionally, financially, and socially immature. Low socioeconomic status may be the major reason for the high incidence of LBW infants and other complications of adolescent pregnancy.
- May not have adequate nutrient stores because they need large amounts of nutrients for their own growth and development. Although female adolescent growth is usually complete by the age of 15 years, physical maturity is not reached until 4 years after menarche, which usually occurs by age 17 years.
- Have eating practices that may not provide adequate nourishment to support their own growth, pregnancy, and fetal development. Voluntary calorie restriction to control weight, erratic eating patterns, reliance on fast foods and convenience foods, and meal skipping (especially breakfast) are common adolescent practices.
- Must gain weight early and steadily to maximize the chance of giving birth to an optimal-weight infant.
- Are more concerned with body image and confused about weight gain recommendations. Many do not understand why they should gain 30 pounds when the average baby weighs only about 7 pounds.
- Are more likely to smoke during pregnancy.
- Seek prenatal care later and have fewer total visits during pregnancy.

Proper nutrition is one of the most important controllable factors that determine the overall outcome of pregnancy. Good nutrition has the potential to decrease the incidence of LBW infants and to improve the health of infants born to adolescents. Teenagers within the healthy BMI range should gain about 30 pounds. The MyPyramid recommendations in Table 11.3 can also be used by pregnant teens; MyPyramid is useful both in assessing dietary strengths and weaknesses and in providing a framework for implementing dietary changes in a way the teenager can understand.

Because teens living with one or more adults may have little control over what food is available to them, parents and significant others should also be encouraged to attend counseling sessions.

LACTATION

Breast-feeding provides significant nutritional, health, and psychological benefits to both mother and infant (Box 11.5). Breast milk is uniquely and specifically designed to support optimal growth and development in the newborn. It provides optimal amounts and forms of nutrients the infant can easily tolerate and digest, with added

BOX 11.5

BENEFITS OF BREAST-FEEDING

For the Mother

- Breast-feeding promotes optimal maternal–infant bonding.
- Breast-feeding can mobilize fat stores to help women lose weight particularly in the lower body.
- Early breast-feeding stimulates uterine contractions to help control blood loss and regain prepregnant size.
- Breast milk is readily available and requires no mixing or dilution.
- Breast-feeding is less expensive than purchasing bottles, nipples, sterilizing equipment, and formula.
- Breast-feeding may decrease the risk of thromboembolism especially after operative deliveries.
- Childbirth and breast-feeding may be protective against breast cancer.
- Although not reliable for birth control, breast-feeding does afford some contraceptive protection.

For the Infant

- Breast milk is a “natural” food that contains no artificial colorings, flavorings, preservatives, or additives.
- Breast milk contains many components that impart active and passive protection to infants against viral and bacterial pathogens such as specific T and B lymphocytes and nonspecific macrophages and neutrophils.
- Breast milk is sterile, is at the proper temperature, and is readily available.
- Breast-feeding promotes better tooth and jaw development than bottle-feeding because the infant has to suck harder.
- Breast-feeding avoids nursing-bottle caries.
- Breast-feeding is protective against food allergies.
- Overfeeding is not likely with breast-feeding.
- Breast-feeding is associated with decreased frequency of certain chronic diseases later in life such as non–insulin-dependent diabetes mellitus, lymphoma, and Crohn’s disease.

benefits in the form of enzymes, hormones, growth factors, host resistance factors, inducers/modulators of the immune system, and antiinflammatory agents. The benefits of breast-feeding are especially important to infants born of low-income mothers because they are at higher risk for health problems that could be minimized by breast-feeding. Because of the unquestionable benefits to both mother and infant, the American Academy of Pediatrics recommends exclusive breast-feeding for full-term infants for the first 6 months of life and that infants receive breast milk for at least the first 12 months of age.

Composition of Breast Milk

Breast milk is said to have more than 200 known components, with more being identified all the time. Its dynamic composition is uniquely suited to support the growth and development of human infants.

Protein

Protein provides a mere 4% to 5% of total calories of mature milk, an amount adequate to support growth and development without contributing to an excessive renal solute load. The majority of the protein is whey, which is easy to digest. Breast milk contains small amounts of amino acids that may be harmful in large amounts (e.g., phenylalanine) and high levels of amino acids that infants cannot synthesize well (e.g., taurine).

Fat

Approximately 58% of the total calories in mature milk are from fat, yet it is easily digested because of fat-digesting enzymes contained in the milk. The content of linoleic acid (the essential fatty acid) is high. Long-chain polyunsaturated fatty acids, especially docosahexaenoic acid (an omega 3 fatty acid), promote optimal central nervous system development. The high level of cholesterol is believed to help infants develop enzyme systems capable of handling cholesterol later in life.

Carbohydrate

Lactose, which stimulates the growth of friendly gastrointestinal bacteria and promotes calcium absorption, provides 35% to 41% of total calories of mature milk. Only trace amounts of glucose and other carbohydrates are present. Breast milk contains amylase (a starch-digesting enzyme), which may promote starch digestion in early infancy, when pancreatic amylase is low or absent.

Minerals

Breast milk contains enough minerals to support adequate growth and development, but not excessive amounts that would burden immature kidneys with a high renal solute load. The minerals are mostly protein-bound and balanced to enhance bioavailability. For instance, the rate of iron absorption from breast milk is approximately 50%

compared with about 4% for iron-fortified formulas. Zinc absorption is better from breast milk than from either cow's milk or formula. Breast milk is low in sodium, allowing fluid needs to be met while keeping renal solute load low.

Vitamins

All vitamins needed for growth and health are supplied in breast milk, but the vitamin content of breast milk varies with the mother's diet. The two vitamins of greatest concern are vitamin D and vitamin B_{12} (in vegan mothers). Although vitamin D content varies with maternal intake and exposure to the sun, the concentration of active vitamin D is generally low in breast milk. The American Academy of Pediatrics recommends that all infants consume at least 200 IU of vitamin D to prevent rickets. Breastfed infants born to complete vegans may need a vitamin B_{12} supplement if maternal diet is inadequate.

Renal Solute Load

The renal solute load of breast milk is approximately one-half that of commercial formulas and one-quarter that of cow's milk. The low renal solute load is suited to the immature kidneys' inability to concentrate urine.

Other Compounds

Although they are more abundant in colostrum, antibodies and antiinfective factors are present in mature breast milk. Existing resistance factors include bifidus factor, which promotes the growth of friendly gastrointestinal bacteria (e.g., *Lactobacillus bifidus*) that protect the infant against harmful gastrointestinal bacteria. Breast milk also contains several enzymes (e.g., lipases, amylase) and numerous hormones and hormone-like substances such as melatonin, thyroid gland hormones, adrenal gland hormones, estrogen, insulin, and prostaglandins.

Variables Affecting Breast Milk Composition

The composition of breast milk is constantly changing with the stage of lactation, the mother's diet, and the duration of the feeding.

Stage of Lactation

Colostrum: a thick, yellowish fluid milk secreted during the first few postpartum days.

The composition of breast milk varies considerably with the stage of lactation. Colostrum is higher in protein, minerals, and sodium than mature milk but lower in sugar, fat, and calories. It is rich in antibodies and anti-infective factors that protect the infant against various gastrointestinal and nongastrointestinal infections.

Colostrum begins to change to transitional milk about 3 to 6 days after delivery as the protein content decreases and the carbohydrate and fat contents increase. Major changes in the milk take place by the tenth day; mature milk is stable by the end of the first month.

Maternal Diet

Almost all women are capable of producing enough high-quality breast milk to meet the infant's needs. The content of minerals, total fat, and cholesterol is not significantly affected by maternal diet. The content of other nutrients, such as calcium and folate, is maintained at the expense of maternal tissues when maternal intake is inadequate. However, the vitamin content of breast milk declines as a result of inadequate maternal intake, especially B vitamins and vitamins A, C, and D.

Conversely, unusually high intakes of water-soluble vitamins through either food or supplements do not increase their concentration in breast milk, but excessive intakes of fat-soluble vitamins do.

Duration of the Feeding

Foremilk, the milk secreted as each feeding begins, is significantly lower in fat than hindmilk, the milk secreted at the end of each feeding. The increase in fat content may be a physiologic mechanism designed to provide satiety and to signal the infant to stop nursing.

Nutritional Needs During Lactation

Nutritional needs during lactation are based on the nutritional content of breast milk and the nutritional "cost" of producing milk. Compared to pregnancy, the need for some nutrients increases whereas the need for other nutrients falls (Table 11.2).

Calories

Calorie requirements while breast-feeding are proportional to the amount of milk produced and are higher during lactation than during pregnancy. Approximately 650 calories are used daily to produce milk during the first 6 months of breastfeeding. Women who gained the appropriate amount of weight during pregnancy are advised to increase their calorie intake by 500 cal/day for the first 6 months of lactation; because more than 500 cal/day is actually used to produce milk, women draw on fat reserves accumulated during pregnancy to furnish the additional calories needed. This calorie deficit over time may help them to reduce fat stores and body weight to prepregnancy levels. Women who only partially breast-feed use fewer calories.

Because failure to consume enough calories can jeopardize the quantity of milk produced, women should be discouraged from restricting their calorie intake. The average woman should consume a total of 2500 to 3300 cal daily while exclusively breast-feeding. Women who failed to gain enough weight during pregnancy or who have inadequate fat reserves have higher calorie requirements.

Fluid

Another nutritional consideration during lactation is fluid intake. It is suggested that nursing mothers drink 2 to 3 quarts of fluid daily, preferably in the form of water, milk, and fruit juices instead of carbonated beverages, sweetened fruit drinks, and caffeine-containing beverages. Usually women are urged to drink a glass of fluid every time the baby nurses. Thirst is a good indicator of need except among women who live in a dry climate or who exercise in hot weather. Fluids consumed in excess of thirst quenching do not increase milk volume.

Vitamins and Minerals

For many vitamins and minerals, requirements during lactation are higher than during pregnancy. Foods, rather than supplements, are the preferred source of these nutrients because foods provide a plethora of other nutrients and substances important for good health. To obtain adequate amounts of vitamins and minerals, women are encouraged to choose a varied diet that includes enriched and fortified grains and cereals, fresh fruits and vegetables, and lean meats and dairy products.

Multivitamin and mineral supplements are not recommended for routine use. However, specific supplements may be indicated when maternal intake is inadequate. For instance

- A balanced multivitamin and mineral supplement may be necessary for women who consume fewer than 1800 cal/day.
- A calcium supplement is indicated for women who are lactose intolerant or who do not consume enough milk and other calcium-rich foods.
- A vitamin D supplement may be appropriate for women who avoid vitamin D-fortified foods (e.g., milk, cereals) and have limited exposure to the sun.
- A vitamin B_{12} supplement is necessary for vegans if they do not regularly consume vitamin B_{12}-fortified plant products.
- An iron supplement may be needed to replace iron deficits during pregnancy and blood loss during delivery.

Food Guidance During Lactation

A food intake guide for various calorie levels appears in Table 11.3. To meet the increased calorie demands of lactation, a woman needs a calorie level two or three channels higher than her normal calorie requirements. Healthy eating practices followed during pregnancy—namely, emphasizing nutrient-rich foods, eating frequently throughout the day, and consuming adequate fluids—should continue. Limiting calories can impair milk production. Additional recommendations for lactation include

- *Avoid freshwater fish from water contaminated with dioxin, PCBs, or other chemicals.* Women should contact their state health department for recommendations regarding fish consumption during lactation. Women who have been exposed to high levels of environmental toxins should have their milk analyzed for contaminants.
- *Consume little or no alcohol.* Alcohol easily enters breast milk and can adversely affect the production, volume, and composition of breast milk. Although an occasional drink may be within safe limits, alcohol should be avoided.

- *Limit caffeine intake.* Caffeine also enters breast milk but at lower rates. Consumption of one to two cups of coffee daily does not pose any problems. Intakes higher than this may cause the infant to become irritable and restless.
- *Restrict other foods only on an as-needed basis.* It usually is not necessary to eliminate any other foods while breast-feeding unless the infant shows intolerance. For instance, oils from garlic and onion may flavor the taste of breast milk, but they need not be eliminated from the mother's diet unless the taste of the milk is objectionable to the infant. The American Academy of Pediatrics recommends that breast-feeding mothers with a family history of food allergies eliminate peanuts and tree nuts (almonds, walnuts, etc.) from their diets while nursing and consider avoiding eggs, cow's milk, fish, and perhaps other foods.

Lactation in the Diabetic Mother

Breast-feeding complicates blood glucose control in women with type 1 diabetes by inducing hypoglycemia and lowering insulin requirements. Because successful lactation is dependent on adequate blood glucose control, individualized care is needed to balance intake, insulin, exercise, and lactation. Although optimal calorie requirements for lactation for type 1 diabetics have not been determined, 35 cal/kg is usually recommended to achieve optimal glucose and lipid levels and promote moderate weight loss. Other points to consider include

Careful and frequent monitoring of blood glucose levels is essential. Women should be encouraged to check their blood glucose levels immediately before breast-feeding. An acceptable 1-hour postprandial capillary blood glucose level is proposed to be 150 to 160 mg/dL.

Frequent snacks are recommended. Unless breast-feeding occurs within 1 to 2 hours after eating, women should eat a light snack before or during breast-feeding. Milk, fruit, or crackers are sufficient.

Medical concerns may keep mother and baby apart during the critical first few hours after birth. If the child is born with hypoglycemia or the mother has complications, the mother and infant may be separated during the first 60 to 90 minutes after delivery, a time shown to be critical in establishing successful lactation. Mothers can be assisted to pump milk for storage to help initiate lactation and prevent engorgement.

Breast care takes on greater importance. Diabetic women face a higher risk of mastitis because of their elevated blood glucose levels. Measures to prevent mastitis include alternating breasts when feeding, cleaning breasts with water and letting them air dry, making sure the baby's mouth is positioned correctly over the nipple, drinking adequate fluids, and not wearing tight brassieres.

Support groups may be especially helpful. Encourage participation in appropriate programs that provide support and education.

Contraindications to Breast-Feeding

Breast-feeding is contraindicated when the mother is being treated with certain drugs (or uses addictive drugs) that have the potential to enter breast milk and harm the infant. Examples are antiprotozoal compounds, antineoplastic drugs, some antithyroid drugs, and synthetic anticoagulants. If possible, drugs known to pose a risk for infants should be replaced with safer, more acceptable ones. Street drugs such as amphetamines, cocaine, heroin, marijuana, and phencyclidine (PCP) are contraindicated during lactation as are large amounts of alcohol.

Colostrum and breast milk can efficiently transmit HIV from infected mothers to their infants. The Centers for Disease Control and Prevention and the American Academy of Pediatrics recommend that HIV-positive women not breast-feed to avoid postnatal HIV transmission. However, breast-feeding is recommended regardless of HIV status in developing countries where infants are at high risk for death from infectious disease and malnutrition.

Other contraindications to breast-feeding include

- An inborn error of metabolism in the infant such as galactosemia
- Untreated tuberculosis in the mother
- Breast cancer diagnosed during pregnancy
- Pregnancy because the combined demands of pregnancy and lactation on maternal tissues are great

Assessment of Nutritional Needs During Lactation

The reliability and validity of anthropometric and laboratory data for assessing the nutritional status of lactating women have not been proven. The only criteria recommended for routine screening for nutritional problems are maternal weight and dietary intake.

Maternal Weight

- Is the client's weight stable?
- If she is losing weight, how much weight is lost per month? Normal monthly weight loss while breast-feeding is 0.5 to 1 kg, an amount that does not adversely affect milk production. Even among overweight women, it is recommended that weight loss not exceed 2 kg/month.

Dietary Intake

- Is the client's usual 24-hour intake adequate for lactation? Pay particular attention to the total quantity of food consumed; the number of servings consumed from each of the major food groups and from the Fats, Oils, and Sweets group; and the amount of fluids consumed.
- What cultural, religious, and ethnic influences affect food choices?

- Does the client adhere to a modified diet to treat a disease?
- Is the client's exposure to sunlight adequate?
- Does the client use alcohol, tobacco, caffeine, drugs, or artificial sweeteners?

Promotion of Breast-Feeding

Although almost all women have the potential to breast-feed successfully, lactation may fail because of inadequate knowledge, lack of adequate support, or conflict with lifestyle and career. The partner's beliefs and concerns about breast-feeding also directly influence most mothers. To provide the greatest chance for success, preparation for breast-feeding should begin prenatally with counseling, guidance, and support for both the woman and her partner and continue throughout the gestational period.

Postpartum teaching has been shown to have a significant effect on both the ability to breast-feed successfully and the duration of lactation. Individual or small group counseling sessions should first assess the couple's attitudes, fears, expectations, misperceptions, and knowledge. Information can then be provided on how milk is produced and secreted, factors that impair lactation (Box 11.6), breast care, feeding positions, how to express milk manually, how to stimulate the infant, and how to prevent and manage various breast-feeding problems.

Some studies show that the most vulnerable period for lactation is the immediate postpartum period. To establish lactation and promote the best chance of success, the infant should be offered the breast as soon as possible after birth and at frequent intervals thereafter. Hospital procedures should allow for immediate

BOX 11.6

FACTORS THAT IMPAIR LACTATION

Impaired Letdown, Related to

Embarrassment or stress
Fatigue
Negative attitude, lack of desire, lack of family support
Excessive intake of caffeine or alcohol
Smoking
Drugs

Failure to Establish Lactation, Related to

Delayed or infrequent feedings
Weak infant sucking because of anesthesia during labor and delivery
Nipple discomfort or engorgement
Lack of support especially from baby's father

Decreased Demand, Related to

Supplemental bottles of formula or water
Introduction of solid food
Infant's lack of interest

maternal-infant contact after delivery and for true demand feedings preferably through rooming-in. Other practices that facilities can use to promote successful breast-feeding include

- Informing all pregnant women about the benefits and management of breast-feeding
- Showing mothers how to breast-feed and how to maintain lactation even if they are separated from their infants
- Giving newborn infants no food or drink other than breast milk unless medically indicated
- Giving no artificial teats or pacifiers (e.g., dummies, soothers) to breast-feeding infants
- Fostering the establishment of breast-feeding support groups and referring mothers to them upon discharge from the hospital or clinic

Although almost 70% of newborns are breast-fed, only 31% of all infants are still breast-fed at 6 months of age and less than 18% still receive breast milk at 12 months of age. The dramatic decline in breast-feeding after the first few months means significant health benefits are being forfeited.

Instruct the client and partner

About the benefits of breast-feeding. Provide assurance that all women have the ability to breast-feed if given proper instruction and encouragement. Emphasize the benefits of breast-feeding for both mother and infant and point out that even a short period of breast-feeding is better than not nursing at all but that optimal benefits are obtained from sustained breast-feeding. Partners who believe that they will miss opportunities to bond with their exclusively breast-fed infant may benefit from developing skills to comfort the infant that do not involve feeding.

On the mechanics of breast-feeding. Women need basic how-to information especially if they do not have any family members or friends who have successfully breast-fed their infants.

- Discuss breast care, positioning the infant, ways to stimulate the infant, and how to end a feeding. Explain that certain factors may inhibit lactation (Box 11.6). Point out that a warm bath, gentle massage, and a relaxed atmosphere may help to achieve letdown.
- Inform the client that the infant should be allowed to nurse for 5 minutes on each side on the first day to achieve letdown and milk ejection. By the end of the first week, the infant should be nursing up to 15 minutes per side.
- Mothers need to know that the supply of milk is equal to the demand—the more the infant sucks, the more milk is produced. Infants age 6 weeks or 12 weeks who suck more are probably experiencing a growth spurt and so need more milk.
- Advise the client that even though the infant will be able to virtually empty the breast within 5 to 10 minutes once the milk supply is established, the infant needs to nurse beyond that point to satisfy the need to suck and to receive emotional and physical comfort.

- Reassure the client that both feeding the infant more frequently and manually expressing milk will help to increase the milk supply.
- Acknowledge that because breast milk is easier to digest than formula, breast-fed babies usually need to nurse at shorter intervals than bottle-fed babies do.
- Warn that early substitution of formula or introduction of solid foods may decrease the chance of maintaining lactation.

How to pump milk for later use. Breast pumps are available for manual expression of milk. Milk expressed into a sanitary bottle should be refrigerated or frozen immediately. Milk should be used within 24 hours if refrigerated, within 3 months if stored in the freezer compartment of the refrigerator, and within 2 years if maintained at 0°F.

About the importance of eating a varied and balanced diet that is adequate in calories and fluid. Use MyPyramid to illustrate the food group approach to choosing an adequate diet. Appetite and thirst are generally good indicators of need. Excess consumption of either foods or liquids will not produce "better" or more milk. Women should avoid freshwater fish and alcohol and should limit their intake of caffeine to one to two cups of coffee a day or less.

Not to aggressively diet while breast-feeding. Reassure the mother that even if she has adequate fat stores, calorie intake should increase during lactation because fat is mobilized slowly. Lean women may be at risk for impaired lactation if calorie intake is restricted.

Not to take drugs or medications unless approved by the physician.

Where to find additional information. The La Lèche League is an international organization founded for the purpose of helping nursing mothers. The League prints a bimonthly newsletter, holds conventions and monthly group meetings, and is available as a source of information and advice 24 hours a day. Also numerous instructional materials and books on breast-feeding are available from community organizations and bookstores.

NURSING PROCESS

Jana is a well-educated professional who is 33 years old and 20 weeks pregnant with her first baby. Her prepregnancy BMI was 19.2. She has gained 7 pounds and complains of constipation. She plans on returning to work 6 weeks after delivery and wants to limit her weight gain so that she can fit into her clothes by the time she returns to work. She has asked you what she should eat that will be good for the baby but not cause her to get fat.

Assessment

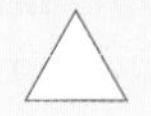

Obtain Clinical Data:

Current weight
Blood pressure
Laboratory data including hemoglobin, hematocrit, albumin, glucose
Interview client to assess:
Medical history such as diabetes, hypertension, anemia, or other chronic disease
Use of prescribed and over-the-counter medications that affect nutrition
Symptoms of constipation including frequency, interventions attempted, and results
Intake information including

- Usual 24-hour intake of food and fluid with focus on calories, protein, calcium, folic acid, fiber, and fluid
- Frequency and pattern of eating
- Pica or unusual eating habits
- Use of vitamin/mineral or dietary supplements: what, how much, and why taken
- Appetite
- Cultural, religious, and ethnic influences on eating habits
- Use of alcohol, tobacco, caffeine, and drugs

Prepregnancy weight history; rate and pattern of 7-pound weight gain
Usual frequency and intensity of physical activity
Psychosocial and economic issues including

- Attitude regarding pregnancy
- Living situation, family support
- Understanding of recommended weight gain during pregnancy and nutritional requirements
- Willingness to change eating behaviors

Nursing Diagnosis

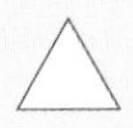

1. Constipation, related to pregnancy and the use of iron supplements.
2. Health-Seeking Behaviors, as evidenced by lack of knowledge of appropriate diet for pregnancy and a desire to learn.
3. Altered Nutrition: Less Than Body Requirements, related to voluntary food restriction to limit weight gain.

Planning and Implementation

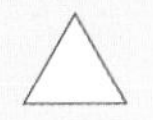

Client Goals

The client will:

Explain the importance of diet for her health and for fetal growth and development.
Explain the amount and pattern of recommended weight gain.
Consume an adequate, varied, and balanced diet based on MyPyramid.
Gain approximately 1 pound of weight per week.
Avoid constipation.

Nursing Interventions

Nutrition Therapy

Promote the intake of a varied, nutrient-dense diet based on MyPyramid.
Increase fiber and fluids to prevent constipation.

Client Teaching

Instruct the client

On the role of nutrition and weight gain in the outcome of pregnancy
On the role of fiber and fluids in preventing and alleviating constipation
On eating plan essentials including
- Choosing a variety of foods within each major food group
- Selecting the appropriate number of servings from each major food group
- Consuming sources of fiber such as bran and whole-grain breads and cereals, dried peas and beans, fresh fruits, and vegetables

On behavioral matters including

- Abandoning the idea of limiting weight gain to fit into clothes after pregnancy
- Eating small, frequent meals
- The importance of maintaining physical activity

On where to find more information (see websites at the end of this chapter)

(continued)

Evaluation

The client:

Explains the importance of diet for her health and for fetal growth and development
Explains the amount and pattern of recommended weight gain
Consumes an adequate, varied, and balanced diet based on MyPyramid
Gains approximately 1 pound of weight per week
Avoids constipation

How Do You Respond?

Is it possible for some infants to be allergic to breast milk? Allergy to breast milk occurs infrequently and some researchers believe it does not exist. However, the infant may develop an allergic reaction to breast milk if the mother ingests a protein that enters the breast milk intact; if this occurs, the protein can be identified and eliminated from the mother's diet.

▲ Focus on Critical Thinking

Respond to the following statements:

1. The fetus is a perfect parasite and will take from the mother what it needs regardless of maternal intake.
2. Pregnancy increases the risk of overweight and obesity in women of childbearing age.
3. If a woman can't commit to breast-feeding exclusively for 6 months, she should be encouraged to do so for as long as she can because the benefits are dose-related.
4. For HIV mothers, the risk of transmitting HIV to their infant through breast milk outweighs any potential health benefit bestowed by breast-feeding.

Key Concepts

- Although proper nutrition before and during pregnancy cannot guarantee a successful pregnancy outcome, it does profoundly affect fetal development and birth.
- A woman's prepregnancy weight status and weight gain during pregnancy are correlated to infant birth weight. Underweight women should gain weight before conception or gain more weight during pregnancy to reduce their risk of adverse pregnancy outcomes.

- Most nutrient requirements increase during pregnancy but can be met with an adequate and varied diet.
- Calorie requirements do not increase until the second trimester of pregnancy. During the last two trimesters, normal-weight women need approximately 300 extra cal/day.
- Women who are capable of becoming pregnant should take a multivitamin containing folic acid or eat folic acid-fortified cereals to ensure an adequate intake.
- Nutrition counseling should be initiated early in prenatal care and continue throughout the pregnancy. It should stress the importance of weight gain, ways to improve overall intake, the adverse effects of smoking, and the benefits of breast-feeding.
- Proper nutrition may help to reduce the incidence of preterm births, pregnancy-induced hypertension, and anemia—three problems common to adolescent pregnancies.
- Breast-feeding is recommended for the first 12 months of life. In addition to being uniquely suited to infant growth and development, it imparts other significant benefits to both infant and mother.
- Almost all women are capable of breast-feeding.
- Generally when maternal intake of nutrients is inadequate, the quantity, not the quality, of breast milk is diminished. The carbohydrate, protein, fat, and mineral contents of milk are relatively stable; vitamin concentrations fluctuate in response to maternal intake.
- For many nutrients, nutritional needs are higher during lactation than during pregnancy.

ANSWER KEY

1. **FALSE** The amount of weight a woman gains during pregnancy is an important indicator of fetal growth. However, adequate weight gain during pregnancy cannot by itself ensure the delivery of a normal-birth-weight infant.
2. **FALSE** Obese women should gain at least 15 pounds during pregnancy.
3. **TRUE** Fortified cereals are a significant source of folic acid. In fact, the recommended amount of folic acid could easily be exceeded with fortified cereal.
4. **TRUE** Excessive weight gain is likely to result in an increase in maternal fat stores, increasing the likelihood that prepregnancy weight will not be restored after delivery.
5. **FALSE** The RDA for calcium does not increase during pregnancy because calcium absorption greatly increases. Calcium needs can be met with the equivalent of three cups of milk daily.
6. **FALSE** Pregnant and lactating women as well as women who may become pregnant are advised to eliminate only shark, swordfish, king mackerel, and tilefish from their diets; other fish and shellfish can be consumed in amounts up to 12 oz/week as long as any one particular type of fish is not eaten more than once a week.
7. **TRUE** Calorie requirements are generally higher during lactation than during pregnancy.

8. **TRUE** The vitamin content of breast milk varies with the mother's diet.
9. **TRUE** Thirst is a good indicator of the need for fluids except among women who live in a dry climate or exercise in hot weather.
10. **TRUE** The Centers for Disease Control and the American Academy of Pediatrics recommend that HIV-positive women not breast-feed to avoid postnatal HIV transmission. However, breast-feeding is recommended regardless of HIV status in developing countries where infants are at high risk for death from infectious disease and malnutrition.

WEBSITES

Information on nutrition as it relates to pregnancy and lactation is available at
March of Dimes at **www.modimes.org**
Government nutrition information center at **www.nutrition.gov**
American Dietetic Association at **www.eatright.org**
LaLèche League International at **www.lalecheleague.org**
American College of Obstetricians and Gynecologists at **www.acog.org**
American Academy of Pediatrics at **www.aap.org**

REFERENCES

American Dietetic Association. (2003). Position of the American Dietetic Association and Dietitians of Canada: Vegetarian diets. *Journal of the American Dietetic Association, 103,* 748–765.

American Dietetic Association. (2002). Position of the American Dietetic Association: Nutrition and lifestyle for a healthy pregnancy outcome. *Journal of the American Dietetic Association, 102,* 1479–1490.

American Dietetic Association. (2001). Position of the American Dietetic Association: Breaking the barriers to breastfeeding. *Journal of the American Dietetic Association, 101,* 1213–1220.

Berg, M., VanDyke, D., Chenard, C., et al. (2001). Folate, zinc, and vitamin B_{12} intake during pregnancy and postpartum. *Journal of the American Dietetic Association, 101,* 242–244.

Brown, J., Murtaugh, M., Jacobs, D., & Margellos, H. (2002). Variation in newborn size according to pregnancy weight change by trimester. *American Journal of Clinical Nutrition, 76,* 205–209.

DiPietro, J., Millet, S., Costigan, K., Gurewitsch, E., & Caulfield, L. (2003). Psychosocial influences on weight gain attitudes and behaviors during pregnancy. *Journal of the American Dietetic Association, 103,* 1314–1319.

French, M., Barr, B., & Levy-Milne, R. (2003). Folate intakes and awareness of folate to prevent neural tube defects: A survey of women living in Vancouver, Canada. *Journal of the American Dietetic Association, 103,* 181–185.

Mangels, A. & Messina, V. (2001). Considerations in planning vegan diets: Infants. *Journal of the American Dietetic Association, 101,* 670–677.

Marcason, W. (2002). Should my client with a family history of food allergies avoid certain foods during pregnancy or lactation? *Journal of the American Dietetic Association, 102,* 936.

March of Dimes Birth Defects Foundation. (2003). *Fact sheet: Herbal supplements: Their safety, a concern for health care providers.* [On-line]. Available at: www.modimes.com/printableArticles/681_1815.asp?printable=true. Accessed November 28, 2003.

March of Dimes Birth Defects Foundation. (2002). *Fact sheet: Food-borne risks in pregnancy.* [On-line]. Available: www.modimes.com/printableArticles/681_1152.asp?printable=true. Accessed November 28, 2003.

March of Dimes Birth Defects Foundation. (2003). *Fact sheet: Caffeine in pregnancy.* [Online]. Available at: www.modimes.com/printableArticles/681_1148.asp?printable=true. Accessed November 28, 2003.

March of Dimes Birth Defects Foundation. (2003). *Fact sheet: Breastfeeding.* Available at: www.modimes.com/printableArticles/681_9148.asp?printable=true. Accessed November 28, 2003.

March of Dimes Birth Defects Foundation. (2003). Quick reference: Birth defects & genetics: PKU. Available at http://search.marchofdimes.com/cgi-bin/MsmGo.exe?grab_id=7&page_id=3279104&que. Accessed on 12/31/03.

McCaffree, J. (2001). Folic acid fortification: Informed mothers, healthy babies. *Journal of the American Dietetic Association, 101,* 872.

Moya, S., McIver, G., Seiter, J., & Bailey, D. (2002). Folic acid fortification: Additional issues. *Journal of the American Dietetic Association, 102,* 346.

National Academy of Sciences. (2002). *Dietary Reference Intakes for energy, carbohydrate, fiber, fat, fatty acids, cholesterol, protein, and amino acids.* Available at www.nap.edu.

Olson, C., & Strawderman, M. (2003). Modifiable behavioral factors in a biopsychosocial model predict inadequate and excessive gestational weight gain. *Journal of the American Dietetic Association, 103,* 48–54.

Turner, R., Langkamp-Henken, B., Littell, R., Lukowski, M., & Suarez, M. (2003). Comparing nutrient intake from food to the estimated average requirements shows middle- to upper-income pregnant women lack iron and possibly magnesium. *Journal of the American Dietetic Association, 103,* 461–466.

For information on the new dietary guidelines 2005 and MyPyramid, visit
http://connection.lww.com/go/dudek

12

Nutrition for Infants, Children, and Adolescents

TRUE	FALSE	
◯	◯	**1** Infants have higher requirements per kilogram of body weight for calories and most nutrients than adults do.
◯	◯	**2** If breast-feeding is discontinued before the infant's first birthday, it should be replaced with iron-fortified infant formula.
◯	◯	**3** Protein is the nutrient of most concern when solids are introduced into the diet.
◯	◯	**4** A potential problem with early introduction of solid foods is overfeeding.
◯	◯	**5** The risk of nutrient deficiencies among American toddlers is negligible.
◯	◯	**6** The Dietary Guidelines for Americans are intended for adults only.
◯	◯	**7** Iron deficiency in young children may be related to drinking too much milk.
◯	◯	**8** Adolescents need to drink more milk than young children.
◯	◯	**9** An overweight child is more likely to become an obese adult than a child of normal weight.
◯	◯	**10** Adolescents consume more soft drinks than milk.

UPON COMPLETION OF THIS CHAPTER, YOU WILL BE ABLE TO

- Discuss how growth and development influence calorie and nutrient requirements in infancy.
- Explain why iron-fortified cereal is usually the first solid food introduced to an infant's diet.
- Explain how adequacy of intake is assessed during infancy.
- Discuss nutritional concerns in infants and toddlers.
- Explain why children are at risk of vitamin D deficiency.
- Explain why children and adolescents are at risk of iron deficiency.
- Name nutritional concerns of childhood.
- Name nutritional concerns of adolescence.
- List food groups most likely to be consumed in inadequate amounts by both children and adolescents.

Although adequate nutrition cannot guarantee that a child will experience normal growth and development, inadequate nutrition can prevent the child from reaching his or her genetic potential for physical and mental growth and development. For instance, general undernutrition can cause growth retardation, and iron deficiency can impair cognitive development. *Weight for height* is the foremost standard used to assess whether or not a child is receiving adequate nutrition.

Actual nutrient requirements vary according to health status, activity pattern, and growth rate. The greater the rate of growth, the more intense the nutritional needs. Although the focus of childhood nutrition has traditionally been on getting enough calories and nutrients, problems related to overconsumption are much more prevalent among today's American children. Nutritional guidance for children has expanded beyond "getting enough" to include recommendations for healthy eating to reduce the risk of chronic disease related to nutritional excesses.

INFANCY (BIRTH TO 1 YEAR)

Excluding fetal growth, growth in the first year of life is more rapid than at any other time in the life cycle. Birthweight doubles by 4 to 6 months of age and triples by the first birthday. To support the rapid rate of growth, the need for calories and nutrients is high. In fact, although the *total* amount of calories and nutrients needed by infants is less than that of adults, the *amount per kg of body weight* for calories and most nutrients is higher at birth than at any other time in the life cycle (Fig. 12.1). After the first

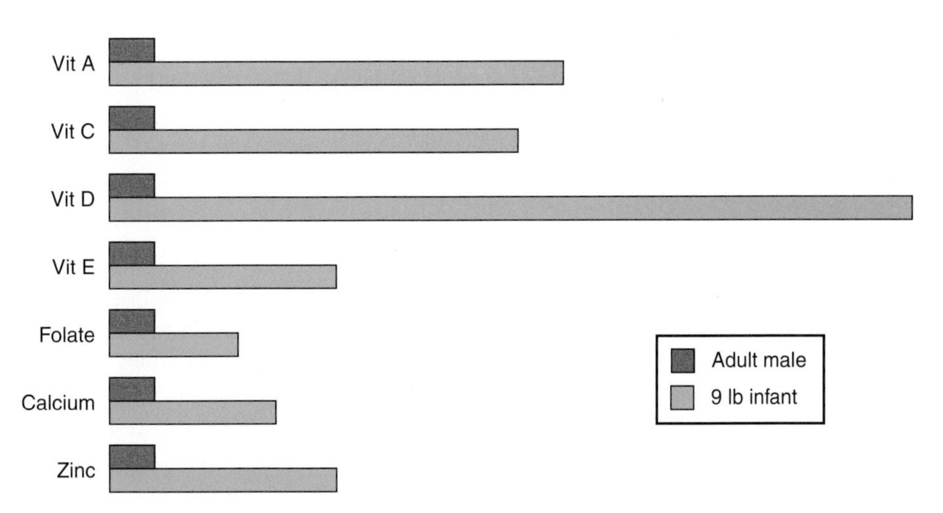

FIGURE 12.1 Comparison of selected nutrient needs between a 9-lb (4-kg) infant and a 154-lb (70-kg) 25-year-old male.

6 months of life, energy requirements increase at a slower rate, reflective of the slowing in the rate of growth.

Up until 4 to 6 months of age, milk—either in the form of breast milk, infant formula, or a combination of the two—is the sole source of nutrition. With the exception of vitamin D and iron (after 4 to 6 months of age), breast milk is nutritionally complete. Iron-fortified infant formulas have nutrient levels at or above those in breast milk, making supplemental nutrients unnecessary. Supplemental water is usually not needed because both breast milk and formula provide 1.5 mL water/cal, the water-to-calorie ratio estimated to be adequate to meet the needs of infants. However, infants are especially prone to dehydration because of their large surface area/kg of body weight and their inability to communicate thirst. Therefore, in unusually hot weather infants may need some additional water. Allowing infants to sip water also may set the stage in teaching them to drink water to quench thirst.

Breast-Feeding

The American Academy of Pediatrics recommends that infants be exclusively breastfed for the first 6 months of life and continue to receive breast milk until the age of 1 year. Nutrition experts throughout the world agree that breastfeeding is superior to formula feeding because it offers unique nutritional and non-nutritional advantages to both infant and mother (see Chapter 11). Although every mother should be encouraged to breast-feed, the final decision is an individual one. Coercion is not appropriate.

The benefits of breast-feeding are dose dependent; 4 months of exclusive breastfeeding are better than 2 months and any duration is better than none at all. A recent study showed that about 75% of children between the ages of 4 and 24 months had been breast-fed to some extent and the average age at which breastfeeding was stopped was 5.5 months. Only about 30% of infants were still breastfeeding at 6 months of age and 16% at 12 months of age. When breast-feeding is discontinued before the age of 12 months, it should be replaced with iron-fortified infant formula.

Infant Formula—An Appropriate Substitute for Breast-Feeding

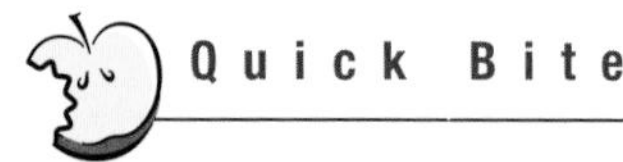

Examples of routine formulas

Similac
Enfamil
SMA
Gerber
Good Start

Iron-fortified infant formula is an appropriate substitute or supplement to breastfeeding. Routine infant formulas made from cow's milk are modified to resemble breast milk and to provide comparable nutritional benefits (Table 12.1). In fact, the levels of many nutrients are higher in formula than breast milk, based on the rationale that some nutrients are less well absorbed from formula.

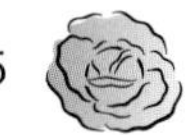

TABLE 12.1 **COMPARISONS BETWEEN BREAST MILK AND INFANT FORMULA**

Nutrient	Mature Breast Milk	Formula
Protein (g/L)	7–9	15
Whey-casein ratio	60:40	60:40
Fat Total (g/L)	34	37
% Linoleic acid calories	14.7–18.8	17.2
Carbohydrate (g/L)	66	71
Minerals (mg/L)		
Sodium	170	200
Calcium	260	470
Phosphorus	140	350
Ca:P ratio	2.4	1.1–2.0
Iron	5	12*
Calories (cal/L)	640	670

*Iron-fortified formula. Unfortified formula is 1.0.

Standards for levels of nutrients in formulas were established by the U.S. Congress in the Infant Formula Act (revised in 1982), based mostly on recommendations of the Committee on Nutrition of the American Academy of Pediatrics. Almost all infant formula used in the United States is iron-fortified.

Formula Varieties

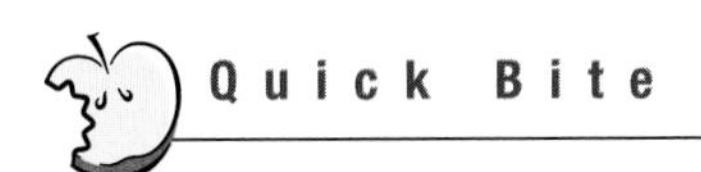

Examples of soy-based formulas

Prosobee
Isomil

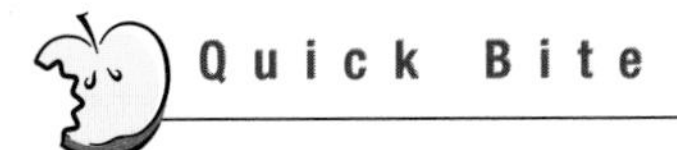

Examples of casein hydrolysate formulas for infants who do not tolerate either routine formulas or soy formulas

Nutramigen
Pregestimil

Infants who are intolerant of the protein or lactose in cow's milk may be given formulas made with soy isolates or casein hydrolysates. A variety of formulas have been developed for infants with special needs. For instance, incomplete formulas are available for infants with inborn errors of metabolism such as phenylketonuria (PKU) or maple syrup urine disease. These specialized formulas are intentionally lacking or deficient in one or more nutrients and, therefore, do not supply adequate nutrition for normal infants. They must be supplemented with small amounts of regular formula. Low birth weight formulas are available for premature infants; they are higher in whey protein, vitamins, and minerals (except iron) and have less lactose than routine formulas. The amount of formula provided per feeding and the frequency of feeding depend on the infant's age and

TABLE 12.2 GENERAL PARAMETERS FOR FORMULA FEEDING

Age	No. of Feedings in 24 h	Amount per Feeding (oz)	Amount per Day (oz)
1 wk–1 mo	6–8	4–5	21–24
1–3 mo	5–6	5–7	24–32
3–6 mo	4–5	6–7	24–32
6–12 mo (feedings from the cup and bottle if the infant is not completely weaned)	3–4	6–8	16–24

individual needs. General parameters are provided in Table 12.2. Caregivers should recognize that infants cry for reasons other than hunger and should not be fed every time they cry. Nor should an infant be forced to finish her or his bottle. Overfeeding is one of the biggest hazards of formula feeding. Teaching points for formula feeding are summarized in Box 12.1.

Formula Preparation

Most caregivers prepare formula a single bottle at a time and powdered formula is the most common form. Formula must be prepared using safe food handling practices that include proper handwashing before making the formula; thorough washing of formula cans, bottles, and nipples; and proper refrigeration. Water must be clean and free of contamination. Care must be taken to prepare formulas to the proper level of dilution. Formulas that are made too dilute can result in inadequate growth and water intoxication; formulas that are made too concentrated can cause hypernatremia, tetany, and excessive weight gain. Formula that remains in the bottle after a feeding is discarded.

Introducing Solids

Because of inborn reflexes, the most appropriate feeding during the first several months of life is milk in the form of breast milk and/or infant formulas. The American Academy of Pediatrics recommends solid foods be introduced when the infant is developmentally ready, that is, when the infant can lift the head, sit with support, and turn the head to indicate that he/she has had enough to eat. Most infants exhibit developmental readiness around 4 to 6 months of age as reflexes disappear, head control develops, and the infant is able to sit, making spoon-feeding possible. Over time, control of the head, neck, jaw, and tongue; hand-eye coordination; and the ability to sit, grasp, chew, drink, and self-feed all develop. The eruption of teeth also indicates readiness to progress from strained to mashed to chopped fine to regular as the ability to chew improves. Box 12.2 features tips for introducing solids.

BOX 12.1

TEACHING POINTS FOR FORMULA FEEDING

One of the greatest hazards of formula feeding is overfeeding. Never force the infant to finish a bottle or to take more than she wants. Signs that an infant is finished include biting the nipple, puckering the face, and turning away from the bottle. Discourage the misconception that "a fat baby = a healthy baby = good parents."

Each feeding should last 20 to 30 minutes.

Formula may be given at room temperature, slightly warmed, or directly from the refrigerator; however, always give formula at approximately the same temperature.

Spitting up of a small amount of formula during or after a feeding is normal. Feed the infant more slowly and burp more frequently to help alleviate spitting up.

Hold the infant closely and securely. Position the infant so that the head is higher than the rest of the body.

Avoid jiggling the bottle and making extra movements that could distract the infant from feeding.

Never prop the bottle or put the infant to bed with a bottle. Giving the infant a bottle of anything but plain water at bedtime can cause nursing bottle caries once the teeth erupt. Nursing bottle caries occur when infants or children are put to bed with a bottle of milk, juice, or any other sweetened liquid (Fig. 12.2). Advise parents that after the teeth erupt the baby should be given only plain water for a bedtime bottle-feeding.

Check the flow of formula by holding the bottle upside down. A steady drip from the nipple should be observed. If the flow is too rapid because of too large a nipple opening, the infant may overfeed and develop indigestion. If the flow rate is too slow because of too small a nipple opening, the infant may tire and fall asleep without taking enough formula. Discard any nipples with holes that are too large; enlarge holes that are too small with a sterilized needle.

Reassure caregivers that there is no danger of "spoiling" an infant by feeding him when he cries for a feeding.

Burp the infant halfway through the feeding, at the end of the feeding, and more often if necessary to help get rid of air swallowed during feeding. Burping can be accomplished by gently rubbing or patting the infant's back as she is held on the shoulder, lies on her stomach over the caregiver's lap, or sits in an upright position.

Approximately 30% of infants begin solids before 4 months of age, frequently based on the unsupported belief that it will help infants to sleep through the night. A major objection to early introduction of solids is that it may interfere with establishing sound eating habits and may contribute to overfeeding because infants less than 4 months old are unable to communicate satiety by turning away and leaning back.

For both breast- and formula-fed infants, iron-fortified infant cereal is generally the first solid food introduced because of its iron content. Breast-fed infants need supplemental iron or high iron foods beginning around 4 months of age when their

BOX 12.2

TIPS FOR INTRODUCING SOLID FOODS

Always feed the infant in an upright position; do not feed the infant solids from a bottle.

Offer iron-fortified infant rice cereal as the first solid feeding; follow with other iron-fortified infant cereals.

Before giving cereal the first few times, give the infant a small amount of formula or breast milk to take the edge off hunger and increase the likelihood of acceptance. After the infant is accustomed to solids, introduce new foods at the beginning of the feeding (when the infant is most hungry) and with a familiar favorite.

Introduce new foods in plain and simple forms one at a time for a period of 5 to 7 days each to observe for possible allergic reactions that may be exhibited as a rash, fussiness, vomiting, diarrhea, or constipation.

Infants differ in the amount of food they want or need at each feeding; let the baby determine how much food she needs. The amount of solids taken at a feeding may vary from 1 to 2 teaspoons initially to ¼ to ½ cup as the infant gets older.

Respect the infant's likes and dislikes; rejected foods may be reintroduced at a later time.

If there is a positive family history for food allergies, delay introduction of milk, eggs, wheat, and citrus fruits that tend to cause allergic reactions in susceptible infants.

Except for mixed dinners (little meat content) and desserts (highly sweetened), commercially prepared baby food is nutritious and safe for infant use (sodium was removed in 1976). Read the label to determine if sugar or fillers have been added.

Homemade baby food can be prepared by blending, mashing, or grinding food to the proper consistency for the infant's stage of development. Do not salt the food, and do not use spicy or high-fat foods. Do not use canned vegetables because their sodium content is high and their water-soluble vitamin content is usually lower than that of fresh or frozen vegetables.

Do not give honey to infants younger than 1 year of age because of the risk of infant botulism.

Avoid peanuts and peanut butter because of the potential for severe allergic reactions.

By 6 to 8 months of age, the infant may be ready for three meals with three planned snacks daily.

When the infant is ready for finger foods, try ripe banana, Cheerios, toast strips, graham or soda crackers, cubes of cheese, noodles, and chunks of peeled apple, pear, or peach.

Avoid foods that are difficult to digest such as bacon, sausage, fatty foods, fried foods, gravy, spicy foods, and whole kernel corn.

iron stores start to become depleted. In infants exclusively fed iron-fortified formula, the food introduced needs to provide iron because it is displacing a source of iron. Iron-fortified infant cereals are recommended until the infant is 12 to 18 months old because the iron in these cereals is absorbed more readily than that in other cereals.

The CDC recommends the consumption of plain meats after 6 months of age to prevent iron deficiency. Although easily chewed red meats such as baby food meat and home-pureed cooked meats are recommended, relatively few infants under the age of 9 months are fed plain meats of any kind. Commercial baby food dinners are more commonly consumed. Chicken and turkey, which provide less heme iron than red meats, are the most popular meats. Other commonly consumed meats are hot dogs, sausages, and cold cuts, all of which are higher in fat and sodium than plain meats and lower in iron and zinc.

Additional infant feeding considerations are as follows:

- Feeding guidance given to parents and caretakers should emphasize the potential impact of early food preferences on long-term eating habits. Because children's diets tend to reflect what the rest of the family eats, getting the family to eat healthier will cause the infant to eat healthier.
- As infants begin eating solid foods, a variety of soft fruits and cooked vegetables should be included on a daily basis with an emphasis on color—dark green, deep yellow vegetables, and red.
- Sweets, desserts, and salty foods should be limited to avoid excessive calorie consumption and to ensure adequate micronutrient intake.
- The American Academy of Pediatrics (AAP) recommends that juices not be introduced into the diets of infants less than 6 months of age. If introduced, only 100% juice should be offered. The AAP guidelines also state that fruit juice consumption should be limited to 4 to 6 ounces/day for children aged 1 to 6 years. Infants can drink the same plain, pure fruit juices as the rest of the family drinks instead of expensive infant juices. Excessive amounts of juice, even if 100% fruit juice, may displace the intake of nutrient-rich food and milk in the diet. Furthermore, some fruit juices are more nutritious that others. For instance, apple juice is widely used although it is inferior to many other

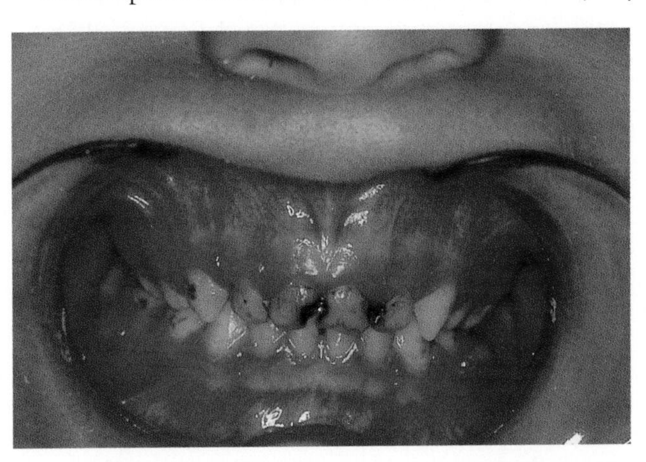

FIGURE 12.2 Nursing bottle caries. Notice the extensive decay in the upper teeth. (© K. L. Boyd, DDS/ Custom Medical Stock Photo.)

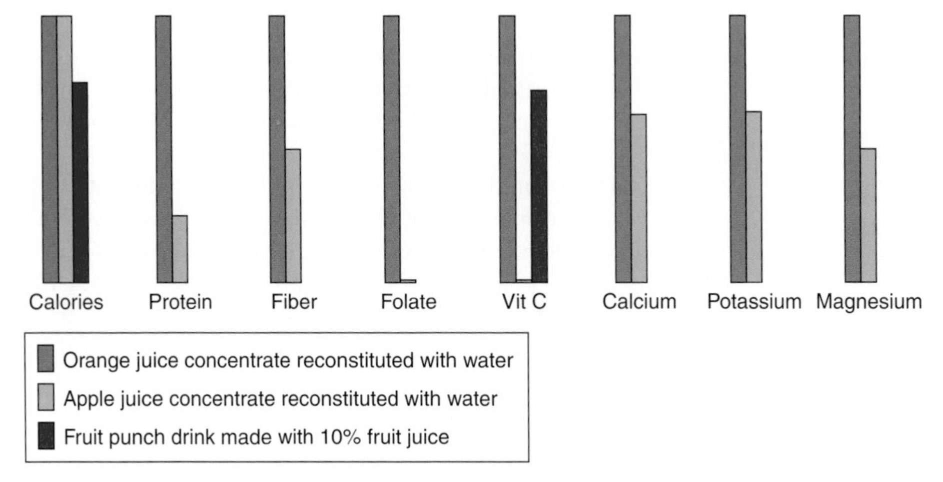

FIGURE 12.3 Nutrient comparison between orange juice, apple juice, and fruit punch drink.

types of fruit juice but is better than fruit drinks (Fig. 12.3). Parents need to understand that fruit drinks are not the equivalent of 100% fruit juice, that the proportion of real juice varies among drink products, and that juices are made with added sugars.

- The introduction of cow's milk should be delayed until the age of 1 year. Cow's milk is a poor source of iron, can cause occult blood loss (possibly from an allergic response to the protein), and provides an unsuitably high potential renal solute load related to its protein, phosphorus, and electrolyte composition. Whole milk should be used until the age of 2 years, because skim and 2% milks do not provide adequate fat or sufficient calories for the amount of protein they contain.

Assessing Adequacy of Intake

Adequacy of growth is the best indicator of whether an infant is receiving sufficient nutrition. However, it should be noted that breast-fed infants usually have a slower growth rate than formula-fed infants. Also infants with impaired growth related to undernutrition or illness experience "catch-up" growth, which usually is completed by 2 years of age. When this occurs, weight gain increases rapidly until the child reaches her normal weight percentile; thereafter, weight and height increase together at a

slower rate. Depending on the timing, severity, nature, and duration of the malnutrition, growth may or may not be permanently affected.

To assess growth percentile for age, height (length) and weight measurements are plotted on the appropriate grids such as on the National Center for Health Statistics growth grids (Appendix). Normally an individual's percentile status for height (length) and weight remains fairly constant throughout childhood. A deviation of more than two percentile channels warrants a more in-depth assessment of growth and nutritional status. An increase in weight percentile may suggest the development of obesity; a decrease may indicate undernutrition, an undiagnosed chronic disease, or the onset of emotional problems.

BETWEEN INFANCY AND CHILDHOOD

The period between age 1 and 2 is a time of transition between infancy and childhood. The dramatic decrease in the growth rate is reflected in a disinterest in food, a "physiologic anorexia" due to lower calorie needs. At age one, the child should be drinking from a cup and eating many of the same foods as the rest of the family although in smaller portions. By the end of the second year, children can completely self-feed and can seek food independently.

Beginning around 15 months of age, food jags may develop as a normal expression of autonomy as the child develops a sense of independence. As long as the diet is adequate but not excessive in water, calories, and all essential nutrients, food jags should not be a cause of concern.

FITS Study: Feeding Infants and Toddlers Study, a dietary intake survey of infants and toddlers 4 to 24 months of age commissioned by Gerber in response to the growing childhood obesity epidemic.

There are no official intake guidelines for this transition period. Data from the FITS study show that American infants and toddlers consume a nutritionally adequate diet with little risk of nutrient deficiencies. One possible exception is of vitamin E, for which the prevalence of apparently inadequate intakes was 58% among toddlers aged 12 to 24 months. However, the rate of low plasma vitamin E levels is very low, indicating that vitamin E intake may be underestimated. Because evidence of biochemical vitamin E deficiency is lacking, there does not appear to be any cause for concern.

Although the risk of nutrient deficiencies appears negligible in American toddlers, there are nutritional concerns:

- Many caregivers may be overfeeding their toddlers based on the new Dietary Reference Intake standard for calories called the estimated energy requirement (EER). According to the FITS data, mean calorie intake exceeded the EER by 10% for infants 4 to 6 months of age, 23% for infants 7 to 12 months of age, and 31% for toddlers 12 to 24 months of age. It is possible that what appears to be an overconsumption of calories is actually an over-reporting of food intake or an underestimation of calorie requirements. However, as the transition from a milk-based diet to table food progresses, the family diet exerts increasing influence; if the family diet is less than ideal, the child's diet will be less than ideal. Because some food preferences seem to be established early life and may predict later eating habits, efforts to cultivate healthy eating habits should begin very early in life.

- Substantial proportions of infants and toddlers consumed no vegetables or fruits as individual food items in a day. In addition, the vegetables most commonly consumed tended to be lower in nutrients and higher in calories (e.g., French fries). Relatively small percentages of children consumed a variety of fruits and vegetables. Studies show that fruit and vegetable variety in the diets of children at 8 years of age is predicted by food-related experiences before the age of 2. Thus efforts should be made to foster the acceptance of a variety of fruits and vegetables in the daily diet.
- Sizable percentages of toddlers consumed high-calorie, high-fat, and salty snacks; and carbonated beverages and sweetened fruit drinks. The FITS study found that approximately 10% of infants 4 to 6 months of age consumed desserts, sweets or sweetened beverages in a day. By age 7 to 8 months, 46% had one or more servings of these foods daily. By age 19 to 24 months, nearly all children consumed one or more of these items in a day. Many of these foods are high in calories and low in nutrients. Considering the increasing prevalence of childhood obesity, the use of these foods should be examined.
- Fiber intake is well below the AI of 19 g/day for 1- to 3-year-olds. However, the AI for adults is set at a level estimated to decrease the risk of chronic disease; this endpoint may not be appropriate for toddlers. A rule of thumb guideline for children age 2 and older is that fiber intake should be ≥ 5 g plus the child's age. With this calculation, a 3-year-old should consume 8 g/day, not the current AI of 19 g.

(*text continues on page 326*)

NURSING INTERVENTIONS AND CONSIDERATIONS FOR DISORDERS UNIQUE TO OR BEGINNING IN INFANCY AND CHILDHOOD

Failure to Thrive

Failure to thrive is generally defined as an inadequate gain in weight and/or height in comparison with growth and development standards. It can be caused by clinical diseases such as central nervous system disorders, endocrine disorders, congenital defects, or intestinal obstructions, or it can occur secondary to an inability to suck, chew, or swallow related to neuromuscular problems. An inadequate calorie intake related to inappropriate formula selection, improper formula dilution, or alterations in digestion or absorption (e.g., lactose intolerance) can lead to failure to thrive. Family problems, such as inadequate nurturing and infant stimulation, may also be implicated.

Nursing Interventions and Considerations

To develop a plan of care, the cause or causes of failure to thrive must first be identified.

Diet interventions depend on the infant's age and stage of development. Usually a high-calorie, high-protein diet is indicated.

NURSING INTERVENTIONS AND CONSIDERATIONS FOR DISORDERS UNIQUE TO OR BEGINNING IN INFANCY AND CHILDHOOD (continued)

Physical, emotional, and intellectual growth may be permanently affected if failure to thrive becomes a chronic problem.

Colic

Colic is characterized by intermittent periods of profuse crying lasting 3 hours or longer per day. It is accompanied by symptoms of irritability, gastrointestinal distention, and abdominal cramping. It most often affects the firstborn child, is more common in formula-fed infants than breast-fed infants, and usually resolves itself by the time the infant is 3 months old. The exact cause of colic is unknown but it may be related to overfeeding, underfeeding, feeding too quickly, swallowed air, or maternal or infant anxiety. Although conclusive evidence is lacking, some studies suggest that cruciferous vegetables (broccoli, cauliflower, brussels sprouts), cow's milk, onion, and chocolate in the diets of women who exclusively breast-feed may be related to colic symptoms in infants.

Nursing Interventions and Considerations

Assess feeding practices: frequency of burping; type of feeding used; volume, concentration, and frequency of feedings; and size of nipple opening (formula-fed infants).

Assess maternal diet for intake of cruciferous vegetables, cow's milk, onion, and chocolate; advise the mother to eliminate these food items and observe for improvement. Women who eliminate cow's milk may need supplemental calcium.

If no feeding problems are identified, reassure the caregivers that colic is transient and does not indicate health problems or parental ineptness.

Cleft Palate

Numerous combinations of developmental defects involving the lip and palate can occur and result in an opening in the roof of the mouth or incompletely formed lips. Feeding difficulties begin at birth. The cause may be hereditary or unknown.

Nursing Interventions and Considerations

Depending on the type of defects, infants with a cleft palate may be unable to suck. A squeezable cleft lip/palate nurser and a crosscut nipple with rigid bottle are effective methods of feeding.

Infants with cleft palates may achieve normal growth when caregivers are educated about feeding techniques, formula volume goals, and use of energy-dense solids.

Advise caregivers

- To feed the infant in an upright position and direct the formula to the side of the mouth to prevent formula from entering the nasal passage.
- To feed the infant slowly and burp the infant frequently. Feeding can be a long and tiring process for both infant and caregivers.
- To follow the normal diet progression and introduction of solids based on the child's development and nutritional needs. Reassure the caregivers that children with a cleft palate can handle solids better than liquids.

(box continues on page 324)

Pyloric Stenosis

Pyloric stenosis is characterized by an obstructive narrowing of the pyloric opening, which results in projectile vomiting within 30 minutes after feeding, weight loss, dehydration, and poor nutritional status. Excessive thickening of the pyloric muscle or hypertrophy and hyperplasia of mucosa and submucosa cause it.

Nursing Interventions and Considerations

The major goal of nutritional therapy is to achieve fluid and electrolyte balance so that the infant can undergo surgery.

After surgery, the infant is given glucose water then advanced to full-strength formula as tolerated, after which the infant can be breast-fed if desired.

Phenylketonuria

PKU is an inborn error of metabolism (autosomal recessive hereditary trait) characterized by a defect in the metabolism of phenylalanine (an essential amino acid) that prevents the conversion of phenylalanine to tyrosine (a nonessential amino acid), which is normally converted to thyroxine, melanin, and catecholamines. Tyrosine becomes an essential amino acid. PKU causes the accumulation of toxic phenylalanine in the tissues, bloodstream, and the central nervous system, resulting in mental retardation and urinary excretion of phenylketones.

Nursing Interventions and Considerations

Because early diagnosis and initiation of the diet can prevent mental retardation, all infants are tested for PKU immediately after birth. Diet cannot reverse brain damage after it occurs.

The diet for PKU is low in phenylalanine but it is not phenylalanine-free. Because phenylalanine is an essential amino acid, it must be supplied in the diet for tissue growth and repair to occur. If the phenylalanine content of the diet is inadequate, the body will catabolize its own protein to supply the missing amino acid; the effect is the same as cheating on the diet, namely an increase in blood and urine phenylalanine levels. Therefore, the phenylalanine content of the diet, as well as the child's blood and urine phenylalanine levels and physical and mental growth and development, must be closely monitored and evaluated. The diet is continuously modified to provide enough phenylalanine to support growth and development without causing a buildup of phenylketones.

The diet must be adequate in protein-sparing calories to prevent the use of protein for energy, which would also result in body protein catabolism. Because protein foods are excluded, it is virtually impossible to provide adequate calories and nutrients without the use of special supplemental formulas. These formulas, either low in phenylalanine or phenylalanine-free, are vital to ensuring nutritional adequacy.

In the past, it was common practice to discontinue the diet when the child enters school (4 to 6 years of age) because brain growth is at least 90% completed. However, children who discontinued the diet performed less well in school, which could be as damaging to overall development as a decrease in IQ. Research has shown that the diet should be followed for life to prevent impairments in attention span, concentration, and memory.

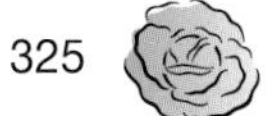

NURSING INTERVENTIONS AND CONSIDERATIONS FOR DISORDERS UNIQUE TO OR BEGINNING IN INFANCY AND CHILDHOOD (continued)

Women with PKU who do not follow the diet before conception and during pregnancy have a high incidence of aborted pregnancies and infants born with mental handicaps (see Chapter 11).

PKU 1, PKU2, and PKU3 (Mead Johnson) are incomplete formulas made from phenylalanine-free amino acids enriched with vitamins and minerals intended for use by infants, children, and adolescents/pregnant women, respectively. They must be supplemented with adequate amounts of fat, carbohydrate, and phenylalanine from other foods or formulas. Phenyl-Free (Mead) is a phenylalanine-free formula that provides protein, vitamins, minerals, and calories.

Once solid foods are added to the infant's diet (at 4 to 6 months of age), caregivers may be given meal patterns and exchange lists of foods grouped according to their phenylalanine content to aid in diet planning.

Comprehensive and frequent diet counseling is necessary to assess the child's intake, monitor progress, and allay caregivers' fears.

Advise caregivers

- That following the diet can effectively prevent mental retardation and other problems of PKU.
- That although other infant formulas or milk may be used to *supplement* phenylalanine-free formulas, they cannot *replace* phenylalanine-free formulas in the infant's diet.
- That the diet is low in phenylalanine, not phenylalanine-free, and must provide adequate calories.
- That phenylalanine is an amino acid and, therefore, is found in greatest concentrations in high-protein foods such as meat, fish, poultry, nuts, dried peas and beans, milk, dairy products, and eggs. These products are eliminated from the diet. Also excluded are breads, pasta, and pastries made from regular flour.
- Foods with low phenylalanine content are vegetables, fruits, fruit juices, and low-protein bread and pasta. Foods that are phenylalanine free are fats, sugars, jellies, and some candies. These foods, along with special phenylalanine-free or reduced phenylalanine formulas, form the diet.
- That label reading is essential; for example, aspartame (NutraSweet) is not appropriate for phenylketonurics because it contains phenylalanine.

Cystic Fibrosis

Cystic fibrosis (CF), inherited as a recessive trait, is a metabolic disease characterized by excessive exocrine secretions (especially mucus) that form plugs. The sites most commonly affected by mucous plugs are the bronchi, which leads to chronic pulmonary infections and fibrosis of the lung tissue; the intestines, which creates problems with nutrient absorption; and the pancreatic and bile ducts, which impairs pancreatic enzyme secretion and results in protein and fat malabsorption (steatorrhea), secondary nutrient deficiencies, malnutrition with possible growth retardation, and glucose intolerance related to impaired insulin secretion. In addition, sweat gland secretions contain excessive amounts of sodium and chloride. Research suggests that nutritional status may be associated with long-term survival and pulmonary function. Nutritional interventions should begin as soon as CF is diagnosed.

(box continues on page 326)

Nursing Interventions and Considerations

Diet recommendations for CF are designed with the goal of promoting normal growth and development. Calorie needs are estimated to be a minimum of 120% RDA for calories with 35 to 40% of total calories from fat. Most children with CF are meeting DRI values for most micronutrients through their diet but are not meeting their calorie needs. Optimal energy is necessary to maximize growth and development.

Fat malabsorption (leading to steatorrhea, malabsorption syndrome, and malnutrition) is the greatest nutritional problem of CF. Clients with CF need to take pancreatic enzyme supplements with all meals and snacks to enhance fat digestion and absorption.

Because protein requirements are greatest during the first year of life, infants are particularly susceptible to protein deficiency and malnutrition. Protein-calorie malnutrition impairs immune function and increases the risk of pulmonary infection.

Anorexia, nausea, and early satiety may occur during periods of decreased pulmonary function and infection and may impair intake.

Clients with CF excrete high concentrations of sodium in their sweat. Addition of table salt to formula or food may be needed to prevent hyponatremia especially in summer months.

Increasing calorie intake and weight seems to improve clinical and respiratory status. Advise caregivers

- That good nutritional status can influence long-term survival and quality of life.
- That a high-protein, high-calorie diet is necessary to replace losses. The Daily Food Guide can be used to plan a varied, balanced diet.
- That although fats are a concentrated source of calories and are needed for their essential fatty acids, tolerance varies. Medium-chain triglycerides (MCTs) are readily absorbed and may be given for additional calories (see Chapter 4).
- That simple sugars are better tolerated than starches.
- To give the child water-soluble supplements of the fat-soluble vitamins and a multivitamin, as prescribed.
- To give the child pancreatic enzyme supplements with all meals and snacks.
- That children with CF need more fluid and sodium than other children do; encourage a liberal intake of both.
- When CF is complicated by diabetes, the diet is adjusted. Nutrition guidelines recommend adequate calories (100% to 200% of RDA), with 30% to 40% of total calories from fat. Simple sugars are not restricted. Carbohydrate counting may be used to achieve glycemic control without limiting calories or sacrificing preferences.

NUTRITION FOR CHILDREN (2 TO 12 YEARS OF AGE)

Growth rate during childhood is much slower than during infancy and adolescence. Before puberty, children generally grow 2 to 3 inches in height annually and gain about 5 pounds. Although there are individual differences, usually a larger child eats more than a smaller one, an active child eats more than a quiet one, and a happy, content child eats more than an anxious one. School-age children maintain a relatively constant intake in relation to their age group; that is, children who are considered big eaters in

second grade are also big eaters in sixth grade. Toward the end of the school-age period, nutrient needs increase in preparation for the adolescent growth spurt. Girls are usually well into puberty by the end of this period.

Calorie and Nutrient Needs

Although total calorie needs steadily rise during childhood, calorie needs *per kilogram of body weight* progressively fall. Generally, a 1 year old needs approximately 1000 calories/day and a 4 year old needs about 1400 cal/day. By age 10, the average child needs about 2000 calories. An individual child's calorie requirements are influenced by growth rate and the amount of physical activity.

For children, the Dietary Reference Intakes are divided into 2 age groups: 1 to 3 year olds and 4 to 8 year olds. Thereafter, age groups are further divided by gender: for males and females, the age groupings through adolescence are 9 to 13 and 14 to 18. Generally, nutrient needs increase with each age grouping and most nutrient requirements reach their adult levels at the 14 to 18 age group. Nutrients that do not fit this pattern are vitamin D, calcium, and iron.

Vitamin D

From birth through age 50 the Adequate Intake for vitamin D is 5 micrograms/day. This is the amount estimated to prevent rickets in children and osteomalacia in adults. On a pound per pound basis, infants and children need substantially more vitamin D than adults because their bones are growing, not simply maintaining. In the absence of adequate sun exposure, 5 micrograms of vitamin D can be obtained from consuming 2 (8 oz) servings of nonfat or low fat milk or fortified soy milk daily and 2 to 3 servings/week (a total of 12 oz) of fatty fish. Most children rarely eat fatty fish.

With few good natural food sources of vitamin D, decreased sun exposure (related to more video games and less outdoor play and the increased use of sunscreen that blocks vitamin D synthesis on the skin), and the substitution of carbonated beverages for vitamin D fortified milk, rickets is making a resurgence in the United States. Because vitamin D has other roles beyond assisting with calcium metabolism, a subclinical deficiency may increase other health risks. For instance, there is growing evidence that a lack of vitamin D increases the risk of colon, breast, and prostate cancers and may increase the risk of hypertension and heart failure. In addition, type 1 diabetes and multiple sclerosis are more common as the distance from the equator increases, causing many researchers to speculate that a lack of vitamin D may be involved.

Calcium

The highest AI for calcium is 1300 mg/day, which is set for both males and females from the ages 9 to 18, a threshold intake believed necessary to attain peak bone mass (Fig. 12.4). The greater the peak bone mass attained during this period, the less damaging the subsequent loss of bone that occurs naturally after about age 35 in all men and women. Like vitamin D, researchers are discovering that calcium has physiologic roles beyond bone health. For instance, calcium appears to be involved in controlling body weight: studies in both children and adults have found an inverse relationship

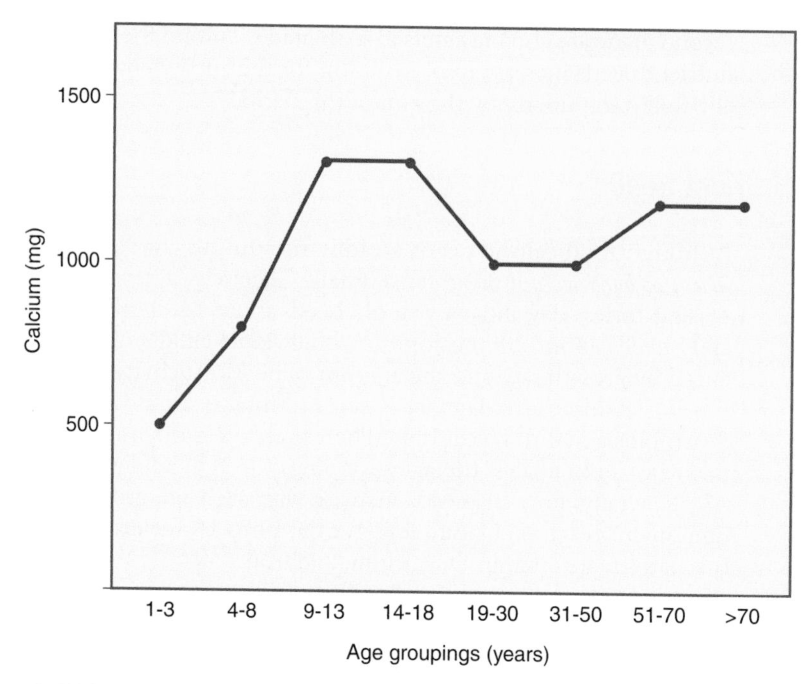

FIGURE 12.4 Adequate intake for calcium for both males and females.

between calcium intake and body fat. An adequate calcium intake may also decrease the risk of hypertension and insulin resistance.

To obtain adequate calcium, two servings of milk are recommended up to age 6 and 3 cups/day from 6 to 12 years of age. To help establish healthy eating practices, milk should be served with every meal. Whole milk is recommended up to the age of 2; thereafter, low-fat or non-fat milk is appropriate.

Iron

The major components of iron need in children and adolescents are the increase in blood volume, increase in hemoglobin concentration, and the increase in tissue iron (e.g., myoglobin and enzymes) related to muscle growth. Menstruating girls have increased iron losses. The peak RDA for males occurs during the 14- to 18-year-old age grouping; for females, peak iron need is between ages 19 and 50 (Fig. 12.5).

In the United States, iron deficiency anemia is the most common nutritional

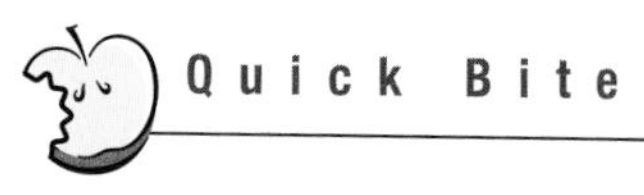

Sources of non-heme iron

Iron-fortified, ready-to-eat cereals
Whole wheat, enriched, or fortified bread
Noodles, rice or barley
Canned plums
Cooked dried apricots
Raisins
Bean dip
Peanut butter

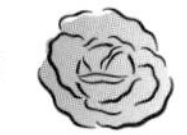

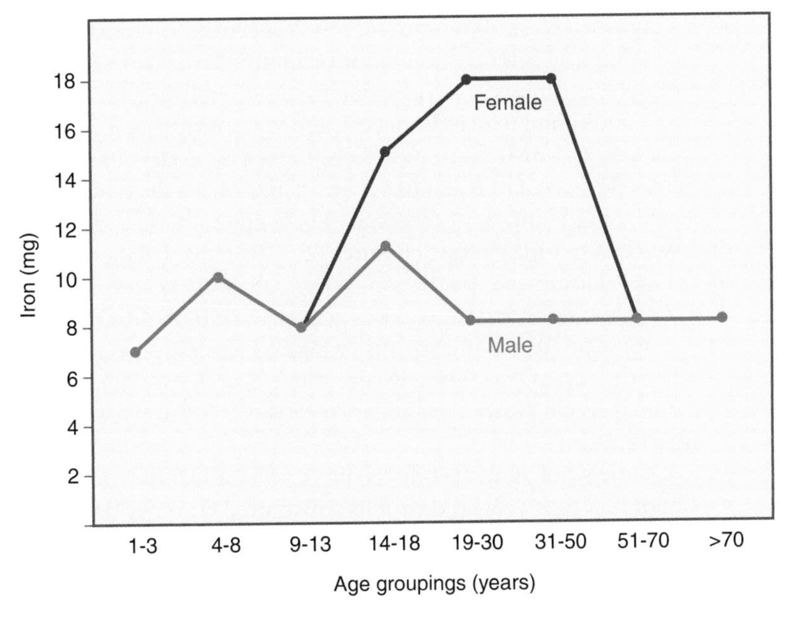

FIGURE 12.5 RDA for iron.

disorder among children and adolescents. Even before the symptoms of anemia (e.g., fatigue) become apparent, inadequate iron can cause intellectual or behavioral symptoms, such as decreased attention span and lowered intellectual performance, which may be mistaken for learning disabilities.

To prevent iron deficiency, milk should be limited to the quantities stated above because milk is a poor source of iron and can displace the intake of iron rich foods. Lean red meats provide readily absorbable heme iron. A rich source of vitamin C (e.g., orange juice, tomatoes) consumed with plant sources of iron help to maximize nonheme iron absorption.

Choosing a Healthy Diet

Dietary Guidelines for Americans provide dietary advice for all people over the age of 2. Studies show that children can follow the Dietary Guidelines without compromising calorie and essential nutrient intake. The 2005 edition of the Guidelines makes specific key recommendations for children and adolescents:

- To maintain body weight in a healthy range, balance calories from foods and beverages with calories expended. Parents should set an example of healthy "thin" eating habits because young children tend to imitate their parents. Subtle changes such as eating baked instead of fried foods; substituting fresh fruits and nutritious desserts for pies, cakes, and cookies; and eliminating traditional empty-calorie snack foods are strategies aimed at preventing excess weight gain.

- Engage in at least 60 minutes of physical activity on most, preferably all, days of the week. Physical activity should not be limited to organized sports but should include a more active lifestyle such as walking the dog, flying a kite, joining the marching band, and riding a bike. Because there is a positive association between television/video use and BMI, limiting television viewing to less than 2 hours daily is prudent. High television and video use is associated with a decrease in physical activity and an increase in the intake of carbonated beverages, fried foods, and snacks.
- Use MyPyramid for Kids (Figure 12.6) to make balanced choices. Although young children can eat the same types of foods as adults, they cannot and should not eat the same serving sizes as adults. A rule-of-thumb guideline to determine age-appropriate serving sizes is to allow 1 tablespoon of food per year of age (e.g., the serving size for a 3-year-old is 3 tablespoons). By age 4 to 6, recommended serving sizes are similar to those for adults. A sample menu is featured in Box 12.3.
- Consume whole grain products often; at least half the grains should be whole grain.
- Children 2 to 8 years old should consume 2 cups per day of fat-free or low-fat milk or equivalent milk products. That amount increases to 3 cups/day for children aged 9 and older.
- Children aged 2 to 3 should keep total fat intake between 30% and 35% of total calories. Between the ages of 4 and 18, fat intake should be between 25% and 33% of total calories, with most fats coming from unsaturated sources such as fish, nuts, and vegetable oils.
- Choose and prepare foods and beverages with little added sugars or caloric sweeteners.
- Choose and prepare foods with less salt.

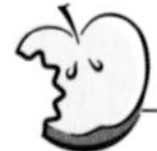

Quick Bite

Foods that are most often the cause of choking

Hot dogs
Candy
Nuts
Grapes
Raw carrots
Tough meat
Watermelon with seeds
Celery
Popcorn
Peanut butter

Up until the age of 4, young children are at risk of choking. To decrease the risk of choking, avoid foods that are difficult to chew and swallow; supervise meals and snacks; prepare foods in forms that are easy to chew and swallow (e.g., cut grapes into small pieces and spread peanut butter thinly); and do not allow the infant to eat or drink from a cup while lying down, playing, or strapped in a car seat.

Establishing Healthy Eating Habits

Childhood eating patterns can have long-term health effects. In other words, food served at home in the early years sets a pattern for the rest of the child's life. For instance, preschoolers whose households have an abundance of fruits and vegetables tend

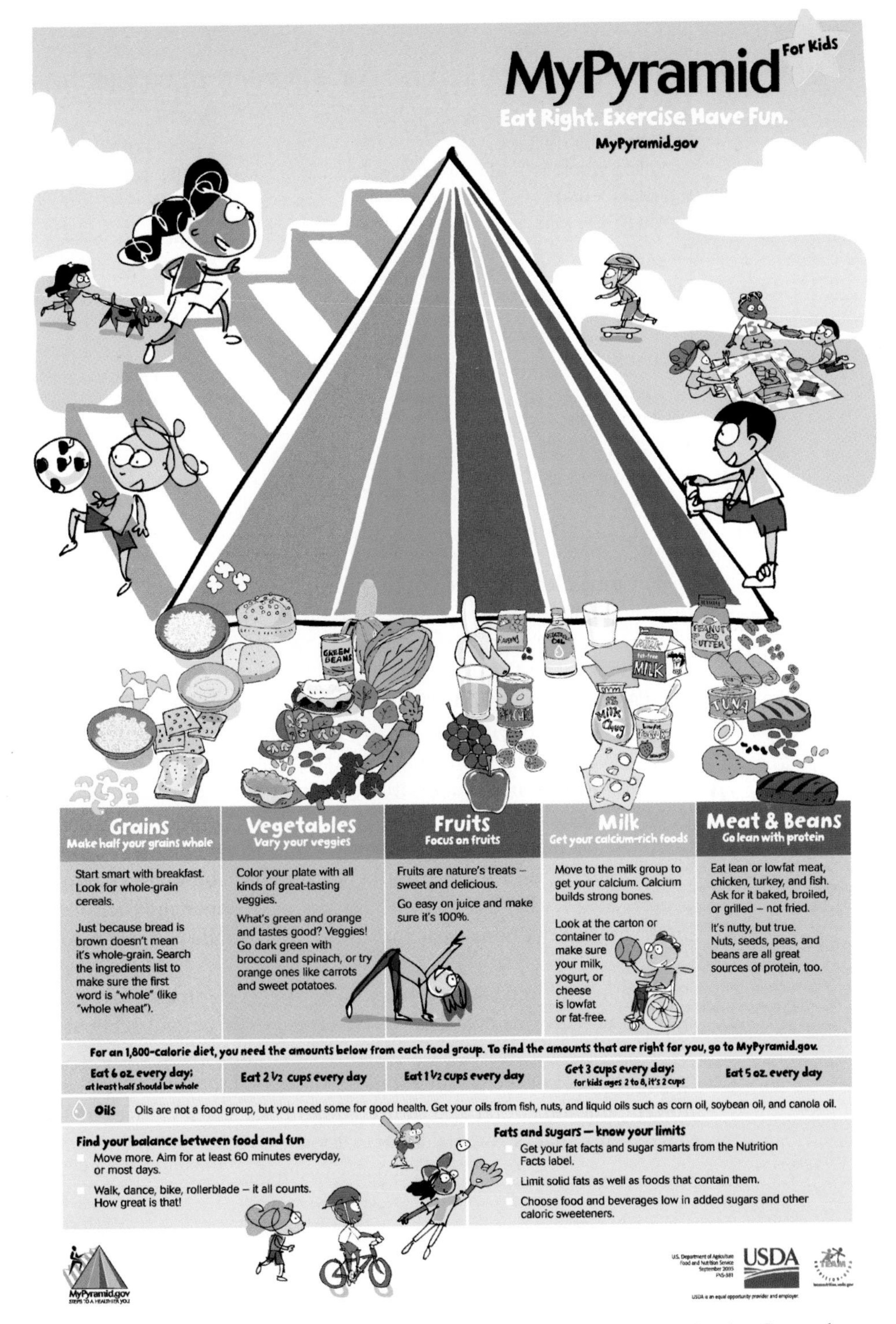

FIGURE 12.6 MyPyramid for Kids. (USDA, Food and Nutrition Service, September 2005. FNS-381.)

BOX 12.3 **SAMPLE MEAL PATTERN FOR 4–6-YEAR-OLD CHILDREN**

Breakfast

¾ cup orange juice
1 slice whole wheat toast with jelly
1 oz Cheerios
½ cup 1% milk

Snack

2 graham crackers
½ cup 1% milk

Lunch

Cheese taco
Fresh apple
½ cup 1% milk

Snack

5 whole grain crackers
1 Tbsp peanut butter
water

Dinner

2½ oz roast chicken breast
½ cup mashed potatoes
½ cup green beans
1 cup tossed salad with dressing
1 small piece cornbread
½ cup milk

to consume more of these foods during the school years. Likewise, milk consumption during childhood is the strongest predictor of milk intake in older adults. Childhood is seen as a time to establish healthy eating habits before patterns become inflexible and difficult to change.

Parents are the primary gatekeepers and role models of their young children's food intake and habits. Parents can promote healthy eating habits by making healthy foods available and setting a good example in eating and activity habits. To help children develop a sense of appropriate-sized portions and meals, parents should decide *what* young children should eat and the child should decide *how much*. It is better to offer second helpings than to overwhelm the child with too much food. Instead of "clean your plate," the rule should be "try a little bit of everything." Conversely, some experts believe that parents who restrict or overmanage their infant's or child's food intake for fear of obesity may impair the child's ability to self-regulate food intake later in life.

Young children eat an average of five to seven times a day, and 82% of 6 to 11 year olds eat at least one snack daily. Healthy snacks are an excellent way to provide protein, calories, and essential nutrients to children who cannot eat a lot at mealtime (Fig. 12.7). However, depending on the actual foods chosen, snacks can provide significant amounts of fat and saturated fat. Poor snack choices include carbonated beverages, salty snacks, sweets, and fast foods.

Nutrition Concerns

The health status of American children has improved over the last 30 years. For instance, the incidence of iron deficiency anemia has decreased in recent years and

Career Connection

The most frequent nutritional concerns of parents of young children are that their children are not eating enough and that they have limited variety in their food choices. However, feeding problems often occur because parents overestimate the amount of food children need and force them to overeat. Reassure parents that if the child's growth chart shows a consistent and reasonable rate of growth, nutritional intake is probably adequate. Encourage parents to

- Keep in mind that it is not important if a child refuses to eat a particular food (e.g., spinach), so long as the child has a reasonable intake from each major food group.
- Offer a variety of foods. However, it may take 8 to 15 exposures before a child accepts a new food.
- Never force a child to eat; if a healthy child is hungry, he will eat.
- Not use food to reward, punish, bribe, or convey love.
- Keep mealtime relaxed, pleasant, and unhurried, allowing 20 to 30 minutes per meal.
- Eat with the child.
- Avoid common pitfalls. Children may refuse to eat because they are (1) too excited or distracted, (2) seeking attention, (3) expressing independence, (4) too tired, or (5) simply not hungry. In that cause, the child's plate should be removed without comment. If the child wants a snack later, make it nutritious. Space meals further apart and limit snacking so the child will be hungry at mealtime.

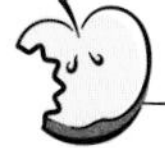

Quick Bite

Healthy snack ideas

Unsweetened cereal with or without milk
Meat or cheese on whole-grain bread or crackers
Graham crackers, fig bars
Whole-grain cookies or muffins made with oatmeal, dried fruit, or iron-fortified cereal
Quick breads such as banana, date, pumpkin
Raw vegetables, vegetable juices
Fresh, dried, or canned fruits without sugar
Pure fruit juice as a drink or frozen on a stick
Low-fat yogurt with or without fresh fruit added
Air-popped popcorn (not before age 3), pretzels
Peanut butter on bread, crackers, celery, apple slices
Milk shakes made with fruit and ice milk or frozen yogurt
Low-fat ice cream, frozen yogurt, ice milk, sherbet, sorbet, fruit ice
Animal crackers, ginger snaps
Skim or 1% milk (after age 2)
Low-fat cheese, low-fat cottage cheese

the average intake of most vitamins and minerals exceeds 100% of the previously used RDAs. Underweight and growth retardation are not the concerns they once were.

Despite improvements in health status, there are critical nutritional concerns facing American children. The Healthy Eating Index indicates that among 2 to 8 year olds, the percentage of children whose diet "needs improvement" ranges from 60% to 80%. The food choices of most children do not meet the food group serving recommendations for fruits, grains, and dairy products. Children's diets typically need more calcium and fiber and less total fat and saturated fat. Also the number of overweight children has more than doubled over the last 30 years. Nutritional concerns discussed below are breakfast skipping, the increased consumption of soft drinks, and overweight.

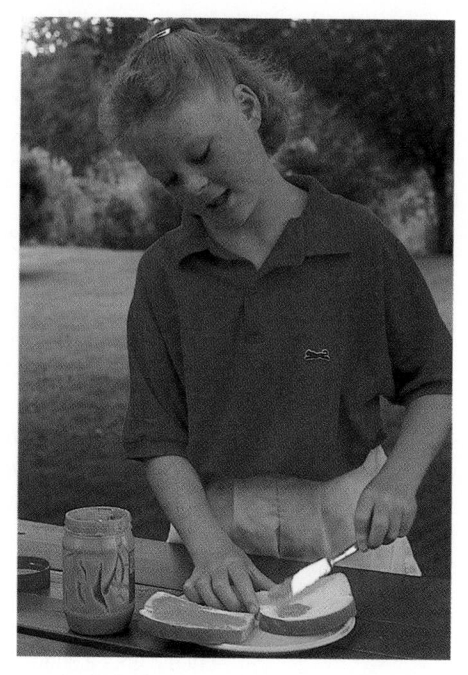

FIGURE 12.7 Good nutritional habits, such as eating healthy snacks, develop early in life. (© Bob Kramer.)

Breakfast Skipping

Approximately 10% of children skip breakfast. Studies suggest that cognition and learning are adversely affected when children skip breakfast. The effect is more striking in children at risk for poor nutritional status than in well-nourished children. Breakfast eating is correlated with improved school attendance; adds significantly to a child's total intake of calories, protein, carbohydrate, and micronutrients; and increases the likelihood of meeting nutritional requirements.

Although virtually any food at breakfast is better than no food at all, studies point to the positive effect ready-to-eat breakfast cereals have on weight status and overall nutrient intake. Children who regularly eat cereal tend to have the most appropriate age-related BMI and are least likely to be at risk of overweight. It is not known if eating breakfast cereals exerts a positive effect on weight management because cereals are 1) simply correlated to a healthful lifestyle (eating breakfast), 2) provide calcium either from fortified cereal and/or milk added to the cereal, or 3) are associated with a lower intake of fat.

Increased Consumption of Soft Drinks

Between the late 1970s and 1994, soft drink consumption increased 41% in the United States. During that same period, milk consumption decreased 24% among boys and 32% among girls 6 to 11 years of age. As soft drink intake increases, milk consumption

 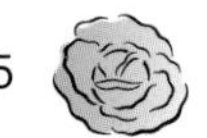

Career Connection

Identifying what motivates kids to eat healthy was the focus of a recent study. While appearance, weight control, immunity, longevity, and future health were all considered moderately important benefits of healthful eating, the most important benefits cited by study participants, in descending order of importance, were as follows:

- Improvements in cognitive function such as improved ability to concentrate, increased mental alertness, and better performance in school.
- Desirable physical sensations such as feeling physically "clean" and "refreshed" and not "clogged up."
- Psychological benefits such as improved self-esteem, reduced guilt and anxiety, and cleared mental function.
- Improvements in physical performance such as improved fitness, better performance in sports, and enhanced strength.
- Enhanced or sustained energy and endurance.

Focusing on these perceived benefits may help wellness educators to motivate children and adolescents to eat healthfully—the rationale for *why* healthful eating is a good idea. The *how to* may be just as important and should include

- Enlisting parental support. Even though adolescence is a period of increasing independence, parents still have a major impact on food intake. The vast majority of children and adolescents eat what is available at home.
- Encouraging family meals. Studies show a strong positive association between the frequency of family meals and the quality of food intake particularly in the intake of fruits, vegetables, grains, and calcium-rich foods. Family meals are negatively associated with the intake of carbonated beverages. Family meals may also contribute to the establishment of "regular" eating patterns and normal psychosocial development.
- Planning to eat healthfully such as taking healthful food to school and not taking money to school to eliminate the temptation to buy junk food.
- Using self-motivating strategies such as reminding oneself about the potential benefits of healthful eating.
- Promoting healthy habits such as eating when hungry, but not too hungry, and eating until full but not stuffed.

and the intake of calcium, folate, vitamin A, and vitamin C tend to decrease. Soft drinks provide empty calories and they contribute to dental caries because sugars are fermentable carbohydrates.

Overweight

In the past several decades, the prevalence of childhood obesity has risen dramatically in the United States. An estimated one in five children is overweight, and 10 million American children are obese. Increases in the rate of childhood obesity are seen in both males and females and across socioeconomic, racial, and ethnic populations. Overweight children are more likely to become obese adults than are children of normal weight.

Although multifactorial in origin, the bottom line is that overweight and obesity result from an imbalance between caloric intake and caloric expenditure. Over the last 25 years, the average calorie intake of American children has increased and portion sizes have grown. On the other side of the energy equation, physical inactivity is seen as a major contributor to weight gain in children.

The social and psychological impacts of obesity are greater on children than on adults. For instance, overweight or obese children tend to have poorer academic performance than normal-weight children of the same intellectual ability. They may be discriminated against in school and later in college and at work. Studies have found that most preschoolers believe a fat child is ugly, stupid, mean, sloppy, lazy, dishonest, forgetful, naughty, sad, lonely, and poor at sports. Both children and adults ranked a chubby child lower on a scale of preference than a child with crutches and a brace, a child in a wheelchair, a child missing the left hand, or a child with a facial disfigurement. Teasing and psychological abuse by peers and adults leads to social isolation, depression, and low self-esteem. Overweight children may actually consume fewer calories than their thin counterparts; because they are social outcasts though, a perpetuating cycle of weight gain, inactivity, and further weight gain makes weight control difficult.

Healthy Lifestyles and Obesity Prevention

Parental support for a more healthful lifestyle is vital to initiating and sustaining changes in eating and exercise behaviors. Parents often recognize that they need to set

Career Connection

Before a child is labeled as obese or overweight, assess

- Age at onset. Fat stores that increase before puberty in preparation for the adolescent growth spurt may cause transient excess body weight and resolve themselves as the child grows taller while maintaining body weight.
- Family history for genetic or endocrine problems that may be the cause of obesity.
- Health status for medical complications. In children, obesity is the major cause of hypertension and increases the risk of cardiovascular disease, diabetes mellitus, joint diseases, and other chronic illnesses.
- Family dynamics. Unresolved crises and conflicts within the family may contribute to eating problems and complicate weight control.
- Body image and attitudes toward body weight. Tolerance toward body weight varies considerably among families and ethnic groups. For instance, African-American women prefer a larger body size. One study found that African-American girls were two times more likely to describe themselves as thinner than other girls their age and seven times more likely to say that they were not overweight. African-American girls were more satisfied with their size than Caucasian girls were.

an example for their children but lack the time to do so. Still other parents who are overweight may feel they cannot set a good example because they do not practice what they preach. Other barriers to parents taking action are (1) many parents believe that children will outgrow their excess weight, (2) a lack of knowledge about how to help children control their weight, and (3) a fear they will cause eating disorders in their children. Studies show that direct involvement of at least one parent improves short- and long-term weight regulation. The key is implementing programs in the home by both parents and children. What parents and children want are

- Positive, realistic approaches to healthful lifestyles. Some parents and children recognize the problem of overweight but do not know what to do about it. Parents need to be positive and encouraging, not negative and critical.
- Ideas for physical games and activities for the whole family.
- Attainable goals to sustain motivation. Ensuring success with small victories helps boost self-esteem and keeps children interested. Goals should be behaviorally based, never linked to weight loss. For instance, a behavior goal may be to eat three vegetables/day for 5 out of 7 days.
- Healthful meal, snack, and recipe suggestions particularly for working moms who are pressed for time.
- Incentive ideas for increasing kids' activity. Fun and variety are critical factors in maintaining children's long-term involvement.
- Referral services for local support groups.

NUTRITION AND ADOLESCENCE (12 TO 18 YEARS OF AGE)

The slow growth of childhood abruptly and dramatically increases with pubescence until the rate is as rapid as that of early infancy. Adolescence is a period of physical, emotional, social, and sexual maturation. Approximately 15 to 20% of adult height and 50% of adult weight are gained during adolescence. Subsequently calorie and nutrient needs increase, but exactly when those increases occur depends on the timing and duration of the growth spurt. Because there are huge variations in the timing of the growth spurt among individuals, chronological age is a poor indicator of physiological maturity and nutritional needs.

Gender differences are obvious. For instance, girls

- Generally begin the growth spurt at 10 to 11 years of age and peak at 12 years. Stature growth ceases at a median age of 17.3 years. Because peak weight occurs before peak height, many girls and parents become concerned about what appears to be excess weight. Weight loss during this period may affect ultimate adult height.
- Experience a disproportionate deposition of fat compared to muscle tissue due to the effects of estrogen. Girls also experience less bone growth than boys do. These differences account for the difference in calorie requirements. An inactive 15-year-old girl may need fewer than 2000 calories/day to avoid weight gain.

In contrast, boys

- Usually begin the growth spurt at about 12 to 13 years of age and peak at 14 years. Stature growth ceases at a median age of 21.2 years. Nutritional needs increase later for boys than for girls.
- Experience a greater increase in muscle mass, lean body tissue, and bones, accounting for their higher calorie requirements than girls. An active 15-year-old boy may need 4000 calories or more per day just to maintain his weight.

Nutrient Needs

Specific experimental data on which to determine the nutrient needs of adolescents is lacking. Because the RDAs are based on chronologic, not physiologic age, they may be invalid for some or many adolescents depending on when the growth spurt begins. Generally, nutrient requirements are higher during adolescence than at any other time in the lifecycle with the exception of pregnancy and lactation. Surveys consistently show that calcium and iron intake among adolescents is marginal.

Calcium

Forty-five percent of the skeletal mass is added during adolescence, making the need for calcium greater during this time than during childhood or early adulthood. For both male and female adolescents, the AI for calcium is 1300 mg, or about three to four glasses of milk or yogurt daily (see Fig. 12.3).

Calcium intake tends to decline among girls from 10 to 17 years of age and surveys show that adolescent girls are at high risk of inadequate calcium intake. On average, adolescent girls consume 720 to 820 mg calcium/day and boys average 800 to 920 mg calcium/day. For both girls and boys, calcium intake has dropped over the last 30 years. The substitution of soft drinks for milk appears to contribute to an inadequate calcium intake among adolescents. In addition, the phosphoric acid in soft drinks works against calcification and may lead to bone resorption.

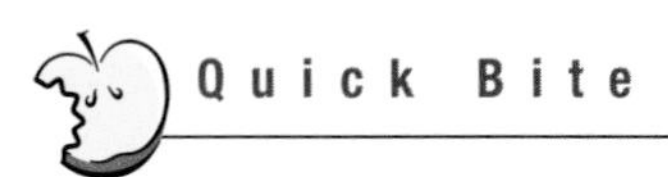

A comparison between soft drink consumption and milk intake among adolescents

	Average soft drink consumption/day	*Average milk intake/day*
Boys	30 oz	12 oz
Girls	21 oz	<8 oz

Iron

Adolescents have increased needs for iron related to an expanding blood volume, the rise in hemoglobin concentration, and the growth of muscle mass. In boys, iron requirement quickly decreases after the growth spurt, allowing for recovery if a deficiency developed during the growth spurt. Adolescent girls tend to develop iron deficiency slowly after pu-

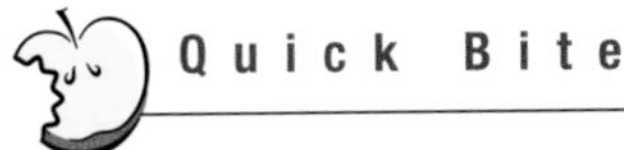

Barriers to healthful eating as identified by children and adolescents

Lack of sense of urgency about personal health
Undesirable taste
Appearance and smell of healthful food
Lack of time
Limited availability of choice
Convenience

berty related to poor eating habits, chronic fad dieting, and menstrual losses. The requirement for iron in girls almost doubles between the 9- to 13-year-old age grouping and the 14 to 18-year-old age grouping (see Fig. 12.4). The requirement for iron remains high until menopause.

Studies indicate iron intakes are between 12.5 and 14.2 mg/day for adolescent girls and 13.6 and 18.0 mg/day for adolescent boys. Iron deficiency is found in approximately 14% of girls aged 14 to 18 and 12% of boys aged 11 to 14. Iron deficiency is prevalent in both genders and in all races and socioeconomic levels.

Nutrition Concerns

Evidence suggests that dietary quality decreases from childhood to adolescence. Specifically, the intake of milk, fruit, and vegetables decreases and soft drink consumption increases with negative effects on calcium and fiber intakes. Sodium intake in 12 to 19 year olds is approximately 4000 to 5000 mg/day for males and 3000 mg/day for females, both significantly higher than the UL for adults of 2300 mg/day. As a group, adolescents have poor eating habits related to their high intake of fast foods and high fat foods and erratic eating behaviors. The prevalence of breakfast skipping increases from childhood to adolescence. Additional concerns discussed below include unhealthful dieting, chronic disease risk, and adolescent pregnancy.

Unhealthful Dieting

Dieting is a common and widespread practice among adolescents, especially adolescent females. In 1999, 59% of high school girls and 26% of males nationwide reported dieting to lose weight in the 30 days prior to the survey. Unhealthy weight loss strategies include fasting for 24 hours or longer, the use of diet pills, self-induced vomiting, and laxative abuse. Counting calories often results in an inadequate intake of nutrients essential for normal growth and development. Adolescents should be counseled on realistic views of desirable weight and on the importance of increasing physical activity and decreasing sedentary pursuits. Parental influence is critical. The nutrition goals to improve eating habits and manage weight are to

- Manage hunger to prevent meal skipping. Balanced meals and regular snacking are encouraged.
- Control portion sizes to control overeating.
- Eat less high-fat food. *Less* is realistic, *eliminating* high-fat foods and fast foods is not. Adolescents eat at a fast-food outlet an average of twice per week. Fast food

use is associated with higher intakes of fried potatoes, hamburger, pizza, and soft drinks and lower intakes of fruits, vegetables, and milk.
- Consume fewer empty calorie soft drinks. Diet soft drinks are safe and provide sweetness without calories. They are a *compromise* to regular soft drinks, not the optimal nutritional alternative.
- Eat more fruits and vegetables. Fruit and vegetable intake is inversely related to the intake of fat. Fruits and vegetables are also a good source of fiber.
- Ensure healthy foods are available at home.

Chronic Disease Risk

National nutrition surveillance data suggest adolescents are at risk for chronic disease based on what they eat. Their low-calcium, high-soft-drink intake may increase the risk for osteoporosis. Their high intakes of saturated fat and sodium and low intakes of fruit, vegetables, and fiber may increase the risk of cardiovascular disease. Cancer risk is influenced by the low intake of fruits, vegetables, and fiber. Alarmingly, the negative health effects of obesity are not confined to the adult population but are appearing in children and adolescents. For instance, the prevalence of type 2 diabetes, once unheard of in young people, is high among overweight adolescents. With the mean age of diagnosis of 13.5 years, the long-term ramifications are great: the longer a person has diabetes, the greater the risk of complications. The dismal success rate of curing obesity underscores the importance of prevention.

Adolescent Pregnancy

Adolescent pregnancy is associated with increased medical, nutritional, social, and economic risks depending on biologic maturity, ethnic background, economic status, prenatal care, and lifestyle (see Chapter 11).

NURSING PROCESS

Amanda is a 24-month-old girl who is regularly brought to the Well Baby Clinic for her checkups and immunizations. At this visit you discover that her height and weight are in the 25th percentile for her age; records indicate that previously she had consistently ranked in the 75th percentile for weight and 50th percentile for height. The change has occurred over the last 6 months. Her mother complains that Amanda is "fussy" and has lost interest in eating.

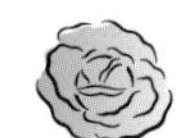

Assessment

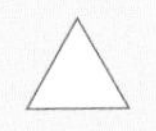

Obtain Clinical Data:

Laboratory values including hemoglobin, hematocrit, serum albumin, and the significance of any other values that are abnormal
Level of development for age
Elimination and reflux patterns, if applicable
Use of medications that can cause side effects such as delayed gastric emptying, diarrhea, constipation, or decreased appetite
Length for age, weight for age, head circumference for age, and weight for length
Food records, if available
Interview the primary caregiver to assess:
Amanda's usual 24-hour intake including portion sizes, frequency and pattern of eating, and texture of foods eaten. Assess caloric and nutritional adequacy of usual intake based on MyPyramid. Assess appropriateness of texture and meal frequency. Are self-feeding skills appropriate for Amanda's age? Is the mealtime environment positive?
Weight history
Pattern of elimination including history of vomiting or reflux
Caregiver's attitude about Amanda's current weight, recent weight loss, and eating behaviors. Are the caregiver's expectations about how much Amanda should eat reasonable and appropriate? What is the problem according to the caregiver?
Caregiver's ability to understand, attitude toward health and nutrition, and readiness to learn
Medical history including prenatal, perinatal, and birth history. Specifically assess for gastrointestinal problems such as slow gastric emptying, constipation, diarrhea, and allergies.
Cultural, religious, and ethnic influences on the family's eating habits
Psychosocial and economic issues such as the living situation, who does the shopping and cooking, adequacy of food budget, need for food assistance, and level of family and social support
Usual activity patterns
Use of prescribed and over-the-counter drugs
Use of vitamins, minerals, and nutritional supplements: what, how much, and why they are given

Nursing Diagnosis

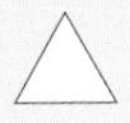

1. Altered Nutrition, Less Than Body Requirements, related to inadequate intake as evidenced by change of two percentile channels in growth charts.

(continued)

Planning and Implementation

Client Goals

The client will

Experience appropriate growth in height and weight
Consume, on average, adequate calories, protein, vitamins, and minerals for her age
Achieve or progress toward age-appropriate feeding skills

Nursing Interventions

Client Teaching

Instruct the caregiver on the role of nutrition in maintaining health and promoting adequate growth and development including
The importance of adequate calories, protein, and other nutrients to support growth
The importance of frequent feedings of nutrient-dense foods to help maximize intake
Eating plan essentials, including the importance of

- Providing adequate calories and protein to meet needs for growth
- Choosing a varied diet to help ensure an average adequate intake
- Providing foods of appropriate texture for age
- Providing three meals plus three or more planned snacks to maximize intake
- Providing liquids after meals, instead of with meals, to avoid displacing food intake

The importance of limiting low-nutrient-density foods (e.g., fruit drinks, carbonated beverages, sweetened cereals) because they displace the intake of more nutritious foods
The need to modify the diet, as appropriate, to improve elimination patterns
The need to address behavioral matters, including the importance of

- Providing a positive mealtime environment (e.g., limiting distractions, having the child well rested before mealtime)
- Not using food to punish, reward, or bribe the child
- Promoting eating behaviors and skills appropriate for this age

The value in keeping accurate food records
How to modify foods to increase their nutrient density such as fortifying milk with skim milk powder; using milk in place of water in recipes; melting cheese on potatoes, rice, or noodles; and so on.

Evaluation

The client

Experiences appropriate growth in height and weight
Consumes, on average, adequate calories, protein, vitamins, and minerals for her age
Achieves or progresses toward age-appropriate feeding skills

How Do You Respond?

What foods are most likely to cause allergies? Ninety percent of food allergy reactions are caused by these eight foods: milk, eggs, soy, peanuts, nuts (cashews, almonds), wheat, fish, and shellfish. Most people who have a food allergy are allergic to only one food.

Does chocolate cause or aggravate acne? There is no scientific evidence to correlate any dietary factors with the appearance or severity of acne. Although vitamin A is important for normal skin integrity, vitamin A supplements are not effective in treating acne and are toxic in large amounts. A compound related to vitamin A (13-*cis*-retinoic acid or Accutane) has been approved for treatment of severe cystic acne but is available only through prescription and must be used with caution.

Do food additives cause attention-deficit disorder or hyperactivity? In the 1970s, the late Dr. Ben Feingold proposed that food additives and salicylates may be responsible for about 25% of cases of hyperactivity with learning disability among school-age children. Numerous studies indicate that the Feingold diet (a diet devoid of artificial colors and flavors; the preservatives beta-hydroxytheophylline [BHT] and butylated hydroxyanisole [BHA]; and salicylate-containing fruits, vegetables, and spices) rarely helps to control hyperactivity. However, the Feingold diet is probably not nutritionally harmful so long as fruits and vegetables containing vitamin C are allowed, and it may have a placebo effect on behavior.

▲ Focus on Critical Thinking

Respond to the following statements:

1. In a growing child, it is better to wait for the child to outgrow obesity than to promote actual weight loss through dieting.
2. To ensure that sweets do not displace healthy foods, dessert should be a reward only after the child "cleans the plate."
3. Which factor is more important for managing weight in children: a healthy eating plan or increased activity?

Key Concepts

- An optimal diet is necessary to support normal growth and development.
- Because of varying rates of growth and activity, nutritional requirements are less precise for children and adolescents than they are for adults.
- Exclusive breast-feeding is the recommended for the first 6 months of life and should continue up to the age of 1 year.
- Iron-fortified infant formula is an acceptable alternative or supplement to breast-feeding.
- Adequacy of growth (height and weight) is the best indicator of whether or not an infant's intake is nutritionally adequate.
- Solid foods should not be introduced before the infant is developmentally ready, usually around 4 to 6 months of age. Iron-fortified infant cereal is usually the first food introduced. New foods should be introduced one at a time for a period of 5 to 7 days so that any allergic reaction can be easily identified.
- Infants and toddlers are at negligible risk of nutrient deficiencies. Nutritional concerns regarding this age group are overfeeding; the inadequate intake of fruits and vegetables; and the intake of high-calorie, high-fat, and salty snacks as well as the intake of soft drinks and sweetened fruit drinks.
- The food groups most likely to be consumed in inadequate amounts by children and adolescents are fruits, vegetables, and dairy products; this inadequacy negatively impacts calcium and fiber intakes.
- The Dietary Guidelines are intended for all healthy Americans over the age of 2. MyPyramid for Kids, crafted from the 2005 Dietary Guidelines for Americans, incorporates the principles of variety, moderation, proportionality, and activity.
- Children who skip breakfast tend to have a lower quality diet, perform less well in school, and are less likely to be within healthy BMI range than children who regularly eat breakfast. Approximately 10% of children skip breakfast.
- The rise in soft drink consumption occurs with a decrease in milk intake. Soft drinks are empty calories that may contribute to a positive calorie balance.
- One in five children is overweight. Children suffer greater social and psychological effects of obesity than adults. Overweight children are more likely to become obese adults than are children of normal weight. Prevention programs should focus on managing hunger, increasing fruits and vegetables, decreasing high fat foods, and increasing activity.
- Childhood nutrition problems often worsen during adolescence. Calcium and iron intakes tend to be marginal. The prevalence of breakfast skipping increases from childhood to adolescence.
- Dieting is common and widespread among adolescents. Girls are more likely to diet than boys. Unhealthy diet practices include fasting, use of diet pills, self-induced vomiting, and laxative abuse. Realistic expectations about weight, dieting, and physical activity should be promoted.
- Adolescents may be at increased risk of chronic disease because of what they eat. Additionally obesity increases the risk of type 2 diabetes among young people, previously a disease of middle age.

- The risks associated with adolescent pregnancy depend on the mother's biologic maturity, ethnic background, prenatal care, and lifestyle.

ANSWER KEY

1. **TRUE** The amount of calories and protein needed per unit of body weight is greater for infants than for adults because growth in the first year of life is more rapid than at any other time in the life cycle (excluding the fetal period).
2. **TRUE** If breast-feeding is discontinued before the infant's first birthday, it should be replaced with iron-fortified infant formula. Cow's milk is not recommended before the age of 1 year.
3. **FALSE** Iron is the nutrient of most concern when solids are introduced into the diet.
4. **TRUE** Overfeeding is a potential problem with early introduction of solid foods because young infants are unable to communicate satiety, the feeling of fullness.
5. **TRUE** The risk of nutrient deficiencies among American toddlers is negligible. However, the risks of overfeeding and eating empty calories are real.
6. **FALSE** The Dietary Guidelines for Americans are intended for all Americans over the age of 2 years.
7. **TRUE** Milk can displace the intake of iron rich foods, increasing the risk of iron deficiency.
8. **TRUE** Adolescents need to drink the equivalent of three to four glasses of milk daily, up from three glasses in children aged 6 to 12 years.
9. **TRUE** An overweight child is more likely to become an obese adult than a child of normal weight.
10. **TRUE** Adolescents consume approximately 2.5 to 3 times more soft drinks than milk.

WEBSITES

American Academy of Pediatrics at **www.aap.org**
Children's Nutrition Research Center at Baylor College of Medicine at **www.bcn.tcm.edu/cnrc**
Food and Nutrition Information Center for information on child care nutrition, WIC, and healthy school meals at **www.nal.usda.gov/fnic**
Kids Food CyberClub at **www.kidsfood.org**
Nutrition Explorations at **www.nutritionexplorations.org**
KidsHealth at **www.kidshealth.org**

REFERENCES

Albertson, A., Anderson H., Crockett, S., & Goebel, M. (2003). Ready-to-eat cereal consumption: Its relationship with BMI and nutrient intake of children aged 4 to 12 years. *Journal of the American Dietetic Association, 103,* 1613–1619.

American Dietetic Association. (2004). Position of the American Dietetic Association: Dietary guidance for healthy children ages 2–11 years. *Journal of the American Dietetic Association, 104,* 660–677.

Borra, S., Kelly, L., Shirreffs, M., et al. (2003). Developing health messages: Qualitative studies with children, parents, and teachers help identify communications opportunities for healthful lifestyles and the prevention of obesity. *Journal of the American Dietetic Association, 103,* 721–728.

Briefel, R., Reidy, K., Karwe, V., & Devaney, B. (2004). Feeding infants and toddlers study: Improvements needed in meeting infant feeding recommendations. *Journal of the American Dietetic Association, 104,* S31–S37.

Briefel, R., Reidy, K., Karwe, V., et al. (2004). Toddlers' transition to table foods: Impact on nutrient intakes and food patterns. *Journal of the American Dietetic Association, 104,* S38–S44.

Carruth, B., Ziegler, P., Gordon, A., & Barr, S. (2004). Prevalence of picky eaters among infants and toddlers and their caregivers' decisions about offering a new food. *Journal of the American Dietetic Association, 104,* S57–S64.

Coulston, A. (2004). A new look at nutrient recommendations: Calcium & vitamin D. *Health Connections 1(2).*

Devaney, B., Ziegler, P., Pac, S., et al. (2004). Nutrient intakes of infants and toddlers. *Journal of the American Dietetic Association, 104,* S14–S21.

Fleischhacker, S., & Achterberg, C. (2003). Ensuring a healthy start is part of Head Start. *Journal of the American Dietetic Association, 103,* 1583–1586.

Fomon, S. (2001). Feeding normal infants: Rationale for recommendations. *Journal of the American Dietetic Association, 101,* 1002–1005.

Fox, M., Pac, S., Devancy, B., & Jankowski, L. (2004). Feeding infants and toddlers study: What foods are infants and toddlers eating? *Journal of the American Dietetic Association, 104,* S22–S30.

Lytle, L. (2002). Nutritional issues for adolescents. *Journal of the American Dietetic Association, 102,* S8–12.

McCaffree, J. (2003). Childhood eating patterns: The roles parents play. *Journal of the American Dietetic Association, 103,* 1587–1588.

Neumark-Sztainer, D., Hannan, P., Story, M., et al. (2003). Family meal patterns: Associations with sociodemographic characteristics and improved dietary intake among adolescents. *Journal of the American Dietetic Association, 103,* 317–322.

O'Dea, J. (2003). Why do kids eat healthful food? Perceived benefits of and carriers to healthful eating and physical activity among children and adolescents. *Journal of the American Dietetic Association, 103,* 497–501.

Ogden, C., Flegal, K., & Johnson, C. (2002). Prevalence and trends in overweight among United States Children and Adolescents, 1999–2000. *Journal of the American Medical Association, 288,* 1728–1732.

Paeratakul, S., Ferdinand, D., Champagne, C., et al. (2003). Fast-food consumption among U.S. adults and children: Dietary and nutrient intake profile. *Journal of the American Dietetic Association, 103,* 1332–1338.

Powers, S., & Patton, S. (2003). A comparison of nutrient intake between infants and toddlers with and without cystic fibrosis. *Journal of the American Dietetic Association, 103,* 1620–1625.

Skinner, J., Ziegler, P., Pac, S., & Devaney, B. (2004). Meal and snack patterns of infants and toddlers. *Journal of the American Dietetic Association, 104,* S65–S70.

Skinner, J., Ziegler, P., & Ponza, M. (2004). Transitions in infants' and toddlers' beverage patterns. *Journal of the American Dietetic Association, 104,* S45–S50.

Spear, B. (2002). Adolescent growth and development. *Journal of the American Dietetic Association, 102,* S23–S29.

United States Department of Agriculture, Food and Nutrition Service. (2005). MyPyramid for Kids. Available at www.mypyramid.gov/kids.

University of Washington, PKU Clinic. (2000). What is the diet for PKU? Available at http://depts.washington.edu/pku/diet.html. Accessed on 3/30/04.

Utter, J., Neumark-Sztainer, D., & Jeffery, R. (2003). Couch potatoes of French fries: Are sedentary behaviors associated with body mass index, physical activity, and dietary behaviors among adolescents? *Journal of the American Dietetic Association, 103,* 1298–1305.

For information on the new dietary guidelines 2005 and MyPyramid, visit
http://connection.lww.com/go/dudek

13

Nutrition for Adults and Older Adults

TRUE	FALSE	
⬭	⬭	**1** Differences in biology account for the longer longevity in women compared to men.
⬭	⬭	**2** In general, calorie needs in older adults decrease while the need for other nutrients stays the same or increases.
⬭	⬭	**3** Older adults should drink at least eight 8-ounce glasses of fluid daily.
⬭	⬭	**4** An all-purpose multivitamin and mineral supplement may be a good idea for older adults.
⬭	⬭	**5** Older adults absorb natural vitamin B_{12} better than synthetic vitamin B_{12} found in supplements and fortified food.
⬭	⬭	**6** The dietary supplement glucosamine sulfate may help to improve symptoms of osteoarthritis.
⬭	⬭	**7** On average, adults consume only about half the recommendation for calcium.
⬭	⬭	**8** Peak calcium retention occurs in older adults.
⬭	⬭	**9** Long-term care residents are more likely to be malnourished than independently living older adults.
⬭	⬭	**10** Obesity is the most common nutritional problem among older adults.

UPON COMPLETION OF THIS CHAPTER, YOU WILL BE ABLE TO

- Identify leading health issues for women.
- List possible reasons why men have shorter longevity than women do.
- Explain how nutritional requirements change with aging.
- Describe how older adults can choose a nutritionally adequate diet without exceeding their calorie needs.
- Name criteria that may indicate nutritional risk among older adults.
- Discuss the advantages of using a liberal diet over restrictive diets in long-term care.
- List strategies for enhancing food intake in long-term care residents.

Genetic and environmental "life advantages"—such as genetic potential for longevity, intelligence, motivation, curiosity, good socialization, religious affiliation, marriage and family, physical activity, avoidance of substance abuse, availability of health care, adequate sleep, sufficient rest and relaxation, and good eating habits—have positive effects on both length and quality of life. Studies suggest that good eating habits established early in life promote health maintenance throughout adulthood. Clearly, the development and progression of certain degenerative disorders associated with aging, such as diabetes mellitus, atherosclerosis, hypertension, and obesity, are influenced by lifelong eating habits.

This chapter discusses differences in adult health issues related to gender. Nutritional implications of aging, the nutritional needs of older adults, and nutrition interventions for selected physiological problems associated with aging are presented. Finally, nutrition in long-term care is addressed.

WOMEN'S HEALTH ISSUES

It has long been recognized that women have more health problems than men do, even though women live approximately 7 years longer than men do on average. Women are more likely than men to develop acute symptoms, chronic health problems, and chronic disabilities. Women members of minority groups are at even greater risk for health problems related to higher rates of poverty, lack of education, and limited or no access to health care. For instance, minority women have shorter life expectancies, higher rates of maternal and infant mortality, higher rates of acquired immunodeficiency syndrome (AIDS), and a higher incidence of chronic disease such as hypertension and diabetes.

The term "women's health issues" refers to the prevention, diagnosis, and management of health concerns that

- Are unique to women such as menstruation, pregnancy, and reproductive diseases
- Are more prevalent in women than in men; for instance, osteoporosis, autoimmune diseases, eating disorders, breast cancer, certain gastrointestinal diseases (e.g., irritable bowel syndrome) and psychiatric conditions (e.g., depression) afflict women disproportionately
- Manifest differently in women than in men such as heart disease and AIDS

Women's health issues have emerged as both political and public health concerns. As food and nutrition providers, women influence not only their own health and well-being but also that of their children. Interventions to help women achieve better health through improved nutrition have the potential to positively affect future generations.

According to data compiled by the National Women's Health Information Center, heart disease and cancer are respectively the first and second leading causes of death among American and Canadian women. Diabetes, stroke, osteoporosis, and obesity are other leading causes of death and disability with nutritional implications. (For more information, visit the National Women's Health Information Center, a project of the office on women's health in the U.S. Department of Health and Human Services, on the World Wide Web, available at http://www.4women.org.) Dietary recommendations to

Career Connection

Prescriptions for hormone replacement therapy have dropped by two thirds since the announcement was made in 2003 that post menopausal use of HRT significantly increases the risk for heart disease and breast cancer. Without HRT, hot flashes are left unchecked—a mild inconvenience for some, a debilitating effect for others. Lifestyle changes and nutrition may provide relief in some cases:

- Eating cold food and drinking cold liquids may help; so may keeping the house cooler than normal.
- Exercise regularly. Exercisers report fewer and less severe hot flashes than nonexercisers.
- Lose excess weight. Excess weight increases the risk of more frequent and more severe hot flashes.
- Quit smoking.
- Try one or two servings/day of soy foods, which may not help but won't hurt. The safety of soy *supplements* is less clear, particularly the long-term risks. Some researchers speculate that high amounts of isoflavones, the active ingredient in soy, may be dangerous for women at risk of breast cancer or who have a personal history of breast cancer.
- Black cohosh. Although recent results of studies using black cohosh have been negative, the North American Menopause Society states that a black cohosh supplement taken for less than 6 months may help mild hot flashes and is likely to do no harm.
- Vitamin E. Evidence is inconclusive but 400 to 800 IU/day may help particularly if used with soy foods. Alone, vitamin E may have little impact.
- Products that are *not recommended* for hot flashes include Dong quai, evening primrose oil, ginseng, licorice, Chinese herb mixtures, acupuncture, and magnet therapy.

reduce the risk of chronic diseases are remarkably similar from disease to disease: Avoid obesity, eat less saturated fat, and eat more fruits, vegetables, and whole grains. Box 13.1 highlights women's health issues.

MEN'S HEALTH ISSUES

Men have shorter life spans than women do, partly because men are greater risk takers. Rates of accidental death and disability are greater among men and such outcomes are associated with both voluntary activities (e.g., driving) and involuntary activities (e.g., serving in combat). Nutritional interventions can do little to change these risks.

In terms of lifestyle, men generally smoke and drink more than women, are less physically active, and do not seek medical care as often as women. Because men tend to define themselves by their work, they may feel more stress and emotionally disconnected in their relationships. Interestingly, men live as long as women among some groups of Mormons, which points to lifestyle, not biology, as the basis for gender

BOX 13.1 **ON WOMEN'S HEALTH**

- Even though heart disease is commonly considered a disease of men, more women die each year from heart disease than do men.
- Heart disease usually appears 10 to 15 years later in women than in men because of the protective effect of estrogen. As estrogen levels decline during menopause, concentrations of total and low-density lipoprotein ("bad") cholesterol rise and those of high-density lipoprotein ("good") cholesterol decline. The increased ratio of "bad" to "good" cholesterol increases the risk of cardiovascular disease. After 50 years of age, women die from heart disease at the same rate as men.
- Myocardial symptoms are different in women than men, which can lead to misdiagnosis of the disease in women.
- Compared with men, women tend to have poorer outcomes of heart disease. For instance, women who recover from a myocardial infarction are more likely to have another MI or stroke than are men.
- Approximately 50% of American women are overweight or obese. Among African American, Native American, and Mexican American, the prevalence is even higher.
- Teenage girls often start to smoke to prevent weight gain.
- 50% of strokes occur in women but women account for 61% of stroke deaths.
- 80% of people with osteoporosis are women.
- 75% of all autoimmune diseases occur in women.
- 60% of arthritis cases occur in women.
- More than twice as many women die from Alzheimer's disease than men, possibly because women live longer and the risk increases with aging.
- Almost twice as many women (12%) as men (6.6%) are affected by a depressive disorder each year.
- 85 to 95% of people with eating disorders are women.
- Women are 5 to 8 times more likely than men to develop a thyroid disorder.

differences in longevity. For instance, Mormons do not use coffee, tea, alcohol, or tobacco, and followers are encouraged to limit meats and consume mostly grains.

As for women, heart disease and cancer are, respectively, the first and second leading causes of death in men. The remaining leading causes of death for all men appear in Box 13.2.

AGING AND OLDER ADULTS

Aging is a gradual, inevitable, complex process of progressive physiologic, cellular, cultural, and psychosocial changes that begin at conception and end at death. As cells age, they undergo degenerative changes in structure and function that eventually lead to impairment of organs, tissues, and body functioning. Exactly how and why aging occurs is unknown, although most theories are based on genetic or environmental causes.

BOX 13.2

THE 10 LEADING CAUSES OF DEATH AMONG ALL AMERICAN MALES, 2001

1. Heart disease
2. Cancer
3. Unintentional injuries
4. Stroke
5. Chronic lower respiratory diseases
6. Diabetes
7. Influenza and pneumonia
8. Suicide
9. Kidney disease
10. Chronic liver disease

CDC, Office of Women's Health (2004). Leading causes of death. Males—United States, 2001. Available at www.cdc.gov/of/spotlight/nmhw/lcod.htm. Accessed on 3/24/04.

Older adults, especially those older than 85 years of age, represent the fastest-growing segment of the American population. By the year 2030, an estimated 71 million Americans (20% of the population) will be over 65, up from 35 million (13% of the population) in 2000. The number of Americans over 85 years of age is expected to increase from 1.6% of the population in 2000 to about 2.5% of the population in 2030. Currently life expectancy is 77 years compared with 47 years in 1900. The increase can be attributed to improved health care, greater use of immunizations, better hygiene, and the development of nutritional practices that promote well-being.

Despite the misconceptions and stereotypes that people have of older adults, they are a heterogeneous group that varies in age, marital status, social background, financial status, living arrangements, and health status. The majority of adults older than 65 years of age suffer from one or more of the following chronic health problems: arthritis, hypertension, heart disease, and diabetes. Yet the majority of older people consider their health to be good to excellent, possibly because people define wellness and illness differently as they age and may accept changes in health as a normal aspect of aging. Certainly differences exist between the "well" and the "frail" elderly, the latter group consisting of those with defined needs for support for activities of daily living. Only 6% of older adults live in nursing care facilities.

Nutritional Implications of Aging

Predictable changes in physiology and function, income, health, and psychosocial well-being are associated with aging, although the rate and timing with which they occur vary among individuals. Changes with a potential impact on diet and nutritional status are as follows:

- Changes in body systems including gastrointestinal, cardiovascular, respiratory, renal, hepatic, musculoskeletal, endocrine, central, and peripheral nervous systems

- Changes in body composition with a decrease in lean body mass and decrease or increase in fat tissue
- Lowered basal metabolic rate
- Changes in fine and gross motor skills
- Change in functional status
- Changes in dental and oral status
- Sensory losses such as hearing loss, loss of visual acuity, decreased sense of smell, and taste alterations
- Social isolation
- Change in economic status

Nutritional Needs of Older Adults

Knowledge of the nutritional needs of older adults is growing. However, health status, physiologic functioning, physical activity, and nutritional status vary more among older adults (especially people older than 70 years of age) than among individuals in any other age group; therefore, recommendations and generalizations about nutritional needs may be less valid for this age group. In general, calorie needs decrease while the need for other nutrients stays the same or increases.

Calories

Calorie needs are generally lower among older adults because basal metabolic rate (BMR) declines as a result of the decrease in lean body mass that occurs with aging. Physical activity also declines with aging, although this too is neither desirable nor inevitable. However, because energy expenditure changes occur at varying times among individuals, chronologic age may not necessarily be a valid predictor of energy requirements. The rule-of-thumb guideline of approximately 25 to 30 cal/kg is a starting point that is adjusted upward or downward based on the individual's need.

Protein

The protein requirement of older adults is controversial. Whereas some studies based on nitrogen balance have shown that older adults require more protein, other studies indicate decreased protein requirements resulting from the reduction in muscle mass and the decrease in renal function that characterize the aging process. Although the newest edition of the RDA for protein for older adults remained at the adult level of .8 g/kg, many nutrition experts believe protein requirement increases to 1.0 to 1.25 g/kg in older adults.

Fluid

Fluid needs of older adults are approximately 30 mL/kg, the same as those of younger adults, with a minimum of 1500 mL/day for adequate urine output. Fluid needs increase with heat, fever, vomiting, diarrhea, and drug-induced fluid losses. Fluid restrictions are used in the treatment of some renal disorders and liver diseases. Most adults can maintain homeostasis over a wide range of intakes.

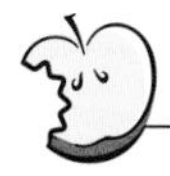

Quick Bite

Estimated needs for an older adult weighing 165 pounds (75 kg) are as follows:

Calories: 1875 to 2250 cal/day

75 kg × 25 cal/kg = 1875 cal   75 kg × 30 cal/kg = 2250 cal

Protein: 60–94 g/day

75 kg × 0.8 g/kg (actual RDA) = 60 g/day

but some researchers say protein need may be as high as . . .

75 × 1.0 g/kg = 75 g/day

75 × 1.25 g/kg = 94 g/day

Fluid: 2250 mL/day

75 kg × 30 mL/kg = 2250 mL/day

Vitamins and Minerals

Most recommended levels of intake for vitamins and minerals do not change with aging. Exceptions to this generalization are calcium, vitamin D, and vitamin B_6, which increase approximately 20%, 300%, and 30%, respectively. These increases are related to changes in nutrient absorption or metabolism. A mineral requirement that decreases with aging is iron but only among women related to the cessation of menstruation. Although the total amount of vitamin B_{12} recommended does not change with aging, people over 50 are advised to consume most of their requirement from fortified food or supplements because absorption of natural vitamin B_{12} may be impaired. Table 13.1 summarizes the nutrient recommendations that change for older adults.

Subclinical: without producing clinical signs and symptoms.

With lower calorie requirements and frequently a drop in appetite, older people are at risk for subclinical nutrient deficiencies. For instance, a below-normal vitamin C status may impair immune system functioning but not be so low as to produce the deficiency disease scurvy. Table 13.2 lists potential benefits from obtaining adequate amounts of various vitamins even in the absence of full-blown deficiency diseases. Nutrients most likely to be consumed in inadequate amounts include the following:

- Calcium. Average adult intake of all ages is approximately one-half the AI.
- Folate. Although estimates vary, 10% or more adults fail to consume adequate amounts of folate.
- Riboflavin. One in three older adults regularly consumes less than two-thirds the recommended amount of riboflavin. Riboflavin is unique among water-soluble vitamins in that milk and dairy products contribute the most riboflavin to the diet.

TABLE 13.1 **NUTRIENT NEEDS THAT CHANGE WITH AGING**

	Age			
	Age 31–50 y	**Age 51–70 y**	**Age >70 y**	**Rationale for Change**
Iron (mg)				
Men	**8**	**8**	**8**	
Women	**18**	**8**	**8**	Cessation of menses
Calcium (mg)				
Men	1000	1200	1200	Efficiency of Ca absorption
Women	1000	1200	1200	decreases with age.
Vitamin D (microgram)				
Men	5	10	15	Ability to synthesize vitamin D from
Women	5	10	15	sunlight decreases with age.
Vitamin B_{12} (micrograms)				
Men	**2.4**	**2.4***	**2.4***	The *amount* of vitamin B_{12} doesn't
Women	**2.4**	**2.4***	**2.4***	change but the recommended *source* does. Because many older adults have impaired absorption of food-bound vitamin B_{12}, it is recommended people over 50 meet their RDA mainly from B_{12} fortified foods or vitamin supplements.
Vitamin B_6 (mg)				
Men	**1.3**	**1.7**	**1.7**	Aging alters vitamin B_6 metabolism
Women	**1.3**	**1.5**	**1.5**	to increase need.

Bold items are Recommended Dietary Allowances (RDA), whereas Adequate Intakes (AI) appear in ordinary type.

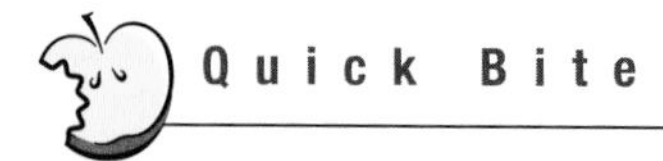

Sources of vitamin B_6 are

Liver
Banana
Salmon
Chicken
Fortified ready-to-eat cereals
Potatoes

- Vitamin B_6. Fifty percent to 90% of older adults fail to consume adequate amounts of vitamin B_6.
- Vitamin D. Older adults average 25% or less of the recommended amount of vitamin D.
- Magnesium. Adults over 70 years old consume 65 to 70% of the recommended intake of magnesium. They also tend to absorb less and excrete more, placing them at risk of magnesium deficiency.

TABLE 13.2 POTENTIAL IMPROVEMENTS IN AGE-RELATED CHANGES FROM OBTAINING ADEQUATE AMOUNTS OF VARIOUS VITAMINS

Potential benefit	From obtaining enough
Improved cognition; better memory and reasoning ability	Folic acid, vitamin B_6, vitamin B_{12}
Decreased levels of homocysteine, which may decrease the risk of heart disease and Alzheimer's disease	Folic acid, vitamin B_6, vitamin B_{12}
Improved muscle strength and decreased risk of falls	Vitamin D
Decreased risk of cataract formation	Vitamin E, beta-carotene, vitamin C
Decreased risk of macular degeneration	Caroteinoids (lutein, zeaxanthin), vitamin E, vitamin C
Decreased risk of osteopenia	Vitamin K

Choosing an Adequate Diet

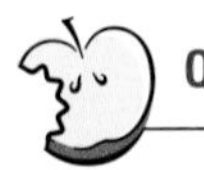

Quick Bite

Sources of vitamin D are

Vitamin D-fortified milk or soy milk
Fatty fish such as salmon, mackerel, and sardines
Some fortified ready-to-eat cereals
Sunshine

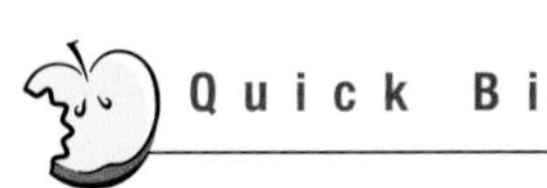

Quick Bite

Sources of magnesium include

Spinach
Yogurt
Brown rice
Almonds
Kidney beans
Banana
Milk
Salmon
Lean beef and pork
Chicken

To obtain adequate amounts of vitamins and minerals in the context of fewer calories, older adults need to concentrate on fruits, vegetables, whole grains, low-fat and nonfat dairy foods, and lean meats while minimizing their intake of foods high in fat and/or sugar. Although actual needs vary according to the individual's activity level and health status, a general guide is as follows:

- **Choose whole grains over refined grains; the amount varies with individual calorie needs.** Whole grains offer more vitamins, minerals, phytochemicals, and fiber than refined grains. Fibers in grains are especially beneficial in preventing constipation, a common problem among older adults.
- **Eat a variety of fruits and vegetables.** Variety is important because each fruit and vegetable provides a unique array

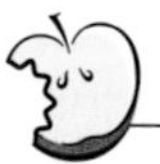

Quick Bite

Fruits and vegetables that are easily consumed by people who have difficulty chewing

Ripe bananas
Baked winter squash
Mashed potatoes
Stewed tomatoes
Baked apples
Canned fruit
Soft melon
Citrus sections
Cooked carrots

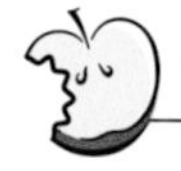

Quick Bite

Sources of calcium

Milk, yogurt, aged cheese
Low-oxalate greens such as bok choy, broccoli, Chinese/Napa cabbage, collards, kale, okra, turnip greens
Calcium-set tofu
Fortified fruit juices
Calcium-fortified foods such as tomato juice and certain ready-to-eat breakfast cereals

of vitamins, minerals, fibers, and phytochemicals in a low-calorie package. Studies show that fruit and vegetable variety is positively associated with the intake of fiber, vitamin C, and vitamin B_6 and inversely associated with the intake of fat. Clients should be encouraged to eat at least one serving daily from each of these categories:

Dark green, leafy vegetables
Yellow or orange fruits and vegetables
Red fruits and vegetables
Dried peas and beans
Citrus fruits

- **Consume at least three servings of low-fat or nonfat milk or yogurt.** Although there are rich nondairy sources of calcium, it is often difficult to meet calcium requirements when the intake of dairy products is limited. People who cannot or will not consume the equivalent of at least three 8-ounce glasses of milk daily need calcium supplements to ensure an adequate intake.
- **Eat two to three servings of lean meat, fish, skinless white meat poultry, dried peas and beans, or nuts daily.** Fish provide health-enhancing n-3 fatty acids; dried peas and beans are excellent sources of fiber that are virtually fat-free.
- **Use fats, oils, and sweets sparingly.** Heart-healthy fats are canola oil, olive oil, and trans fat free margarines.
- **Drink adequate fluids.** New recommendations on fluid intake eschew the old adage of drinking 8 eight-ounce glasses of fluid daily, even among older adults whose sense of thirst is blunted. A recent study showed that even when less than 64 oz of fluid was consumed, there was no evidence of dehydration, even among adults aged 70 and older. In fact, adults aged 70 to 79 who drank eight glasses of water or more per day showed signs of over-hydration, possibly due to diminished ability to handle water. Another consideration is that solid food supplies varying amounts of water; depending on food selections, it is possible to obtain adequate fluid even when beverage intake is low. For *healthy* adults, the newer guideline is to let normal drinking and eating habits guide fluid intake.

 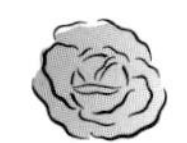

- **Individualize sodium intake.** Younger adults are advised to reduce their intake of sodium because excessive sodium increases the risk of developing hypertension. While older adults who are treated for hypertension can maximize the effectiveness of their treatment by following a low-sodium diet, restricting sodium may compromise calorie intake, an undesirable effect in someone with a marginal calorie intake. Lowering sodium intake is particularly problematic in older adults who live alone and rely on convenience foods. Individual considerations should determine sodium allowance.

Vitamin and Mineral Supplements

In theory, older adults should be able to obtain adequate amounts of all essential nutrients through well-chosen foods. In practice, between 50 to 90% of older adults have diets lacking one or more nutrients. Although a wide variety of foods is considered the best way to obtain adequate amounts of essential nutrients, a low-dose multivitamin and mineral supplement is useful for meeting recommended nutrient levels when intake is less than ideal. A study among relatively healthy older adults living in the community found that multivitamin supplementation improved lymphocyte function and reduced the incidence of infection. Certainly a multivitamin and mineral supplement that provides 100% of the DV has the potential to enhance health and well-being with little risk and for nominal cost. Depending on calcium intake from food, additional calcium supplements may also be needed.

Older Adults at Risk

Older adults at greatest risk of consuming an inadequate diet are those who are less educated, live alone, and have low incomes. Frequently, food choices of older adults are based on considerations other than food preferences such as income; the client's physical ability to shop, prepare, chew, and swallow food; and the occurrence of food intolerances related to chronic disease or side effects of medications.

Identifying nutritional problems in older adults can be a challenge. Traditional assessment findings may be unreliable or invalid in older adults due to changes related to aging. For instance, accurate weights are difficult to obtain in clients who are bedridden, and curvature of the spine interferes with accurate measurement of height. Likewise, age-related changes in physiology and function may mimic signs of a nutritional deficiency. For instance, loss of visual acuity in dim light occurs with aging and may not indicate a deficiency of vitamin A. Historical data are difficult to obtain from clients who have hearing loss or cognitive impairments. Box 13.3 lists screening criteria that may indicate nutritional risk.

Nutrition for Health Issues in Older Adults

Rather than using a textbook approach, nutrition therapy for older adults should be client-centered and based on the individual's physiologic, pathologic, and psychosocial

BOX 13.3

SCREENING CRITERIA THAT MAY INDICATE NUTRITIONAL RISK IN OLDER ADULTS

- The presence of illness or chronic disease, including depression or dementia, that may alter nutrient needs or intake.
- An excessive or inadequate intake of limited variety with missing food groups or compromised by alcohol.
- Dental problems such as missing or decayed teeth or ill-fitting dentures. Loss of teeth impairs chewing, leading to avoidance of foods that are difficult to chew such as fruits, vegetables, and whole grains. Studies show that people with self-perceived ill-fitting dentures also tend to eat fewer fruits and vegetables and have less variety in their diet.
- Low economic status, which can compromise a food budget.
- Social isolation. Older adults living alone are more likely to experience hunger than households with more than one older adult member.
- The use of three or more prescribed or over-the-counter daily medications. Drugs may affect nutritional status by altering appetite; the ability to taste and smell; or the digestion, absorption, metabolism, and excretion of nutrients. Also if a large percentage of a fixed income is spent on medications, less money is available to purchase food.
- Significant unintentional weight change. Significant weight loss is defined as 5% or more in 30 days, 10% or more in 180 days.
- Self-care deficits that may complicate food purchasing, food preparation, and eating.
- Age over 80 years old. The risk of health problems and frailty increases with increasing age.

conditions. Overall goals of nutrition therapy for older adults are to maintain or restore maximal independent functioning and health and to maintain the client's sense of dignity and quality of life by imposing as few dietary restrictions as possible. Any necessary dietary changes should be incorporated into the client's existing food pattern because attempting to impose a completely new approach to eating could be counterproductive. Special health concerns in older adults with nutritional implications include osteoarthritis, osteoporosis, Alzheimer's disease, obesity, and social isolation.

Osteoarthritis

Osteoarthritis (OA), the most common form of arthritis, is a major cause of pain and disability in older adults. Obesity is a modifiable risk factor for OA; studies show that a modest weight loss of 11 pounds can lower a woman's risk of developing OA of the knee by 50% over the next 10 years. Also, additional studies show that older adults who are overweight or obese experience improvements in knee pain and disability from modest weight loss through diet and exercise. Low intakes and low serum concentrations of vitamin D appear to increase the risk of knee OA

progression. Weight loss, exercise, and adequate intakes of vitamin D may prevent and alleviate OA.

A multitude of unorthodox or unproven dietary remedies are touted to "cure" arthritis, ranging from fasting, amino acid supplements, vitamin megadoses, and raw liver to watercress, garlic, vinegar, and honey. Most are useless, some potentially dangerous. However, clinical studies show that two supplements *do* improve pain, function, and may reduce joint space narrowing of the knee in OA sufferers. They are glucosamine sulfate and chondroitin sulfate. Glucosamine appears safe and has few side effects such as nausea, diarrhea, heartburn, drowsiness, rash, and headache. Despite popular belief, glucosamine has not been shown to elevate blood glucose levels. Chondroitin has blood-thinning effects similar to warfarin, heparin, and aspirin. The recommended daily doses are 1500 mg of glucosamine sulfate in divided doses three times daily and 1200 mg of chondroitin sulfate either in one dose or as 400 mg three times a day. If improvement is not seen within 3 months, the supplements should be discontinued.

Osteoporosis

Peak Bone Mass: the most bone mass a person will ever have.

Throughout life, bone tissue is constantly being destroyed and rebuilt, a process known as remodeling. In the first few decades of life, net gain exceeds net loss as bone mass is accrued. Between 30 and 35 years of age, peak bone mass is attained. Thereafter, more bone is lost than is gained. During the first 5 years or so after onset of menopause, women experience rapid bone loss related to estrogen deficiency. After that, bone loss continues at a slower rate.

Osteoporosis is a disease characterized by a decrease in total bone mass and deterioration of bone tissue which leads to increased bone fragility and risk of fracture. It affects one in five white American women (figures are not available for blacks or Asians) and another one out of two white women are at risk due to low bone density of the hip. As many as 20% of people who experience a hip fracture die from complications, making osteoporosis a serious disease.

Although osteoporosis manifests itself in older adults, the process actually begins much earlier in life. The peak period for calcium retention—and, therefore, the period during which measures to prevent osteoporosis can have their greatest impact—is between 4 and 20 years of age. The greater the peak bone mass, the less damaging the inevitable loss of bone mass. However, at any age, an adequate calcium and vitamin D intake along with regular weight-bearing exercise is important for maximizing bone density. Specific recommendations are to

- Consume adequate calcium. For younger adults, that means 1000 mg/day; for those older than 50, the recommendation increases to 1200 mg. That is the equivalent of approximately three to four servings of nonfat or low-fat milk or yogurt.
- Consume 10 to 25 micrograms of vitamin D. Supplements of vitamin D are essential for people older than 70, especially during the winter months and for those who live in northern climates.
- Engage in weight-bearing exercises most days of the week and strength training exercises two to three times/week. Weight-bearing exercises promote the uptake

of calcium into the bone and strength-training exercises restore or maintain muscle mass to improve strength and mobility.
- Avoid excessive alcohol and all tobacco, both of which can weaken bones.

Alzheimer's Disease

Alzheimer's disease is the most common cause of dementia in Americans 65 years of age and older; it affects an estimated 4 million people. Although researchers do not fully understand what causes Alzheimer's disease, it appears to result from a complex series of events in the brain that occur over time. Disruptions in nerve cell communication, metabolism, and repair eventually cause many nerve cells to stop functioning, lose connections with other nerve cells, and die. Genetic and nongenetic factors (e.g., inflammation of the brain, stroke) have been identified in the etiology of Alzheimer's disease. Like coronary heart disease, dementia is at least partially a vascular problem, but plaques that form with Alzheimer's disease are filled with beta-amyloid, not fat and cholesterol. However, researchers speculate that risk factors for coronary heart disease may also increase the risk of Alzheimer's disease. For instance, elevated homocysteine levels, known to increase the risk of CHD, have recently been identified as a strong risk factor for Alzheimer's disease. New research also suggests that being overweight at age 70 is strongly associated with developing Alzheimer's disease from ages 79 to 88. Also, researchers theorize that large doses of the antioxidant vitamin E may keep free radicals from accumulating and causing damage. Studies are promising but incomplete.

At present, there is no clear evidence that Alzheimer's disease alters nutritional requirements. However, it can have a devastating impact on the nutritional status. Early in the disease, impairments in memory and judgment may make shopping, storing, and cooking food difficult. The client may forget to eat or may forget that he or she has already eaten and consequently eat again. Changes in the sense of smell and in food preferences may also develop. A preference for sweet and salty foods is noted and unusual food choices may occur. Agitation increases energy expenditure and calorie requirements may increase by as much as 1600 cal/day. Weight loss is common. Choking may occur if the client forgets to chew food sufficiently before swallowing or hoards food in the mouth. Eating of nonfood items may occur, and eventually self-feeding ability is lost.

Nutritional interventions that may be appropriate for clients with Alzheimer's disease include the following recommendations:

- Closely supervise mealtime; check food temperatures to prevent accidental mouth burns.
- Serve meals in the same place at the same time each day and keep distractions to a minimum.
- Minimize confusion by providing a nonselected menu based on the patient's likes and dislikes, if known.
- Provide one food at a time; a whole tray of foods may be overwhelming.
- Provide between-meal snacks that are easy to consume such as sandwiches, beverages, and finger foods.

- Modify food consistency as needed, cutting food into small pieces and reminding the client to chew to avoid choking. Physical assistance (e.g., lightly stroking the underside of the chin) may be needed to promote swallowing.
- Monitor weight closely.
- Clients in the latter stage of Alzheimer's disease are not only unable to feed themselves but also no longer know what to do when food is placed in the mouth. When this occurs, a decision regarding the use of other means of nutritional support (i.e., nasogastric or percutaneous endoscopic gastrostomy tube feedings) must be made.

Obesity

Obesity in older adults is a serious nutritional risk and is associated with chronic diseases. In addition, obesity may significantly diminish quality of life by impairing mobility and function. According to the Institute of Medicine, obesity is the most common nutritional disorder in older adults with 27% of females and 24% of men aged 65 to 74 considered obese. Yet the healthiest BMI for older adults is controversial. For instance, a longitudinal cohort study of more than 7000 people revealed that a high BMI (30 to 35 for women and 27 to 30 for men) was associated with minimal risk for mortality in adults over the age of 70. Another study found that the association between high BMI and mortality seen in younger adults was not observed in people aged 65 to 100. However, no benefits have been shown for severe obesity, although a higher BMI may help older adults to withstand the metabolic demands of illness. Complicating the issue is that loss of weight is not synonymous with, nor does it have the same prognostic value as, loss of fat.

Promoting weight loss in obese older adults presents unique challenges. Many older people may not feel a need to make changes at this point in life. Active participation in physical activity may be difficult because of medical problems, financial limitations, or impaired hearing or vision. Diminished sense of taste, living alone, and limited food budget may impede changes in intake. However, small changes in intake and activity can produce significant benefits in terms of function, health, and quality of life, even if weight loss is only modest.

A nutrient-dense diet with adequate protein and fiber is recommended to promote weight loss in older adults. A nonstructured approach that simply limits sweets, desserts, and "extras" promotes greater compliance than a rigid plan and so may yield better overall results. Increasing activity is encouraged. Appetite suppressants and herbal remedies are not recommended.

Social Isolation

Eating alone is a risk factor for poor nutritional status among older adults; therefore, efforts should be made to eat with friends and relatives whenever possible. Other potential options are the federally funded nutrition programs, congregate meals, and Meals on Wheels. These programs are designed to provide low-cost, nutritious hot meals; education about food and nutrition; opportunities for socialization and recreation; and information on other health and social assistance programs. The congregate meal program provides a hot, balanced, midday meal and the opportunity to socialize in senior citizen centers and other public or private facilities. Those who choose to pay may do so; otherwise, the meal is free. Meals on Wheels is a home-delivered meal program for elderly persons who are unable to get to congregate meal centers because they live in an isolated area or have a chronic illness or disability. Usually a hot meal is served at midday and a bagged lunch is included to be used as the evening meal. Modified diets, such as diabetic diets and low-sodium diets, are provided as needed.

Long-Term Care

The typical resident of a long-term care facility has numerous psychosocial, functional, and medical problems that often are complicated by poor nutritional status. An estimated 35% to 85% of long-term care residents suffer from malnutrition or dehydration that sometimes existed prior to admission or may have developed after admission. Both malnutrition and dehydration are associated with higher prevalence of pressure sores, delayed wound healing, increased rates of infection, hospitalization, and mortality.

Nutritional interventions aimed at maintaining quality of life by preventing overt malnutrition are economically, medically, and ethically desirable. Specifically quality of life issues include *preventing* unintentional weight loss and pressure ulcers via the provision of adequate calories and protein. Small, frequent feedings may help to maximize intake. A low serum albumin concentration is associated with both unintentional weight loss and pressure ulcers and should be monitored.

For the *treatment* of pressure ulcers, a high-calorie (30 to 35 cal/kg), high-protein (1.2 to 1.5 g/kg or more) diet with adequate fluid (25 to 30 mL/kg) is recommended. Supplemental vitamin C and zinc may be indicated to promote healing. Frequent and accurate monitoring of the resident's intake, weight, and hydration status is vital.

Commercial supplements are often given between meals to increase the calorie and protein contents of a resident's diet. Although they may be temporarily useful, these supplements are generally not well accepted or tolerated on a long-term basis. Taste fatigue and lack of hunger for the meal that follows often occur. Use of supplements as a *substitute* for food deprives residents of the enjoyment of eating foods of their choice. The potential benefits must be weighed against the potential negative consequences. Another option is to increase the nutrient density of foods served with commercial modules or added ingredients: the nutritional value increases while the volume of food served remains the same.

To promote optimal intake in an institutional setting, the nurse should make mealtime as enjoyable an experience as possible. Encourage independence in eating, and supervise dining areas so that proper feeding techniques are used when residents are assisted or fed by certified nursing assistants. Food preferences should be honored whenever possible. Family involvement increases residents' intake. Encourage adequate fluid intake. Although protein and calories are frequently the focus of intervention

Career Connection

Unrecognized anorexia can lead to weight loss and depletion of essential nutrients, which increases the risk of illness and infection. If an infection does develop, metabolic rate increases and so does the demand for calories and nutrients. Undernutrition is exacerbated and a downward spiral ensues.

Timely identification of inadequate food intake should lead to prompt nutrition action that may prevent the decline in nutritional status. In theory, food intake records can identify residents at risk (e.g., eating <75% of food at most meals) and evaluate the nutritional interventions. In fact, the Minimum Data Set requires food intake be assessed. Usually nursing assistants assess food items on a meal tray as a whole and assign a value to the amount eaten, such as 0%, 25%, 50%, or 100%. In practice, this system is fraught with many shortcomings such as

- Food intake records may be neglected because of time constraints or personnel shortages.
- Lack of skill in accurately judging percentage of food consumed. Without adequate training, the reliability of a judgment cannot be guaranteed. One study showed that only 44% of intake records were accurate and that intake estimates failed to identify almost 40% of residents who consume less than 75% of their meals.
- A practical approach to convert individual item estimates into meaningful estimates of overall meal intake has yet to be determined. For instance, 50% may mean the resident ate half of everything served *or* ate all of half the items served (e.g., all the fruit punch, diced peaches, and green beans) and none of the other half (e.g., chicken rice casserole, milk, and whole grain muffin). In terms of estimating calories and nutrients consumed, there are significant differences between these two scenarios.

Although the system is far from perfect, it has the potential to yield accurate estimations of individual food and fluid intake when staff is adequately trained and the importance of monitoring intake is understood by the whole health care team. One study found that adequate training and the use of diagrams depicting representations of meal items on the actual intake record improved accuracy to 85%.

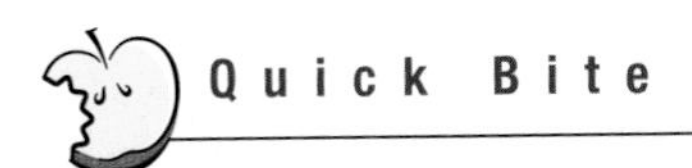

Quick Bite

Examples of foods made more nutrient/calorie dense

Mashed potatoes made with a glucose module
Milk fortified with nonfat dry milk powder
Oatmeal made with added butter, nonfat dry milk, and sugar
Coffee with a commercial supplement similar to cream that adds calories and protein
Scrambled eggs with added cheese
Fruit juice with a glucose module added

Career Connection

Significant weight change is defined as 5% or more in 30 days or 10% or more in 180 days. Most often, significant unintentional *weight gain* reflects fluid accumulation, not weight per se, and although it may indicate a serious health threat, eating too many calories is not to blame. Conversely, significant unintentional *weight loss* is much more common, and even if nutrition is not the cause, it is certainly part of the solution. Because weight loss is one of the most important and sensitive indicators of malnutrition, accurate monthly weighing is vital. More frequent weighings may be necessary if a nutritional problem is suspected.

- Weights should be measured at approximately the same time of day, using the same scale, and after the resident has voided. If the resident is weighed in a wheel chair, the chair's weight must be known and subtracted from the total to ensure accuracy.
- Scales must be accurately calibrated.
- A re-weight is recommended for all residents who appear to have a significant weight change.

efforts, supplemental vitamins and minerals are prudent to ensure optimal intake. Additional strategies to promote food intake appear in Box 13.4.

Restrictive Diets

The use of restrictive diets as part of medical care in long-term care facilities is controversial. Although carbohydrate- or calorie-controlled diets may be theoretically beneficial for older adults with diabetes or obesity, the goals of preventing malnutrition and maintaining quality of life are of greater priority for most long-term care residents.

BOX 13.4

STRATEGIES TO PROMOTE INTAKE IN LONG-TERM CARE RESIDENTS

Provide neat and comfortable dining environment.
Use simple verbal prompts to eat.
Provide small frequent meals rather than three large meals.
Provide specialized utensils such as a scoop plate, nosey cup, etc.
Place food on placemat directly in front of resident.
Avoid staff interruptions during feeding of residents.
Minimize noise and distractions in the dining room.
Use tactile prompt such as hand-over-hand.
Offer finger foods.

Clusky, M., & Kim, Y. (2001). Use and perceived effectiveness of strategies for enhancing food and nutrient intakes among elderly persons in long-term care. *Journal of the American Dietetic Association, 101*, 111–114.

Restrictive diets have the potential to negatively affect quality of life by eliminating personal choice in meals, dampening appetite, and promoting unintentional weight loss, thereby compromising functional status. Restrictive diets should be used only when a significant improvement in health can be expected as in cases of severe hypertension, ascites, or constipation.

A Liberal Diet Approach

It is the position of the American Dietetic Association that the quality of life and nutritional status of older adults living in long-term care facilities may be enhanced by a liberal diet. Residents in long-term care facilities who receive a liberal diet (Box 13.5) similar to what they were eating at home tend to eat better, have fewer bowel problems, enjoy their meals more, are more alert, and are generally happier than residents receiving restrictive diets. The risks of a restrictive diet (e.g., decreased intake and weight loss) must be weighed against the potential benefits especially when potential benefits may be lacking in older adults. Consider the following:

- Studies on the effects of liberalizing therapeutic diets in older adults with hypertension (e.g., allowing 4 g of sodium per day instead of 2 g) revealed no notable or unacceptable changes in edema, blood pressure, or weight. Likewise congestive heart failure in older adults could be controlled with drug therapy and a mild sodium restriction (4 g) instead of the more restrictive 2 g sodium diet.

BOX 13.5

SAMPLE LIBERAL DIET FOR OLDER ADULTS

Breakfast

Orange juice
Oatmeal
1 soft-cooked egg
1 slice buttered whole wheat toast
Low-fat milk
Coffee/tea
Salt/pepper/sugar*

Lunch

Turkey sandwich made with two slices whole wheat bread, tomato, romaine, and low-fat salad dressing
Vegetable soup
Sliced strawberries over angel food cake
1 cup low-fat milk
Coffee/tea
Salt/pepper/sugar*

Dinner

Roast pork
Oven roasted potatoes
Baked acorn squash
Fresh fruit salad
Ice cream
Coffee/tea
Salt/pepper/sugar*

Snack

1 cup low-fat yogurt

*Packages of salt or sugar may be omitted if a restriction of either is appropriate.

- According to the American Diabetes Association, imposing dietary restrictions on long-term care residents is unwarranted nor does it support the use of "no concentrated sweets" or "no sugar added" diets. It is preferable to achieve glycemic control with medication changes rather than dietary restrictions.
- Epidemiological studies indicate that the importance of hypercholesterolemia as a risk factor for CHD decreases after age 44 and virtually disappears after the age of 65. Thus the validity of a low cholesterol diet in treating long-term care residents is questionable. Malnutrition is a greater threat to the majority of older adults than is hypercholesterolemia. Prudent measures for long-term residents with cardiac disease include using 1% or lower fat milk; substituting trans fat free margarines for regular margarine and butter; providing lean cuts of meat in place of fatty meats.

To meet the needs of individual residents, a holistic approach is advocated that includes the individual's personal goals, overall prognosis, the risk/benefit ratio, and quality of life. For many residents, a liberal diet enhances quality of life, nutrient intake, and resident satisfaction while reducing the risks of malnutrition and weight loss.

NURSING PROCESS

Harold Hausman is a regular participant of the monthly congregational nursing program sponsored at his church. He is an 80-year-old widower who lives alone. You have noticed that he has lost weight over the last several months. He has asked you to answer a few questions he has about the low-sodium, low-cholesterol diet his doctor gave him.

Assessment

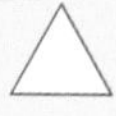

Obtain Clinical Data:

Because a medical record is not available, clinical data are limited to Mr. Hausman's weight, height, and blood pressure. Determine BMI.

Interview the Client to Assess:

Understanding the rationale for the diet the physician gave him and how it can be implemented in his lifestyle

Ability to understand, attitude toward health and nutrition, and readiness to learn

Attitude about his present weight and recent weight loss

Medical history including hyperlipidemia, hypertension, cardiovascular disease, or gastrointestinal complaints. Does he know his cholesterol level?

Dentition and ability to swallow

Manner of implementing the low-sodium, low-cholesterol diet. For instance, did he simply not use the saltshaker at the table or did he begin reading labels for sodium content? What sources of fat did he eliminate from his usual diet?

Usual 24-hour intake including portion size, frequency and pattern of eating, and method of food preparation. Assess appropriateness of usual calorie intake and overall nutritional adequacy based on MyPyramid. Assess the appropriateness of the low-sodium, low-cholesterol diet.

Cultural, religious, and ethnic influences on eating habits

Appetite

Functional disabilities such as impaired ability to shop, cook, and eat. Frequent disabling conditions include arthritis, dementia, heart disease, hip fractures, lung disease, Parkinson's disease, and stroke.

Psychosocial and economic issues such as the client's living situation, who does the shopping and cooking, adequacy of food budget, need for food assistance, and level of family and social support

Usual activity patterns

Use of prescribed and over-the-counter drugs

Use of vitamins, minerals, and nutritional supplements: which ones, how much, and why they are taken

Use of alcohol, tobacco, and caffeine

Nursing Diagnosis

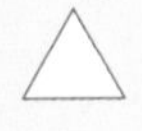

1. Altered Nutrition: Less Than Body Requirements, related to inadequate intake as evidenced by weight loss.

Planning and Implementation

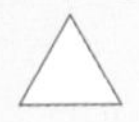

Client Goals

The client will

Attain/maintain a "healthy" weight

Consume, on average, a varied and balanced diet that meets the recommended number of servings from each of the major food groups

Nursing Interventions

Client Teaching

Instruct the client

On the role of nutrition in maintaining health and quality of life, including

- A balanced diet based on the major food groups can help to maximize the quality of life

(continued)

- Avoiding excess salt is prudent for all people; recommendations on sodium intake should be made on an individual basis according to the client's cardiac and renal status, appetite, and use of medications
- Although it is wise to avoid high-fat, nutrient-poor foods such as most cakes, cookies, pastries, pies, chips, full-fat dairy products, and fried foods, observing too severe a fat restriction compromises calorie intake and may result in undesirable weight loss.

On eating plan essentials, including the importance of

- Choosing a varied diet to help ensure an average adequate intake; limiting food choices or skipping a food group increases the risk of both nutrient deficiencies and excesses
- Eating enough food to avoid unfavorable weight loss
- Eating enough high-fiber foods such as whole-grain breads and cereals, dried peas and beans, and fresh fruits and vegetables
- Drinking adequate fluid

On behavioral matters, including

- It is important for the client to discuss the rationale for the low-sodium, low-cholesterol diet with his physician particularly because he has had an unfavorable weight loss
- How to read labels to identify low-sodium foods

On physical activity goals

Evaluation

The client

Attains/maintains "healthy" weight
Consumes on average a varied and balanced diet that meets the recommended number of servings from each of the major food groups

How Do You Respond?

Can gingko biloba help prevent memory loss? Although manufacturers would have you believe gingko can keep your memory intact, no conclusive studies show that it improves memory, thinking, or learning.

Does eating fish lower the risk of Alzheimer's disease? Maybe. An unexpected discovery of the Framingham Heart study was that people with the highest blood levels of DHA, one of the omega-3 fatty acids found in fish, were only about half as likely to develop dementia by the time they were in their 80s as those with the lowest levels of DHA. In terms of fish intake, that means eating three servings of fish per week. Another study found that older adults at particularly

high risk for dementia who ate fish at least once a week lowered their risk of Alzheimer's disease and similar conditions by 60%. Although how fish oils may lower the risk of dementia is not yet known, researchers conclude that eating more fish can't hurt the brain and provides other known health benefits.

▲ Focus on Critical Thinking

Respond to the following statements:

1. Good nutrition throughout life can slow the aging process.
2. It is better for older adults to weigh more than the healthy BMI range than to weigh less.
3. In older adults who have already outlived their life expectancy, there is no convincing argument to persuade them to make healthier food choices.

Key Concepts

- Although women live longer than men do, they have more acute and chronic health problems. Helping women to make healthier food choices has the potential to positively impact the whole family.
- Men have shorter life expectancies than women. This may be related to lifestyle, not simply a matter of biology.
- Aging begins at birth and ends in death. Exactly how and why aging occurs is not known.
- Good eating habits developed early in life promote health in old age.
- As a group, older adults are at risk for nutritional problems because of changes in physiology (including changes in body composition, gastrointestinal tract, metabolism, central nervous system, renal system, and the senses), changes in income, changes in health, and psychosocial changes.
- Older adults represent a heterogeneous population that varies in health, activity, and nutritional status. Generalizations about nutritional requirements are less accurate for this age group than for others.
- Generally, calorie needs decrease but the need for nutrients stays the same or increases with aging. Older adults should choose whole grain bread and cereals, eat a variety of fruits and vegetables, consume the equivalent of three glasses of low-fat or non-fat milk, and choose lean protein foods. Sweets, desserts, and snacks should be limited because they provide calories with few nutrients.
- Calcium, vitamin D, and vitamin B_{12} are the nutrients most likely to be needed through supplements. An all-purpose multivitamin and mineral supplement is prudent but additional calcium supplements may be needed depending on the amount of calcium consumed through food.
- Goals of diet intervention for older adults are to maintain or restore maximal independent functioning and to maintain quality of life. Restrictive diets may not be appropriate for older adults and may actually promote malnutrition except when a significant improvement in health can be expected.

- Long-term care residents are at high risk for malnutrition. Preventive efforts should focus on maintaining an adequate calorie and protein intake. Honor special requests, encourage food from home, and provide assistance with eating as needed.
- Weight loss, low serum albumin, and impaired skin integrity increase the need for calories and protein. Increasing nutrient density without increasing the volume of food served may be the most effective method of delivering additional nutrients. However, between-meal supplements may also be needed to maximize intake.

ANSWER KEY

1. **FALSE** It appears that lifestyle, not biology, is the basis for longevity differences between the genders.
2. **TRUE** In general, calorie needs in older adults decrease due to a decrease in lean body mass and physical activity while the need for other nutrients stays the same or increases.
3. **FALSE** A defined prescription for water intake has not been made by the Institute of Medicine, even for older adults whose thirst mechanism is blunted. Fluid homeostasis is maintained over a wide range of intakes.
4. **TRUE** An all-purpose multivitamin and mineral supplement may be a good idea for older adults because suboptimal intakes over time may negatively impact health even if full blown deficiency diseases do not develop. Older adults in particular may not get adequate calcium, vitamin D, and vitamin B_{12} without supplements.
5. **FALSE** Older adults absorb synthetic vitamin B_{12} found in supplements and fortified food better than natural vitamin B_{12}. Many older adults lack sufficient gastric acid to liberate natural vitamin B_{12} bound to protein in foods whereas synthetic vitamin B_{12} is not bound and so is readily absorbed.
6. **TRUE** Glucosamine sulfate may help to improve pain and function in people with osteoarthritis.
7. **TRUE** On average, adults of any age consume only about half the recommendation for calcium.
8. **FALSE** Peak calcium retention—the period when calcium intake has the greatest impact on bone density—occurs between the ages of 4 and 20.
9. **TRUE** Long-term care residents are more likely to be malnourished than independently living older adults.
10. **TRUE** According to the Institute of Medicine, obesity is the most common nutritional problem among older adults. However, healthy BMI in older adults may differ than that in younger adults.

WEBSITES

Alzheimer's Association at **www.alz.org**
American Association of Retired Persons at **www.aarp.org**
American Geriatrics Society at **www.americangeriatrics.org**
Arthritis Foundation at **www.arthritis.org**
National Institute of Aging Information Office at **www.nih.gov/nia**

REFERENCES

American Dietetic Association. (2002). Position of the American Dietetic Association: Liberalized diets for older adults in long-term care. *Journal of the American Dietetic Association, 102,* 1316–1323.

American Dietetic Association. (2000). Position of the American Dietetic Association: Nutrition, aging, and the continuum of care. *Journal of the American Dietetic Association, 100,* 580–595.

Andrews, Y., & Castellanos, V. (2003). Development of a method for estimation of food and fluid intakes by nursing assistants in long-term care facilities: A pilot study. *Journal of the American Dietetic Association, 103,* 873–877.

Bernstein, M., Tucker, K., Ryan, N., et al. (2002). Higher dietary variety is associated with better nutritional status in frail elderly people. *Journal of the American Dietetic Association, 102,* 1096–1104.

Centers for Disease Control and Prevention, Office of Women's Health. (2004). *Leading causes of death. Males–United States, 2001.* Available at www.cdc.gov/od/spotlight/nmhw/lcod.htm. Accessed on 3/24/04.

Cluskey, M., & Kim, Y. (2001). Use and perceived effectiveness of strategies for enhancing food and nutrient intakes among elderly persons in long-term care. *Journal of the American Dietetic Association, 101,* 111–114.

Dausch, J. (2003). Aging issues moving mainstream. *Journal of the American Dietetic Association, 103,* 683–684.

Henderson, C. (2004). *Dietary outcomes in osteoarthritis disease management.* Available at www.arthritis.org/research/bulletin/vot52no12.htm. Accessed on 3/24/04.

LeBoeuf, R. (2003). Homocysteine and Alzheimer's disease. *Journal of the American Dietetic Association, 103,* 304–307.

Mayo Foundation for Medical Education and Research. (2003). *Men's top health threats.* Available at www.mayoclinic.com/invoke.cfm?id=MC00013. Accessed on 3/24/04.

National Women's Health Information Center, U.S. Department of Heath and Human Services, Office on Women's Health. *Women's health statistical information.* Available at www.4women.org/media/statistics.htm. Accessed on 2/28/04.

Rosenberg, I. (Ed.) (2004). If not hormone therapy for hot flashes, then what? *Tufts University Health & Nutrition Letter, 22*(1), 8.

Rosenberg, I. (Ed.) (2004). Tufts nutrition: Translating the research for use at your table. *Tufts University Health & Nutrition Letter, 22*(1), (Suppl.).

Rosenberg, I. (Ed.) (2003). Growing older presents new nutrition challenges. *Tufts University Health & Nutrition Letter, 21*(8), 1, 8.

Rosenberg, I. (Ed.) (2003). Medical community far behind in preventing osteoporosis. *Tufts University Health & Nutrition Letter, 21*(8), 3.

Sahyoun, N., Lin, C., & Krall, E. (2003). Nutritional status of the older adult is associated with dentition status. *Journal of the American Dietetic Association, 103,* 61–66.

Sahyoun, N. & Krall, E. (2003). Low dietary quality among older adults with self-perceived ill-fitting dentures. *Journal of the American Dietetic Association, 103,* 1494–1499.

Trumbo, P., Schlicker, S., Yates, A., & Poos, M. (2002). Dietary Reference Intakes for energy, carbohydrate, fiber, fat, fatty acids, cholesterol, protein and amino acids. *Journal of the American Dietetic Association, 102,* 1621–1630.

For information on the new dietary guidelines 2005 and MyPyramid, visit **http://connection.lww.com/go/dudek**

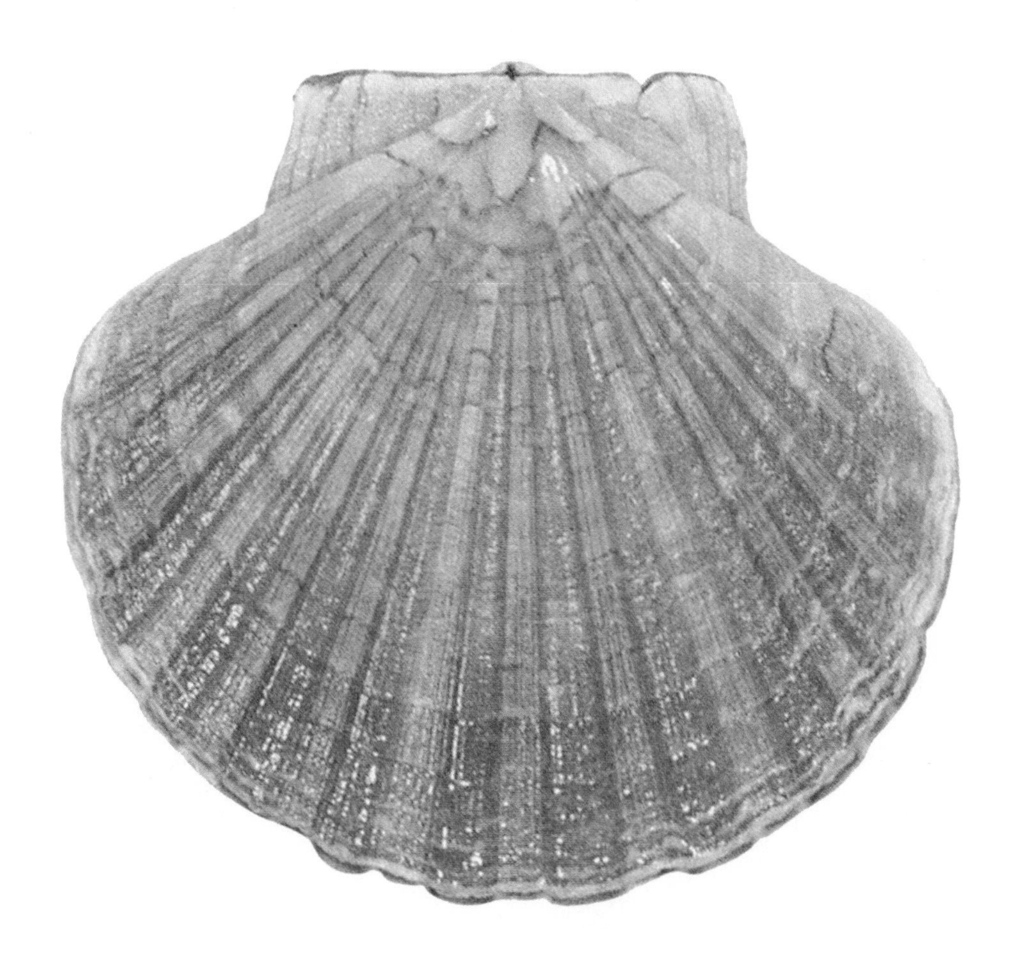

UNIT THREE

Nutrition in Clinical Practice

14

Obesity and Eating Disorders

TRUE	FALSE	
○	○	1 Carbohydrates make people fat.
○	○	2 People shaped like "apples" have greater health risks than people shaped like "pears."
○	○	3 Anyone with a high body mass index (BMI) is at risk for health problems.
○	○	4 Inactivity is a major cause of obesity in Americans.
○	○	5 Obesity-related health problems improve only after BMI is lowered to normal.
○	○	6 If a person will try only one strategy, lowering calories is more effective at promoting short-term weight loss than increasing activity is.
○	○	7 Even if weight loss does not occur, increasing activity helps to lower blood pressure and improves glucose tolerance.
○	○	8 People who eat fewer than 1200 cal may need a multivitamin and mineral supplement.
○	○	9 For weight loss, it is better to cut carbohydrates than to cut fat grams.
○	○	10 Bulimia poses fewer nutritional problems than anorexia does.

UPON COMPLETION OF THIS CHAPTER, YOU WILL BE ABLE TO

- Describe the following standards used to evaluate weight: BMI, waist circumference, and risk status.
- Define overweight and obesity.
- List etiologic factors that may be involved in the development of obesity.
- Discuss the role of each of the following in the treatment of obesity: exercise, behavior therapy, medication, and surgery.
- Explain why drastic calorie-controlled diets are counterproductive to long-term weight management.
- Compare and contrast low-carbohydrate and low-fat weight loss plans.
- List five behavior modification ideas.
- Describe nutritional interventions used in the treatment of eating disorders.

Issues of weight are a pervasive concern in American culture. Recent data indicate that 64.5% of American adults are overweight with 30.9% classified as obese. The proliferation of "diet" foods, "diet" books, and "diet" programs adds up to a business of more than $30 billion annually. From the best sellers list to television talk shows, weight is a hot topic in the United States.

A far less common weight issue is disordered eating manifested as anorexia nervosa or bulimia. Historically the study of obesity and eating disorders has been separate: The former has been rooted in medicine, and the latter has been the focus of psychiatry and psychology. Yet there are commonalities between them such as questions of appetite regulation, concerns with body image, and similar etiologic risk factors.

This chapter explores the concept of "normal" weight and how weight is evaluated. The complications, prevalence, and treatment of obesity are presented. Eating disorders and their nutritional management are described.

WHAT IS "NORMAL" WEIGHT?

How much should a person weigh? From a health perspective, "normal" or "desirable" weight is that which is statistically correlated to good health. However, the relationship between body weight and good health is more complicated than simply the number on the scale. The amount of body *fat* a person has and where a person's weight is distributed also influence health risks. For instance, someone with a well-developed muscle mass who is very lean, as is the case with many athletes, may be technically overweight but not overfat and, therefore, does not at have higher health risks. Also, the presence of certain diseases or conditions (comorbidities) affects overall health risks related to weight. Ideally body mass index (BMI), waist circumference (weight distribution), and overall risk status are all considered when evaluating a client's weight status and identifying who might benefit from treatment.

Body Mass Index

Body Mass Index (BMI): an index of weight in relation to height, calculated mathematically by dividing weight in kilograms by the square of the height in meters.

In the clinical setting, body mass index (BMI) has replaced traditional height and weight tables as the best method of assessing a person's weight. Using pounds and inches, BMI can be determined by using the following equation:

$$\text{BMI} = \frac{\text{weight (lb)}}{\text{height (in) squared}} \times 705$$

Nomograms and tables have been developed to eliminate complicated mathematical calculations (Table 14.1). A BMI of 18.5 and 24.9 is considered a "healthy" or "normal" weight; that is, a weight with low risk of health problems related to weight.

Using BMI to evaluate body weight is inexpensive, nonthreatening, and noninvasive to clients and requires minimal equipment and skill. The major limitation of using BMI

 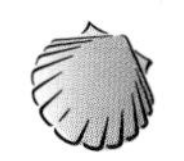

is that it can be elevated for reasons other than excess fat such as large muscle mass or edema. The BMI levels assigned to define overweight and obesity are somewhat arbitrary in that the relationship between increasing weight and risk of disease is continuous.

Waist Circumference

Waist Circumference: waistline measurement in inches.

Central Adiposity: excess fat carried in the abdomen and trunk.

Where excess body fat is deposited may be a more important and reliable indicator of disease risk than the degree of total body fatness. Storing a disproportionate amount of total body fat in the abdomen increases risks for type 2 diabetes, dyslipidemia, hypertension, and cardiovascular disease. Generally, men and postmenopausal women tend to store fat in the upper body, particularly in the abdominal area, whereas premenopausal women tend to store fat in the lower body, particularly in the hips and thighs. Regardless of gender, people with a high distribution of abdominal fat (i.e., "apples") have a greater health risk than people with excess fat in the hips and thighs (i.e., "pears") (Fig. 14.1).

Waist circumference is a common measure to assess abdominal fat. Men with a waist circumference greater than 40 inches and women with a waist circumference greater than 35 inches are at increased risk for health problems associated with central adiposity. However, in people with a BMI of 35 or higher, waist measurement is unnecessary because health risk is already high based on BMI alone. At very high BMIs, waist measurements lose their predictive power.

Evaluating Risk Status

Overweight: a BMI greater than or equal to 25.

The presence of existing health problems impacts a person's absolute risk related to weight. People with established coronary heart disease, other atherosclerotic diseases, type 2 diabetes, and sleep apnea are classified as being at very high risk for disease complications and mortality related to overweight and obesity. Also, a high absolute risk for obesity-related disorders occurs when a person has three or more of the following risk factors: cigarette smoking, hypertension, high concentration of low-density lipoprotein (LDL)-cholesterol, low concentration of high-density lipoprotein (HDL)-cholesterol, impaired fasting glucose, family history of premature heart disease, and age (45 years or older for men, 55 years or older for women). Physical inactivity and high serum triglyceride levels each represents a higher absolute risk above that estimated from the preceding risk factors.

▶ OVERWEIGHT AND OBESITY

Obese: a BMI greater than or equal to 30.

Overweight and obese are terms frequently used interchangeably even though they vary by degree. The terms are not mutually exclusive because obese people are also overweight.

TABLE 14.1

BODY MASS INDEX

	Normal						Overweight					Obese					
BMI	**19**	**20**	**21**	**22**	**23**	**24**	**25**	**26**	**27**	**28**	**29**	**30**	**31**	**32**	**33**	**34**	**35**
Height (inches)	**Body Weight (pounds)**																
58	91	96	100	105	110	115	119	124	129	134	138	143	148	153	158	162	167
59	94	99	104	109	114	119	124	128	133	138	143	148	153	158	163	168	173
60	97	102	107	112	118	123	128	133	138	143	148	153	158	163	168	174	179
61	100	106	111	116	122	127	132	137	143	148	153	158	164	169	174	180	185
62	104	109	115	120	126	131	136	142	147	153	158	164	169	175	180	186	191
63	107	113	118	124	130	135	141	146	152	158	163	169	175	180	186	191	197
64	110	116	122	128	134	140	145	151	157	163	169	174	180	186	192	197	204
65	114	120	126	132	138	144	150	156	162	168	174	180	186	192	198	204	210
66	118	124	130	136	142	148	155	161	167	173	179	186	192	198	204	210	216
67	121	127	134	140	146	153	159	166	172	178	185	191	198	204	211	217	223
68	125	131	138	144	151	158	164	171	177	184	190	197	203	210	216	223	230
69	128	135	142	149	155	162	169	176	182	189	196	203	209	216	223	230	236
70	132	139	146	153	160	167	174	181	188	195	202	209	216	222	229	236	243
71	136	143	150	157	165	172	179	186	193	200	208	215	222	229	236	243	250
72	140	147	154	162	169	177	184	191	199	206	213	221	228	235	242	250	258
73	144	151	159	166	174	182	189	197	204	212	219	227	235	242	250	257	265
74	148	155	163	171	179	186	194	202	210	218	225	233	241	249	256	264	272
75	152	160	168	176	184	192	200	208	216	224	232	240	248	256	264	272	279
76	156	164	172	180	189	197	205	213	221	230	238	246	254	263	271	279	287

Adapted from U.S. Department of Health and Human Services (1998). *Clinical guidelines on the identification, evaluation, and treatment of overweight and obesity in adults: The evidence report.* Rockville, MD: Author.

Etiologic Factors

The basic mechanism of overweight and obesity is an imbalance between calorie intake and calorie expenditure. When more calories are consumed than are burned, a positive calorie balance results, leading to weight gain over time. This positive balance can be caused by overeating, inactivity, or, most often, a combination of both. For instance, 1 pound of body fat equals 3500 cal; therefore, eating 500 extra calories per day for 7 days will produce a 1-pound weight gain. A person will gain 2 pounds in 1 week if

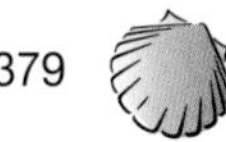

Extreme Obesity																		
36	**37**	**38**	**39**	**40**	**41**	**42**	**43**	**44**	**45**	**46**	**47**	**48**	**49**	**50**	**51**	**52**	**53**	**54**
Body Weight (pounds)																		
172	177	181	186	191	196	201	205	210	215	220	224	229	234	239	244	248	253	258
178	183	188	193	198	203	208	212	217	222	227	232	237	242	247	252	257	262	267
184	189	194	199	204	209	215	220	225	230	235	240	245	250	255	261	266	271	276
190	195	201	206	211	217	222	227	232	238	243	248	254	259	264	269	275	280	285
196	202	207	213	218	224	229	235	240	246	251	256	262	267	273	278	284	289	295
203	208	214	220	225	231	237	242	248	254	259	265	270	278	282	287	293	299	304
209	215	221	227	232	238	244	250	256	262	267	273	279	285	291	296	302	308	314
216	222	228	234	240	246	252	258	264	270	276	282	288	294	300	306	312	318	324
223	229	235	241	247	253	260	266	272	278	284	291	297	303	309	315	322	328	334
230	236	242	249	255	261	268	274	280	287	293	299	306	312	319	325	331	338	344
236	243	249	256	262	269	276	282	289	295	302	308	315	322	328	335	341	348	354
243	250	257	263	270	277	284	291	297	304	311	318	324	331	338	345	351	358	365
250	257	264	271	278	285	292	299	306	313	320	327	334	341	348	355	362	369	376
257	265	272	279	286	293	301	308	315	322	329	338	343	351	358	365	372	379	386
265	272	279	287	294	302	309	316	324	331	338	346	353	361	368	375	383	390	397
272	280	288	295	302	310	318	325	333	340	348	355	363	371	378	386	393	401	408
280	287	295	303	311	319	326	334	342	350	358	365	373	381	389	396	404	412	420
287	295	303	311	319	327	335	343	351	359	367	375	383	391	399	407	415	423	431
295	304	312	320	328	336	344	353	361	369	377	385	394	402	410	418	426	435	443

daily intake exceeds expenditure by 1000 cal/day. Even a seemingly insignificant 1 ounce of cheddar cheese that supplies 100 cal will produce a 10-pound weight gain in a year if consumed daily and not offset by an increase in activity:

$$100 \text{ cal} \times 365 \text{ d/y} = 36{,}500 \text{ excess cal/y}$$

$$36{,}500 \text{ cal/y divided by } 3500 \text{ cal/lb} = \text{slightly over } 10 \text{ lb/y weight gain}$$

Conversely, reducing calories by 500/day will lead to a 1-pound weight loss/week; a 1000 calorie deficit/day results in a 2-pound loss/week.

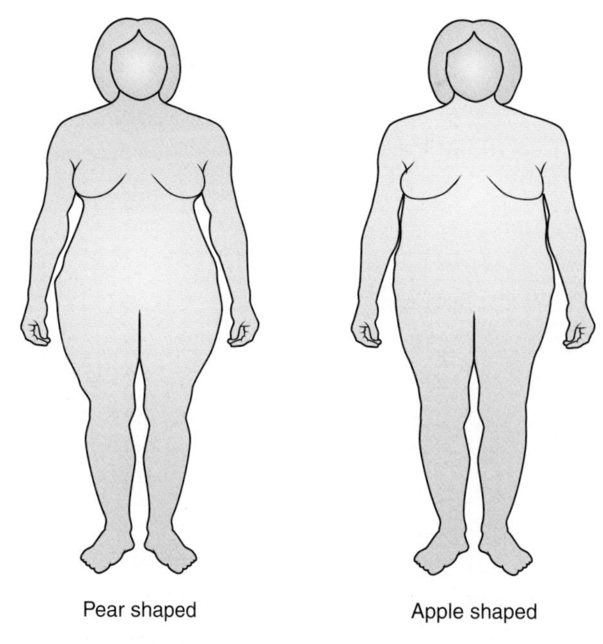

FIGURE 14.1 "Pear" shape versus "apple" shape.

In reality, the relationship between calorie intake and weight status is much more complex. For instance, in some people the body seemingly compensates for variations in calorie intake by adjusting the rate at which it burns calories during inactivity. The "set point" theory of weight control has long proposed that when weight falls below what the body has determined to be "ideal," metabolic rate is adjusted downward to reduce energy expenditure and conserve fat stores. Conversely, when calorie intake increases, some people are able to burn hundreds of extra calories in the activities of daily living to help control weight. These results suggest that the reason some people gain weight from overeating and others do not is related to whether this compensatory increase in nonexercise energy expenditure occurs.

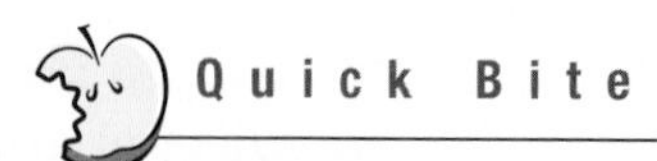

Quick Bite

What 100 calories looks like

12 oz light beer
5 oz white wine
8 oz soft drink
3 Buffalo wings
½ cup sweetened applesauce
1 medium size cookie
½ cup diet chocolate pudding
1 fun size Almond Joy
½ small McDonald's French fries
12 cashews

Although we know *how* obesity occurs, *why* it occurs is not fully understood. It is likely that a combination of factors is involved such as

- **Genetics.** Understanding the role of genetics in weight management is incomplete. Studies on twins and families suggest that genetic factors account for 60 to 80% of the predisposition to obesity. Where excess body fat is stored is also influenced by genetics. In addition, genetic defects have been found to alter levels of leptin. It is not known if manipulating leptin levels can be an effective treatment for obesity.

Leptin: a protein that helps to regulate metabolism and appetite.

- **Nutrition factors.** Excessive food intake contributes to obesity. With the proliferation of fast and convenience foods, food availability and caloric density have increased. Several trends, such as an increasing consumption of soft drinks and snacks; a greater proportion of food expenditures spent on food away from

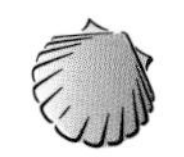

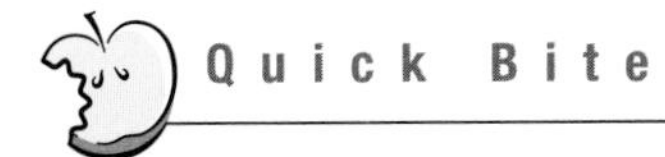

Compare the serving size and calories from food eaten outside the home vs. the official FDA serving size.

	Serving size	*calories*
Large movie theater popcorn	20 cups	1160
FDA official serving	3 cups	160
Typical order of spaghetti with tomato sauce	3½ cups	850
FDA official serving	1 cup	250
Coca-Cola, 7-Eleven double gulp	64 oz	800
FDA official serving	8 oz	100
McDonald's super size French fries	7 oz	610
FDA official serving size	3 oz	220

home; and the growing portion size of restaurant meals, may be at least partially responsible for the increase in obesity among Americans.

- **Level of activity.** Inactivity has been identified as a major cause of obesity among Americans. Only 22% of American adults claim to be regularly active for 30 minutes/day. The proliferation of labor-saving devices and decreased leisure time are among the factors contributing to the overall decline in physical activity. Whether inactivity leads to weight gain or weight gain leads to inactivity, the snowball effect perpetuates obesity, that is, inactivity can lead to increased weight and weight gain can lead to social isolation and further reduction in activity (Fig. 14.2).
- **Psychological status.** Altered mood states and weight status are frequently related. Research shows that depression plays a significant role in patterns of weight change. People who gain weight with one depressive episode are likely to gain weight with subsequent bouts of depression. Also, because serotonin is involved in controlling mood and eating affects serotonin levels, some people learn how to eat to reduce the symptoms of depression.
- **Medication.** Certain medications including antipsychotics, antidepressants, mood stabilizers, steroids, cyproheptadine, and insulin cause weight gain.
- **Sociocultural factors.** Sociocultural factors, such as ethnicity, race, gender, income, and education, are important influences on the prevalence of obesity.

Prevalence of Overweight and Obesity

Thirty-one percent of Americans between the ages of 20 to 74 are obese. This level represents a 100% increase over the prevalence of adult obesity from 1976 to 1980. The rate of obesity has climbed in both men and women, in all age groups, and in all racial and ethnic groups.

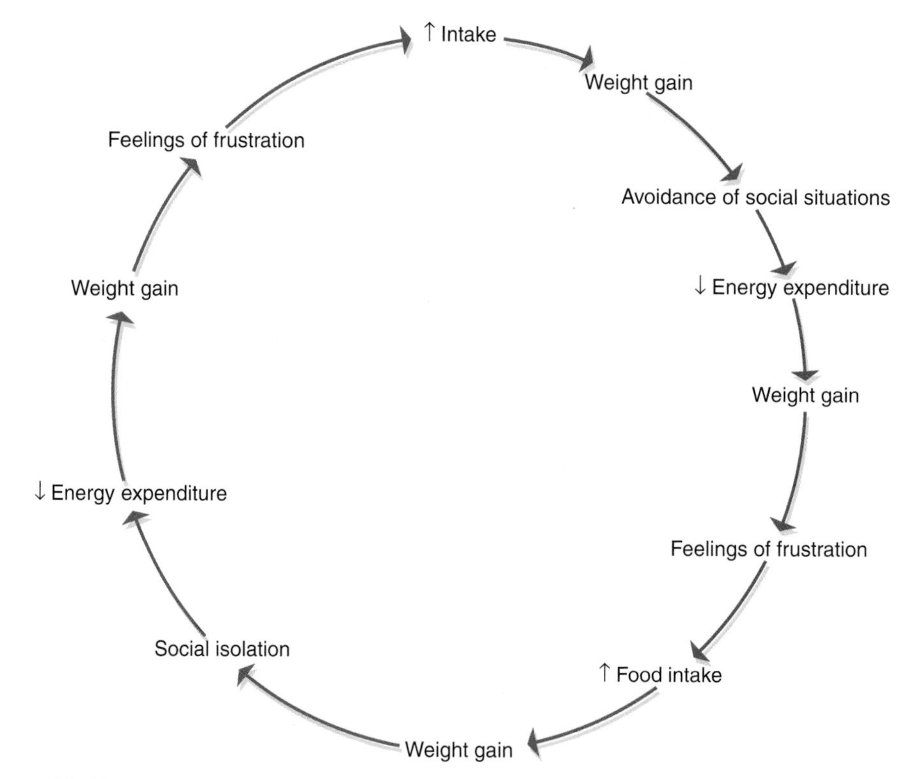

FIGURE 14.2 Perpetuating the cycle of inactivity and weight gain.

A variety of demographic and behavioral factors, such as age, gender, socioeconomic status, race, and ethnic background, influence the rate of obesity in the United States. Obesity is more prevalent among women than men. Generally, lower income and lower education are associated with higher BMI in women. The relationship between socioeconomic status and obesity in men is less consistent. By racial groups, obesity occurs in 23% of white women, 31% of Hispanic women, and 37% of Black women. The prevalence of obesity also rises with parity.

Complications of Obesity

Obesity significantly increases mortality and morbidity. The most common complications of obesity are insulin resistance, type 2 diabetes, hypertension, dyslipidemia, cardiovascular disease, stroke, gallstones and cholecystitis, sleep apnea, respiratory dysfunction, and increased incidence of certain cancers. Obesity increases the risk of complications during and after surgery and the risk of complications during pregnancy, labor, and delivery. Higher weights are associated with higher mortality from all causes. Obesity is considered to be a major contributor to preventable deaths in the United States today.

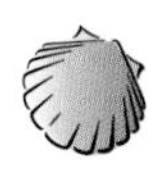

Obesity presents psychological and social disadvantages. In a society that emphasizes thinness, obesity leads to feelings of low self-esteem, negative self-image, and hopelessness. Negative social consequences include stereotyping, prejudice, stigmatization, social isolation, and discrimination in social, educational, and employment settings.

Benefits of Weight Loss

The potential benefits from losing excess weight can be realized with modest weight loss of 5% to 10% of initial weight. Immediate and significant improvements in sense of well-being, self-esteem, energy level, and quality of sleep occur. Risk factors associated with metabolic syndrome, namely hyperinsulinemia, hypertension, glucose intolerance, and dyslipidemia, are improved or resolved with weight loss. Weight loss reverses insulin resistance, protects against certain cancers, and improves or reverses osteoarthritis, diabetes, and cardiovascular disease. Weight loss is the single, most cost-effective treatment for disorders related to obesity.

Evaluating Motivation to Lose Weight

Objectively identifying who may benefit from weight loss is not the only criterion to be considered before beginning treatment; assessing the client's level of motivation is crucial because weight loss is not likely to occur in people who are not motivated or committed to lifestyle change. Even worse, imposing treatment on an unmotivated or unwilling client may preclude subsequent attempts at weight loss when the client may be more likely to succeed. Therefore, it is essential to assess the client's level of motivation before beginning weight loss therapy. Assess the following factors:

Reasons and motivation for weight loss. Is the client ready to make a lifelong commitment to lifestyle change? What is motivating the client to lose weight? Is it for health reasons, cosmetic reasons, or societal pressures? Is the client's goal realistic or based on an "ideal" weight that may never be achieved?

Previous history of successful and unsuccessful attempts at weight loss. What does the client see as reasons why previous attempts failed or succeeded?

Family, friends, and worksite support. Does the client have a social support system that may help the client to achieve his or her goals?

Understanding the causes of obesity and its impact on disease risk. Is the client aware of how obesity influences overall health? Is the client concerned about disease risks?

Attitude toward physical activity. What is the client's current level of physical activity (frequency, intensity, duration)? Is the client motivated to increase activity? Is the client willing to commit time to exercise consistently?

Capacity to participate in physical activity. In what activities is the client physically capable of participating?

Time available for weight loss intervention. Is the client able to commit the time necessary to interact with health professionals for weight loss therapy?

Financial considerations. Is the client able and willing to pay for weight loss therapy that is not covered by health insurance?

Barriers to success. What or who does the client anticipate will hinder his or her ability to succeed? For instance, overweight friends may not support the client's lifestyle change efforts because of their own fears or insecurities. Other barriers include depression, post-traumatic stress disorder, anxiety, bipolar disorder, addictions, binge eating disorder, and bulimia.

Goals of Weight Management

Ideally, treatment would "cure" overweight and obesity; that is, weight would fall to the healthy BMI category and would be maintained there permanently. This would be gradually accomplished with a 1- to 2-pound loss every week for the first 6 months of weight loss therapy. After 6 months, when the rate of weight loss usually decreases, then plateaus, the focus would shift to maintaining that weight loss. After 6 months of weight maintenance, weight loss efforts would be repeated. The cycle would continue until healthy weight is achieved.

In reality, this ideal is seldom achieved. The goal of losing large amounts of weight is unrealistic and overwhelming and from a health perspective does not appear necessary to achieve health benefits. A more appropriate goal is a modest weight loss of 5 to 10% of initial body weight, or a drop of 1 or 2 BMI units (approximately 10 to 16 lbs below current weight) even if "healthy" weight is not achieved. Compared with dramatic weight loss, modest weight loss (1) is more attainable, (2) is easier to maintain over the long term, and (3) sets the stage for subsequent weight loss.

Setting a modest weight loss goal and keeping that weight off are far more realistic than striving for thinness. Yet for some people, even modest weight loss may be unattainable. A more appropriate weight management goal for clients unable to lose weight is to prevent additional weight gain. Although this may sound like a passive approach, it requires active intervention, not simply maintaining the status quo.

Strategies for Weight Loss and Maintenance

Simply stated, to lose weight daily calorie intake must be less than calories expended over a period of time. Options to manage weight include nutritional therapy, increased physical activity, behavior therapy, pharmacotherapy, surgery, and combinations of these options.

Nutritional Therapy

Devising the most appropriate nutrition therapy for an individual begins by answering the following questions: How many calories should the client consume to lose weight? How is a lower calorie intake achieved? What is the optimal breakdown of carbohydrates, protein, and fat for weight loss? And finally what does it mean in terms of food?

How Many Calories?

From a strictly mathematical standpoint, losing 1 to 2 pounds/week means cutting daily calories by 500 to 1000 respectively. For overweight clients with a BMI of 27 to 35, a decrease of calories 300 to 500/day will lead to a ½- to 1-pound loss/week. For

 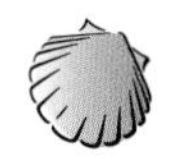

clients with a BMI > 35, a calorie deficit of 500 to 1000/day will result in a 1 to 2 pound weight loss/week. To put that in perspective, an overweight woman who requires 2000 calories to maintain her weight needs to limit calories to 1500 to 1700/day to lose ½ to 1 pound/week. If that woman is classified as obese, a daily deficit of 500 to 1000 calories/day limits her to a total of 1000 to 1500 calories/day. Instead of doing the math, a standard calorie level may be chosen such as 1200 to 1500 calories for women and 1800 calories for men.

If 1500 calories can promote a 1/2 to 1 pound loss/week, will a bigger cut in calories speed the weight loss process? Clients often think that the more drastically they cut calories, the quicker they'll lose weight. In reality, cutting calories too much—for instance, below the estimated basal calorie requirement—becomes counterproductive. First, very low-calorie diets leave clients feeling hungry, so compliance is difficult and often short-term. Also, very low-calorie diets are likely to be deficient in one or more nutrients; supplements can compensate to some extent but cannot fully replace the myriad of essential and nonessential components found in whole foods. Last, a drastic reduction in calories results in loss of lean body tissue as the body seeks to lower its total calorie needs by slowing metabolism. A slowed metabolism makes weight loss more difficult and is counter to long-term weight management.

Despite the counterproductive effects of cutting calories too drastically, severe calorie deficit plans are sometimes used such as fasting, very low-calorie diets, and low-calorie diets (Box 14.1). At best, these diets may be appropriate on a short-term basis for a select group of clients who medically require rapid weight loss or who may emotionally benefit from a "jump start" to their weight loss efforts. At worst, these diets are potentially dangerous stopgap measures.

How Is a Lower Calorie Intake Achieved?

Diets

Diet: In its most common usage, diet is a restricted calorie eating plan designed to achieve weight loss. In a broad sense, diet refers to what a person normally eats.

Satiety: the feeling of fullness.

People react negatively to the word "diet:" it is a four-letter word; it is restrictive and feels like punishment; it interferes with the pleasure of eating and lacks satiety; the only sure thing about going "on" a diet is that eventually the client will go "off" a diet. As such, most "diets" are viewed as short-term hurdles to endure before resuming a "normal" intake. Consider other downfalls of "dieting."

- Counting calories can take precedence over healthy eating. Counting 1200 calories from French fries and soda will promote weight loss but does not provide all the nutrients needed for good health.
- Most "diets" fail, as evidenced in the growing prevalence of obesity despite the widespread practice of "being on a diet."
- Research shows that "diets" (food restriction) can leave people feeling unsatisfied and hungry; this may lead to binge eating once food is available. Restrictive eating also promotes preoccupation with food and eating and other psychological manifestations.
- Highly restrictive diets lack flexibility in food choices and generally do not address the problematic behaviors that lead to weight gain.

See the Connection website for information on commercial weight loss diets such as Weight Watchers and Slim Fast.

BOX 14.1 **EXTREME LOW-CALORIE DIETS**

Total Fasting

Fasting or starvation (<200 calories/day) is a drastic strategy not recommended for anyone. Wasting of vital organs and muscle mass and a lowering of metabolic rate occurs as the body breaks down lean tissue to convert certain amino acids into glucose to maintain blood glucose levels. Fasting also carries the risk of rebound bulimia, or compensatory binging.

Very-Low-Calorie Diets

Very-low-calorie diets, also known as protein-sparing modified fasts, are a medically supervised aggressive, "jump-start" approach for severely obese clients (BMI > 30) who have failed to lose weight by other methods and who whose health is so jeopardized by obesity that the risk of a modified fast is less than the risk of remaining obese. These diets provide 600 to 800 cal, are high in protein (70 to 100 g/day), contain little or no fat, and little carbohydrate. Meals consist of a small variety of lean meats, a powdered protein formula available by prescription, or a combination of the two. VLCD are generally safe when used under medical supervision but are not appropriate for people under the age of 18, the elderly, clients who are ill, and those with emotional problems. Although short-term weight loss is dramatic (approximately 20 to 25% of initial body weight during 12 to 16 weeks of treatment), it is almost certainly regained. Studies suggest that the short-term effectiveness of very-low-calorie diets is related more to the choice-free menu of portion-controlled meals than to their severe calorie restriction. A maintenance program is crucial.

Low-Calorie Diets

Low calorie diets provide 800 to 1000 calories/day. They are most appropriate for clients who need to lose weight quickly for medical reasons such as those with type 2 diabetes, hypertension, hypercholesterolemia, or hypertriglyceridemia. Calories may be provided in the form of regular food augmented with vitamin and mineral supplements or from specially formulated food products or meal replacements. With either type of low-calorie diet, choice is restricted, boredom is common, and skills for changing food behaviors are not addressed.

A Lifestyle

A better alternative to a "diet" is a commitment to a lifestyle change that is permanent; as old habits are replaced with a healthier way of eating, the "new" way becomes the norm. Devising a plan for lifestyle changes first requires examining *what, how much, when,* and *why* the client eats and determining what changes could improve those parameters. Actively involving the client in deciding what changes he/she is willing and able to make is vital for long lasting change.

What. Foods that are nutrient dense in relation to the number of calories provided form the foundation of a healthy intake. Choosing foods with a high satiety value per calorie will enable clients to avoid hunger while controlling calorie intake. High-satiety foods tend to be those that are minimally processed, high in fiber, and high in protein—in other words, fruit, vegetables, legumes, whole grains, and lean protein.

 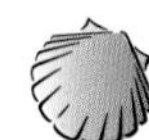

Career Connection

People desperate for weight loss are vulnerable to deceptive diet ads, including the lure of a "money back guarantee." Although this claim appears in almost 50% of weight loss ads studied, it should not inspire confidence. Consumers erroneously conclude that the product or diet must work; after all, why would companies deliberately market something that doesn't work if they had to refund customers' money? In truth, "money back guarantee" claims are simply a marketing ploy used to convince consumers that the product or diet must work or the guarantee would not be made. Actually, the FTC frequently sues companies that do not honor their "guarantees." Warn clients about other deceptive promises to watch out for such as

- Lose weight rapidly
- Lose weight without dietary restrictions or exercise
- Leads to permanent weight loss
- Lose weight despite past failures
- Scientifically proven or doctor-approved

Career Connection

Feeling chronically hungry is a common complaint among dieters and usually leads to abandoning the weight loss plan. But hunger is not an obligatory component of a weight loss plan. Concentrating on minimally processed, high-satiety foods can enable clients to fill full *and* lose weight. Here are some ideas for creating nutrient-dense, high-satiety meals that are reasonable in calories:

Breakfast ideas
- Peanut butter and banana sandwich on whole wheat bread with skim milk
- Breakfast parfait made with low-fat vanilla yogurt layered with fresh strawberries and rolled oats
- A smoothie made with skim milk, vanilla yogurt, frozen blueberries, and a banana

Lunch ideas
- Vegetarian chili, whole grain crackers, fresh salad
- Baked potato topped with salsa and a large salad
- Black beans and rice with sliced tomatoes

Dinner ideas
- Baked, broiled or grilled fish, baked potato, steamed vegetables
- Salmon sushi roll with large green salad
- Chicken stir-fry over brown rice

How much. Studies show that portion sizes in America have become much larger than standard serving sizes. Many people have a distorted perception of a "normal" serving. Reorienting clients to the appropriate serving size can greatly decrease calories.
When. Skipping meals often leads to ravenous hunger that increases the risk of overeating later. Also, people who are starving are less likely to be discriminating when they finally eat and may make poor food choices. Small frequent meals and snacks may be optimal for fueling metabolism and avoiding hunger.
Why. For many people, what and how much they eat are less important than why. Because eating cures hunger and nothing else, eating for reasons other than hunger—anxiety, stress, boredom, loneliness, anger—not only fails to relieve those feelings but also usually contributes to excess calorie intake. *Mindful* eating done only after the questions of "am I really hungry?" and "is this what I really want?" should replace *mindless* eating done as habit or in response to nonhunger cues.

Lifestyle changes can be implemented by using a food group approach. By counting servings/day from each food group and focusing on the size of those servings, intake is balanced and calories are relatively controlled. Exchange lists that detail items within each food and appropriate serving sizes ensure freedom of choice and variety. An accompanying meal pattern similar to those used by diabetics specifies the number of servings from each food group "allowed" for each meal and snack. This approach helps to reorient clients toward eating appropriate-sized servings and appropriate-sized meals at regular, frequent intervals. Compared to a "diet" or counting calories, this method is more likely to ensure a balanced intake yet provides a sense of structure that many clients want. A sample 1500-cal meal pattern and menu appear in Table 14.2.

Another eating plan approach that eliminates calorie counting while focusing on balance is to use MyPyramid. Specifying total servings to be eaten daily from each food group can approximate a chosen calorie level. This is a more lax approach than the exchange list system because caloric differences between items within a food group can be significant, as can nutrient density and satiety value. Counseling can help clients to choose healthy foods within each group. Table 14.3 represents sample plans for various calorie levels using MyPyramid food groups.

Nondiet Approach

The virtual obsession Americans have with "dieting" presents many concerns, including

- The physical and psychological impacts of the pressure to continually diet, especially for women
- The impact of the American ideal of beauty (e.g., extremely thin models) on the incidence of eating disorders
- The changes in food preferences that occur in chronic dieters, namely the increased preference for high-fat, high-sugar foods
- The increased tendency for chronic dieters and restrained eaters to binge eat
- The psychological consequences a failed diet has on the dieter
- Discrimination against fat children and adults
- Long-term health problems associated with certain weight reduction methods

These concerns have led to a relatively new conceptual approach to the nutritional management of obesity: the nondiet paradigm. The nondiet approach contends that the negative consequences of "dieting" outweigh the temporary benefits of weight loss. Its

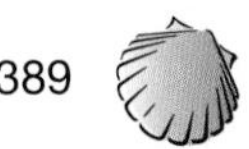

TABLE 14.2 SAMPLE MEAL PLAN AND MENU FOR A 1500-CALORIE INTAKE BASED ON THE AMERICAN DIABETES ASSOCIATION EXCHANGE LISTS

Exchange	No. of Exchanges (Servings)	Sample Menu
Breakfast		
Fruit	1	½ cup orange juice
Starch	3	½ cup shredded wheat ½ of a 4 oz bagel
Fat	1	1½ tbsp reduced-fat cream cheese
Milk, skim	1	1 cup skim milk
Free foods	as desired	coffee, tea 2 tsp light jelly
Lunch		
Starch	2	1 hamburger bun
Meat, lean	3	3 oz ground-round hamburger
Vegetable	1	1 cup salad made with greens, carrots, onions, mushrooms, and green peppers
Fat	1	1 tbsp regular salad dressing
Fruit	1	1 small apple
Free foods	as desired	1 tbsp ketchup mustard 1 large dill pickle coffee, tea
Dinner		
Meat, lean	3	3 oz grilled skinless chicken breast
Starch	2	⅓ cup rice 1 cup winter squash
Vegetable	1	½ cup steamed broccoli
Fruit	1	1¼ cup watermelon cubes
Fat	1	1 tsp margarine
Free foods	as desired	sugar-free gelatin
High-starch Snack		
Milk, skim	1	1 cup skim milk
Starch	1	3 cups microwave popcorn (1 starch, 1 fat)
Fat	1	

Contains approximately 1482 calories: 54% carbohydrate, 23% protein, 23% fat.

TABLE 14.3

DAILY AMOUNTS OF FOOD FOR VARIOUS CALORIE LEVELS USING MYPYRAMID GROUPS

	Total calories/day				
Group	**1200**	**1400**	**1600**	**1800**	**2000**
Grains	4 oz equivalents	5 oz equivalents	5 oz equivalents	6 oz equivalents	6 oz equivalents
Vegetables	1.5 cups	1.5 cups	2 cups	2.5 cups	2.5 cups
Fruits	1 cup	1.5 cups	1.5 cups	1.5 cups	2 cups
Milk	2 cups	2 cups	3 cups	3 cups	3 cups
Meat and Beans	3 oz equivalents	4 oz equivalents	5 oz equivalents	5 oz equivalents	5.5 oz equivalents
Oils	4 tsp	4 tsp	5 tsp	5 tsp	6 tsp
Discretionary Calorie Allowance*	171	171	132	195	267

The following are considered 1 oz grain equivalent:
- 1 slice bread
- 1 cup of ready-to-eat cereal
- ½ cup cooked rice, pasta, or cooked cereal

1 oz meat and beans equivalent:
- 1 ounce of lean meat, poultry, or fish
- 1 egg
- 1 tbsp peanut butter
- ¼ cup cooked dry beans
- ½ ounce nuts or seeds

*Discretionary Calorie Allowance is the remaining amount of calories in a food intake pattern after accounting for the calories needed for all for all food groups, using forms of foods that are fat-free or low-fat and with no added sugars.

process-oriented approach addresses size acceptance, disordered eating, eating in response to hunger and satiety, finding pleasure in healthful eating, and enjoying movement without the pressure to follow a precise exercise prescription. Clients most suited to the nondiet approach are those who are basically healthy and are able to invest time and financial resources in the process. See the Connection website for further information.

What Is the Optimal Distribution of Carbohydrates, Protein, and Fat?

What is the optimal breakdown of calories for weight loss? The most popular diets today fall into the category of either low fat or low carbohydrate (Table 14.4). The question of which type is best for weight loss is hotly debated among health experts, diet book authors, and dieters. Studies suggest that *any diet that creates a calorie deficit leads to weight loss.* When the issue is solely weight loss, eating fewer calories than the amount expended is the key: *the relative contribution and types of fat and carbohydrate eaten influence overall health but may not be important for weight loss per se.* Unambiguous conclusions drawn from a review of the literature and analysis of CSFII data are that

 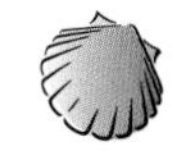

Career Connection

"What about the Atkins Diet?" This is a question of hot debate. The Atkins diet *does* cause weight loss because it is lower in calories—how could it not be with virtual elimination of approximately two thirds of MyPyramid? And it does help to lower cholesterol because of that weight loss, not because the foods promoted are inherently cholesterol-lowering. However, it is a short-term solution at best because over time the diet gets boring and situations occur that challenge compliance such as birthday parties, potluck dinners, and family vacations. The Atkins diet is high in saturated fat and red meat, which may increase the risk of heart disease and certain cancers—not just from what they contain but also from what they lack, namely fiber, essential nutrients, and phytochemicals. Although the initial weight loss with the Atkins Diet is quick and significant, it is because glycogen stores are depleted and with it the water glycogen holds; the "weight" loss is not synonymous with "fat" loss. And when carbohydrates are reintroduced into the diet, glycogen storage is replenished and with it the water it holds, making "weight" gain (even though it's not *fat* gain) significant and rapid. So while the Atkins diet may help some people to get motivated to commit to weight loss, it is not a long-term solution to weight management and health promotion.

(1) weight loss occurs independently of macronutrient composition and (2) metabolic benefits (e.g., improved glucose tolerance, lower cholesterol levels) result from weight loss not from inherent superiority of any particular macronutrient composition. In other words, the Atkins diet produces a drop in cholesterol because weight loss decreases serum cholesterol levels, not because the high-protein, high-fat diet is inherently cholesterol-lowering. Table 14.5 features sample low-fat and low-carbohydrate menus.

The arguments for a low-carbohydrate diet are that

People got heavier on the low-fat diets promoted during the 1980s and 1990s. People caught up in the low-fat diet craze erroneously believed that as long as fat intake was low, weight loss was guaranteed. They substituted low-fat cookies for regular cookies and ignored sugar, refined grains, and total calories. In fact, since 1985 average calorie intake has gone up by about 300/day, approximately one-half of which is from refined grains, one-quarter from added fats, and about one-

TABLE 14.4 **MACRONUTRIENT COMPARISON OF POPULAR DIETS**

	% of Total Calories		
Diet	**Carbohydrate**	**Protein**	**Fat**
Average U.S. intake	51–53%	15%	32–34%
NAS recommendation	45–65%	10–35%	20–35%
Ornish diet	Unrestricted	Unrestricted	<10%
Atkins diet	<10% (excluding fiber)	Unrestricted	Unrestricted
The Zone diet	40%	30%	30%

TABLE 14.5 SAMPLE LOW-FAT (<10% FROM FAT) AND LOW-CARBOHYDRATE (<10% OF CALORIES) MENUS

Low-Fat Menu	Low-Carbohydrate Menu
Breakfast	
Fresh orange sections Grape juice Whole wheat bagel with jelly and nonfat cream cheese Scrambled egg whites	Canadian bacon Cheese omelet 1 slice low-carbohydrate toast Margarine
Midmorning Snack	
Nonfat yogurt Fresh apple	Cottage cheese
Lunch	
Minestrone soup Grilled vegetable sandwich on whole wheat bread Tossed salad with fat-free dressing Nonfat milk Fat-free chocolate pudding	Shrimp salad with herb-dill dressing Sliced tomatoes with mozzarella cheese, fresh basil, and olive oil Sugar-free gelatin
Mid-afternoon Snack	
Fat-free rye crackers Low-fat hummus Banana	Sliced ham with cream cheese rolls
Dinner	
Lentil soup Vegetarian shish kebab Brown rice Winter squash Whole grain roll Nonfat milk Strawberries over fat-free frozen vanilla yogurt	Steak with sautéed mushrooms ½ cup broccoli Tossed salad with hard cooked egg, olives, and Italian dressing Chocolate dipped strawberries
Evening Snack	
Air-popped popcorn Nonfat milk	Cheese cubes

quarter from added sugars. Although the percentage of fat in the average American diet has declined, it is because total calories have increased, not from a decrease in total fat intake. Reducing fat intake alone does not cause weight loss unless total calories also are restricted.

Low-carbohydrate diets are easier and more comfortable to achieve than low-fat diets. Very low-fat diets often lack satiety; with hunger comes the temptation

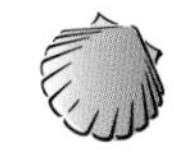

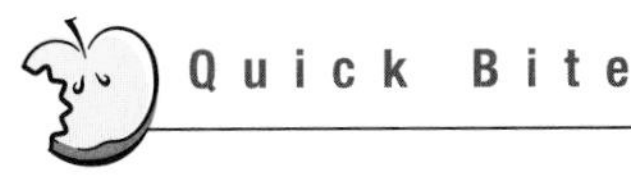

A closer look at reduced-fat cookies shows they are not a calorie bargain

	Serving size	*Fat (gm)*	*Calories*
Chips Ahoy! chocolate chip	3	8	160
Chips Ahoy! Reduced fat	3	5	140
Fig Newtons	2	3	110
Fat-free Fig Newtons	2	0	90
Oatmeal Raisin	1	4	110
Fat-free oatmeal raisin	1	0	105
Raspberry filled cookies	1	4	100
Raspberry oatmeal fat-free cookies	1	0	110

to give up on the diet. In contrast, low-carbohydrate diets rely heavily on protein foods, which are high in satiety value. For many, the guideline to eat as much protein as desired, including eggs, steaks, and other fatty meats, is irresistible.

Initial weight loss is significant. And immediate gratification fuels motivation. Yet the initial rapid weight loss occurs through the diuretic effect of low-carbohydrate diets: the weight loss is from loss of water, not fat. When a normal carbohydrate intake resumes, the water is replaced and weight regained.

Limiting carbohydrates limits insulin secretion. Advocates claim that carbohydrates are the only thing that raise insulin levels and that an overproduction of insulin is responsible for making excess fat that results in obesity. In truth, both protein and fat stimulate insulin secretion and a high postprandial insulin level is from eating excess calories, not carbohydrates. Second, high-carbohydrate diets do not cause prolonged rises in insulin. Even if a high carbohydrate intake *did* raise insulin levels, it wouldn't make people fat: only an excess of calories does that.

Arguments for controlling fat intake are that:

People who consume low- to moderate-fat intakes are more likely to consume fewer total calories. Fat is energy dense, providing more than double the calories as an equivalent amount of carbohydrate or protein. The tendency for calorie intake to rise as fat is increased or drop if fat is lowered is consistent with most clinical trials and epidemiological studies.

Diets high in fat are associated with increased serum cholesterol, heart disease, and some cancers. Also a high intake of red meat may increase the risk of prostate and colon cancers.

A low-carbohydrate intake lacks health-enhancing compounds. Fiber, which is found only in plants, helps to lower serum cholesterol, improve glucose tolerance, prevent constipation, and may help to reduce the risk of colon cancer. Phytochemicals, literally "plant chemicals," represent a varied group of compounds credited with the potential to reduce the risk of several chronic health problems ranging from macular degeneration and impaired memory to cancer and heart disease. Restricting the sources of fiber and phytochemicals, namely "carbs" such as fruits, vegetables, whole grains, and beans, has the potential to adversely impact health.

Controlling fat may be optimal for weight maintenance. Although losing weight is hard, keeping weight off may be even more difficult. The National Weight Registry tracks people who have lost at least 30 pounds and have kept the weight off for at least 6 years. According to their data, 90% of long-term weight maintainers consume a diet with 20 to 30% of calories from fat, limit total calorie intake, and exercise regularly. People on low-carbohydrate diets are rare in the registry.

What to Eat

Although the question of what is the optimal distribution of calories for weight loss has not been determined, most health authorities agree that the following measures improve health and/or weight:

Replace "bad" fats with "good" fats but use "good" fats in moderation. Unsaturated fats found in poultry, fish, nuts, salad dressings, and cooking oils are "good" fats because they do not raise serum LDL-cholesterol (the "bad" cholesterol) levels. Saturated and trans fats found in red meats, dairy products, stick margarine, shortening, butter, and foods made with these items are "bad" because they raise LDL-cholesterol, which increases the risk of coronary heart disease. Because all fats are calorically dense, neither healthy nor unhealthy fats should be eaten in unlimited quantities.

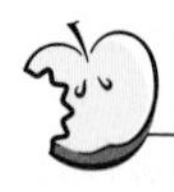

Quick Bite

Sources of trans fats

Fried foods from restaurants, fast food restaurants, bakeries
Stick margarine
Packaged foods such as crackers, chips, cookies, cake mixes, biscuit mixes
Frozen foods made with partially hydrogenated oils such as pies and entrees
Desserts and sweets such as candy, baked goods, toppings, icings, cakes, pie, and cookies

Choose carbohydrates carefully. Not all carbohydrates are created equally. Fruits, vegetables, and whole grains are rich in fiber and phytochemicals; provide high satiety; and are low in calories and are much healthier than refined carbohydrates like white bread, white sugar, soft drinks, and sweets. The type of carbohydrate eaten is as important as the type of fat. Just as the low-fat craze of the 1990s spurred the proliferation of low-fat versions of everything from peanut butter to ice cream toppings, today's low-carbohydrate creations are all the rage. Cutting carbohydrates means reducing starch and/or sugar content but not necessarily calories. Just as low-fat products failed to guarantee weight loss in the 1990s, the new manufactured low-carbohydrate foods will also likely be a disappointment.

Get enough calcium. Recent studies suggest that calcium plays a role in fat metabolism and that fat breakdown is impaired when calcium intake is inadequate. By

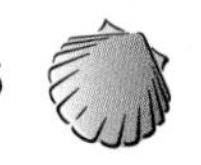

suppressing the active form of vitamin D, calcium may work to increase fat breakdown and reduce fat storage. Other studies in children and adults link increased calcium intake with lower body weight or body fat.

Be flexible in the approach. Some clients find that cutting down on bread, pasta, and rice is easiest for them while others may prefer to curtail intake of margarine, mayonnaise, salad dressings, and fried foods. As long as total calories are reduced and healthy sources of fats and carbohydrates are chosen, the actual percentage of fat and carbohydrate consumed becomes moot.

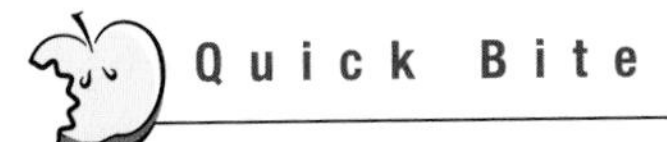

Quick Bite

Compare the calories in sugar-free varieties to their original counterparts

	Calories
Archway chocolate chip cookie, 1	
Original	130
Sugar-free	110
Peanut butter, 2 tbsp	
Original	190
Sugar-free	190
Nature's Own bread, 1 slice	
Original	50
Sugar-free	50
Mrs. Smith Frozen pies, ⅛th pie	
Original	340
Sugar-free	350

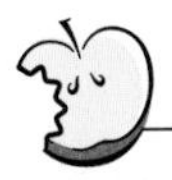

Quick Bite

Although calcium is important, so is limiting excess calories

All the following have approximately 300 mg calcium per serving but notice the serving size and calories.

	Calories
8 oz nonfat milk	90
8 oz whole milk	150
6 oz low-fat vanilla yogurt	160
1½ oz cheddar cheese	160
1¾ cup regular vanilla ice cream	235
2 cups 1% cottage cheese	324

Increasing Physical Activity

Physical activity is a vital component of weight loss therapy, even though it is not likely to produce short-term weight loss unless used in conjunction with a hypocaloric eating plan. Increasing activity is most helpful in maintaining weight loss.

Benefits of Increasing Activity

Physical activity affects obesity in several ways. Increasing activity favorably affects body composition during weight loss by preserving or increasing lean body mass while promoting loss of fat. These changes in body composition result in improved body dimensions and maintenance or an increase in metabolic rate or both. Activity also reduces abdominal fat, favorably altering the distribution of body fat. Finally, physical activity affects the rate of weight loss in a dose-response manner based on the frequency and duration of activity.

With or without weight loss, increasing activity lowers blood pressure and triglycerides, increases HDL-cholesterol, and improves glucose tolerance. Subjectively, increased activity improves the sense of well-being, reduces tension, increases agility, and improves alertness. Even without weight loss, an increase in activity improves cardiorespiratory fitness.

Recommendations for Increasing Activity

Obese clients should change their activity patterns slowly, gradually increasing the frequency, duration, and intensity of exercise. A variety of aerobic activities are suitable, but walking is almost always the most appropriate form of physical activity for obese individuals. An initial goal may be to walk 30 minutes/day for 3 days a week, building to 45 minutes/day of more intense walking at least 5 days/week. This may be accomplished all at once or intermittently throughout the day. In addition, the "everyday" level of activity should be increased, such as taking the stairs instead of the elevator and walking short distances instead of driving. Activity that burns 1500 to 2000 cal/week is suggested as optimal for maintaining weight loss.

Behavior Therapy

Some behavior modification ideas appear in Box 14.2.

No single strategy or combination of methods has proven best in changing behaviors. One or more of the following strategies may be helpful:

- **Self-monitoring eating** involves recording the how, what, when, where, and why of eating to provide an objective tool to help identify eating behaviors that need improvement. Also, the act of recording food eaten causes people to alter their intake. Self-monitoring activity, which includes the frequency, intensity, and type of activity performed, is also useful.
- **Stress management** involves using strategies such as meditation and relaxation techniques to lower stress, which may improve eating behaviors.
- **Stimulus control** involves avoiding or changing cues that trigger undesirable behaviors (e.g., keeping "problem" foods out of sight or out of the house) or instituting new cues to elicit positive behaviors (e.g., putting walking shoes by the front door as a reminder to go walking).
- **Problem solving** involves identifying eating problems or high-risk situations, planning alternative behaviors, implementing the alternative behaviors, and evaluating the plan to determine whether or not it reduces problem eating behaviors.
- **Contingency management** involves rewarding changes in eating or activity behaviors with desirable nonfood dividends.
- **Cognitive restructuring** involves reducing negative self-talk, increasing positive self-talk, setting reasonable goals, and changing inaccurate beliefs. Thoughts precede behavior; changing thoughts and attitude can change behavior.
- **Social support** involves getting others to participate in or provide emotional and physical support of weight loss efforts.

BOX 14.2

BEHAVIOR MODIFICATION IDEAS

Think Thin

- Make a list of reasons why you want to lose weight.
- Set long-term goals; avoid crash dieting based on getting into a particular dress or weighing a certain weight for an upcoming event or occasion.
- Give yourself a nonfood reward (e.g., new clothes, a night of entertainment) for losing weight.
- Don't talk about food.
- Enlist the support of family and friends.
- Learn to distinguish hunger from cravings.

Plan Ahead

- Keep food only in the kitchen, not scattered around the house.
- Stay out of the kitchen except when preparing meals and cleaning up.
- Avoid tasting food while cooking; don't take extra portions to get rid of a food.
- Place the low-calorie foods in the front of the refrigerator; keep the high-calorie foods hidden.
- Remove temptation to better resist it: "Out of sight, out of mind."
- Keep forbidden foods to a minimum.
- Plan meals, snacks, and grocery shopping to help eliminate hasty decisions and impulses that may sabotage dieting.

Eat Wisely

- Wait 10 minutes before eating when you feel the urge; hunger pangs may go away if you delay eating.
- Never skip meals.
- Eat before you're starving and stop when satisfied, not stuffed.
- Eat only in one designated place and devote all your attention to eating. Activities such as reading and watching television can be so distracting that you may not even realize you ate.
- Serve food directly from the stove to the plate instead of family style, which can lead to large portions and second helpings.
- Eat the low-calorie foods first.
- Drink water with meals.
- Use a small plate to give the appearance of eating a full plate of food.
- Chew food thoroughly and eat slowly.
- Put utensils down between mouthfuls.
- Leave some food on your plate to help you feel in control of food rather than feeling that food controls you.
- Eat before attending a social function that features food; while there, select low-calorie foods to nibble on.
- Don't eat within 3 hours of bedtime.
- Eat satisfying foods and do not restrict particular foods.

Shop Smart

- Never shop while hungry.
- Shop only from a list; resist impulse buying.

(box continues on page 398)

BOX 14.2 (continued)

BEHAVIOR MODIFICATION IDEAS

- Buy food only in the quantity you need.
- Don't buy foods you find tempting.
- Buy low-calorie foods for snacking.

Change Your Lifestyle

- Keep busy with hobbies or projects that are incompatible with eating to take your mind off eating.
- Brush your teeth immediately after eating.
- Trim recipes of extra fat and sugar.
- Don't weigh yourself too often.
- Keep food and activity records.
- Keep hunger records.
- Give yourself permission to enjoy an occasional planned indulgence and do so without guilt; don't let disappointment lure you into a real eating binge.
- Exercise.
- Get more sleep if fatigue triggers eating.

Pharmacotherapy

Historically, drug therapy has been used as a short-term intervention to initiate weight loss in clients with resistant obesity. After weight loss was achieved, drug therapy was discontinued. However, the drugs worked only while they were being taken, so the benefits stopped when drug therapy stopped.

Today drug therapy is considered an adjunct to comprehensive weight loss therapy that includes nutritional therapy, increased activity, and behavior therapy. Although drug therapy is currently reserved for selected obese clients, in the future drug therapy likely will be standard in the treatment of obesity as it is for other chronic diseases such as hypertension and diabetes. Drug therapy is not effective as a sole treatment nor do the benefits continue after the drug is stopped.

The use of drug therapy should be considered after 6 months of weight loss therapy that fails to produce a 1-pound weight loss per week. Drug therapy should not be used for "cosmetic" weight loss but only by clients at increased medical risk because of their weight, specifically those with a BMI of 30 or greater with no obesity-related comorbidities (i.e., hypertension, dyslipidemia, coronary heart disease, type 2 diabetes, and sleep apnea) and those with a BMI of 27 or greater if comorbid conditions exist. Clients whose waist circumference is greater than 35 inches (women) and 40 inches (men) are also candidates from pharmacotherapy if comorbidities are present.

Drugs tend to produce a modest weight loss (4.4 to 22 lbs), usually within the first 6 months of use, and may help to maintain weight loss. Additional benefits may also be gained, such as improvement in blood lipid levels, lowered blood pressure, and improved glucose tolerance. When drug therapy effectively promotes or maintains weight loss and the adverse side effects are manageable and not serious, it should continue in the long term, given the chronic nature of obesity. However, it is not known how long drug therapy may be safely used because of the lack of long-term data on the available drugs.

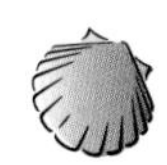

Not all clients benefit from drug therapy. Usually clients who respond initially continue to respond, and nonresponders are not likely to respond even with higher doses. Clients who fail to lose 4.4 pounds in the first 4 weeks of treatment are not likely to respond to drug therapy. Drug therapy should be discontinued if it is not effective or if the side effects are unmanageable or serious.

Phentermine (Ionamin, Fastin, Adipex), diethylpropion (Tenuate), and the over-the-counter drug phenylpropanolamine (Dexatrim, Accutrim) are approved for short-term use. Although they are better than placebo in short-term studies, no large-scale, long-term studies of weight loss or health benefits have been conducted. Drugs approved for long-term use appear in Table 14.6.

Surgery

Morbid Obesity: BMI > 40, or about 100 pounds of excess weight for men, 80 pounds for women.

Surgical intervention is the only proven effective therapy for long-term control of morbid obesity. It results in sustained (>10 years) and substantial (>15%) weight loss in the obese. Surgical candidates are those with severe BMI >40 or >35 with comorbid conditions who fail to lose weight by other methods and are experiencing complications from obesity. Contraindications include unacceptably high surgical risk, unresolved substance abuse, high likelihood of noncompliance with postoperative follow-up, significant uncontrolled emotional disease such as depression, failure to understand the procedure, or unrealistic expectations.

TABLE 14.6

DRUGS APPROVED FOR LONG-TERM USE IN THE TREATMENT OF OBESITY

Drug	Effect	Common Side Effects	Contraindications	Nutritional Considerations
Sibutramine (Meridia)	↓ food intake; May ↑ thermogenesis in some people; May inhibit weight regain after VLCD	Constipation, dry mouth, headache, insomnia May ↑ heart rate and blood pressure	CVD Uncontrolled HTN Use of MAO inhibitors Relative contraindication: use of other SSRI	May need ↑ fluid, ↑ fiber, ↓ Na, ↓ fat Avoid ↑ tryptophan foods
Orlistat (ZENICAL)	↓ fat absorption from GI tract by inhibiting pancreatic lipase ↓ LDL-cholesterol independent of weight loss Improves fasting glucose and glycohemoglobin in Type 2 diabetics	↓ absorption of fat-soluble vitamins Oily stools Anal leakage (initial side effects tend to ↓ over first several months)	Malabsorption syndromes Caution with hyperoxaluria, calcium oxalate renal stones, and diabetes.	Limit total fat Distribute fat evenly throughout the day Multivitamins may be needed; should not be taken within 2 hr of eating.

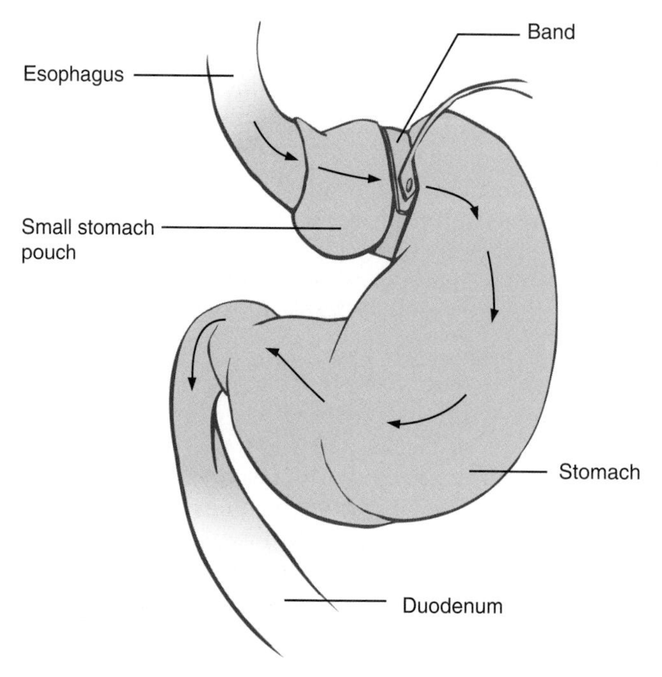

FIGURE 14.3 Adjustable gastric banding.

Surgical procedures for obesity work by (1) restricting the stomach's capacity, (2) creating malabsorption of nutrients and calories, or (3) a combination of both. Intensive nutritional counseling is needed to help clients minimize GI distress after eating and optimize effectiveness of the surgery. Gastric banding and gastric bypass are discussed below.

Gastric Restriction

Gastric banding drastically limits the stomach's capacity to hold food by creating a small, proximal pouch with a limited outlet (Fig. 14.3). The outlet diameter can be adjusted by inflating or deflating a small bladder inside the "belt" through a small subcutaneous reservoir. The surgery can be performed with a laparoscope, and the size of the outlet can be repeatedly changed as needed. Clients must understand the importance of eating small meals, eating slowly, chewing food thoroughly, and progressing the diet gradually from liquids, to puréed foods, to soft foods.

The mortality rate for gastric banding is low at 0 to <1% and weight loss may be as high as 55 to 65% after 3 years. Intolerance to solid food is an early complication relieved by band deflation. Another complication is slipping of the band, which occurs when the expanding proximal pouch pulls additional stomach above the belt, eventually causing occlusion of the outlet. Resurgery is often indicated. Overall, results of this relatively new procedure are encouraging.

Gastric Bypass (Roux-en-Y)

Gastric bypass combines gastric restriction to limit food intake with the construction of bypasses of the duodenum and the first portion of the jejunum, which creates malabsorption of calories and nutrients (Fig. 14.4). Rapid emptying of the stomach pouch contents into the small intestine may produce the "dumping syndrome" characterized by nausea, flushing, lightheadedness, diarrhea, and abdominal cramping that improve over time. This procedure is superior to gastric resection in both promoting and maintaining significant weight loss. After 5 years, average weight loss is 60% of excess body weight. Early complications include perioperative mortality, wound infections, anastomotic stenosis, and subphrenic abscess. The most common late complication is vitamin B_{12} deficiency and anemia.

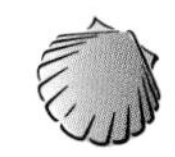

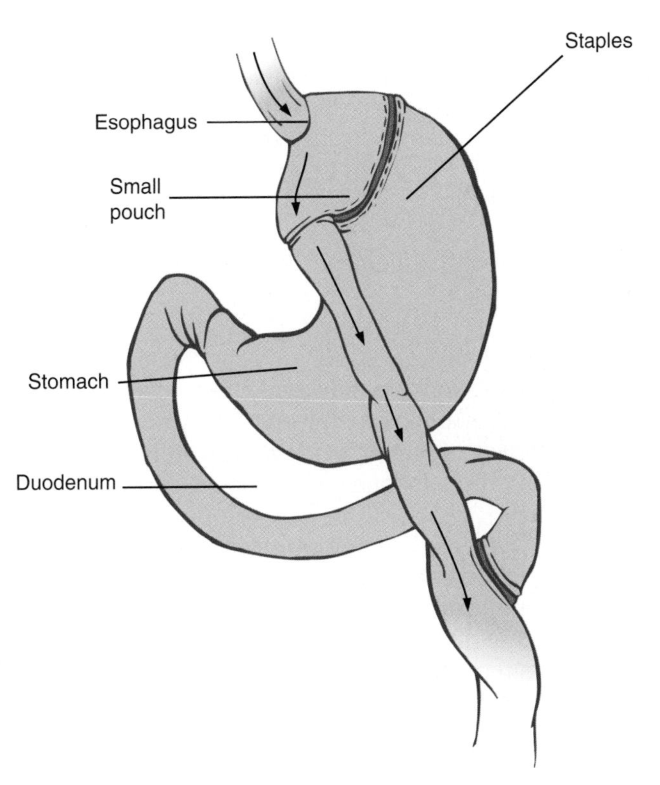

FIGURE 14.4 Roux-en-Y gastric bypass.

NURSING PROCESS

Thirty-three-year-old Megan Jackson has been "chunky" all her life. She weighs 189 pounds, the heaviest her 5-foot 7-inch frame has ever weighed. Her doctor has advised her to lose weight to bring down her blood glucose levels and blood pressure. She complains of frequent heartburn. She has been on and off "diets" for years without any long-lasting success at weight control. The doctor wants you to talk to her about dieting.

Assessment

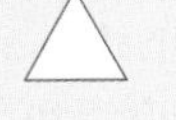

Obtain Clinical Data:

Current BMI and waist circumference
Recent weight history

(continued)

Medical history and comorbidities such as hypertension, dyslipidemia, cardiovascular disease, diabetes, sleep apnea, osteoarthritis, esophageal reflux
Abnormal laboratory values especially serum cholesterol, triglycerides, glucose, triiodothyronine (T_3), and thyroxine (T_4)
Ability to increase activity
Blood pressure
Medications that affect nutrition such as oral hypoglycemic agents, antihypertensives, and antacids

Interview Client to Assess:

Understanding the relationship between intake, activity, and weight
Understanding the relationship between obesity and health
Motivation to lose weight including previous history of successful and unsuccessful attempts to lose weight, social support, and perceived barriers to success
Usual 24-hour intake including portion sizes, frequency and pattern of eating, method of food preparation, intake of high-fat foods, intake of high-sugar foods, and fiber intake
"Problem" foods that may trigger overeating
Emotional triggers that stimulate overeating, such as depression, boredom, anger, guilt, frustration, or self-hate. People who are identified as compulsive overeaters may benefit from participation in Overeaters Anonymous (OA), a self-help group that uses a 12-step program similar to that of Alcoholics Anonymous. See website for additional information on OA.
Cultural, religious, and ethnic influences on eating habits
Psychosocial and economic issues such as living situation, cooking facilities, finances, employment, education level, and food assistance (if applicable)
Usual activity patterns and attitude toward increasing activity
Sense of body image and weight expectations
Use of vitamins, minerals, and nutritional supplements: what, how much, and why taken
Use of alcohol, nicotine, and caffeine

Nursing Diagnosis

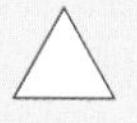

1. Altered Nutrition: More Than Body Requirements, related to excessive intake in relation to metabolic need.

Planning and Implementation

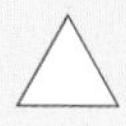

A positive, supportive approach is needed to establish rapport with the client and develop an atmosphere conducive to weight loss therapy. The nurse may not have the opportunity to discuss weight management with the client on a regular, ongoing basis. If time and follow-up opportunities are limited, it is important to focus on one or two changes the client is willing to make.

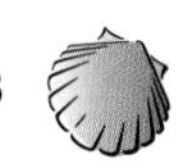

Remember that the objective of promoting weight loss is to improve health, which can be measured by criteria other than numbers of pounds lost such as decrease in blood pressure, improvement in serum lipid levels, or subjective improvements in quality of life (e.g., increased self-confidence, feeling more energetic). Involve the client in developing eating and exercise goals and plans to increase the likelihood of achieving success.

Goals must be specific, measurable, attainable, and individualized. Small sequential changes in intake and activity are easier to make and usually last longer than a complete overhaul. For instance, an initial goal may be to eat three servings of vegetables daily. After that goal is achieved, a goal of using light margarine in place of regular margarine may be added.

A balanced weight-reduction meal plan may be based on the "normal" recommended pattern of approximately 20% of calories from protein, less than 30% from fat, and the remainder from carbohydrate. The carbohydrate and fat can be adjusted according to the client's preference as long as total calories are controlled. Healthy fats should replace unhealthy fats; unrefined carbohydrates should replace refined grains and sugars. Include all major food groups in the plan. Discourage empty "liquid calories" such as from soda, fruit punches, and sweetened tea and coffee. Studies show that per equal calorie intake, foods in liquid form are less satisfying than solid form.

Hypocaloric eating plans usually do not provide less than 1200 calories for women and 1500 calories for men. Although extremely low-calorie diets can speed weight loss, they also make compliance more difficult, may be nutritionally inadequate, and may accelerate loss of lean body mass. Multivitamins and mineral supplements are indicated when intake falls below 1200 calories.

Dispel the myth that foods are either "good" or "bad." Forbidden or "bad" foods take on mystical qualities and become increasingly appealing. Rather than forbidding certain foods, emphasize portion control.

Weight-loss plateaus are to be expected because of the temporary increase in body water that results from the oxidation of fat tissue. Eventually an increase in urine output rids the body of excess water and weight loss continues.

Studies show that people who monitor their intake are more likely to be successful at weight management or weight loss than people who do not. Recording intake raises awareness of eating and portion sizes and is a useful tool for identifying patterns or choices in need of improvement. Encourage clients to diligently document everything they eat and drink for at least 2 to 3 days per week, more if possible. See websites at the end of the chapter for online diet analysis programs clients can use to analyze their food intake.

(continued)

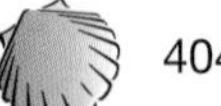

Client Goals

The client will

Increase physical activity to ___ minutes daily on ___ days of the week.

Explain the relationship between calorie intake, physical activity, and weight control.

Consume a nutritionally adequate, hypocaloric diet consisting of healthy carbohydrates, healthy fats, and lean protein.

Practice behavior therapy techniques to change undesirable eating habits.

Not skip meals.

Lose 1 pound/week on average until ___ pounds of total weight loss is achieved after 6 months.

Improve health status as evidenced by a decrease in total cholesterol, LDL-cholesterol, and glucose; an increase in HDL-cholesterol; and improved blood pressure, as appropriate.

Maintain weight loss by regaining less than 6.6 pounds in 2 years and sustaining a reduction in waist circumference of at least 4 cm.

Nursing Interventions

Nutrition Therapy

Decrease calorie intake by 500 to 1000 cal/day from calculated requirements to promote gradual weight loss.

Individualize the eating plan as much as possible to correspond with the client's likes, dislikes, and eating pattern because standard plans rarely fit into a person's lifestyle and eating habits.

Limit total fat because it is calorically dense and change to healthy fats. Encourage an adequate intake of lean protein and unrefined carbohydrates.

Encourage unrefined, high-fiber carbohydrates in place of foods made with white flour and sugar. Fiber contributes to satiety and is found in foods that are nutrient dense and relatively low in calories. Excellent sources of fiber include whole-grain breads and cereals especially wheat bran; dried peas and beans; and fresh fruits and vegetables.

Encourage a pattern of three meals plus two to three snacks throughout the day to prevent intense hunger and subsequent overeating. Breakfast is particularly important because it "breaks the fast" experienced while sleeping.

Encourage ample fluid intake to promote excretion of metabolic wastes. Water and other noncalorie drinks are preferred over sweetened beverages. Drinking fluid with meals contributes to a feeling of fullness.

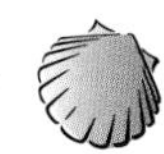

Client Teaching

Instruct the client

On the role of a low-calorie eating plan, increased physical activity, and behavior change in weight loss therapy and maintaining weight loss

On the eating plan essentials, including

- The importance of eating at least three times per day to avoid hunger, which often leads to snacking and a higher calorie intake
- The emphasis on high-satiety foods
- Tips for eating out, food preparation techniques, and the basics of food purchasing and label reading (see Chapter 9)
- The benefits of reducing fat intake to limit calories and improve blood lipid levels.
- The concept that "all foods can fit" as long as portion size and frequency are considered
- Maintaining adequate fluid intake
- Limiting alcohol consumption

On behavioral matters, including

- Eating only in one place and while sitting down
- Putting utensils down between mouthfuls
- Monitoring hunger on a scale of 1 to 10 with 1 corresponding to "famished" and 10 corresponding to "stuffed." Encourage clients to eat when the hunger scale is at about 3 and to stop when satisfied (not full) at about 6 or 7.
- Not getting weighed too frequently because weight losses that are less than anticipated are discouraging. Some clinicians recommend getting rid of the scale because it has too much power to make or break the client's day.
- Periodic record-keeping of food and fluid intake
- "Planned" splurges instead of eating on impulse. Planned splurges involve making a conscious decision to eat something, enjoying every mouthful of the food, then moving on from the experience without feelings of guilt or failure.

On changing eating attitudes

- Replacing negative self-talk with positive talk
- Replacing the attitude of "always being on a diet" with an acceptance of eating lighter and less as a way of life

To consult her physician or dietitian if questions concerning the eating plan or weight loss arise

(continued)

Evaluation

The client

Increases physical activity to ___ minutes daily on ___ days of the week
Explains the relationship among calorie intake, physical activity, and weight control
Consumes a nutritionally adequate, hypocaloric diet consisting of healthy carbohydrates, healthy fats, and lean protein
Practices behavior therapy techniques to change eating habits that lead to weight gain
Does not skip meals
Loses 1 to 2 pounds/week until ___ pounds total weight loss is achieved after 6 months
Improves health status as evidenced by a decrease in total cholesterol, LDL-cholesterol, and glucose; an increase in HDL-cholesterol; and improved blood pressure as appropriate
Maintains weight loss by regaining less than 6.6 pounds in 2 years and sustaining a reduction in waist circumference of at least 4 cm

EATING DISORDERS: ANOREXIA NERVOSA (AN), BULIMIA NERVOSA (BN), AND EATING DISORDERS NOT OTHERWISE SPECIFIED (EDNOS)

Eating disorders are defined psychiatric illnesses that can have a profound impact on nutritional status and health. They are generally characterized by abnormal eating patterns and distorted perceptions of food and weight that result in nutritional and medical complications.

Over a lifetime, an individual may meet the diagnostic criteria for more than one of these disorders, suggesting a continuum of disordered eating. Despite the dissimilarities in attitudes and behaviors among these eating disorders, each has distinctive patterns of comorbidity and risk factors. As such, the nutritional and medical complications as well as therapy can differ greatly.

Description

Anorexia Nervosa (AN): a condition of self-imposed fasting or severe self-imposed dieting.

Clients with AN pursue thinness compulsively through semistarvation and compulsive exercise. They are intensely preoccupied with weight and food, and their distorted perception causes them to see themselves as fat when they are emaciated.

Critical to the diagnosis of AN is that clients weigh less than 85% of expected weight, which translates to a BMI of 17.5 or less for adults (>20 years old) or a BMI of less than the 5th percentile for children and adolescents. Physical symptoms include

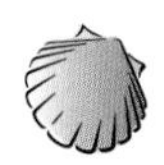

lanugo hair on the face and trunk, brittle listless hair, cyanosis of the hands and feet, and dry skin. Cardiovascular changes, including bradycardia, hypotension, and orthostatic hypotension, are sometimes fatal. Starvation leads to GI changes that include delayed gastric emptying, decreased motility, and severe constipation. Structural brain changes related to tissue loss may occur with chronic starvation. While some brain changes may be reversible with recovery, it is not known if complete recovery is possible. Amenorrhea is a cardinal characteristic. Osteopenia and osteoporosis may be serious and irreversible. Permanent sterility, damage to vital organs, and heart failure may occur. As many as one of every five to seven clients with chronic anorexia dies from complications.

Bulimia Nervosa (BN): an eating disorder characterized by recurrent episodes of bingeing and purging.

Clients with BN may quickly eat large amounts of food (e.g., 1200 to 11,500 cal) and feel unable to stop or control the binge. After gorging, clients purge to prevent weight gain, which may take the form of self-induced vomiting; excessive exercise; abuse of laxatives, emetics, diuretics, or diet pills; or fasting. Binges may occur several times a day and are frequently planned, with the client stockpiling food for a time when the binge can proceed uninterrupted. Binge foods are easy to swallow and regurgitate and usually consist of the fatty, sweet, high-calorie foods that the client denies himself or herself at other times.

Like anorexics, bulimics are preoccupied with body shape, weight, and food and have an irrational fear of becoming fat. Much of the time, bulimics are "dieting." In fact, dietary restriction can be the physiological or psychological trigger to bingeing as can "cheating" on their diet. Just the feeling of fullness, whether real or imagined, may be enough to trigger purging. Purging may bring initial relief, but it is often followed by guilt and shame. When normal eating is resumed, clients may complain of bloating, constipation, and flatulence. The physical discomfort after eating may motivate the client to resume dieting, thus a perpetuating cycle of restriction, bingeing, and purging. Although food is the vehicle, the binge/purge behavior is a means to manage emotions and ease psychological pain.

Unlike anorexics, bulimics experience weight fluctuations and are of normal or slightly above-normal weight. It is estimated that, on average, 1200 calories may be retained from a binge because purging does not completely prevent the absorption of calories and nutrients. Bulimics tend to have fewer serious medical complications than anorexics because their undernutrition is less severe. Muscle weakness, fatigue, cardiac arrhythmias, dehydration and electrolyte imbalance may develop secondary to vomiting and laxative abuse. Dental erosion can be severe. Gastric dilation, with its risk of rupture, may be the most frequent cause of death among bulimics.

Eating Disorders Not Otherwise Specified (EDNOS) account for 50% of the population with eating disorders. This group represents subacute cases of AN or BN. For instance, these clients may meet all the criteria for anorexia except that they have not missed three consecutive menstrual periods, or they may be of normal weight and purge without bingeing. Binge eating disorder, in which bingeing occurs without purging, is also classified as an EDNOS. Bingeing must occur at least twice a week over at least 6 months. Most clients are overweight and present with concerns about weight management, not disordered eating. Left untreated, binge eating may develop into BN or AN.

Etiology

Eating disorders are considered to be multifactorial in origin. Although numerous psychological, physical, social, and cultural risk factors have been identified, it is not known how or why these factors interact to cause eating disorders. People with eating disorders are prone to depression, irritability, passivity, sadness, and suicidal tendencies. The incidence of alcohol and drug abuse may be four to five times higher among women with eating disorders than in the general population. Psychological and social factors, especially problems with family dynamics, are usually considered to be central to the problem. Abuse and trauma may precede eating disorders in some clients.

An estimated 85% of eating disorders have their onset during adolescence; they are almost always preceded by "dieting." Major stressors, such as onset of puberty, parents' divorce, death of a family member, broken relationships, and ridicule because of being or becoming fat are frequent precipitating factors. Athletes (e.g., dancers, gymnasts) may develop eating disorders to improve their performance. Binge eating is often related to anxiety, tension, boredom, drinking alcohol or smoking cannabis, and fatigue. Hunger is rarely cited as a reason for binge eating, even when the gorging follows a 24-hour fast.

Approximately 90% to 95% of cases of anorexia and bulimia occur in females with two peak ages at onset: 12 to 13 years and 19 to 20 years. Anorexics are often described as "model" children although they tend to be immature, require parental approval, and lack independence. They typically are from white, middle- to upper-middle-class families that place heavy emphasis on high achievement, perfection, and physical appearance. Bulimia nervosa is more common than anorexia, with as many as one in five female college students admitting bulimic symptoms. Because bulimics are secretive about their binge-purge episodes, the behaviors may go undetected by family members for years and many cases go unnoticed. Eighty-five percent of bulimics are college-educated women. As many as 30% of bulimics have a previous history of anorexia; however, bulimia in persons of normal weight rarely develops into anorexia nervosa.

Assessment

Numerous physical and mental signs and symptoms may be observed in people with eating disorders.

Historical Data

- What are the client's current, usual, and ideal weights? What is the client's recent weight history?
- Does the client complain of fatigue, tooth sensitivity, indigestion, nausea, dizziness, intolerance to cold, constipation, or feeling bloated after eating? Does the client self-induce vomiting or abuse laxatives, diet pills, or diuretics? Is menstruation irregular or absent?
- What is the client's usual 24-hour intake? Which foods are best and least tolerated? What cultural, religious, or ethnic influences affect the client's food choices?

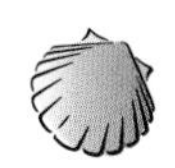

Does the client admit to food phobias? Does the client practice abnormal eating behaviors? For instance, anorexics may refuse to eat high-calorie foods, cut food into tiny pieces, choose inappropriate utensils, eat extremely slowly, use excessive condiments, drink too much or too little fluid, dispose of food secretly, binge eat, or exhibit ritualistic eating behaviors. Bulimics may eat large amounts of food when not physically hungry, eat rapidly, regurgitate (spit out) food, eat in secrecy, and eat until feeling uncomfortably full.

- What vitamins, minerals, or nutritional supplements does the client use and for what purpose?
- Does the client have a significant medical history?
- What over-the-counter and prescription medications does the client use? Does the client use alcohol or street drugs?
- What is the client's emotional state?
- What is the client's sense of body image? What are her weight expectations?
- What is the client's usual physical activity pattern?
- Does the client have family and social support?

Physical Findings

- Does the client have edema in the legs and feet?
- Is the client's tooth enamel damaged?
- Does the client have a wasted appearance?
- Is there growth of lanugo hair, alopecia, dry skin, thinning hair, decreased heart rate, or low blood pressure?
- Does the client have puffy cheeks as a result of enlarged salivary glands, particularly the parotid glands?

Laboratory Data

Evaluate serum electrolytes, protein status (e.g., serum albumin), and abnormal laboratory values.

Management

Each person's recovery process is unique; therefore, treatment plans are highly individualized. A multidisciplinary approach that includes nutrition counseling, behavior modification, psychotherapy, family counseling, and group therapy is most effective. Antidepressant drugs effectively reduce the frequency of problematic eating behaviors but do not eliminate them. Most eating disorders are treated on an outpatient basis; however, severe cases of anorexia nervosa may necessitate hospitalization. Bulimia tends to be easier to treat than anorexia because bulimics know their behavior is abnormal and many are willing to cooperate with treatment. Treatment is often time-consuming and frustrating.

Nutritional intervention seeks to reestablish and maintain normal eating behaviors; correct signs, symptoms, and complications of the eating disorder; and promote long-term maintenance of reasonable weight.

Nutrition Therapy for Anorexia

The goal of nutritional intervention is to gradually restore normal eating behaviors and nutritional status. Step-by-step goals are (1) to prevent further weight loss, (2) to gradually reestablish normal eating behaviors, (3) to gradually increase weight, and (4) to maintain agreed-upon weight goals. Sometimes a lower-than-normal weight is selected as the initial weight goal (i.e., enough weight to regain normal physiologic function and menstruation). When this has been achieved, the goal may be reevaluated. Many recovered clients have chronic problems with eating and weight.

Involving the client in formulating individualized goals and plans promotes compliance and feelings of trust. Offer rewards linked to the quantity of calories consumed, not to weight gain. Initially it may be beneficial to have the client record food intake and exercise activity.

Even though calorie needs are high to restore body weight, the initial eating plan offered is low in calories to avoid overwhelming the client. Also, large amounts of food may not be well tolerated or accepted after prolonged semistarvation. Generally, initial intake should not go below 1200 cal/day with calories gradually added each week until the appropriate level is achieved. Small, frequent meals help to maximize intake and tolerance. The diet is advanced only when the client is able to complete a full meal. Calories may eventually be increased to 3000 or more per day.

- Because gastrointestinal intolerance may exist, limit gassy and high-fat foods in the early stages of treatment.
- Monitor for signs of refeeding syndrome early in the refeeding process.
- Serve small, attractive meals based on individual food preferences. Foods that are nutritionally dense help to minimize the volume of food needed. Finger foods served cold or at room temperature help to minimize satiety sensations.
- Never force the client to eat, and minimize the emphasis on food. Initially clients may respond to nutritional therapy better if they are allowed to exclude high-risk binge foods from their diet. However, the binge foods should be reintroduced later so that the "feared food" (trigger food) idea is not promoted.
- A high-fiber or low-sodium diet may be helpful in controlling symptoms of constipation and fluid retention respectively.
- A multivitamin and mineral supplement may be prescribed.
- Caffeine is avoided because it is both a stimulant and a mild diuretic.

Refeeding Syndrome: a reaction to overfeeding characterized by sudden and sometimes severe hypophosphatemia, sudden drops in potassium and magnesium, glucose intolerance, hypokalemia, GI dysfunction, and cardiac arrhythmias.

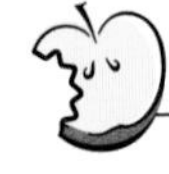

Quick Bite

"Gassy" foods

Cruciferous vegetables: broccoli, cauliflower, Brussels sprouts, cabbage
Dried peas and beans such as kidney beans, garbanzo beans, lentils
Dried fruit such as prunes and raisins
Carbonated beverages
Garlic and onions
Fried foods
Melon
Products containing sorbitol

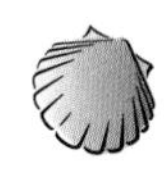

- Tube feedings or parenteral nutrition is used only if necessary to stabilize the client medically. Overly aggressive nutritional repletion carries medical risks of fluid retention and refeeding syndrome; psychological risks may include a perceived loss of control, loss of identity, increased body distortion, and mistrust of the treatment team. Enteral support should never be used as punishment for difficult clients.

Nutrition Therapy for Bulimia

Nutrition education and dietary guidance are an integral component of therapy. Nutritional counseling focuses on identifying and correcting food misinformation and fears and includes discussion on meal planning, establishing a normal pattern of eating, and the dangers of dieting. Bulimics must understand that gorging is only one aspect of a complex pattern of altered behavior; in fact, excessive dietary restriction is a major contributor to the disorder. Although most clients with BN want to lose weight, dieting and recovery from an eating disorder are incompatible. Normalization of eating behaviors is a primary goal.

Initially, nutrition therapy for bulimia is structured and relatively inflexible to promote the client's sense of control. Meal patterns similar to those used for diabetics can be used to specify portion sizes, food groups to include with each meal and snack, and the frequency of eating. Having the client record intake *before* eating adds to a sense of control.

- To increase awareness of eating and satiety, meals and snacks should be eaten while sitting down; finger foods and foods that are cold or at room temperature should be avoided; and the meal duration should be of appropriate length.
- Eating strategies that may help to regulate intake include not skipping meals or snacks and using the appropriately sized utensils.
- Encourage clients to gradually introduce forbidden binge foods into their diets. This is a key step in changing the all-or-none behavior of bingeing/purging.
- Clients who are laxative-dependent are at risk of bowel obstruction if the protocol for laxative withdrawal is not implemented. A high-fiber diet with plenty of fluids helps to normalize bowel movements while the use of laxatives is gradually decreased. Stool softeners may be ordered.

The initial meal plan provides adequate calories for weight maintenance so as to avoid hunger, which can precipitate a binge—usually not less than 1500 calories distributed among three balanced meals plus snacks. Adequate fat is provided to help delay gastric emptying and contribute to satiety. Calories are gradually increased as needed.

Expect minor relapses, especially after therapy is discontinued. When relapse occurs, the structured meal plan should be resumed immediately.

Teaching Points

Promote self-esteem in clients with eating disorders by using a positive approach, providing support and encouragement, fostering decision making, and offering the client choices. Avoid preaching rules and reinforcing the client's preoccupation with food.

Instruct the client

On the role of calories and nutrition in promoting optimal health and weight management

On the eating plan essentials, including

- The rationale for the particular eating plan used
- The characteristics of a healthy diet and the recommended servings from each food group. MyPyramid or exchange lists may serve as a teaching aid
- Appropriate food intake patterns such as not skipping meals

On behavioral matters, including

- Food- and weight-related behaviors
- Body image
- The dangers of dieting, bingeing, and purging
- How to recognize signs of hunger and satiety
- The likelihood that relapse will occur but should not be viewed as failure

How Do You Respond?

Is it a good idea to substitute special low-carbohydrate products for regular foods? Choosing reduced carbohydrate versions of "empty calorie" foods ignores the big picture: to lose weight, calories have to be cut. Substituting reduced carbohydrate muffins or beer over their regular carbohydrate counterparts is likely to have little or no impact on calorie intake. In addition, specially prepared low-carbohydrate foods do not taste like the original food and may cost two to four times more. A better alternative to choosing low-carbohydrate items is to avoid foods made with white flour and sugar and switch to carbohydrates that provide satiety, namely whole grain breads and cereals, fruit, vegetables, and dried peas and beans.

What are "net carbs"? Specially formulated low carbohydrate products have starch and regular sweeteners removed and fiber and sugar alcohols added. Food manufacturers have created the "net carb" concept to show consumers that their products are carbohydrate savers. They reason that because fiber is not digested and, therefore, provides no calories, grams of fiber should not be counted as carbohydrates. While it is true that fiber is generally "calorie-free," it is common practice among diabetes educators to subtract fiber grams from total carbohydrate grams *only when* the fiber content is greater than 5 grams/serving; for lesser amounts, no adjustment is needed. Food manufacturers also contend that the grams of sugar alcohols should be ignored even though they do provide calories, albeit about one-half the amount in regular sweeteners. Using their rationale, a product that has 10 grams of total carbohydrates with 3 grams of fiber and 4 grams of maltitol would have a

 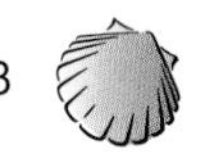

"net carb" content of only 3 grams [10 gm – (3 gm + 4 gm) = 3 gm.] Unfortunately, the same math does not apply to calories available to the body. Advise clients to ignore "net carbs" and instead evaluate a product on the basis of calories, serving size, and taste.

What is "yo-yo dieting"? The repeated loss and regain of weight is known as yo-yo dieting or weight cycling. It was once thought to be more harmful than static obesity; however, there is no convincing evidence that weight cycling has adverse effects on body composition, energy expenditure, risk factors for cardiovascular disease, or the effectiveness of future weight loss attempts. Fears about weight cycling should not deter overweight people from trying to lose weight.

▲ Focus on Critical Thinking

Respond to the following statements:

1. A client who needs to lose weight and wants to use the Atkins diet should be encouraged to do so.
2. Promoting size acceptance is like giving obese people permission to remain obese.
3. Because gastric surgery is the only proven effective treatment for obesity, it should be made available to more people.
4. Health care professionals have a professional obligation to point out the health risks associated with obesity.

Key Concepts

- The BMI may be the best method of evaluating weight status but it does not account for how weight is distributed. Overweight is defined as a BMI of 25 to 29.9; obesity is defined as a BMI of 30 or higher.
- Waist circumference is a tool to assess for visceral fatness. "Apples" (people with upper-body obesity) appear to have more health risks than "pears" (people with lower-body obesity).
- Beginning at a BMI of 25, the risk for development of certain diseases increases as does morbidity from existing disorders.
- Obesity is a chronic disease of multifactorial origin. It is likely that a combination of genetic and environmental factors is involved in its development.
- Approximately 61% of American adults are overweight or obese. Obesity is more prevalent among women than men and in racial-ethnic minority groups with the exception of Asian-Americans. Black and Hispanic women have the highest prevalence of obesity.
- Obesity is resistant to treatment when success is measured by weight loss alone. Rather than concentrating solely on weight loss to measure success, other health benefits, such as lowered blood pressure and lowered serum lipids, should also be considered. A modest weight loss of 5 to 10% of initial body weight usually effectively lowers disease risks.

- A hypocaloric intake, increased activity, and behavior therapy are the cornerstones to weight-loss therapy. Pharmacotherapy and surgery are additional options for some people.
- Calorie intake should be lowered by 500 to 1000 cal/day to promote a gradual weight loss of 1 to 2 pounds/week.
- As long as calories are reduced and healthy sources of fat and carbohydrates are used, the macronutrient composition of the diet does not impact weight loss.
- The nondiet approach to weight management promotes self-regulated eating instead of restrained dieting. It is founded on the belief that the body will find its own natural weight as the individual eats in response to internal hunger and satiety cues. Its focus is enhancing total health not achieving a specific weight.
- An increase in activity helps to burn calories and has a favorable impact on body composition and weight distribution. Even without weight loss, exercise lowers blood pressure and improves glucose tolerance and blood lipid levels.
- Behavior therapy is essential to promote lifelong changes in eating and activity habits. It is a process that involves identifying behaviors that need improvement, setting specific behavioral goals, modifying "problem" behaviors, and reinforcing the positive changes.
- Pharmacotherapy is adjunctive therapy in the treatment of obesity. Drugs are not effective in all people, and they are only effective for as long as they are used.
- Surgery to promote weight loss therapy involves limiting the capacity of the stomach. Gastric bypass also circumvents a portion of the small intestine to cause malabsorption of calories. Both types effectively promote weight loss but have complications.
- Anorexia nervosa and bulimia nervosa are characterized by preoccupation with body weight and food and usually are preceded by prolonged dieting. Although their cause is unknown, they are considered to be multifactorial in origin.
- Anorexia nervosa is a condition of severe self-imposed starvation, often accompanied by a frantic pursuit of exercise. Although they appear to be severely underweight, anorexics have a distorted self-perception of weight and see themselves as overweight. They may have numerous physical and mental symptoms. Anorexia can be fatal.
- Bulimia, which occurs more frequently than anorexia, is characterized by binge eating (consuming large amounts of food in a short period) and purging (e.g., self-induced vomiting, laxative abuse). Bulimics usually appear to be of normal or slightly above-normal weight, and they experience less severe physical symptoms than anorexics do. Bulimia is rarely fatal.
- Eating disorders are best treated by a team approach that includes nutritional intervention and counseling to restore normal eating behaviors and adequate nutritional status.

ANSWER KEY

1. **FALSE** The body converts calories consumed in excess of need to body fat, whether those calories are from carbohydrates, protein, fat, or alcohol. It is the ratio of calories in vs. calories out that influences weight, not specifically the source of those calories.

2. **TRUE** Although the mechanism is not clear, people of either gender with a high distribution of abdominal fat ("apples") have a greater health risk than people with excess fat in the hips and thighs ("pears").
3. **FALSE** BMI can be elevated for reasons other than excess fat such as large muscle mass.
4. **TRUE** Physical inactivity, as well as overeating, are major contributors to obesity.
5. **FALSE** Obesity-related problems improve or are resolved with a modest weight loss of 5 to 10% of initial weight even if healthy weight is not achieved.
6. **TRUE** Most short-term weight loss occurs from a decrease in total calorie intake. Physical activity helps to maintain weight loss.
7. **TRUE** With or without weight loss, an increase in physical activity helps to lower blood pressure and improve glucose tolerance.
8. **TRUE** Eating plans that provide less than 1200 calories may not provide adequate amounts of essential nutrients.
9. **FALSE** Neither cutting carbohydrates nor cutting fat grams ensures weight loss unless total calories are reduced. There is no magic combination of nutrients that causes weight loss independent of reducing calories.
10. **TRUE** People affected by bulimia tend to have fewer medical complications than those affected by anorexia because the undernutrition is less severe.

WEBSITES

For reliable information on weight, dieting, physical fitness, and obesity
- American Obesity Association at **www.obesity.org/**
- Calorie Control Council at **www.caloriecontrol.org**
- Centers for Obesity Research and Education at **www.uchse.edu/core/**
- Council on Size and Weight Discrimination, Inc. at **www.cswd.org**
- Division of Nutrition and Physical Activity, National Center for Chronic Disease Prevention and Health Promotion at **www.cdc.gov/nccdphp/dnpa**
- International Obesity Task Force at **www.iotf.org**
- NHLBI Obesity Education Initiative at **www.nhlbi.nih.gov/about/oei/index.htm**
- North American Association for the Study of Obesity at **www.naaso.org**
- Partnership for Healthy Weight Management at **www.consumer.gov/weightloss**
- Shape Up America at **www.shapeup.org**
- U.S. Department of Agriculture site for a Symposium on the Great Nutrition Debate at **www.usda.gov**
- Weight Control Information Network: **www.niddk.nih.gov/health/nutrit/win.htm**

For free intake/diet analysis
- **www.fitday.com**
- **www.dietsite.com**
- **www.foodcount.com** (offers both free and fee-based subscriptions)
- **www.nat.uiuc.edu/mynat**

For eating disorders
- Anorexia Nervosa and Related Eating Disorders (ANRED) at **www.anred.com**
- National Eating Disorders Organization at **www.laureate.com/aboutned.html**
- The Renfrew Center at **www.renfrew.org**
- Search "eating disorders" at **www.nal.usda.gov/fnic** for *Eating Disorders—A Food and Nutrition Resource List*
- Something Fishy on Eating Disorders at **www.somethingfishy.org**
- Overeaters Anonymous, Inc. at **www.oa.org**

REFERENCES

American Dietetic Association. (2002). Position of the American Dietetic Association: Weight management. *Journal of the American Dietetic Association, 102,* 1145–1155.

American Dietetic Association. (2001). Position of the American Dietetic Association: Nutrition intervention in the treatment of anorexia nervosa, bulimia nervosa, and eating disorders not otherwise specified (EDNOS). *Journal of the American Dietetic Association, 101,* 810–819.

Brownell, K., & Fairburn, C. (Eds.). (2002). *Eating disorders and obesity: A comprehensive handbook* (2nd ed.). New York: The Guilford Press.

Federal Trade Commission (2002). Tipping the scales? Weight-loss ads found heavy on deception. *Consumer Features.* Available at www.ftc.gov/bcp/conline/features/wgtloss.htm. Accessed on 9/22/03.

Flegal, K., Carroll, M., Ogden, C., & Johnson, C. (2002). Prevalence and trend in obesity among US adults, 1999–2000. *Journal of the American Medical Association, 288,* 1723–1727.

Gentry, M. (Ed). (2002). Growing evidence confirms that Americans eat too much. *American Institute for Cancer Research Newsletter,* (75), 4.

Harnack, L., & French, S. (2003). Fattening up on fast food. *Journal of the American Dietetic Association, 103,* 1296–1297.

Kennedy, E., Bowman, S., Spence, J., et al. (2001) Popular diets: Correlation to health, nutrition, and obesity. *Journal of the American Dietetic Association, 101,* 411–420.

Kenney, J. (2003). Weight loss: What's working? *Communicating Food for Health,* January, 1, 5.

Liebman, B. (2002). Big fat lies. The truth about the Atkins diet. *Nutrition Action Health Letter, 29*(9), 1, 3–7.

Marcason, W. (2002). Nutrition therapy and eating disorders: What is the correct calorie level for clients with anorexia? *Journal of the American Dietetic Association, 102,* 644.

McBean, L. (2002). Weight control: An emerging beneficial role for dairy. *Dairy Council Digest, 74*(4), 19–24.

National Heart, Lung, and Blood Institute Expert Panel on the Identification, Evaluation, and Treatment of Overweight and Obesity in Adults. (1998). *Executive summary of the clinical guidelines on the identification, evaluation, and treatment of overweight and obesity in adults.* Rockville, MD: Author.

Neighbors-Dembereckyj, L. (2002). Online diet analysis tools: A functional comparison. *Journal of the American Dietetic Association, 102,* 1738–1742.

Paeratakul, S., York-Crowe, E., Williamson, D., et al. (2002). Americans on diet: Results from the 1994–1996 continuing survey of food intakes by individuals. *Journal of the American Dietetic Association, 102,* 1247–1251.

Putnam, J., Allshouse, J., & Kantor, L. (2002). US per capital food supply trends: More calories, refined carbohydrates, and fats. *FoodReview 25,* 2–15. (Economic Research Service, U.S. Department of Agriculture).

Rosenberg, I. (Ed.). (2003). Low-carb craze, or low-carb crazy? *Tufts University Health and Nutrition Letter, 21*(8), 4–5.

Rosenberg, I. (Ed.). (2003). Carbohydrates vindicated. *Tufts University Health and Nutrition Letter, 21*(5), 1.

U.S. Department of Health and Human Services, Public Health Service, National Institutes of Health, National Heart, Lung, and Blood Institute. (1998). *Clinical guidelines on the identification, evaluation, and treatment of overweight and obesity in adults: The evidence report.* (NIH Publication No. 98-4083). Rockville, MD: Author.

Variyam, J. (2002). Patterns of caloric intake and body mass index among US adults. *FoodReview 25,* 16–20.

Young, L., & Nestle, M. (2003). Expanding portion sizes in the US marketplace: Implications for counseling. *Journal of the American Dietetic Association, 103,* 231–234.

For information on the new dietary guidelines 2005 and MyPyramid, visit
http://connection.lww.com/go/dudek

15

Feeding Patients: Hospital Food and Enteral and Parenteral Nutrition

TRUE	FALSE	
⬭	⬭	**1** Routine hospital diets generally meet the recommendations put forth in the *Dietary Guidelines for Americans.*
⬭	⬭	**2** Full liquid diets that are planned or supplemented are nutritionally adequate and can be suitable for long-term use.
⬭	⬭	**3** Tube feedings can be made more nutrient dense by adding one or more modular products.
⬭	⬭	**4** The more digested the protein is in a formula, the greater the osmolality.
⬭	⬭	**5** The terms *fiber* and *residue* are synonymous.
⬭	⬭	**6** The patient's digestive and absorptive capacities are the primary considerations when deciding the type of tube feeding to use.
⬭	⬭	**7** Peripheral parenteral nutrition (PPN) is not suitable for patients who need more than 2500 cal/daily.
⬭	⬭	**8** Intermittent feedings should take 20 to 30 minutes to infuse.
⬭	⬭	**9** Diarrhea in tube-fed patients may be caused by giving too much formula or administering the formula too rapidly.
⬭	⬭	**10** Coloring tube feeding formulas with food dye helps to prevent aspiration.

UPON COMPLETION OF THIS CHAPTER, YOU WILL BE ABLE TO

- Describe ways to promote the patient's acceptance of hospital food.
- Describe the characteristics, indications, and contraindications for liquid and soft diets.
- Define enteral nutrition.
- List indications for using enteral nutrition.
- Compare the two major types of enteral formulas.
- Define the two types of parenteral nutrition
- Describe the uses of each type of parenteral nutrition.
- Discuss possible causes of diarrhea in tube-fed patients.
- Describe possible interventions for diarrhea in tube-fed patients.
- Outline teaching points for patients using home enteral nutrition.

Feeding patients who are acutely or chronically ill presents many challenges. A common problem is inadequate intake, which may occur for a variety of reasons. Appetite may be impaired or lacking because of physical or emotional stress of illness or hospitalization. For instance, eating alone, physical pain, and facing an uncertain prognosis all affect appetite. Hospital food may be refused because it is unfamiliar, tasteless (e.g., cooked without salt), inappropriate in texture (e.g., pureed meat), religiously or culturally unacceptable, or served at times when the patient is unaccustomed to eating. Meals may be withheld or missed because of diagnostic procedures or medical treatments. Inadequate liquid diets may not be advanced in a timely manner.

In addition to inadequate intake, altered nutrient use or increased nutrient requirements may complicate patient feeding. Digestion, absorption, metabolism, or excretion may be impaired by illness or treatments, making it necessary to restrict the intake of certain foods or to provide "artificial" nutrition. Requirements for protein, calories, fluid, and other nutrients may be increased because of stress, illness, fever, infection, or wound healing. It is essential that the nourishment provided be such that the patient is able to consume it, tolerate it, use it, and meet individual nutrient requirements. Figure 15.1 depicts a decision-making model for choosing the appropriate type and method of feeding.

Patients who do not meet their nutritional requirements are at risk for malnutrition, which is seen in all age groups and across the continuum of care. As many as 40% to 55% of hospitalized patients have malnutrition or are at risk for developing malnutrition. Consequences of malnutrition include longer hospital stays, higher costs, and higher rates of complications. Impaired wound healing and susceptibility to infection are well-known outcomes, both of which increase morbidity and mortality. Preventing malnutrition is easier and more effective than treatment.

This chapter explores hospital diets and how nurses can help to promote an adequate intake in their patients. Oral supplements and modular products are discussed. For patients who are unable or unwilling to consume an adequate oral diet, the use of enteral and parenteral nutrition is presented.

HOSPITAL FOOD

Hospital food rarely has a positive image, despite its importance to the patient's health and recovery and overall satisfaction. Although the nurse has no control over the quality of the food, nursing actions can greatly affect the patient's satisfaction with the food. Delivering the tray in a courteous manner, showing a positive attitude toward the food, and explaining the diet to the patient are acts that increase patient satisfaction. Patients who are satisfied are more likely to eat well than patients who are dissatisfied.

Private and government regulatory agencies require that hospital menus be supervised by a qualified dietitian and that they meet the Recommended Dietary Allowances. These stipulations are intended to prevent deficiency diseases, not to prevent chronic diseases. Because of this focus, "regular" diets in hospitals (i.e., the default menu sent to patients who do not select their own food) often fail to meet the *Dietary Guidelines for Americans* recommendations to limit fat, saturated fat, cholesterol, and sodium (see

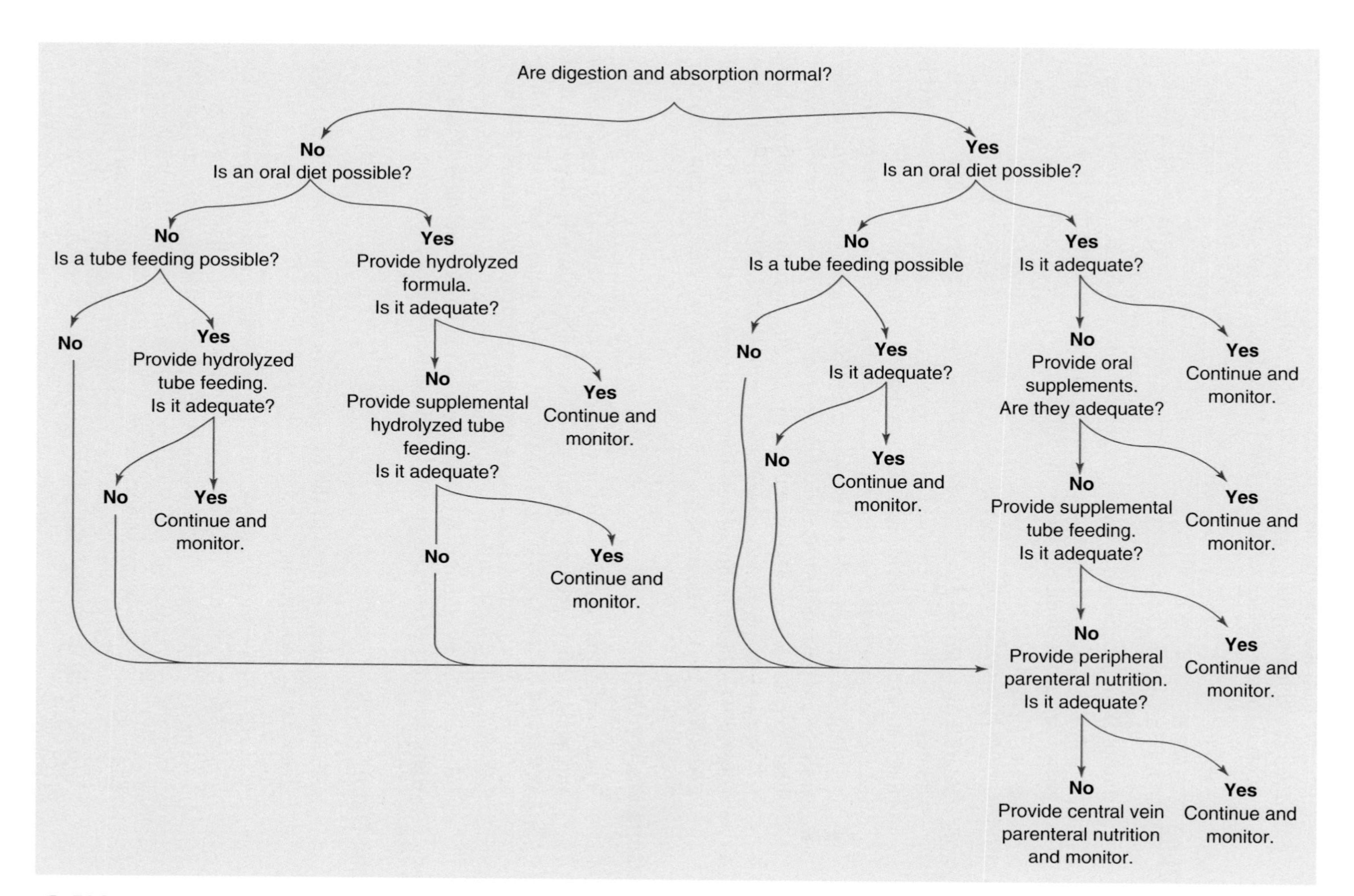

FIGURE 15.1 Selecting the appropriate type and method of feeding.

Chapter 8). Likewise, the fiber content is often less than recommended. An argument against making routine hospital diets "heart-healthy" is that the objective of feeding patients is to meet increased needs, not to avoid nutritional excesses.

Types of Diets

Hospital food comes in a variety of regular and modified oral diets. Often combination diets are ordered such as a 1500-calorie, low-sodium diet or a high-protein, soft diet. Categories of diets include the following.

Normal, Regular, and House Diets

Regular diets are used to achieve or maintain optimal nutritional status in patients who do not have altered nutritional needs related to illness, injury or impaired health. No foods are excluded; portion sizes are not limited on a normal diet. The nutritional value of the diet varies significantly with the actual foods chosen by the patient.

Regular diets are adjusted to meet age-specific needs throughout the life cycle. For instance, a regular diet for a child differs from one for a pregnant woman or an elderly patient. Regular diets are also altered to meet specifications for vegetarian or kosher eating.

Sometimes physicians order a *diet as tolerated (DAT)* on admission or after surgery. This order is interpreted according to the patient's appetite and ability to eat and tolerate food. The nurse has the authority to advance the diet as tolerated.

Modified Consistency Diets

The following diets are modified in consistency and texture: clear liquid, full liquid, soft, mechanical soft, pureed, low-residue, and high-fiber. Usually, after acute illness or when oral intake resumes after a prolonged period, clear liquids are ordered and progressed to full liquids, then to a soft diet, and finally to a normal or modified diet as appropriate. Depending on the patient's tolerance and condition, this routine progression may be accelerated by eliminating one or more of the transitional diets. Table 15.1 outlines the characteristics, indications, and contraindications of consistency modified diets.

Therapeutic Diets

Therapeutic diets are used in the treatment of disease or illness. Types of therapeutic diets may be modified in

Calories. Diets with specific calorie levels are ordered to promote weight loss or to provide a consistent calorie intake as indicated (e.g., in the treatment of diabetes). The specified calorie levels usually range from 1000 to 3000 cal/day. When weight gain is desired, the physician may simply order a "high-calorie" diet without specifying a desired calorie level.

The concentration of macronutrients. For instance, the amount of carbohydrate, protein, or fat in the diet may be increased or decreased depending on need. The

(*text continues on page 425*)

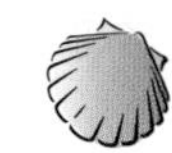

TABLE 15.1

CHARACTERISTICS, INDICATIONS, AND CONTRAINDICATIONS FOR LIQUID AND SOFT DIETS

Diet Characteristics	Foods Allowed	Indications	Contraindications
Clear Liquid			
A short-term, highly restrictive diet composed only of clear fluids or foods that become fluid at body temperature (e.g., gelatin). It requires minimal digestion and leaves a minimum of residue. Although they provide some electrolytes and carbohydrates, clear liquid diets are inadequate in calories and all nutrients (except vitamin C if vitamin C–fortified juices are used). Be sure to include bouillon in the diet if electrolyte replacement is needed; eliminate bouillon if the client requires sodium restriction (one bouillon cube provides 424 mg of sodium).	Clear broth or bouillon Coffee, tea, and carbonated beverages, as allowed and as tolerated Fruit juices, clear (apple, cranberry, grape) and strained (orange, lemonade, grapefruit) Fruit ice made from clear fruit juice Gelatin Popsicles Sugar, honey, hard candy Commercially prepared low residue, lactose-free supplements	In preparation for bowel surgery or colonoscopy; acute GI disorders; transitional feeding after parenteral nutrition. Practice of using clear liquids as initial feeding after surgery may not be warranted.	Long-term use
Full Liquid			
Composed of foods that are liquid or liquefy at body temperature (e.g., ice cream). Full liquid diets can be carefully planned or supplemented to approximate the nutritional value of a regular of high-calorie, high-protein diet, making them suitable for long-term use. Full liquid diets may be inade-	All items on the clear liquid diet plus: All milk and milk drinks, puddings, and custards All vegetable juices All fruit juices Refined or strained cereals Eggs in custard Butter, margarine, cream	Used as a transition between a clear liquid diet and a soft diet and by clients who have difficulty chewing or swallowing	Severe lactose intolerance (diet relies heavily on milk and dairy products for protein and calories) Unless modified to decrease the cholesterol content, a liquid diet is not suitable for long-term use by clients

(table continues on page 422)

TABLE 15.1
(continued)

CHARACTERISTICS, INDICATIONS, AND CONTRAINDICATIONS FOR LIQUID AND SOFT DIETS

Diet Characteristics	Foods Allowed	Indications	Contraindications
quate in folic acid, iron, vitamin B_6, and fiber. If the diet is used longer than 2–3 d, the following modifications may be needed to increase calories and protein: Add sugar and syrups whenever possible. Use whole-fat milk unless the client has hypercholesterolemia. Melt butter or margarine on soup and cereal. Add glucose supplements to fruit juices, milk, and milk drinks. Add skim milk powder to milk, milk drinks, soup, custard, puddings, and cereal. Add instant breakfast mix or commercial supplements. Lactose-reduced milk is available for clients with lactose intolerance. Adapt the diet for clients with diabetes mellitus, renal disease, and other disorders. Low-sodium soups, eggnogs, and custards should be used by clients who require sodium restriction. To avoid salmonella infection, raw eggs should not be used.			with hypercholesterolemia.

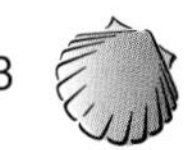

TABLE 15.1
(continued)

CHARACTERISTICS, INDICATIONS, AND CONTRAINDICATIONS FOR LIQUID AND SOFT DIETS

Diet Characteristics	Foods Allowed	Indications	Contraindications
Blenderized Liquid Diet (also known as pureed diet)			
A diet composed of liquids and foods blenderized to liquid form. Thickness/viscosity depends on patient tolerance. Most foods can be liquified by combining equal parts of solids and liquids; fruits and vegetables need less liquid. Broth, gravy, cream soups, cheese, tomato sauce, milk, and fruit juice are preferable to water for blenderizing due to their higher calorie and nutritional value.	All foods are allowed, but consistency is changed to liquid	Used after oral or facial surgery; for wired jaws; chewing and swallowing problems	None
Soft Diet Other Common Names: Bland Diet, Low Fiber Diet			
An adequate diet that is moderately low in fiber and lightly seasoned. Food textures range from smooth and creamy to moderately crisp. Restrictions vary considerably among institutions, but most raw fruits and vegetables, coarse breads and cereals, and potentially gas-forming foods are excluded.	All items on the full liquid diet plus: Cooked vegetables as tolerated Lettuce in small amounts Cooked or canned fruit Avocado Banana Grapefruit and orange sections without membranes	Used for patients who are unable to tolerate a regular diet after surgery or because of mild gastrointestinal distress Used as a transition between liquids and a regular diet	None

(table continues on page 424)

TABLE 15.1
(continued)

CHARACTERISTICS, INDICATIONS, AND CONTRAINDICATIONS FOR LIQUID AND SOFT DIETS

Diet Characteristics	Foods Allowed	Indications	Contraindications
	Melon White, refined-wheat, or light-rye enriched breads and cereals Potatoes Enriched rice, barley, pasta All lean, tender meats; fish; poultry Eggs, mild cheese, smooth peanut butter Soybeans and other meat alternatives Flavored or plain yogurt Butter, margarine, mild salad dressings Cakes, cookies, and pies made with allowed foods		
Mechanical Soft Diet			
A regular diet modified in texture only. Excludes most raw fruits and vegetables and foods containing seeds, nuts, and dried fruit.	Chopped, ground, mashed, and pureed foods Foods soaked in gelatin or commercial thickener slurry (e.g., for breads, cakes, cookies) Mashed, soft ripened fruit (peaches, pears, bananas) Cooked, mashed soft vegetables (peas, carrots, yams)	Used for patients who have limited chewing ability, such as patients who are edentulous, have ill-fitting dentures, or have undergone surgery to the head, neck, or mouth	None

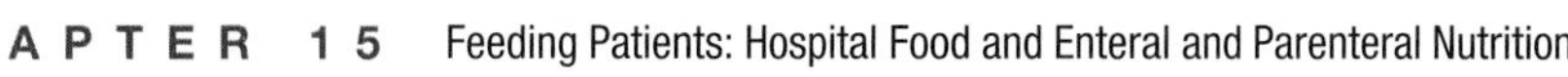

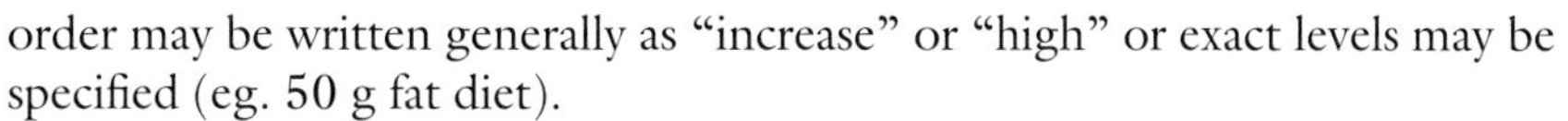

order may be written generally as "increase" or "high" or exact levels may be specified (eg. 50 g fat diet).

The concentration of micronutrients. The amounts of micronutrients, such as sodium, potassium, and iron, may be restricted or encouraged as part of a therapeutic regimen.

Fluid content. "Push fluids" is written to encourage, not force, fluid intake. Fluid restricted diets specify the amount of total fluid allowed per day including fluids served with meals and fluids provided by nursing for medication passes.

Particular food components. For instance, gluten (the protein portion of wheat flour) is eliminated from the diets of people with celiac disease, so wheat and other gluten-containing grains must be avoided.

A combination of any of the above. For instance, a diet order for a diabetic with hypertension may specify 1500 calorie, low sodium.

Nutritional Supplements

Some patients are unable or unwilling to eat enough food to meet their requirements either because intake is poor or because their nutritional needs are so high that it is difficult to meet requirements in a normal volume of food. For these patients, liquid supplements with or between meals can significantly boost protein and calorie intakes.

Liquid supplements are easy to consume, are generally well accepted, and tend to leave the stomach quickly, making them a good choice for between-meal snacks. Different brands taste different. If a patient refuses a supplement because of its taste, offer a nutritionally comparable alternative. Studies suggest that patient knowledge of the brand name of the supplement (i.e., "the power of advertising") increases acceptability. With any supplement, taste fatigue may occur over time. To maximize acceptance, serve oral supplements cold and experiment with different flavors.

Categories of supplements include clear liquid supplements, milk-based drinks, prepared liquid supplements, and specially prepared foods. Modular products are a special category of single-nutrient supplements that are used to enhance the nutrient density of food or tube feedings. A sampling of products follows.

Clear Liquid Supplements

Clear liquid supplements come in a ready-to-use form or as a powder mixed with water. They provide protein, calories, or both for patients on clear liquid diets. They are extremely low in fat and have little residue. Although they come in flavors, they are not as well accepted as the other categories of supplements.

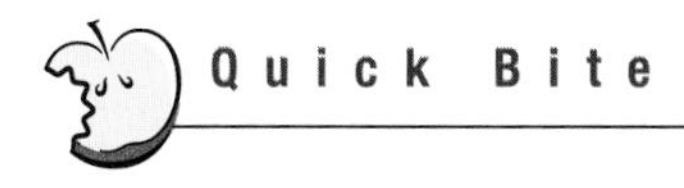

Quick Bite

Examples of supplements suitable for a clear liquid diet

Enlive!
Forta Drink
Resource Fruit Beverage

Career Connection

Giving the right food to the patient is one thing; getting the patient to eat (most of it) is another. The nurse plays a key role in promoting an adequate intake and bridging the gap between the dietary department and the patient. Attention to details can make a big difference in the patient's acceptance of hospital food.

- Let the patient select his or her own menu whenever possible. This gives the patient a greater sense of control, increases the likelihood that the food will be consumed, and may prompt the patient to ask questions about the particular diet or provide information about his or her personal food and nutrition history.
- Offer patients who do not like menu selections the daily "standby" or choices as alternatives. Be aware that "hospital food" is frequently used as a vehicle for patients to vent anger and frustration over their loss of control.
- Be aggressive about diet progressions. Keep in mind that advancing the diet as quickly as possible allows the patient to meet nutritional requirements sooner and increases patient satisfaction.
- Set the stage for a pleasant meal. Be sure trays are delivered promptly to ensure foods are at the proper temperatures. Adjust the lighting and make sure the patient is in an appropriate sitting position. Screen the patient from offensive sights and remove unpleasant odors from the room. Encourage family to visit at mealtime, if appropriate. Offer mouth care to improve appetite, if appropriate.
- Be positive. Refrain from negative comments about the food. Also be aware of what your body language is saying to the patient. A frown or raised eyebrows can speak volumes.
- Provide assistance when necessary. Encourage the patient to self-feed to the greatest extent possible. Some patients may benefit from minor help such as opening milk cartons or buttering bread; others may need to be completely fed. Monitor the patient's ability to self-feed and adjust the intensity of help accordingly.
- Gently motivate the patient to eat. Sometimes encouragement is all that is needed to get the patient to eat. For other patients, motivation comes from being made aware of the importance of food in the recovery process. Thinking of food as part of treatment instead of a social function may improve intake even when appetite is compromised.
- Identify eating problems. Patients who feel full quickly should be encouraged to eat the most nutritious items first (meat, milk) and save the less dense items for last (juice, soup, coffee). Patients who have difficulty chewing benefit from a mechanical soft diet. Determine if the patient would accept between-meal supplements and a bedtime snack to help maximize intake.

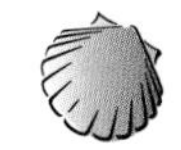

Milk-Based Supplements

Homemade milk-based supplements may be prepared "from scratch" or with the use of powdered commercial mixes; a few milk-based drinks come prepared and individually packaged. Milk-based drinks provide significant amounts of protein and calories, are palatable, and are relatively inexpensive. However, these drinks are not appropriate for patients with lactose intolerance (i.e., those unable to digest milk sugar) or for those who need complete nutritional support.

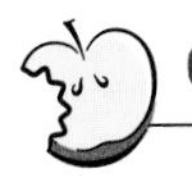

Quick Bite

Examples of commercial milk-based supplements

Forta Shake
Carnation Instant Breakfast
Boost (only regular Boost is made with milk protein)

Commercially Prepared Liquid Supplements

A wide variety of all-purpose, commercially prepared supplements are available that vary in composition, taste, and cost. They are quick and easy, consistent in quality, varied in flavor, and often available in grocery stores. Most are also suitable as tube feedings because they provide complete nutrition: Because they are generally sweet and flavored, they are primarily intended for oral use. Standard supplements usually provide 1.0 to 1.2 cal/mL, and 14% to 16% of the total calories are from protein. They are low in residue and lactose free. Variations of the standard formulas include high-protein, high-calorie, light, and added-fiber types.

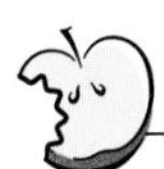

Quick Bite

Examples of routine oral supplements providing approximately 8 g of protein and 250 cal/8 oz
- Ensure
- NuBasics

High protein versions with 12 to 15 g protein/8 oz
- Ensure High Protein
- Boost High Protein

For both protein (approximately 14 g/8oz) and calories (approximately 360/8 oz)
- Ensure Plus
- Boost Plus

Supplements with fiber added (about 3 g/8 oz)
- Boost with Fiber
- Ensure with Fiber

Commercially Prepared Supplemental Foods

As an alternative to liquid supplements, manufacturers offer a variety of foods specially designed to provide a concentrated source of protein and calories.

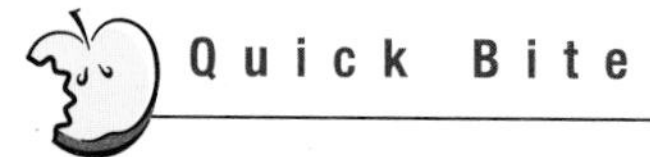

Types of supplemental foods

Bars Coffee creamer Pudding
Broth Gelatin Soup
Coffee

Modular Products

Modular products are a way of boosting nutrient intake without increasing volume. They are generally composed of a single nutrient, either carbohydrate (e.g., hydrolyzed cornstarch), protein (e.g., whey protein), or fat (e.g., medium-chain triglycerides [MCT oil]). Used individually or in combination, they increase nutrient density of foods or enteral formulas. For instance, a protein module may be added to a tube feeding to increase protein density without significantly affecting volume. Likewise, clients with chronic renal failure may receive carbohydrate-fortified mashed potatoes and juices to increase calorie intake without increasing protein content. Disadvantages of using modular products are quality control (calculation errors), bacterial contamination, higher costs than standard formulas, and possible nutrient imbalances when modules are added to tube feedings.

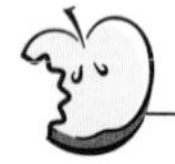

Quick Bite

Examples of carbohydrate modules
- Moducal
- Polycose

Examples of protein modules
- Casec
- ProMod

A fat module is
MCT oil

ENTERAL NUTRITION

Enteral Nutrition (EN): the delivery of nutrients by tube into the gastrointestinal tract; commonly known as tube feeding.

Enteral nutrition (EN) is a way of providing nutrition for patients who are unable to consume an adequate oral intake but have at least a partially functional GI tract that is accessible and safe to use. EN may augment an oral diet or may be the sole source of nutrition. Patients who have problems chewing and swallowing; have prolonged lack of appetite; have an obstruction, fistula, or altered motility in the upper gastrointestinal tract; are in a coma; or have very high nutrient requirements are candidates for a tube feeding. Although they are not routinely prescribed, tube feedings may be beneficial in cases of major trauma, acute or chronic liver failure, malabsorption syndromes, chemotherapy, or radiotherapy

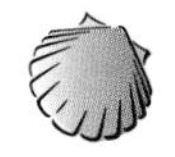

and as a transition between parenteral nutrition and an oral diet. Tube feedings are contraindicated when the gastrointestinal tract is nonfunctional as in gastric or intestinal obstruction, paralytic ileus, intractable vomiting, and severe diarrhea.

Tube feedings are significantly less costly than parenteral nutrition and provide the psychological benefit of a more "normal" intake than feeding by vein. Other long-held beliefs, such as that EN has fewer complication and better outcomes than parenteral nutrition, are being challenged. Recent comparative studies suggest that there is no significant difference in outcome between the two nutritional support methods and that it is more difficult to achieve full feeding rates with EN than with PN. Also, procedure-related complications may be slightly higher with EN than with PN.

Parenteral Nutrition (PN): the delivery of nutrients by vein.

Types of Formulas

There is a vast array of EN formulas available in ready-to-use or powdered mixes specially designed to meet the needs of virtually any patient. The most common way to categorize formulas is by the complexity of protein they contain. The two major types of formulas available are standard and hydrolyzed (Table 15.2).

Standard Formulas

Standard formulas, also known as polymeric or intact formulas, are made from whole proteins as found in foods. (e.g., milk, meat, eggs) or protein isolates. Because they contain complex molecules of protein, carbohydrate, and fat, standard formulas are intended for patients who have normal digestive and absorptive capacity. They are complete with regard to vitamins, minerals, and trace elements. Like oral supplements, standard tube feedings come in a wide variety such as standard, high protein, high calorie, and disease specific.

Standard Formulas: tube feeding formulas that contain whole molecules of protein; also known as intact or polymeric formulas.

Protein Isolates: semipurified, high-biologic-value proteins that have been extracted from milk, soybean, or eggs.

Career Connection

The use of artificial nutrition is not always clear-cut, especially in elderly or terminal patients. The number one priority is to honor the patient's wishes regarding the extent of medical care desired. Some ethical considerations include the following:

- Once the decision to forgo nutrition is made, the effects may be irreversible.
- Food and hydration are considered medical interventions. However, the decision to forgo "heroic" medical treatment does not include baseline nutrition support. "Do not resuscitate" does not mean "do not feed."
- Quality of life issues. Will food or nutrition improve what is left of the patient's life? Nutrition support for some may provide emotional comfort, ease anxiety, improve family interaction, or relieve fear of abandonment even if nutritional status does not improve.
- If death is imminent, will nutritional support be burdensome?
- If an oral therapeutic diet is used, can it liberalized? Some patients who religiously adhere to a therapeutic diet may not want to eat foods they normally avoid.

TABLE 15.2 A COMPARISON BETWEEN STANDARD AND HYDROLYZED ENTERAL FORMULAS

	Standard	Hydrolyzed
Cal/mL	Most are 1.0–1.2	1.0–1.5
Sources of:		
Protein	Casein hydrolysates	Hydrolyzed casein, whey, or soy protein; amino acids
Carbohydrate	Maltodextrin, sucrose, corn syrup solids	Maltodextrin, modified corn starch
Fat	Vegetable oil	Vegetable oil, MCT, fish oil
Macronutrient composition	Similar to oral diet	Many are higher in CHO and much lower in fat than usual mixed diet
Osmolality	Many are isotonic	Most are hypertonic
Residue	Most are low	Virtually residue-free
Fiber	Fiber-enriched formulas are available	Fiber-free
Cost	Relatively inexpensive	Relatively expensive

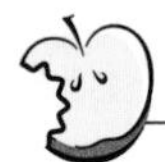

Quick Bite

Examples of routine standard formulas

Isocal
Nutren
Isosource Standard
Osmolite

Examples of high-calorie standard formulas

Deliver 2.0
Nutren 2.0
TwoCal HN

Hydrolyzed Formulas

Hydrolyzed: broken down.

Partially hydrolyzed formulas contain proteins that are partially digested into small peptides. The protein in completely hydrolyzed formulas, frequently referred to as elemental formulas, is in its simplest form: free amino acids. Hydrolyzed formulas also provide other nutrients in simpler forms that require little or no digestion. For instance, the fat content is very low and in the form of medium-chain triglycerides (MCT). Hydrolyzed formulas are intended for patients with impaired digestion or absorption such as people with inflammatory bowel disease, short-gut syndrome, cystic fibrosis, and pancreatic disorders.

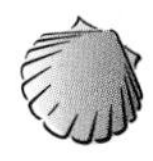

Additional Factors to Consider When Choosing a Formula

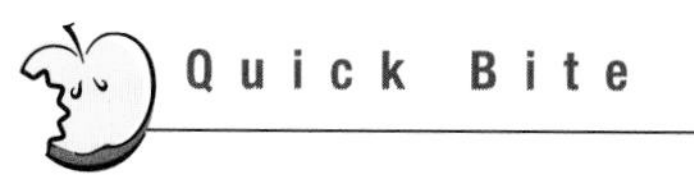

Examples of hydrolyzed formulas

Criticare HN
Reabilan
Vital HN
Vivonex T.E.N.

The first step in choosing a formula is to select either a standard or hydrolyzed formula based on the patient's ability to digest and absorb foodstuffs. Other characteristics of the formula to evaluate when choosing a formula are the nutrient density, osmolality, fiber and residue content, and the feeding equipment available.

Calorie Density

Routine formulas provide 1.0 to 1.2 cal/mL, whereas high calorie formulas provide 1.5 to 2.0 cal/mL. The calorie density of a product determines the volume of formula needed to meet the patient's estimated needs. For instance, a patient who needs 2000 calories can meet her or his calorie needs with 2000 mL of a 1.0 cal/mL formula. However, if that patient is volume- or fluid-restricted, a better option is 1000 mL of a 2.0 cal/mL formula. The following guidelines are useful for evaluating calorie density:

Calories/mL	Best for
0.5 cal/mL	Elevated fluid need
1.0 cal/mL	Volume limitations
2.0 cal/mL	Strict volume limitations

Although the Harris-Benedict equation is commonly used to calculate calorie requirements based on the patient's age, gender, height, weight, level of physiologic stress, and activity level, a short-cut method often yielding similar results with fewer calculations is to simply multiply the patient's weight in kilograms by

25 to 35 cal/kg for most adults
21 cal/kg for critically ill obese adults

Water Content

The water content of tube feedings varies with the caloric concentration and is generally as follows:

Calories/mL	mL of Water/Liter
1.0	850 mL
1.2–1.5	690–820 mL
1.5–2.0	690–720 mL

Adults in general need approximately 1 mL/cal consumed daily, or urine output + 500 mL/day. Patients with fever, vomiting, diarrhea, blood loss, draining fistulas, or burns have higher fluid requirements. Whether or not the patient needs additional water to meet fluid requirements depends on his or her medical status and how much fluid is given through the tube feeding and flushing.

When calculating volume, it is important to note the volume of formula required to obtain 100% of the recommended intake for vitamins and minerals. If the tube feeding is the patient's sole source of nutrition, the volume provided must furnish adequate levels of essential nutrients.

Protein Density

Protein density ranges from low to high. Low-protein formulas designed for patients with chronic renal failure may provide as little as 30 g protein/liter of formula. Conversely, the protein content of high nitrogen formulas ranges from 44 to 63 g protein/liter. "Routine" standard formulas provide 34 to 43 g protein/liter. Adding a protein module to a tube feeding can increase protein density without significantly impacting the volume of formula needed.

Healthy adults need 0.8 gm/kg of protein daily. Protein needs increase in response to surgery, stress, trauma, burns, and catabolic states. Patients with renal impairments need to restrict protein intake.

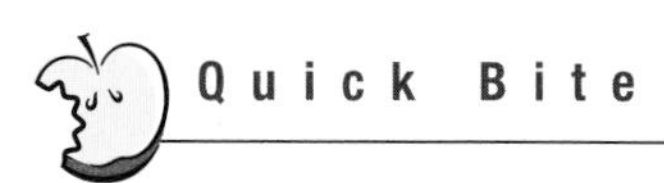

Examples of high-protein standard formulas (>16% of calories from protein) are

Isocal HN
Isosource HN
Osmolite HN
Promote

Other Nutrients

Although the concentrations of fat and carbohydrate also vary among formulas, they are usually not considered unless they are important because of disease. For instance, high-fat formulas are available for patients with respiratory disease and modified-fat formulas are designed for patients with malabsorption. A number of diabetic formulas are available, as are electrolyte-modified formulas for renal disease.

Osmolality

Osmolality: the measure of the number of particles in solution; expressed as milliosmoles per kilogram (mOsm/kg).

In enteral formulas, osmolality is determined by the concentration of sugars, amino acids, and electrolytes. Isotonic formulas have approximately the same osmolality as blood and are well tolerated. Generally, the more digested the protein, the greater the osmolality; thus, hydrolyzed formulas are higher in osmolality than standard formulas. For most people, osmolality does not impact tolerance. However, some patients develop diarrhea when a hypertonic formula is infused into the small intestines. Initiating the formula at a slow rate and advancing the rate gradually and slowly improves tolerance.

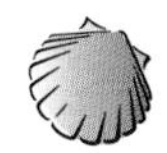

Isotonic: a formula that has approximately the same osmolality as blood, about 300 mOsm/kg.

Hypertonic: a formula with an osmolality greater than blood (>300 mOsm/kg).

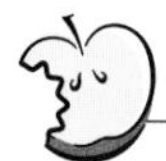

Quick Bite

Examples of disease-specific formulas

High fat, low carbohydrate for pulmonary patients
Respalor, Pulmocare, NutriVent

Modified fat, reduced carbohydrate, fiber-containing for patients with glucose intolerance
Choice DM, Diabetisource, Glucerna, Glytrol

Enriched with arginine and/or glutamine to for metabolically stressed patients
Alitraq, Perative

Protein and electrolyte restricted formulas for predialyzed patients with renal insufficiency
Suplena, Renalcal Diet

Formulas intended for patients on dialysis
Magnacal Renal, Nepro, NutriRenal

Altered amino acid composition formulas for hepatic patients
NutriHep, Hepatic Aid II

High protein with increased levels of certain vitamins and minerals to support wound healing
Protain XL, Replete

Fiber and Residue Content

Fiber: the group name for carbohydrates that are not digested in the human gastrointestinal tract.

Residue: what remains in the GI tract after digestion, namely fiber, undigested food, intestinal secretions, bacterial cell bodies, and cells shed from the intestinal lining.

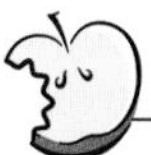

QUICK Bite

Compare the osmolality of selected enteral formulas to various oral supplements and common beverages.

Item	*Osmolality (mOsm/kg H_2O)*
Tube feedings	
Jevity	300
Nutren 1.0	315
Vital	500
Criticare HN	650
Oral Supplements	
Ensure	470
Boost Plus (vanilla)	670
Forta Shake (vanilla)	808
Common Beverages	
Apple juice	705
Cola	714
Cranberry juice	836
Ginger ale	565
Prune juice	1076
Ice cream	1150

Although they are not synonymous, the terms fiber and residue are frequently used interchangeably. Fiber stimulates peristalsis, increases stool bulk, and is degraded by gastrointestinal bacteria to short-chain fatty acids that promote repair and maintenance of the intestinal lining. Fiber combines with undigested food, intestinal secretions, and other cells to make residue. Fiber is one component of residue, but residue encompasses other substances as well.

The residue content of enteral formulas varies greatly. Hydrolyzed formulas are essentially residue free because they are completely absorbed. Most standard formulas are low in residue; because low-residue formulas are not likely to cause gas or abdominal distention, they are most suited as an initial feeding in patients who have been on bowel rest, in patients with certain gastrointestinal disorders, or in patients who have had gastrointestinal surgery.

Blenderized Formula: a type of standard formula made from blenderized whole foods.

Some standard formulas contain fiber. Blenderized formulas, a source of natural fiber, have approximately 4 g of fiber/L. The fiber content of fiber-enriched formulas is generally 10 to 14 g/L. Fiber-enriched formulas may help to normalize bowel function in people with constipation or diarrhea but may cause gas and bloating. Because fiber helps to maintain GI integrity, formulas with added fiber should be considered when EN is to be used for a long period.

Feeding Equipment

Viscosity: resistance to flow.

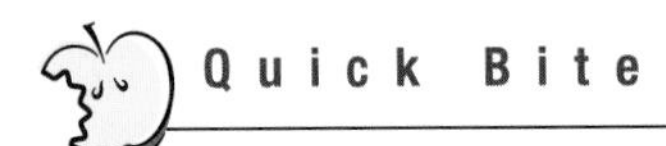

Examples of fiber enriched formulas

Fibersource
Jevity
Promote with Fiber
Relete with Fiber
Ultracal

Tubing size and pump availability may impact formula selection. Generally, high-fiber formulas have a high viscosity and require a large bore tube (8F or greater) to prevent clogging. Adding a modular product to a formula to increase the nutrient or calorie density may also necessitate the use of a larger tube. Hydrolyzed formulas have very low viscosity but should be delivered by pump to ensure controlled administration.

Feeding Routes

Transnasal Tubes: feeding tubes that extend from the nose to either the stomach or small intestine.

Ostomy: a surgically created opening (stoma) made to deliver feedings directly into the stomach or intestines.

The feeding route, or placement of the feeding tube, depends on the patient's medical status and the anticipated length of time the tube feeding will be used. Transnasal tubes, of which the nasogastric (NG) tube is the most common, are generally used for tube feedings of relatively short duration (i.e., less than 3 to 4 weeks). Ostomy feedings are preferred for permanent or long-term feedings because they can be hidden under clothing and eliminate irritation to the mucous membranes. Percutaneous endoscopic gastrostomy (PEG) tubes are placed with the aid of an endoscope. The correct placement of any feeding tube should be determined by radiographs of the chest taken before the first feeding is initiated. Table 15.3 summarizes the advantages and disadvantages of various feeding routes.

Delivery Methods

Formulas may be given intermittently or continuously over a period of 8 to 24 hours. The rates may be regulated either by a pump or by gravity drip. The type of delivery method to be used depends on the type and location of the feeding tube, the type of formula being administered, and the patient's tolerance.

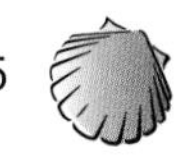

TABLE 15.3

ADVANTAGES AND DISADVANTAGES OF VARIOUS FEEDING ROUTES

Route	Indications	Advantages	Disadvantages
Nasogastric (NG)	Inability to safely and adequately consume oral intake Short-term feeding (<6 wk) with functional gastrointestinal tract	Easy to place and remove tube Uses stomach as reservoir Can use intermittent feedings Dumping syndrome less likely than with NI feedings	Contraindicated for clients at high risk for aspiration Potentially irritating to the nose and esophagus May be removed by uncooperative or confused patients Not appropriate for long-term use Unaesthetic for patient
Nasointestinal (NI)	Short-term feeding for patients at high risk of aspiration, delayed gastric emptying, or gastroesophageal reflux disease (GERD)	Less risk of aspiration, especially important for patients who have impaired gag or cough reflex, decreased consciousness, ventilator dependence, or a history of aspiration pneumonia	Increased risk of dumping syndrome Not appropriate for intermittent or bolus feedings Not appropriate for long-term use Unaesthetic for patient
Gastrostomy	For long-term use in patients with a functional gastrointestinal tract Frequently used for patients with impaired ability to swallow	Same advantages as NG, but more comfortable and aesthetic for patient Confirmation of tube placement easier Cannot be misplaced into the trachea	PEG insertion contraindicated for clients who cannot have an endoscopy Risk of aspiration pneumonia in clients with GERD Stoma care required Danger of peritonitis Potential for tube dislodgment
Jejunostomy	For long-term use in patients at high risk for aspiration pneumonia and in clients with altered gastrointestinal integrity above the jejunum For short-term use after gastrointestinal surgery	Low risk of aspiration No risk of misplacing tube into the trachea More comfortable and aesthetic for clients than transnasal tubes Because motility resumes more quickly in the intestines than in the stomach after gastrointestinal surgery, feedings can begin sooner than other feedings	Small-diameter tubes easily become clogged Peritonitis can occur from tube dislodgment Cannot be used for intermittent or bolus feedings Stoma care required

Intermittent Tube Feedings

Percutaneous Endoscopic Gastrostomy (PEG) Tubes: a feeding tube placed through an opening in the stomach made surgically or under local anesthesia with the aid of an endoscope.

Intermittent feedings are administered throughout the day in equal portions of 200 mL to 300 mL of formula over 30 to 60 minutes every 4 to 6 hours, usually by gravity drip. The number of feedings given per day depends on the total volume of feeding needed. Feedings may be spaced throughout an entire 24-hour period or may be scheduled only during waking hours to give patients time for uninterrupted sleep. Intermittent feedings are generally used for noncritical patients, home-tube feedings, and patients in rehabilitation. They offer the advantage of resembling a more normal pattern of intake and they allow the client more freedom of movement between feedings. Tolerance of intermittent feedings is optimized by infusing the formula at room temperature. To decrease the risk of aspiration, gastric residuals are checked before each feeding until tolerance is clearly established. Residuals should be less than 150 mL before each intermittent feeding; replace aspirate to reduce the loss of electrolytes and gastric juices.

Bolus Feedings

Intermittent Feedings: tube feedings administered in equal portions at selected intervals.

Bolus feedings are a variation of intermittent feedings. The formula is poured into the barrel of a large syringe attached to the feeding tube. A large volume of formula (500 mL maximum; usual volume is 250 to 400 mL) is delivered relatively quickly, usually in less than 15 minutes. These rapid feedings are given four to six times per day. They are used only for feedings into the stomach. Bolus feedings may be poorly tolerated and often cause *dumping syndrome:* nausea, diarrhea, glucosuria, distention, cramps, vomiting, and increased risk of aspiration.

Continuous Drip Method

Gastric Residuals: the volume of feeding remaining in the stomach from a previous feeding.

Bolus Feedings: rapid administration of a large volume of formula.

Continuous drip feedings are given at a constant rate over a 16- to 24-hour period to maximize tolerance and nutrient absorption. Infusion pumps are used to ensure consistent flow rates. This method is recommended for feeding of critically ill clients because it is associated with smaller residual volumes, lower risk for aspiration, a decrease in the severity of diarrhea, and a decrease in the hypermetabolic response to stress when compared to other delivery methods. Continuous feeding is also preferred for feedings delivered into the jejunum; it is frequently used to begin a feeding into the stomach (i.e., NG, gastrostomy, or PEG).

Continuous feedings should be interrupted every 4 hours so that water can be infused into the line to clear the tubing and hydrate the client. Gastric residuals are measured every 4 to 6 hours. If the volume of gastric residual exceeds the volume of formula given over the previous 2 hours, it may be necessary to reduce the rate of feeding.

Cyclic Feedings

A variation of continuous drip feedings, cyclic feedings deliver a constant rate of formula over 8 to 16 hours often during sleeping hours although extra care must be taken to keep the head of the bed continuously elevated more than 30° to avoid aspiration. Because there is "time off," the rate of infusion tends to be higher than for continu-

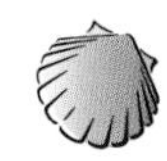

ous feedings. Cyclic feedings are usually well tolerated and are often used to maintain a reliable source of nutrition while transitioning from total EN to an oral intake or in noncritical, undernourished patients unable to meet their nutritional needs orally.

Initiating and Advancing the Feeding

Before initiating a feeding, tube placement is verified ideally by radiography and bowel sounds are confirmed to be present. Other common verification methods, such as aspirating gastric contents and pH testing, are less reliable. Elevate the patient's upper body to at least a 30° angle during the feeding and for at least 30 minutes afterward to reduce the risk of aspiration.

Regardless of the access route, tube feeding formulas are initiated at full strength. The previous practice of diluting hypertonic feedings has not been shown to improve tolerance, prolongs the period of inadequate nutrition support, and may increase the risk of bacterial contamination. Initiating feedings at full strength has not been found to cause tube feeding intolerance or diarrhea.

Although facility policies vary, initial feedings may begin at 10 to 40 mL/hour and advance by 10 to 20 mL/hour every 8 to 12 hours as tolerated until the desired rate is achieved. The commonly recommended maximum flow rate for gastric feedings is 125 mL/hr; higher volumes may increase the risk of aspiration. The maximum flow rate for small bowel feedings is determined by individual tolerance. Usually, rates of 140 to 160 mL/hr are well tolerated. Using a standard feeding progression schedule helps to ensure timely progression of feedings to the goal rate: the sooner the goal rate is achieved, the sooner the patient's nutritional needs are met.

Tolerance may be a problem for patients who are malnourished, who are under severe stress, who have not eaten in a long time, or who are given hypertonic formulas. Starting the feeding at the lower end of the recommended range and progressing slowly generally improves tolerance.

Tolerance and Safety Issues

Tolerance and safety can be maximized by careful attention to details.

Avoiding Bacterial Contamination

Improper handling of formulas increases the risk of bacterial contamination, which causes what is commonly known as *food poisoning*. In a population of patients who are malnourished and, therefore, immunologically compromised, food poisoning is a serious tube feeding complication. To reduce the risk of bacterial contamination, closed feeding systems are recommended. Precautions to take when open feeding systems are used include

Closed Feeding System: a system whereby the formula comes in a container made to be attached to the tubing for administration.

- Use clean equipment.
- Wash hands thoroughly before handling the formula.
- Clean the top of the formula can before opening.
- Label unemptied cans with the date and time of opening.

Open Feeding System: a system whereby the formula must be poured from its original container into a feeding container to which the tubing connects for formula administration.

- Cover opened cans; store mixed or diluted formulas in clean containers.
- Refrigerate unused formula promptly.
- Discard unlabeled formula and all opened cans within 24 hours.
- Rinse the feeding container and extension tubing with water before adding new formula.
- Never add a supply of new formula to old formula.
- Flush the tube with water before and after each use.
- Hang feeding solutions for less than 6 hours.
- Change the feeding container and extension tubing every 24 hours.

Preventing Aspiration

Aspiration is one of the most dangerous complications of EN. Patients with inhibited cough reflex related to debilitation, unconsciousness, or pulmonary complications are at high risk for aspiration as are those with delayed gastric emptying or gastroesophageal reflux. Preventative measures to avoid aspiration are to

- Confirm proper placement of the feeding tube by radiograph prior to initiating a feeding so that formula is not mistakenly infused into the lungs.
- Elevate the head of the bed 30 to 45° during the feeding and for approximately 1 hour afterwards to help maintain normal functioning of the lower esophageal sphincter.
- Monitor gastric residuals to identify delayed gastric emptying, which places the patient at risk for aspiration. A continuous drip method of deliver may be necessary to control gastric residuals.
- Use the smallest diameter feeding tube possible.
- Consider a nasointestinal or jejunostomy feeding for patients with impaired cough reflex.

Maintaining Tube Patency

Patency: openness.

Periodic flushing of the tube with water helps to ensure patency. The often cited standard for maintaining patency is to flush with

- 15 to 30 mL of water before and after medications
- 20 to 60 mL of water every 4 hours during continuous feedings
- 20 to 60 mL of water after each intermittent feeding
- 20 to 60 mL of water any time the feeding is interrupted

If the tube becomes clogged, a 60 mL syringe containing 30 to 60 mL of warm water is recommended.

Giving Medications by Tube

Although many medications are frequently given through feeding tubes to patients who are unable to swallow, they should never be given while a feeding is being infused. Some drugs become ineffective if added directly to the enteral formula; also, adding drugs to the formula may result in a clogged tube. It is important to stop the feeding

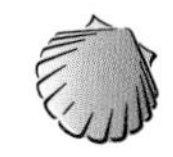

before administering drugs and to make sure the tube is flushed with 15 to 30 mL of water before and after the drug is given. If more than one drug is given, flush the tube between doses with 5 mL of water.

Other drug considerations include the following:

- Drugs absorbed from the stomach should never be given through a nasointestinal tube.
- The liquid form of a medication diluted with 30 mL of water should be used for feeding tube administration. If there is no alternative, a drug can be crushed to a fine powder and mixed with water before it is administered. Slow-release drugs should never be crushed.
- Dilute highly viscous and hyperosmolar liquid medications with 10 to 30 mL of water before administering.
- Drugs should be given orally whenever possible.
- Tube feeding may need to be temporarily stopped to permit drug administration on an empty stomach or to avoid drug–nutrient interaction. Some experts recommend stopping a continuous feeding for 15 minutes before and after the delivery of the medication.

Monitoring

Close monitoring is essential to ensure that the patient is tolerating the EN regimen and that it is adequately meeting the patient's needs. In the hospitalized patient, monitor

- Daily weight to detect fluid shifts.
- Daily intake and output.
- Gastric residuals every 4 hours. Return all aspiration secretions to the stomach because they contain nutrients, electrolytes, and digestive enzymes.
- The character and frequency of bowel movements.
- For signs and symptoms of intolerance: vomiting, nausea, diarrhea, constipation.
- Daily electrolyte levels, BUN, and creatinine until goal rate is achieved; thereafter 2 to 3 times/week. Minerals and a weekly blood count may be ordered.
- Tube site for placement, infection.

Transition to Oral Diet

The goal of diet intervention during the transition period between enteral nutrition and an oral diet is to ensure an adequate nutritional intake while promoting an oral diet. To begin the transition process, the tube feeding should be stopped for 1 hour before each meal. Gradually increase meal frequency until six small oral feedings are accepted. Actual intake should be recorded and evaluated daily. When oral calorie intake consistently includes 500 to 750 cal/day, tube feedings may be given only during the night. When the client consistently consumes two thirds of protein and calorie needs orally for 3 to 5 days, the tube feeding may be totally discontinued.

NURSING PROCESS

The following care plan assumes that the health care team assessed the patient's need for tube feeding and the appropriate order was written to meet the patient's nutritional requirements and goals.

The indicated nursing diagnosis is an example of only one potential problem associated with tube feedings. Other potential problems and their nursing management appear in Box 15.1.

Assessment

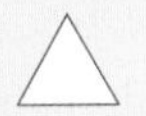

Because most patients who are receiving tube feedings have had feeding difficulties or medical problems that place them at increased risk, initial and periodic nutritional assessments are vital to the success of a tube feeding.

Obtain clinical data:

Current nutrition prescription (name of formula, amount, frequency, volume per 24 hours)
Current height, weight, body mass index (BMI), percentage of usual weight
Laboratory values especially serum albumin, hemoglobin, hematocrit, glucose, electrolytes, and any other abnormal values for their nutritional significance
Clinical signs and symptoms: bowel function, aspiration risk, blood pressure, lactose intolerance, presence of steatorrhea, difficulty swallowing, clinical signs of malnutrition, signs of dehydration or fluid overload
Fluid status: ability to consume oral liquids, intake and output records

Interview client to assess:

Knowledge, willingness, and readiness to learn tube-feeding regimen
Ability to perform activities of daily living
Physical complaints associated with oral food intake or tube feeding such as fatigue, constipation, diarrhea, nausea, vomiting, early satiety, cramping, or bloating
Psychosocial and economic issues especially for patients who are candidates for home enteral nutrition: living situation (availability of running water, electricity, refrigeration), cooking and storage facilities, employment, social support system, and financial status

Nursing Diagnosis

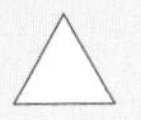

Altered Nutrition: Less Than Body Requirements, related to diarrhea secondary to tube feeding.

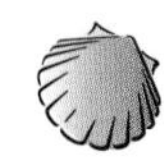

BOX 15.1

TROUBLE-SHOOTING FOR NUTRITION-RELATED PROBLEMS IN TUBE-FED PATIENTS

Potential Problem	Rationale	Nursing Interventions and Considerations
Nausea (Discontinue the feeding. Administer antiemetics if ordered by the physician.)	Malplacement of feeding tube	Check the position of the tube.
	Feeding rate too rapid	Slow the rate of feeding; switch to a continuous drip method of delivery.
	Volume of formula too great → delayed gastric emptying	Check gastric residual and notify the physician if >100 mL. Reduce the volume, then increase gradually. If distention is contributing to nausea, encourage ambulation.
	Feeding too soon after intubation	Allow approximately 1 h between intubation and the first feeding.
	Anxiety	Explain the procedures to the client and encourage questions. Allow client to verbalize his or her feelings; provide emotional support.
	Intolerance to a specific formula, especially high-fat formulas	Switch to a different formula.
Distention and bloating	High fat content of formula	Switch to lower-fat formula.
	Decrease in gastrointestinal function, especially among critically ill clients	Check for active bowel sounds; switch to a hydrolyzed formula if bowel sounds are hypoactive.
	Diarrhea	See Nursing Process section of text.
Dehydration	Excessive protein intake → compensatory increase in urine output to excrete nitrogenous wastes	Switch to a formula with less protein. Increase water intake, if possible.
	Inadequate fluid intake	Provide more additional water.

(box continues on page 442)

BOX 15.1 (continued)

TROUBLE-SHOOTING FOR NUTRITION-RELATED PROBLEMS IN TUBE-FED PATIENTS

Potential Problem	Rationale	Nursing Interventions and Considerations
	Glycosuria (glucose in urine)	Test for glucose in the urine; notify physician of glucosuria of 3+ or 4+. Administer insulin if ordered by physician. Switch to a continuous drip method to avoid giving a high-carbohydrate load with each feeding.
Fluid overload	Excessive use of water to flush tube	Use only 30–50 mL of water to rinse tubing after each feeding.
	Formula too dilute	Check formula preparation for proper dilution.
Constipation	Low residue content of formula	Increase residue content if appropriate (i.e., change to a formula with added fiber or increase fruits and vegetables in a blenderized diet).
	Inactivity	Encourage ambulation as much as possible.
	Dehydration	Monitor intake and output. Add free water if intake is not greater than output by 500 to 1000 mL.
	Obstruction	Stop feeding and notify physician.
Gastric rupture	Dangerous retention of feeding in the stomach related to gastric atony or obstruction	Check for residual before beginning each feeding. Observe for signs of impending gastric rupture: distention, epigastric and upper quadrant pain, nausea, a large residual. If observed, discontinue feeding immediately and notify the physician.

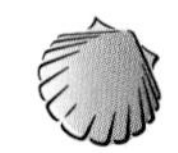

BOX 15.1 (continued)

TROUBLE-SHOOTING FOR NUTRITION-RELATED PROBLEMS IN TUBE-FED PATIENTS

Potential Problem	Rationale	Nursing Interventions and Considerations
Clogged tube	Feeding heated formulas Improper cleaning of tube	Do not heat formula. Replace the feeding tube and bag every 12–24 h. Flush the tube before and after each infusion (regardless of method) with 30–50 mL of water. If flushing fails to remove clog, the tube must be removed and replaced. High-viscosity formulas (i.e., blenderized tube feedings or commercial formulas that provide 1.5–2 cal/mL) should be infused by pump and possibly through a large-bore feeding tube to prevent clogging. If possible, consider switching to a less calorically dense formula. Because it is desirable to use the smallest size tube, viscous formulas may be delivered by a pump to help prevent clogging.
Anxiety	Deprivation of food → lack of sensory, social, and cultural satisfaction from eating	Allow oral intake of food that the client requests, if possible. If oral intake is contraindicated, allow the client to chew his or her favorite food without swallowing. If possible, liquefy and add the client's favorite food to the tube feeding.

(box continues on page 444)

BOX 15.1 (continued)

TROUBLE-SHOOTING FOR NUTRITION-RELATED PROBLEMS IN TUBE-FED PATIENTS

Potential Problem	Rationale	Nursing Interventions and Considerations
		Encourage the client to leave the room when others are eating and find other enjoyable activities. Encourage client and family to view tube feeding as another way of eating, rather than a form of treatment.
	Altered body image	Encourage client to verbalize his or her feelings. Stress positive aspects of tube feeding.
	Loss of control; fear	Encourage client to become involved in preparation and administration of the formula, if possible. Inform client of problems that may occur and how to prevent or cope with them. Encourage socialization with other well-adapted tube-fed clients.
	Limited mobility	Encourage normal activity. Control gastrointestinal symptoms, such as diarrhea, nausea, vomiting, and constipation, that interfere with normal activity.
	Discomfort related to tube or formula intolerance	Observe for intolerances; alleviate with appropriate interventions. Be sure to inspect and properly care for the tube exit site to avoid potential complications.

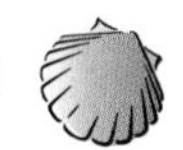

BOX 15.1 (continued)

TROUBLE-SHOOTING FOR NUTRITION-RELATED PROBLEMS IN TUBE-FED PATIENTS

Potential Problem	Rationale	Nursing Interventions and Considerations
Dry mouth	Irritation of the mucous membranes related to lack of oral intake	Encourage good oral hygiene to alleviate soreness and dryness: mouthwash, warm water rinses, regular brushing. Apply petroleum jelly to the lips to prevent cracking. Allow ice chips, sugarless gum, and hard candies, if possible, to stimulate salivation.
	Breathing through the mouth	Encourage client to breathe through the nose as much as possible.

Planning and Implementation

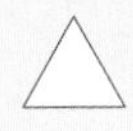

Although properly administered tube feedings do not cause diarrhea, diarrhea frequently develops in tube-fed clients. Clients fed low-residue formulas cannot be expected to have firm stools; rather their stools are likely to be pasty or gruel-like. However, if it is established that the client is truly having diarrhea, investigate the probable cause, which could be

- **Infusion of formula that is cold.** Give canned formulas at room temperature. Warm refrigerated formulas to room temperature in a basin of warm water.
- **Bacterially contaminated formula.** Handwashing and strict sanitation are required for formula preparation. Equipment and utensils used in preparation should be washed in an automatic dishwasher or cleaned with hot, soapy water; rinsed thoroughly in boiling water; and dried upside down. Practice proper techniques for handling formula (see previous discussion).
- **Lactose intolerance,** if milk-based formula is used. Switch to a lactose-free formula.

(continued)

- **Feeding rate too rapid.** Adhere to facility protocol when initiating and advancing tube feedings. For existing feedings, decrease the rate to the level tolerated then advance the feeding at a rate of half the original increment (e.g., by 12 instead of 25 mL/hour).
- **Volume of formula too great.** Feed smaller volumes of formula at more frequent intervals or switch to a continuous drip method of feeding. Consider a high-calorie formula if problem persists.
- **Dumping syndrome related to hypertonic formula.** Decrease the feeding rate to a level tolerated by the client, then gradually increase as tolerated. Use the continuous drip method. Switch to an isotonic formula, if possible.
- **Nasogastric feeding tube misplaced into the duodenum, causing dumping syndrome.** Check the position of the tube before administering the formula.
- **Low serum albumin** causing decreased oncotic pressure, which increases water within the bowel resulting in diarrhea. A low serum albumin concentration, which may indicate malnutrition, may also be accompanied by a decrease in intestinal border enzymes (protein molecules) and/or a decrease or flattening of the microvilli lining the intestinal tract, both of which lead to diarrhea.
- **Side effect of antibiotics or other drugs.** The overgrowth of certain strains of intestinal flora not affected by antibiotics is believed to cause diarrhea. These flora digest formula, producing excess gas and acid and resulting in diarrhea. Antibiotic-associated diarrhea may also be related to a superinfection with *Clostridium difficile* or *Staphylococcus aureus.* Medications that may produce diarrhea include magnesium-containing antacids, lactulose, histamine-blocking agents (e.g., cimetidine), cardiac medications (e.g., digoxin), electrolyte supplements (e.g., potassium chloride), stool softeners, laxatives, and chemotherapy. Investigate possible alternatives; administer antidiarrheals as ordered.

Client Goals

The client will:

Attain/maintain “healthy” body weight.

Receive ___ calories in ___ mL/day of ___ (product used), as ordered.

Be free of any signs or symptoms of diarrhea or other side effects.

Maintain adequate fluid status.

Nursing Interventions

Nutrition Therapy

Implement appropriate interventions for diarrhea based on probable cause.

Reduce rate of administration to highest level tolerated by patient. After 8 to 12 hours, advance feeding slowly and observe tolerance. Gradually attain desired rate as ordered.

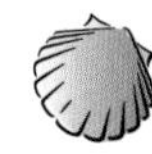

Provide supplemental water as needed based on input and output records and serum sodium concentration, blood urea nitrogen, hematocrit, and urine specific gravity.

Encourage oral intake, if appropriate.

Client Teaching

Instruct the client:

On the importance of tube feedings when oral intake is inadequate or impossible

On the signs and symptoms of intolerance of tube feeding and to alert the nurse if any problems arise

Not to adjust the flow rate unless otherwise instructed

When home enteral nutrition is indicated, discharge teaching should encompass formula preparation, administration, and monitoring as well as the rationales and interventions for tube feeding complications.

Evaluation

The client:

Attains/maintains "healthy" body weight

Receives ___ calories in ___ mL/day of ___ (product used), as ordered

Is free of signs and symptoms of diarrhea and other side effects

Maintains normal fluid status

PARENTERAL NUTRITION

Parenteral nutrition (PN) delivers nutrients directly into the bloodstream, thereby bypassing the gastrointestinal tract. It is used when a patient physically or psychologically cannot consume enough nutrients orally or enterally or when alteration in gastrointestinal function precludes oral and enteral feedings. Indications for use include a nonfunctional GI tract related to obstruction, intractable vomiting or diarrhea, short bowel syndrome, or paralytic ileus. PN may be used pre-operatively to replete patients with severe malnutrition who have been NPO for at least 1 week. PN is contraindicated when there is no central venous access, when EN is a viable option, and for terminal patients.

Depending on the patient's nutritional requirements and anticipated length of need, parenteral nutrition is either administered peripherally (PPN) or centrally (TPN). The basic difference between the two types is the concentration of the solutions infused.

Peripheral Parenteral Nutrition

PPN delivers complete but limited nutrition. Solutions infused into peripheral veins must be isotonic (i.e., they must have low concentrations of dextrose and amino acids) to prevent phlebitis and increased risk of thrombus formation. The final concentration of the solution cannot exceed 10% dextrose and 5% amino acids; 3 L of this 10% dextrose and 5% amino acid solution provide only 1620 calories. Additional lipids contribute the largest portion of calories (50 to 60%) because they are fairly isotonic and tolerated in a peripheral vein. Vitamins, electrolytes, and trace elements are added.

Because the caloric and nutritional value of PPN is limited, it is best suited for patients who need short-term nutritional support but do not require more than 2000 to 2500 cal/day. It is also used when PN is needed but central access is not available and when PN is needed for less than 7 days. Sometimes PPN is used to supplement an oral diet or tube feeding or as a transition from TPN to an enteral intake.

PPN is not adequate for patients who have increased nutritional requirements or who need more than 2500 cal/day, and it is contraindicated in patients with hypertriglyceridemia or volume intolerance (e.g., renal failure, liver failure, congestive heart failure). PPN should not be used when EN is a viable alternative.

Central Total Parenteral Nutrition (TPN)

Central TPN: the infusion into a central vein of a nutritional solution that meets nutrient needs.

Central TPN infuses a hypertonic, nutritionally complete solution through a large-diameter central vein so that it can be quickly diluted. TPN is used when nutritional requirements are high and anticipated length of need is relatively long. For instance, TPN may be used in patients who are being treated aggressively for cancer, and in those with trauma, extensive burns, multiple fractures, sepsis, or bone marrow transplantation. It is lifesaving in patients with gut failure such as those with GI obstruction, peritonitis, malabsorption, enterocutaneous fistulas, chronic vomiting, chronic diarrhea, prolonged paralytic ileus, radiation enteritis, extensive small bowel resection, and severe acute pancreatitis. Although TPN is beneficial in the treatment of malnutrition, it does not cure all illnesses.

Bacterial Translocation: the movement of intestinal bacteria from the gut into lymph nodes and the bloodstream.

Animal studies show that using TPN (i.e., not using the gut) causes significant atrophy of the intestinal mucosa within the first few days. It was theorized that the same is true in people and that atrophied intestinal mucosa allow intestinal bacteria to permeate the bowel wall and infect lymph nodes and blood, causing sepsis and multisystem organ failure in critically ill patients. Studies suggested that providing EN prevented bacterial translocation and sepsis and resulted in lower morbidity and mortality than TPN. However, there is little evidence in humans that TPN and bowel rest cause intestinal mucosa atrophy. And although bacterial translocation does occur, especially in patients with intestinal obstruction, the incidence does not differ between EN and TPN.

Because TPN is expensive, requires constant monitoring, and has potential infectious, metabolic, and mechanical complications (Box 15.2), it should be used only when an enteral intake is inadequate or contraindicated and when prolonged nutritional support is needed. Likewise, TPN should be discontinued as soon as possible. Gradual weaning to enteral nutrition or oral feedings is required to prevent metabolic complications and nutritional inadequacies. TPN is never an emergency procedure and is always accompanied by potential risks.

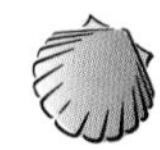

BOX 15.2

POTENTIAL COMPLICATIONS OF TOTAL PARENTERAL NUTRITION

Infection and Sepsis Related to

Catheter contamination during insertion
Long-term indwelling catheter
Catheter seeding from bloodborne or distant infection
Contaminated solution

Metabolic Complications

Dehydration; hypovolemia
Bone demineralization
Hyperglycemia
Rebound hypoglycemia
Hyperosmolar, hyperglycemic, nonketotic coma
Azotemia
Electrolyte disturbances
- Hypocalcemia
- Hypophosphatemia, hyperphosphatemia
- Hypokalemia
- Hypomagnesemia

High serum ammonia levels
Deficiencies of
- Essential fatty acids
- Trace elements
- Vitamins and minerals

Altered acid–base balance
Elevated liver enzymes
Fluid overload

Mechanical Complications Related to Catheterization

Catheter misplacement
Hemothorax (blood in the chest)
Pneumothorax (air or gas in the chest)
Hydrothorax (fluid in the chest)
Hemomediastinum (blood in the mediastinal spaces)
Subcutaneous emphysema
Hematoma
Arterial puncture
Myocardial perforation
Catheter embolism
Cardiac dysrhythmia
Air embolism
Endocarditis
Nerve damage at the insertion site
Laceration of lymphatic duct
Chylothorax
Lymphatic fistula
Thrombosis

Composition

Parenteral nutrition solutions include dextrose, amino acids, lipid emulsion, electrolytes, vitamins, and trace elements in sterile water. The actual composition of the parenteral solution depends on the site of infusion and the patient's fluid and nutrient requirements. Because there are standard concentrations of protein, carbohydrate, and fat in standard volumes, individualization of parenteral solutions is somewhat limited. The usual fluid volume given to adults over a 24-hour period is 1.5 to 3 L.

Carbohydrate

Dextrose: a form of glucose that contains water; dextrose provides 3.4 cal/g, not 4.0 cal/g like glucose.

Refeeding Syndrome: a potentially fatal complication that occurs from an abrupt change from a catabolic state to an anabolic state and an increase in insulin caused by a dramatic increase in calories.

The carbohydrate in parenteral solutions is dextrose. It is available in concentrations ranging from 5% in peripheral solutions to final concentrations of about 70% in total parenteral solutions. It is recommended that dextrose infusion not exceed 4 to 5 mg/kg/minute to prevent hyperglycemia and other complications. For instance, hyperglycemia from excess dextrose and calories is associated with impaired immunity, decreased GI motility, respiratory acidosis, and the deposition of fat in the liver.

Overfeeding also increases the risk of sepsis and of refeeding syndrome in previously catabolic patients. A major manifestation of refeeding syndrome is hypophosphatemia, which may cause anorexia, bone pain, dizziness, muscle weakness, respiratory failure, and cardiac decompensation. Other potential metabolic abnormalities include alterations in sodium balance, possibly leading to congestive heart failure; hypokalemia and arrhythmias as potassium shifts into cells; hypomagnesemia, which can lead to cardiac depression, arrhythmias, tetany, and seizures; fluid intolerance leading to fluid retention and weight gain; and thiamin deficiency due to increased carbohydrate metabolism. It is better to underfeed during critical illness (e.g., less than or equal to 30 cal/kg) rather than overfeed (more than 30 to 35 cal/kg).

Protein

Protein is provided as a solution of crystalline essential and nonessential amino acids ranging in concentration from 3% to 15% of the solution. The amino acid content of PPN typically ranges from 3 to 5%. Amino acids provide 4 cal/gm and should provide 10 to 20% of total calorie intake.

The quantity of amino acids provided depends on the patient's estimated requirements and hepatic and renal function. The suggested limit for protein intake in critically ill patients is 1.2 to 1.5 g/kg; giving higher amounts has not been shown to improve nitrogen accretion and can burden the kidneys. Although specially modified amino acid solutions are available for renal failure and liver failure, their use is controversial because efficacy has not been proven.

Fat

Lipid emulsions, made from safflower and soybean oil with egg phospholipid as an emulsifier, are isotonic. They are available in 10%, 20%, and 30% concentrations, sup-

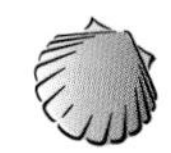

ply 1.1, 2.0, and 3.0 cal/mL, respectively. Lipids are a significant source of calories and so are useful when volume must be restricted or when dextrose must be lowered because of persistent hyperglycemia. Lipids are necessary to correct or prevent fatty acid deficiency; generally, 500 mL of a 10% emulsion given 2 times/week or 500 mL of a 20% emulsion given weekly is adequate to meet essential fatty acid requirement. Because lipids have the potential to impair immune system functioning, fat may be limited to 1 g/kg/day or less than 30% of total calories. Intravenous fat is contraindicated for patients with abnormal lipid metabolism such as hyperlipidemia, severe liver disease, lipid nephrosis, or hypertriglyceridemia-induced pancreatitis. Patients with severe egg allergies may not tolerate lipids because the phospholipids contained in the fat emulsion come from eggs.

Electrolytes, Vitamins, and Trace Elements

Total Nutrient Admixture (TNA): parenteral solutions that contain all nutrients including lipids; also called 3-in-1 admixtures.

The quantity of electrolytes provided is based on the patient's blood chemistry values and physical assessment findings. The electrolyte content can potentially be adjusted three times per day when a 1-L bag is administered over 8 hours. However, total nutrient admixture (TNA) bags may hold a 24-hour quantity of total parenteral nutrition (TPN) solution, which limits flexibility in changing the composition but reduces the risk of contamination.

Parenteral multivitamins, minerals, and trace element preparations containing amounts of nutrients as recommended by the American Medical Association Nutrition Advisory Group are commercially available. Single entity products are also available and may be given to meet increased needs related to illness (e.g., additional zinc may be needed in patients with diarrhea) or because they are not routinely added to PN solutions (e.g., iodine).

Medications

Medications are sometimes added to intravenous solutions by the pharmacist or infused into them through a separate port. Patients receiving TPN may have insulin ordered to help control serum glucose; this intervention is often necessary because of the high glucose concentration of the solution. Heparin may be added to reduce fibrin buildup on the catheter tip. In general, medications should not be added to TPN solutions because of the potential incompatibilities of the medication and nutrients in the solution.

Administration

Before parenteral nutrition begins, the nurse reviews the patient's weight, BMI, nutritional status, diagnosis, and current laboratory data. The patient's educational needs are also assessed.

Strict aseptic procedures are maintained in all techniques to reduce the risk of infection.

Initially TPN is infused slowly (i.e., 1 L in the first 24 hours) to give the body time to adapt to the high concentration of glucose and the hyperosmolality of the solution. Continuous drip by pump infusion is needed to maintain a slow, constant flow rate. After the first 24 hours, the rate of delivery is gradually increased by 1 L/day until the optimal volume is achieved.

Because rapid changes in the infusion rate can cause severe hyperglycemia or hypoglycemia and the potential for coma, convulsions, or death, rate changes must be made incrementally. If the rate of delivery falls behind or speeds up, the drip rate is adjusted to the correct hourly rate only; no attempts are made to "catch up" to the ordered volume.

Cyclic TPN

Cyclic TPN: infusing TPN at a constant rate for 8 to 12 hours/day.

Cyclic TPN is suited for patients receiving TPN at home and when TPN is needed to support an inadequate oral intake. Cyclic TPN allows serum glucose and insulin levels to drop during the periods when TPN is not infused, thus promoting fat and glycogen mobilization and a more normal pattern of intake. When it is given during the night, cyclic TPN frees the patient to participate in normal activities during the day.

During the switch from continuous to cyclic TPN, the infusion time is gradually decreased by several hours each day, as ordered, and assessment is ongoing for signs of glucose intolerance. To give the pancreas time to adjust to the decreasing glucose load, the infusion rate is tapered near the end of each cycle. For instance, during the last hour of infusion the rate may be reduced by one-half to prevent rebound hypoglycemia.

Nursing Management

Once parenteral nutrition solutions are prepared, they must be used immediately or refrigerated. It is recommended that solutions be removed from the refrigerator 1 hour before infusion because they must reach approximately room temperature before they are hung. Once hung, the solution is infused or discarded within 24 hours.

Cracking: the appearance of a layer of fat on top or oily globules in the solution.

Inspect the solution for "cracking," which may occur in TNA mixtures if the calcium or phosphorus content is relatively high or if salt-poor albumin has been added. A "cracked" solution cannot be infused; notify the pharmacy and the physician, who may need to adjust the original TPN order to eliminate or reduce the offending component.

Monitor the flow rate to avoid complications and ensure adequate intake. Solutions that are infused too rapidly can cause hyperosmolar diuresis, leading to seizures, coma, and even death; solutions that are administered too slowly prevent an optimal nutritional intake.

Observe for side effects of parenteral nutrition: weight gain greater than 1 kg/day (indicative of fluid overload), elevated temperature or sepsis, high blood glucose levels, shortness of breath; tightness of chest, anemia, nausea and vomiting, jaundice, allergy to protein content of the solutions, pneumothorax, or cardiac arrhythmias.

Close monitoring of laboratory data and clinical signs is necessary to prevent the development of nutrient deficiencies or toxicities.

 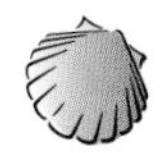

Some patients may feel hungry while receiving TPN and should be allowed to eat, if possible. If oral intake is contraindicated, give mouth care.

Begin weaning the client from TPN to an enteral or oral intake as soon as possible to reduce the risk of bacterial translocation and sepsis. Patients must be weaned off TPN gradually to prevent rebound hypoglycemia. TPN can be discontinued when enteral intake (an oral diet, tube feeding, or combination of the two) provides at least 60% of estimated calorie requirements.

Patients who have permanently nonfunctional gastrointestinal tracts require TPN indefinitely. For home TPN to be successful, clients and their families must be physically and emotionally prepared. Intensive counseling focuses on preparation and administration of the solution, catheter and equipment care, and assessment skills as well as the psychological impact of permanent TPN.

Client and Family Teaching

Instruct the client

- On the importance of TPN when oral or enteral intake is inadequate or impossible
- To alert the nurse if any problems arise
- Not to adjust the flow rate unless otherwise instructed

When home TPN is indicated, discharge teaching includes aseptic preparation and administration techniques, criteria to monitor signs and symptoms of system failure, when to call the doctor, when to call the dietitian, and when to call the pharmacist.

Encourage the client to discuss anxiety, anger, or adaptation to TPN and oral deprivation.

How Do You Respond?

Is it good practice to color tube feedings? Some facilities color tube feedings with blue food dye so that pulmonary secretions can be monitored for aspirated formula. Although this practice can help *detect* aspirate, it does not *protect* against aspiration. In addition, reports of blue dye absorption from enteral feedings in patients with sepsis and other critical illnesses are increasing. The presence of blue and green skin and urine and discolored serum has been linked with death. Instead of tinting formula with blue dye, a better approach is to test pulmonary secretions using a glucose dipstick. Unless they are bloody, pulmonary secretions normally do not contain glucose, whereas enteral formulas do.

My patient claims he can taste his tube feeding. Can he? Except for patients who experience gastric reflux, patients cannot truly taste a tube feeding. However, the appearance and aroma of the formula may influence the patient's acceptance and perception of palatability. If the formula's appearance is offensive, cover the feeding reservoir or remove it from the patient's field of vision, if possible.

▲ Focus on Critical Thinking

Respond to the following statements:

1. The regular diet in the hospital should be made healthier, that is, lower in fat, saturated fat, cholesterol, and sodium to illustrate the concepts of healthy eating.
2. It is better to overfeed than underfeed a malnourished patient.
3. After tolerance to an enteral feeding is established, nutritional problems and tube feeding complications are not likely to develop.
4. Neither enteral nutrition nor parenteral nutrition is appropriate for terminally ill patients.

Key Concepts

- Hospital food is intended to prevent nutrient deficiencies, not to prevent chronic disease. Regular diets may not be consistent with *Dietary Guidelines for Americans,* which recommends limiting intakes of fat, saturated fat, cholesterol, and sodium.
- Depending on the needs of the individual patient, oral diets may be modified in their consistency or in their concentration of certain nutrients or dietary components. Combination diets (e.g., a low-sodium, soft diet) are often ordered.
- Patients with altered appetites or increased needs may benefit from supplements given with or between meals. A variety of supplements are available (clear liquid, milk-based, routine, modified routine, puddings, and bars); they vary in nutritional composition, cost, and taste.
- Enteral nutrition commonly means tube feedings. Tube feedings are preferred to parenteral nutrition whenever the gastrointestinal tract is at least partially functional, accessible, and safe to use. Tube feedings may be delivered through transnasal tubes or through ostomy sites to the gastrointestinal tract.
- The choice of tube feeding method depends on the patient's digestive and absorptive capacities, where the feeding is to be infused, the size of the feeding tube, and the patient's nutritional needs, present and past medical history, and tolerance.
- Standard tube feeding formulas require normal digestion; they contain intact molecules of protein, carbohydrate, and fat. Intact formulas come in several varieties: high-protein, high-calorie, fiber-added, and disease-specific.
- Hydrolyzed formulas are made from partially or totally predigested nutrients; they are higher in cost and osmolality and usually are not well accepted orally. Specially defined formulas are available for specific metabolic disorders (e.g., renal failure, hepatic failure).
- Continuous drip infusion with a pump is the preferred method for delivering tube feedings to critically ill patients and should be used whenever feedings are infused into the jejunum. Intermittent feedings may be preferable for long-term tube feeding and home enteral nutrition because they more closely resemble a normal intake and allow the client freedom between feedings. Bolus feedings are not recommended.

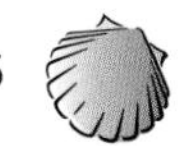

- Diarrhea is a frequent complication of tube feedings that may be caused by bacterial contamination, a feeding rate that is too rapid, giving too much volume of formula, hyperosmolar formula, misplacement of the feeding tube, hypoalbuminemia, or antibiotic therapy.
- Parenteral nutrition delivers nutrients by vein when the gastrointestinal tract is nonfunctional or when oral or enteral intake is inadequate to meet the patient's needs. Amino acids, dextrose, lipid emulsions, electrolytes, multivitamins, and trace elements may be given by vein.
- PPN must be near-isotonic to avoid collapsing small-diameter veins. CVC infusions are hypertonic and are quickly diluted by the rapid blood flow.
- Because parenteral nutrition has numerous potential metabolic, infectious, and mechanical complications, it should be used only when necessary and discontinued as soon as feasible.

ANSWER KEY

1. **FALSE** Hospital menus are intended to prevent deficiency disease, not prevent chronic disease; they often fail to meet the recommendations of the *Dietary Guidelines for Americans.*
2. **TRUE** Full liquid diets can be carefully planned or supplemented to approximate the nutritional value of a regular or high-calorie, high-protein diet. Therefore, they are suitable for long-term use.
3. **TRUE** Modular products, either singly or in combination, can increase the nutrient density of enteral formulas.
4. **TRUE** In general, the more digested a protein is in a formula, the greater the osmolality.
5. **FALSE** Although the terms *fiber* and *residue* are often used interchangeably, they are not synonymous. Fiber refers to carbohydrates not digested in the gastrointestinal tract. Residue is composed of fiber along with undigested food, intestinal secretions, bacterial cell bodies, and cells from the intestinal lining.
6. **TRUE** The individual's capability to absorb and digest food is a primary consideration when choosing a tube feeding method for a patient.
7. **TRUE** PPN cannot supply more than 2000 to 2500 cal/day because hypertonic concentrations of dextrose and amino acids cannot be infused through peripheral veins.
8. **TRUE** Tolerance of intermittent feedings is optimized by infusing the formula at room temperature by slow gravity drip or by pump over a 20- to 30-minute period.
9. **TRUE** Diarrhea may be averted by initiating hypertonic formulas at a slower rate.
10. **FALSE** Coloring tube formulas with food dye may help to detect aspirate but it does not prevent aspiration.

WEBSITES FOR ENTERAL PRODUCT INFORMATION

Ross Laboratories at **www.ross.com** (e.g., Ensure)
Mead Johnson at **www.meadjohnson.com** (e.g., Boost)
Nestlé at **nestleclinicalnutrition.com**
Novartis at **www.novartis.com**

REFERENCES

American Dietetic Association. (2000). *Manual of clinical nutrition* (6th ed.). Chicago: American Dietetic Association.

American Dietetic Association. (2002). Position of the American Dietetic Association: Ethical and legal issues in nutrition, hydration, and feeding. *Journal of the American Dietetic Association, 102,* 716–726.

Bistrian, B. (2001). Update on total parenteral nutrition. *American Journal of Clinical Nutrition, 74,* 153–154.

Braunschweig, C., Levy, P., Sheean, P., & Wang, X. (2001). Enteral compared with parenteral nutrition: A meta-analysis. *American Journal of Clinical Nutrition, 74,* 534–542.

Fuhrman, P. (2001). Parenteral nutrition. *Dietitian's Edge, 2*(1), 53–57.

Harkness, L. (2002). The history of enteral nutrition therapy: From raw eggs and nasal tubes to purified amino acids and early postoperative jejunal delivery. *Journal of the American Dietetic Association, 103,* 399–404.

Jeejeebhoy, K. (2001). Total parenteral nutrition: Potion or poison? *American Journal of Clinical Nutrition, 74,* 160–163.

Maloney, J., Ryan, T., Brasel, K, et al. (2002). Food dye use in enteral feedings: A review and a call for a moratorium. *Nutrition in Clinical Practice, 17,* 169–181.

Pronsky, Z. (2004). *Food–medication interactions* (13th ed.). Birchrunville, PA: Food-Medication Interactions, Inc.

For information on the new dietary guidelines 2005 and MyPyramid, visit **http://connection.lww.com/go/dudek**

16

Critical Illness and Hypermetabolic Conditions

TRUE	FALSE	
○	○	**1** Metabolism slows during acute, severe stress.
○	○	**2** A patient's calorie needs are directly proportional to the degree of trauma or sepsis.
○	○	**3** The Harris–Benedict equations accurately determine energy requirements.
○	○	**4** Protein requirements increase when calorie intake is inadequate.
○	○	**5** After acute stress, the intestines regain motility quicker than the stomach.
○	○	**6** Providing nutrition orally or enterally promotes blood flow to the intestines and may help to preserve intestinal cell function and reduce the risk of sepsis.
○	○	**7** Because calorie and nutrient needs are so high, it is not possible to overfeed a person who has experienced severe stress.
○	○	**8** A clear liquid diet is necessary as the first post-surgical meal.
○	○	**9** Extensive burns are the greatest stress a person can experience.
○	○	**10** People with COPD generally need fewer calories than healthy people because they are less physically active.

UPON COMPLETION OF THIS CHAPTER, YOU WILL BE ABLE TO

- Discuss how metabolism and nutrition are impacted by acute stress.
- Calculate a person's calorie requirements using the Harris–Benedict formula adjusted for activity and injury.
- Describe the roles of the following nutrients in wound healing and recovery: protein, calories, vitamin C, and zinc.
- List ways to increase intake of protein and calories.
- Discuss nutritional considerations for thermal injuries and chronic obstructive pulmonary disease (COPD).

Stress Response: a complex series of hormonal and metabolic changes that occur to enable the body to adapt to stressors.

Hypermetabolic: refers to elevated metabolism; in other words, the sum total of all body processes increases.

According to Hans Selye, stress is the response of the body to demands made on it. Stressors can be physiological, psychological, or both. Physiological stress, a normal part of everyday living, includes events such as marriage, divorce, moving to a new house, and even going on a vacation. Pathologic stress is caused by disease or injury.

The stress response is the body's way of reestablishing homeostasis. The intensity of that response depends on the severity of the stress, the number of stressors, and the individual's ability to adapt to stress. For instance, the stress of minor surgery in a well-nourished patient may have little impact, whereas trauma elicits a rapid and predictable stress response. When sepsis develops in a malnourished patient, the overwhelming burden may prevent adaptation to stress, resulting in multiple organ failure and death.

This chapter reviews how severe stress, or critical illness, impacts metabolism and nutritional requirements. Also presented are additional nutritional considerations of certain other hypermetabolic conditions: surgery, thermal injuries, and COPD.

EFFECT OF ACUTE STRESS ON METABOLISM

Ketones: acidic compounds formed from the breakdown of fat when glucose is unavailable.

Severe, acute stress has a profound impact on metabolism. Unlike starvation, to which the body adapts by lowering metabolic rate and switching to ketones as its major fuel to conserve body protein, hormonal changes resulting from severe stress speed metabolism; mobilize glucose and amino acids; and accelerate loss of lean body tissue.

Hormonal Changes

Resting Energy Expenditure (REE): the calories expended maintaining basic, involuntary activities needed to sustain life such as beating the heart, inflating the lungs, and secreting enzymes. Commonly used interchangeably with basal energy expenditure (BEE), except that REE is measured after a 12-hour fast.

Acute stress causes an immediate spike in circulating levels of catecholamines, cortisol, and glucagon, resulting in a distinct and persistent rise in blood glucose from the breakdown of glycogen and synthesis of glucose from amino acids (Table 16.1). Insulin levels also rise, but because the ratio of glucagon to insulin is increased, it does not effectively lower serum glucose. High levels of glucose are available to provide energy to fight infection, heal wounds, and replenish losses.

These hormonal changes, as well as other factors such as increased activity related to healing, have long been thought to increase resting energy expenditure (REE). In fact, it is commonly believed that energy expenditure increases by about 50% over REE during critical illness. However, at least one study has shown that the REE of critically ill people is close to their normal energy requirement. Actual energy expenditure is highly variable among patients and is influenced by many factors including age, fever, and the stage of recovery.

Protein Catabolism

The overwhelming and unequivocal nutritional concern during acute stress is the catabolism of body protein. The rise in stress hormones promotes the synthesis of glu-

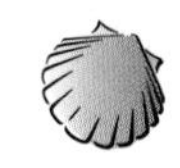

TABLE 16.1 HORMONAL AND METABOLIC CHANGES CHARACTERISTIC OF ACUTE STRESS

Hormonal Change	Metabolic Effect
↑ Catecholamines	↑ Glucagon; ↑ glucagon:insulin ratio ↑ Glycogenolysis ↑ Gluconeogenesis ↑ Mobilization of free fatty acids
↑ Cortisol	↑ Gluconeogenesis ↑ Mobilization of free fatty acids
↑ Glucagon	↑ Glucagon:insulin ratio ↑ Glycogenolysis ↑ Gluconeogenesis Glucose, amino acid, and fatty acid storage is impaired
↑ Insulin	Breakdown of body fat is impaired
Antidiuretic hormone	↑ Fluid retention
Aldosterone	↑ Sodium retention ↑ Urinary excretion of potassium

Glucogenic Amino Acids: amino acids capable of being converted to glucose.

cose from amino acids, which come mostly from the breakdown of skeletal muscle protein. Although only certain amino acids can actually be converted to glucose, whole proteins must be broken down to release those glucogenic amino acids. Although it appears counterproductive, the catabolism of lean tissue also serves to liberate amino acids used for the synthesis of new tissue and immune factors needed to fight infection. The body literally breaks itself down to defend and repair itself.

Potential Complications

Decubitus ulcers or pressure sores: areas where skin and underlying tissues break down because of constant pressure and a lack of oxygen and nutrients.

Ideally, the body adapts: stress hormone levels subside, serum glucose levels fall, metabolism gradually returns to normal, and the patient recovers. Sometimes, however, complications occur especially when nutritional status is compromised. Malnutrition in general and protein deficiency in particular increases the risk of complications such as skin breakdown, infections, multiple organ failure, ulcers, and poor drug tolerance.

Skin Breakdown

People who are protein malnourished are at increased risk of skin breakdown and immobility compounds pressure sore risk. The areas most susceptible to pressure sores are the bony or cartilaginous prominences of the hip, sacrum, elbow, and heels. Pressure ulcers are painful and they increase the risk for infection. Pressure ulcers increase requirements for protein, vitamin C, and zinc to promote healing.

Infections

Systemically, poor nutrition negatively affects immune system functioning by impairing the effectiveness of phagocytes, reducing the number and function of T lymphocytes, and decreasing the production of antibodies. Sepsis occurs when a local infection spreads to the blood.

Multiple Organ Failure

Multiple organ failure refers to a progressive loss of function in two or more organs following major injury. The most common cause is sepsis. Mortality is related to the number of organs that fail and is highest when three or more organs fail (80% to 100%). Multiple organ failure usually begins with pulmonary failure as acute respiratory distress syndrome and progresses quickly to acute renal failure. Acute heart failure can result and liver malfunction is common.

GI Changes

GI motility decreases during acute stress and may result in anorexia, distention, nausea, vomiting, or constipation. A decrease in blood flow to the GI tract increases the risk of ulcers. Malnutrition impairs the gastrointestinal tract's important role in protecting the body from infectious agents. For instance, malnutrition decreases the number and function of intestinal border cells that normally form a protective barrier to prevent the translocation of infectious substances from the bowel to the bloodstream. Researchers speculate that translocation of gut bacteria may be a major factor in the development of sepsis and multiple organ failure. However, the belief that clinically relevant bacterial translocation even exists in humans is being challenged.

Poor Drug Tolerance

Malnutrition can affect the way the body responds to drugs. For instance, patients with malabsorption related to the decreased number and function of intestinal cells may not adequately absorb drugs. A low serum albumin concentration, indicative of protein malnutrition, means that drugs that normally bind to albumin for transport through the blood take longer to be delivered. These drugs also remain in circulation longer because transport to the liver or kidneys for detoxification is delayed.

Nutrition Therapy During Critical Illness

The primary goal of nutrition therapy in critical illness is to protect lean tissue and function; the approach is adequate calories and protein. However, when injury or sepsis is severe and persistent, loss of lean tissue is unavoidable and the goal is to simply minimize losses.

Unfortunately, recommendations regarding calorie and protein requirements during critical illness are imprecise. Estimates are adjusted upward or downward based on the patient's response.

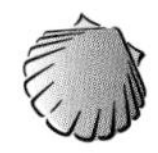

Calories

Refeeding Syndrome: a potentially fatal complication that occurs from an abrupt change from a catabolic state to an anabolic state and increase in insulin caused by a dramatic increase in calories.

It is important to provide enough calories to promote recovery and spare protein yet not too many calories to overwhelm an already stressed system. An excess of calories increases metabolism, oxygen consumption, and carbon dioxide production; this compounds the burden already placed on the heart and lungs to regulate blood gases. In addition, too many calories tax endocrine and thyroid functions and may precipitate dangerous shifts in serum phosphorus and other electrolytes that characterize the refeeding syndrome. In fact, it is believed that overfeeding is the reason why TPN has failed to reduce mortality in critical illness.

Measurement of energy expenditure using indirect calorimetry is ideal but not commonly done. Most often, energy requirements are estimated using predictive equations such as the Harris–Benedict equations to determine resting energy expenditure, which is adjusted for stress and activity factors (Box 16.1).

Some experts contend that the Harris–Benedict equation may generally overestimate basal calorie needs by 5% to 15%, but another author has shown that the equation

BOX 16.1

HARRIS–BENEDICT EQUATIONS FOR ESTIMATING ENERGY EXPENDITURE

Step 1: Calculate basal energy expenditure (BEE) (calories per day) from the actual body weight in kilograms, the height in centimeters, and the age in years.

Men: BEE (cal/d) = 66.47 + (13.75 × weight in kg) + (5 × height in cm) – (6.76 × age in y)

Women: BEE (cal/d) = 655.1 + (9.56 × weight in kg) + (1.85 × height in cm) – (4.68 × age in y)

Step 2: Multiply BEE by the appropriate activity factor:

Confined to bed or chair	1.2 × BEE
Out of bed with little movement and activity	1.4–1.5 × BEE
Seated work with little strenuous activity	1.6–1.7 × BEE
Standing work	1.8–1.9 × BEE
Strenuous work/highly active	2.0–2.4 × BEE

Step 3: Multiply the activity-adjusted BEE by the appropriate stress factor:

Elective surgery	1.0–1.1
Most stress	1.1–1.4
Burns	1.5–2.1

Example: A 20-year-old woman who is 5 feet 5 inches (165 cm) tall and weighs 132 pounds (60 kg) is confined to chair with multiple trauma.

Step 1: BEE = 655.1 + (9.56 × 60) + (1.85 × 165) – (4.68 × 20) = 1440.35

Step 2: 1440.35 × 1.2 (activity factor) = 1728.42

Step 3: 1728.42 × 1.4 (stress factor) = 2419.788

The client's estimated total energy requirement is 2420 cal/d.

Indirect Calorimetry: an indirect estimate of resting energy expenditure that measures the ratio of carbon dioxide expired to the amount of oxygen inspired and uses those values in a mathematical equation.

underestimates the needs of elderly, malnourished patients by 25%. Also of note is that the numbers cited above for the activity and stress factors are not universally agreed upon and, therefore, vary among institutions; they are estimates to be tempered with clinical judgment. From a practical standpoint, the equation is time-consuming and complex.

An alternative method for estimating calorie needs consists of simply multiplying the patient's weight in kilograms by specified calorie level. This is the approach most often given in this text because it is simpler to use and yields similar results to the Harris–Benedict approach. For critically ill people, total calorie needs can be estimated by multiplying weight in kg by

25 to 35 cal for nonobese patients
21 cal for obese patients

But these numbers are not universally agreed upon; sometimes up to 40 cal/kg may be recommended.

Career Connection

A universally agreed upon equation to accurately predict calorie needs does not exist. Calorie requirements are a product of many factors that interact with each other in complicated ways, making estimates truly "best guesses." Variables to consider:

- Because all predictive equations rely on weight, make sure an accurate weight is measured, not estimated, to improve the usefulness of the equations. Optimally, weigh the patient before fluid resuscitation.
- Although it is natural to assume that the greater the severity of trauma or sepsis, the higher the calorie requirements, this is not always true. Factors that may be responsible for this anomaly are fever, age, drug therapy, poor nutritional status, and the duration and phase of the critical illness.
- Burns and head trauma increase resting energy expenditure, but the degree of the increase is highly variable. Paralysis, sedation, and beta-adrenergic blocking agents reduce REE.

Protein

An adequate protein intake is essential to minimize and correct body protein catabolism and to help maintain normal immune functioning. Because the body meets its energy requirements first, dietary protein is used for anabolism only if calorie intake is adequate. Generally, protein requirements (in grams per kilogram body weight) range as follows:

Postoperative	1.0 to 1.5
Sepsis, refeeding syndrome	1.2 to 1.5
Stress, trauma, burns	1.5 to 2.0

If liver or kidney function is impaired, protein intake is adjusted downward to reduce the workload on these organs responsible for metabolizing protein and excreting the by-products. If calorie needs are not met, additional protein is needed.

Besides the total quantity of protein provided, the specific types of amino acids given may influence stress response and recovery. For instance, arginine and glutamine, two nonessential amino acids, may become conditionally essential during periods of stress. Arginine may reduce infectious complications particularly in surgical patients. Glutamine may help to maintain the integrity and function of intestinal cells and improve gut and systemic immune function. Whether glutamine prevents the translocation of gastrointestinal bacteria is widely debated. Other studies suggest that supplementing intake with branch chain amino acids (BCAAs) (leucine, isoleucine, and valine) may minimize protein losses. However, there is not enough evidence to make recommendations about the quantities or percentages of specific amino acids that may be optimal during stress.

Fluid

During periods of stress, fluid requirements are highly individualized according to losses that occur through exudates, hemorrhage, emesis, diuresis, diarrhea, and fever. To accurately assess fluid requirements and status, the fluid intake and output, blood pressure, heart rate, respiratory rate, and body temperature are carefully monitored. Care should be taken to avoid overhydration; decreased renal output is a frequent complication of stress.

Micronutrients

Vitamin, mineral, and electrolyte requirements during stress are unclear and undefined. Because of their role in tissue healing and immune function, supplements of the B-complex vitamins, zinc, vitamin A, and vitamin C may be appropriate.

Type of Feeding

Oral and enteral nutrition are the preferred routes if the gastrointestinal tract is functional. However, an initial response to severe stress is reduced blood flow to the gastrointestinal tract, which slows motility and precludes oral intake. Lack of use of the gastrointestinal tract causes the problems of reduced gastrointestinal blood flow and slower motility to worsen. Even when oral nutrients are provided, they may not be well absorbed because of the loss of gastrointestinal cells and secretions secondary to protein depletion caused by stress or malnutrition.

The actual type of nutrition provided (oral, enteral, or parenteral) depends on the location and extent of the injury. Well-nourished patients who experience mild to moderate stress are given intravenous fluid and electrolytes until gut motility returns to normal usually within a few days. The diet advances as tolerated. Supplements and small, frequent feedings help to maximize intake. Box 16.2 lists methods by which protein and calories can be added to the diet.

Malnourished or severely stressed patients may need enteral or parenteral nutrition. Because motility returns to the intestines much sooner than to the stomach, intestinal feedings can be initiated much sooner than feedings into the stomach and are associated with improved clinical outcomes. For instance, surgeons frequently insert a needle-catheter jejunostomy tube during surgery in patients who are malnourished, hypermetabolic, or not expected to resume oral intake within a few days after surgery. This allows the patient to benefit from feedings several hours after surgery instead of

BOX 16.2 **WAYS TO INCREASE THE PROTEIN AND CALORIE DENSITY OF FOODS**

To Increase Protein and Calories

- Add skim milk powder to milk to make double-strength milk; chill well before serving.
- Use double-strength milk on hot or cold cereals and in scrambled eggs, soups, gravies, casseroles, milk shakes, and milk-based desserts.
- Substitute whole milk or evaporated milk for water in recipes.
- Add grated cheese to soups, casseroles, vegetable dishes, rice, and noodles.
- Use peanut butter as a spread on slices of apple, banana, pear, crackers, or waffles; use as a filling for celery.
- Add finely chopped, hard-cooked eggs to sauces, soups, and casseroles.
- Choose desserts made with eggs or milk such as sponge cake, angel food cake, custard, and puddings.
- Dip meat, poultry, and fish in eggs or milk and coat with bread or cereal crumbs before baking, broiling, or pan frying.
- Use yogurt as a topping for fruit, plain cakes, or other desserts; use in gravies and dips.

To Increase Calories

- Mix cream cheese with butter and spread on hot bread and rolls.
- Whenever possible, add butter to hot foods: breads, pancakes, waffles, soups, vegetables, potatoes, cooked cereal, rice, and pasta.
- Substitute mayonnaise for salad dressing in salads, eggs, casseroles, and sandwiches.
- Add dried fruit, nuts, or granola to desserts and cereal.
- Use whipped cream on pies, fruit, pudding, gelatin, ice cream, and other desserts and in coffee, tea, and hot chocolate.
- Use marshmallows in hot chocolate, on fruit, and in desserts.
- Top baked potatoes, vegetables, and fruits with sour cream.
- Snack frequently on nuts, dried fruit, candy, buttered popcorn, cheese, granola, and ice cream.
- Use honey on toast, cereal, and fruit and in coffee and tea.

waiting 24 to 48 hours for stomach motility to resume. In severely stressed patients, infusing feedings into the intestine within 36 hours after stress stimulates blood flow to the intestine, which may help to preserve intestinal function, promote adaptation, and minimize hypermetabolism. Stress formulas enriched with BCAAs may be appropriate for patients receiving enteral nutritional support. Formulas touted for their immune-enhancing effects provide significant amounts of arginine, omega-3 fatty acids, and nucleotides. Because of the increased risk of infectious, metabolic, and mechanical complications, parenteral nutrition is used only when necessary and is discontinued as soon as possible.

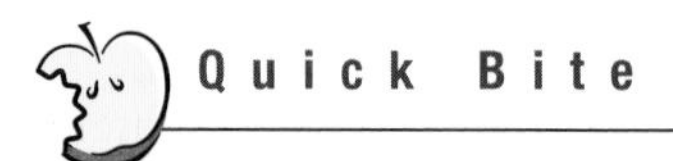

The immunonutrition enteral formulas most commonly used in clinical trials are

Impact
Immun-Aid

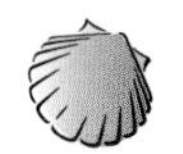

NUTRITION THERAPY FOR CERTAIN HYPERMETABOLIC CONDITIONS

The preceding section that addressed nutrition therapy during critical illness is applicable to a number of conditions, including extensive surgery and burns. However, surgery and burns have additional considerations with nutritional implications that are presented here. Additional considerations for COPD are also included because COPD is a hypermetabolic condition.

Surgery

Ideally, patients who enter into surgery are optimally nourished so they easily tolerate the stress of surgery and the short-term starvation that follows. However, surgical candidates may be malnourished as a result of disease-related symptoms experienced before surgery, such as anorexia, nausea, vomiting, fever, malabsorption, and blood loss. To optimize the chance for a successful surgical outcome, malnourished patients and those at risk for malnutrition should be identified and given preoperative nutritional support that may range from a high-calorie, high-protein diet to enteral or parenteral nutrition.

Patients are restricted to nothing by mouth (NPO) for at least 8 hours before surgery to avoid aspiration related to anesthesia. To minimize fecal residue and postoperative distention after intestinal surgery, a low-residue, residue-free (see Chapter 17), or hydrolyzed formula diet may be used for 2 to 3 days before surgery.

Oral intake is resumed after bowel sounds return usually 24 to 48 hours after surgery. Although the initial feeding after surgery was traditionally limited to clear liquids, this routine may be based more on history and convention than on science, especially for short-stay patients. Studies show that early introduction of solid food is safe and feasible and can enhance recovery and decrease length of stay for certain types of short-stay postsurgical patients. For these types of patients, a meal of simple fluid and solid items (e.g., a sandwich, pudding, dehydrated soup mix that can be prepared later, juice, milk) may be better than traditional liquids.

Usually a high-protein, high-calorie diet is appropriate with a liberal intake of nutrients important for wound healing (Table 16.2). Actual needs depend on the extent of surgery and the patient's nutritional status.

Burns

Extensive burns are the most severe form of stress that a person can experience. Hormonal responses and extensive evaporative water losses may increase metabolism by 100% above normal. The patient is hypercatabolic. Large quantities of fluid, electrolytes, protein, and other nutrients leach through the burned area. Fluid and electrolyte imbalances, paralytic ileus, anorexia, pain, infection or other complications, emotional trauma, and medical-surgical procedures may complicate nutrition support. Weight loss and malnutrition lead to a high incidence of impaired immunocompetence

TABLE 16.2

NUTRIENTS IMPORTANT FOR WOUND HEALING AND RECOVERY

Nutrient	Rationale for Increased Need	Possible Deficiency Outcome
Protein	To replace lean body mass lost during the catabolic phase after stress To restore blood volume and plasma proteins lost during exudates, bleeding from the wound, and possible hemorrhage To replace losses resulting from immobility (increased excretion) To meet increased needs for tissue repair and resistance to infection	Significant weight loss Impaired/delayed wound healing Shock related to decreased blood volume Edema related to decreased serum albumin Diarrhea related to decreased albumin Anemia Increased risk of infection related to decreased antibodies, impaired tissue integrity Decreased lipoprotein synthesis → fatty infiltration of the liver → liver damage Increased mortality
Calories	To replace losses related to lack of oral intake and hypermetabolism during catabolic phase after stress To spare protein To restore normal weight	Signs and symptoms of protein deficiency due to use of protein to meet energy requirements Extensive weight loss
Water	To replace fluid lost through vomiting, hemorrhage, exudates, fever, drainage, diuresis To maintain homeostasis	Signs, symptoms, and complications of dehydration such as poor skin turgor, dry mucous membranes, oliguria, anuria, weight loss, increased pulse rate, decreased central venous pressure
Vitamin C	Important for capillary formation, tissue synthesis, and wound healing through collagen formation Needed for antibody formation	Impaired/delayed wound healing related to impaired collagen formation and increased capillary fragility and permeability Increased risk of infection related to decreased antibodies
Thiamin, niacin, riboflavin	Requirements increase with increased metabolic rate	Decreased enzymes available for energy metabolism
Folic acid, vitamin B_{12}	Needed for cell proliferation and, therefore, tissue synthesis Important for maturation of red blood cells. Impaired folic acid synthesis related to some antibiotics; impaired vitamin B_{12} absorption related to some antibiotics	Decreased or arrested cell division Megaloblastic anemia
Vitamin A	Important for tissue synthesis, wound healing, and immune function Enhances resistance to infection	Impaired/delayed wound healing related to decreased collagen synthesis; impaired immune function Increased risk of infection

TABLE 16.2
(continued)

NUTRIENTS IMPORTANT FOR WOUND HEALING AND RECOVERY

Nutrient	Rationale for Increased Need	Possible Deficiency Outcome
Vitamin K	Important for normal blood clotting Impaired intestinal synthesis related to antibiotics	Prolonged prothrombin time
Iron	To replace iron lost through blood loss	Signs, symptoms, and complications of iron deficiency anemia such as fatigue, weakness, pallor, anorexia, dizziness, headaches, stomatitis, glossitis, cardiovascular and respiratory changes, possible cardiac failure
Zinc	Needed for protein synthesis and wound healing Needed for normal lymphocyte and phagocyte response	Impaired/delayed wound healing Impaired immune response

and increased morbidity and mortality. Sepsis is the most common cause of death among burn victims, followed by pneumonia.

Nutrients of most concern are fluid, calories, and protein. Fluid requirements in the immediate postburn period range from 3 to 5 L daily but up to 10 L/day may be needed for extensive burns. Water losses may continue to be many times greater than normal for the first few postburn weeks. Generally, total calorie needs may range up to 35 to 40 cal/kg. Although the metabolic rate peaks at about the tenth postburn day, metabolism (and, therefore, the calorie requirement) remains high for several weeks or longer depending on the extent of the burn. Protein requirement may be as high as 2.0 g/kg depending upon the total body surface area. Nutritional requirements increase with the development of complications and lessen as wound healing progresses.

To meet increased needs for healing, it is recommended that all burn patients—children and adults, those with minor burns or major burns—receive a multivitamin daily. In addition, all patients over the age of 3 with major burns should receive

500 mg of vitamin C BID
220 mg zinc sulfate daily
10,000 IU per day of vitamin A

Although an oral diet is the preferred method of feeding, it may not be possible or adequate. The use of tube feedings is relatively standard for all patients with major burns, and is also appropriate for intubated patients with a functional GI tract and for patients who are unable to swallow because of facial or neck burns. Nocturnal tube feedings are useful as a supplement to an oral diet when nutritional needs are not met through food alone. Early initiation of tube feedings may prevent a loss in intestinal function and ileus and may reduce the hypermetabolic response to the burn. Protein modules may be added to meet high protein needs.

Total parenteral nutrition is used with extreme caution because of the increased risks for infection and sepsis. TPN may be necessary for patients with

- Adynamic ileus
- Intractable diarrhea
- Bleeding related to Curling's ulcer
- Pancreatitis
- Pseudoobstruction of the colon
- Patients who cannot receive tube feedings for longer than 2 to 3 days

Career Connection

To promote maximum intake among patients whose needs are high and appetite is low

- Work with the client and family to solicit food preferences. Young children may regress in their eating behaviors; adults may prefer foods that they associate with recovery as children (e.g., chicken soup).
- Encourage the family to bring food from home.
- Discourage the intake of empty-calorie food and beverages.
- Provide nutrient-dense liquid supplements between meals.
- Provide emotional support and allow the patient to verbalize feelings.
- If possible, schedule debridement and other medical and surgical procedures at times when they are least likely to interfere with meals.
- Provide pain medication as needed before meals.

Chronic Obstructive Pulmonary Disease

Malnutrition is common among patients with chronic obstructive pulmonary disease even if recent weight loss is not reported. An increase in energy expenditure related to labored breathing and possibly also to a decrease in mechanical and metabolic efficiency can cause weight loss even when intake appears normal. Other factors that may contribute to malnutrition include

- Early satiety related to flattening of the diaphragm and a decrease in abdominal volume
- Abdominal bloating related to swallowed air
- Peptic ulcer disease secondary to steroid therapy
- Dyspnea while eating
- Anorexia related to fatigue
- Anorexia related to excess mucus
- Anorexia related to decreased peristalsis and digestion secondary to inadequate oxygen to gastrointestinal cells

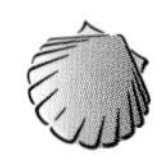

A downhill spiral often occurs: a reduced respiratory rate reduces blood flow to the gastrointestinal tract, thereby decreasing nutrient absorption and increasing risk of malnutrition. Conversely, malnutrition weakens respiratory muscles and reduces exercise capacity, contributing to impaired gas exchange and increasing risk of respiratory mortality. Improving weight and nutritional status in compromised COPD patients improves immune response, respiratory muscle endurance, muscle strength and exercise tolerance, and leads to faster recovery.

Although there is not one single criterion that can reliably identify all COPD patients who are malnourished, it is likely that a BMI < 20 indicates malnutrition. Because BMI is correlated to mortality in patients with COPD, low BMI should be considered a risk factor for mortality. However, patients with COPD may have an increase in total body water that masks malnutrition with an inflated BMI.

Correcting or preventing malnutrition is a priority in the treatment of patients with COPD. A calorie intake of at least 140% to 145% of basal energy expenditure and 1.2 g protein/kg body weight may be sufficient to prevent body protein breakdown. Calorie needs in patients who are nutritionally depleted are higher and their protein requirement may be 1.5 g protein/kg body weight.

Respiratory Quotient (RQ): the ratio of carbon dioxide produced to oxygen consumed; the more carbon dioxide produced, the greater the burden on the lungs to exhale carbon dioxide.

The idea of manipulating carbohydrate and fat intakes to influence the production of carbon dioxide has led to the creation of tube feeding formulas for patients with respiratory disease. Carbon dioxide and water are normal by-products of carbohydrate, protein, and fat metabolism. Because the respiratory quotient (RQ) is higher for carbohydrates than for either proteins or fats, it may be beneficial to limit carbohydrate intake in patients who require ventilator support. Instead of the normal calorie distribution of 50% to 60% carbohydrate, 20% to 30% fat, and 15% to 20% protein, pulmonary formulas provide 25% to 30% of calories from carbohydrates and 50% to 55% of total calories from fat.

Although it has been suggested that ambulatory patients eating an oral diet may also benefit from high-fat oral supplements, this has not been proven. In fact, a recent study compared the use of a high-fat oral supplement to a high-carbohydrate oral supplement and found that the high-carbohydrate product was preferable because lung function increased and there was less shortness of breath.

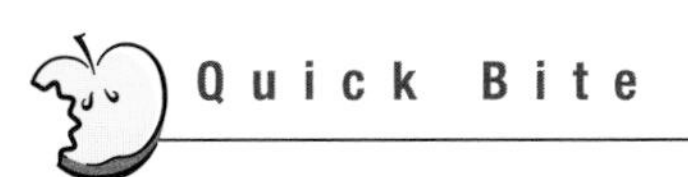

Quick Bite

Enteral formulas designed for respiratory insufficiency

	% of calories from fat
Novasource Pulmonary	41
NutriVent	55
Oxepa	55
Pulmocare	55
Respalor	41

A soft diet may be appropriate for patients who have difficulty chewing and swallowing related to shortness of breath. Fatigued patients may need assistance with cutting food, opening containers, and so forth. Breathing exercises should be avoided for at least 1 hour before and after eating.

Limiting "empty" liquids with meals (e.g., coffee, tea, water, carbonated beverages) and providing small, frequent, nutritionally dense feedings help to maximize intake and reduce gastric distention and pressure on the diaphragm. Gassy foods should be avoided unless they are well tolerated. Consider "feedings" of high-calorie, high-protein eggnogs, shakes, and commercial supplements.

Unless it is contraindicated, a high fluid intake is needed to help thin mucus secretions; fever also increases fluid requirements. Usually 1 mL fluid per calorie consumed is adequate.

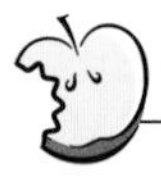

Quick Bite

Although fresh fruits and vegetables with skins and seeds offer fiber, they require effort to chew; dried peas and beans can be gassey. Less taxing sources of fiber are

Hot cereals topped with bran or ground flaxseed
Ready-to-eat bran or whole wheat cereals
Commercially prepared oral supplements with added fiber such as Promote with Fiber and Boost with Fiber

To avoid straining at stool, a high-fiber diet is recommended. Fiber intake should be increased gradually to avoid excessive gas, distention, and diarrhea.

Supplements of B-complex vitamins (for increased energy metabolism) and vitamins A and C (for healing and tissue repair) may be appropriate.

Additional diet modifications may be necessary depending on the patient's drug therapy (see Drug Alert).

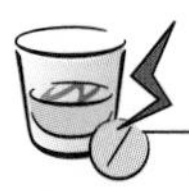

DRUG ALERT

Drugs Commonly Used to Treat COPD

Theophylline (a bronchodilator) commonly causes anorexia. A high-carbohydrate, low-protein diet slows the metabolism of theophylline, thereby increasing the risk of side effects, including dizziness, flushing, and headache. A sudden increase in protein intake may decrease the duration of theophylline action. Caffeine in any form also slows the rate of theophylline elimination; concurrent use of caffeine increases the risk for insomnia and cardiac arrhythmias.

Albuterol (a bronchodilator) may cause hyperglycemia in diabetics.

Prednisone (an anti-inflammatory glucocorticoid) stimulates appetite and, therefore, may cause weight gain. Hyperglycemia may occur in diabetics and nondiabetics. Prednisone promotes sodium retention, potassium excretion, loss of calcium from the bones and may cause gastric ulcers.

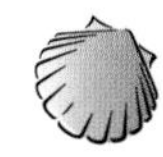

NURSING PROCESS

Mr. Ramirez is a frail, 74-year-old man admitted to the hospital with multiple, non–life-threatening injuries resulting from a car accident. He weighs 128 pounds and is 5 feet, 6 inches tall.

Assessment

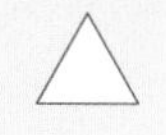

Obtain Clinical Data:

Current body mass index (BMI); recent weight history
Medical history including hyperlipidemia, hypertension, cardiovascular disease, renal impairments, diabetes, gastrointestinal complaints
Extent of injuries; significance of gastrointestinal trauma, if appropriate
Hemodynamic status; signs and symptoms of hemorrhaging
Altered fluid and electrolyte balance particularly sodium and fluid accumulation. Rapid weight gain of more than 1 kg per day indicates fluid retention
Altered neurologic status (e.g., confusion, disorientation); ability to eat, ability to self-feed
Altered gastrointestinal function such as hypoactive bowel sounds, distention, complaints of nausea, anorexia
Abnormal laboratory values especially albumin, transferrin, glucose, and electrolytes. After the initial stress response and peak period of catabolism subside, monitor albumin, transferrin, total lymphocyte count, and creatinine height index to assess protein status. Low serum transferrin and anergy are strongly correlated with the development of wound infection
Diminished renal output; measure intake and output
Clinical signs of malnutrition such as pitting edema, easily pluckable hair, changes in hair or skin pigment, wasted appearance
Medications that affect nutrition such as lipid-lowering medications, cardiac drugs, antihypertensives

Interview the Patient to Assess:

Understanding normal weight and perception of why he is undernourished
Usual 24-hour intake including portion sizes, frequency and pattern of eating, food intolerances, adequacy of protein intake, and adequacy of calorie intake
Cultural, religious, and ethnic influences on eating habits
Psychosocial and economic issues such as if finances, loneliness, or isolation negatively affect food intake. Determine who does food shopping and preparation and if the client is a candidate for the Meals on Wheels program

(continued)

Use of vitamins, minerals, and nutritional supplements: what, how much, and why they are taken
Use of alcohol, nicotine, and caffeine

Nursing Diagnosis

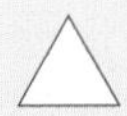

1. Altered Nutrition: Less Than Body Requirements, related to low calorie intake and increased requirements related to injuries.

Planning and Implementation

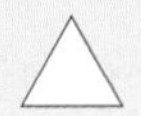

Client Goals

The client will

Maintain normal fluid and electrolyte balance
Avoid complications of malnutrition, stress, and refeeding syndrome, initially by
- Consuming adequate calories to prevent weight loss
- Consuming adequate protein to prevent protein losses

When oral diet is advanced and tolerated by
- Consuming adequate calories to promote weight gain
- Consuming adequate protein to achieve positive nitrogen balance, restore lean body mass, and experience adequate healing and recovery

Describe the principles and rationale of diet management as appropriate and implement the recommended dietary interventions

Nursing Interventions

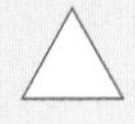

Nutrition Therapy

Initially give intravenous fluid and electrolytes as ordered to maintain hydration until oral intake is resumed.
When oral intake resumes, provide calories based on the basal energy expenditure (BEE) adjusted for activity and injury and adequate protein based on the extent of injury. Gradually increase intake as tolerated to avoid refeeding syndrome.
Adjust fluid intake according to need, based on intake and output and physical findings.
Provide small, frequent feedings as tolerated to maximize intake.

Client Teaching

Instruct the client

On the importance of protein and calories in promoting wound healing and recovery and overall health

 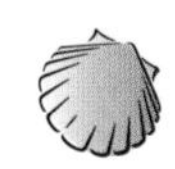

On the eating plan essentials including
- How to increase calories and protein in the diet (see Box 16.2)
- Eating small, frequent meals if anorexia or nausea occurs

Evaluation

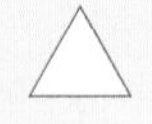

The client

Maintains normal fluid and electrolyte balance
Avoids complications of malnutrition, stress, and refeeding syndrome, initially by
- Consuming adequate calories to prevent weight loss
- Consuming adequate protein to prevent protein losses

When the oral diet is advanced and tolerated by
- Consuming adequate calories to promote weight gain
- Consuming adequate protein to achieve positive nitrogen balance, restore lean body mass, and experience adequate healing and recovery

Describes the principles and rationale of diet management as appropriate and implements the recommended dietary interventions

How Do You Respond?

Are omega-6 fatty acids (predominant in plant oils) bad for the immune system? In amounts that exceed the requirement for essential fatty acids, omega-6 fatty acids may impair immune system functioning. In excess of need, omega-6 fatty acids may also promote the inflammatory process. Because of this, large amounts of omega-6 fatty acids, which are typically found in intravenous lipid emulsions and enteral formulas, may not be appropriate for patients who are severely stressed. Omega-3 fatty acids, commonly referred to as "fish oils," may actually help to slow the inflammatory process and be a better source of fat calories for stressed patients.

How do enteral formulas designed for stress differ from routine formulas? Stress formulas tend to be high in protein and calories and may contain higher than normal amounts of certain nutrients such as vitamin C, the B-complex vitamins, vitamin E, copper, and zinc. Some stress formulas are also fortified with arginine and/or glutamine, omega-3 fatty acids, and nucleotides (components of DNA), all of which may boost immune system functioning. Although the specialized formulas are more expensive than routine formulas, they may help to reduce overall costs by reducing the incidence of infections and the length of hospital stays.

▲ Focus on Critical Thinking

Respond to the following statements:

1. It is prudent to provide vitamin and mineral supplements of nutrients known to promote healing to patients with surgical wounds or burns.
2. During critical illness the body breaks down lean tissue to make other tissues.
3. Your total calorie needs as calculated using the Harris—Benedict equation and factoring in activity are what you expected them to be.

Key Concepts

- The impact of stress on metabolism and nutritional requirements depends on the severity of the stress, the number of stressors, and the individual's ability to adapt to stress.
- Acute stress causes hormonal changes that result in an increase in metabolism, increased blood glucose levels, and body protein catabolism.
- The primary nutritional concern during acute stress is the breakdown of body protein, an effect of the increased levels of stress hormones.
- Protein deficiency increases the risk of complications from critical illness such as skin breakdown, infections, multiple organ failure, ulcers, and poor drug tolerance.
- Preserving lean tissue is the primary goal of nutrition therapy in critical illness but loss of lean tissue is unavoidable when injury or sepsis is severe and persistent.
- Recommendations regarding calorie and protein requirements during critical illness are imprecise. Calories may be estimated by using the Harris–Benedict equations or by multiplying weight by a factor; neither method is guaranteed accurate.
- Protein requirements are generally based on weight and range from 1.0 to 2.0 g/kg or higher depending on the type, severity, and number of stressors as well as the patient's age and prior nutritional status.
- Patients who are well nourished before surgery have a lower incidence of infections and experience fewer complications than malnourished patients. If time allows, nutritional deficits should be corrected before surgery. Healing increases the requirements for calories, protein, vitamin C, and zinc.
- Extensive burns are the most severe form of stress that a person can experience. Nutritional support may be complicated by paralytic ileus, stress ulcers, anorexia, pain, multiple organ failure, and the consequences of medical-surgical treatments.
- Patients with COPD are often underweight and malnourished. Shortness of breath can make eating difficult, and decreased oxygenation of the gastrointestinal cells can impair peristalsis and digestion. Conversely poor nutrition impairs respiratory status.

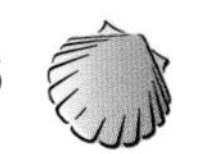

- Nutrition-dense, easy-to-consume foods are preferred for patients with chronic respiratory disorders. Patients on ventilator support may benefit from a restricted carbohydrate intake because carbohydrates produce more carbon dioxide when they are metabolized than do either proteins or fats, creating a greater burden on the lungs.

ANSWER KEY

1. **FALSE** In an attempt to adapt to severe stress, stress hormones accelerate metabolism to supply fuel to meet the high metabolic demands of the stress.
2. **FALSE** It is not always true that the greater the severity of trauma or sepsis the higher the calorie requirements. Factors that may be responsible for this anomaly are fever, age, drug therapy, poor nutritional status, and the duration and phase of the critical illness.
3. **FALSE** The Harris–Benedict equations may under- or over-estimate actual energy expenditure; they are predictive formulas but are not guaranteed to be accurate.
4. **TRUE** Protein requirement increases when calorie intake is inadequate because the body will use protein to help meet its energy need.
5. **TRUE** After trauma, motility returns to the intestines much sooner than to the stomach.
6. **TRUE** Oral and enteral routes are preferred if the gastrointestinal tract is functional. Using the gastrointestinal tract increases the blood flow to the intestines and may reduce the risk of sepsis.
7. **FALSE** A danger of overfeeding is a potentially fatal metabolic complication known as refeeding syndrome. Overfeeding, particularly from TPN, may increase the risk of infection related to hyperglycemia.
8. **FALSE** Providing clear liquid diets postsurgically as a matter of standard practice may not be warranted. Because they are nutritionally inadequate, they should not be used unless absolutely necessary.
9. **TRUE** Extensive burns are the most severe form of stress and dramatically increase the need for calories, protein, and fluid.
10. **FALSE** COPD actually increases calorie expenditure through labored breathing and possibly through impaired metabolic efficiency. Weight loss often occurs even when intake appears normal.

WEBSITES

American Association of Critical Care Nurses at **www.aacn.org**
American Burn Association at **www.americanburn.org**

REFERENCES

Buchman, A. (2001). Glutamine: Commercially essential or conditionally essential? A crucial appraisal of the human data. *American Journal of Clinical Nutrition, 74,* 25–32.

Chicago Dietetic Association & South Suburban Dietetic Association. (2000). *Manual of clinical dietetics* (6th ed.). Chicago: American Dietetic Association.

Dickerson, R., Gervasio, J., & Riley, M. (2002). Accuracy of predictive methods to estimate resting energy expenditure of thermally-injured patients. *Journal of Parenteral and Enteral Nutrition, 26,* 17–29.

Hoffer, L. (2003). Protein and energy provision in critical illness. *American Journal of Clinical Nutrition, 78,* 906–911.

McCowen, K., & Bistrian, B. (2003). Immunonutrition: Problematic or problem solving? *American Journal of Clinical Nutrition, 77,* 764–770.

Thorsdottir, I., & Gunnarsdottir, I. (2002). Energy intake must be increased among recently hospitalized patients with chronic obstructive pulmonary disease to improve nutritional status. *Journal of the American Dietetic Association, 102,* 247–249.

Thorsdottir, I., Gunnarsdottir, I., & Eriksen, B. (2001). Screening method evaluated by nutritional status measurements can be used to detect malnourishment in chronic obstructive pulmonary disease. *Journal of the American Dietetic Association, 101,* 648–654.

Vermeeren, M., Wouters, E., Nelissen, L., et al. (2001). Acute effects of different nutritional supplements on symptoms and functional capacity in patients with chronic obstructive pulmonary disease. *American Journal of Clinical Nutrition, 73,* 295–301.

For information on the new dietary guidelines 2005 and MyPyramid, visit
http://connection.lww.com/go/dudek

17

Nutrition for Patients With Gastrointestinal Disorders

TRUE	FALSE	
⬭	⬭	**1** People who have nausea should limit liquids with meals.
⬭	⬭	**2** Carbonated beverages may contribute to diarrhea.
⬭	⬭	**3** Thin liquids, such as clear juices and clear broths, are usually the easiest items for patients with swallowing disorders to swallow.
⬭	⬭	**4** People with reflux and heartburn should be encouraged to switch from regular coffee to decaffeinated coffee.
⬭	⬭	**5** MCT oil is used to provide calories and essential fatty acids to people who have fat malabsorption.
⬭	⬭	**6** People with lactose intolerance can usually tolerate cheddar cheese.
⬭	⬭	**7** Simple sugars contribute to diarrhea in patients with dumping syndrome.
⬭	⬭	**8** Patients with celiac disease need a gluten-free diet even when they are asymptomatic.
⬭	⬭	**9** Fat is the nutrient most problematic for people with chronic pancreatitis.
⬭	⬭	**10** Most people with gallstones benefit from a low-fat diet.

UPON COMPLETION OF THIS CHAPTER, YOU WILL BE ABLE TO

- Discuss nutritional management of the following conditions: anorexia, nausea and vomiting, diarrhea, constipation, dysphagia, gastroesophageal reflux disease, peptic ulcers, dumping syndrome, malabsorption syndromes, diverticular disease, liver disease, pancreatitis, and gallbladder disease.
- Discuss the characteristics and indications for the following therapeutic diets: low-fiber, high-fiber, dysphagia, gluten-free, low-fat, and lactose-restricted.

Nutrition therapy is a major component in the management of digestive system disorders. For some disorders, diet merely plays a supportive role in alleviating symptoms rather than altering the course of the disease. For other GI disorders, nutrition therapy is the cornerstone of treatment. Frequently, nutrition therapy is needed to restore nutritional status that has been compromised by dysfunction or disease.

ASSESSMENT OF GASTROINTESTINAL STATUS

Before the optimal nutrition therapy can be planned, a nutrition-focused assessment of gastrointestinal status is indicated. Criteria to consider include the following:

- Weight and weight changes
- GI symptoms that interfere with intake such as difficulty chewing and swallowing or nausea and vomiting
- GI symptoms that increase nutritional needs such as diarrhea and malabsorption
- Changes in eating made in response to symptoms
- Use of tobacco, over-the-counter drugs for GI symptoms, alcohol, and caffeine
- Normal bowel habits, change in bowel habits
- Use of nutritional supplements including vitamins, minerals, fiber, and herbs
- Client's willingness to change his or her eating habits
- Abnormal laboratory values that may indicate nutritional problems such as low albumin or altered electrolyte levels

COMMON GASTROINTESTINAL PROBLEMS

Anorexia, nausea and vomiting, diarrhea, and constipation are common symptoms experienced by most people from time to time. Among the "well" population, these problems may simply be related to eating unusual or excessive amounts of specific foods or types of food. These problems may be more severe or long-lasting when they occur as symptoms of underlying gastrointestinal disorders, as a result of viral or bacterial infection, or secondary to medical treatment. GI side effects are the most common adverse reactions occurring from herbal supplements, over the counter medications, and prescription medications. Box 17.1 lists nutritional supplements that may cause GI distress, especially with long-term or excessive use.

Anorexia

Anorexia is a common symptom for numerous physical conditions, not just gastrointestinal problems, and is a side effect of certain drugs. Emotional issues, such as fear, anxiety, and depression, frequently cause anorexia.

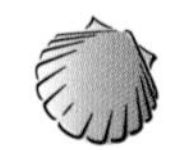

BOX 17.1 **SOME NUTRITIONAL SUPPLEMENTS THAT MAY CAUSE GI DISTRESS**

Aloe	Green tea
Black cohosh	Hydroxycitric acid (HCA)
Brewer's yeast	Iron
Caffeine	Kava
Calcium	Magnesium
Cayenne	Milk thistle
Chromium	Peppermint
Cranberry	Potassium
Fennel	Psyllium
Feverfew	Retinol
Fiber	SAMe
Garlic	Saw Palmetto
Ginger	St. John's Wort
Gingko biloba	Valerian
Ginseng	Vitamin C
Glucosamine	Zinc

Anorexia: lack of appetite; it differs from anorexia nervosa, a psychological condition characterized by denial of appetite.

The aim of nutrition therapy is to stimulate the appetite and attain or maintain adequate nutritional intake. The following interventions may help to maximize intake:

- Serve food attractively and season according to individual taste. If decreased ability to taste is contributing to anorexia, enhance food flavors with tart seasonings (e.g., orange juice, lemonade, vinegar, lemon juice) or strong seasonings (e.g., basil, oregano, rosemary, tarragon, mint).
- If possible, schedule procedures and medications when they are least likely to interfere with appetite.
- Control pain, nausea, or depression with medications as ordered.
- Provide small, frequent meals.
- Provide liquid supplements between meals. These supplements can significantly improve protein and calorie intake and usually are well accepted. In addition, liquids tend to leave the stomach quickly and, therefore, are less likely to interfere with meals.
- Limit fat intake if fat is contributing to early satiety. High-fat foods include fried foods; fatty meats and luncheon meats; whole milk and milk products; butter, margarine, and oils; and rich desserts.
- Solicit food preferences and allow food from home if possible.
- Provide encouragement and a pleasant eating environment. Advise the patient to stay calm at mealtimes and not to hurry through eating.

Nausea and Vomiting

Nausea and vomiting may be related to a decrease in gastric acid secretion, a decrease in digestive enzyme activity, a decrease in gastrointestinal motility, gastric irritation, or acidosis. Other causes include bacterial and viral infection; increased intracranial

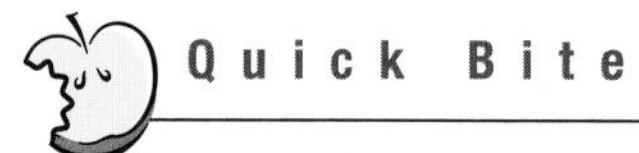

Readily digested carbohydrates that are low in fat:

Dry toast
Saltine crackers
Plain rolls
Pretzels
Angel food cake
Oatmeal
Soft and bland fruit like canned peaches, canned pears, banana

pressure; equilibrium imbalance; liver, pancreatic, and gallbladder disorders; and pyloric or intestinal obstruction. Drugs and certain medical treatments may also contribute to nausea. Prolonged nausea and vomiting can lead to weight loss; vomiting can cause metabolic alkalosis related to the loss of gastric hydrochloric acid.

Food is withheld until nausea or vomiting subsides. If tolerated, clear liquids are used for fluid and electrolytes. Some patients may need intravenous fluid and electrolytes if vomiting is severe or prolonged. Clear liquids are eventually replaced by full liquids, then by diet as tolerated. Small, frequent meals of readily digested carbohydrates are best tolerated. Other interventions include the following:

- Solicit food preferences and observe individual food intolerances.
- Elevate the head of the bed.
- Encourage the patient to eat slowly and not to eat if he or she feels nauseated.
- Promote good oral hygiene with mouthwash and ice chips.
- Limit liquids with meals because they can cause a full, bloated feeling. Encourage a liberal fluid intake between meals with whatever liquids the patient can tolerate, such as clear soup, juice, gelatin, ginger ale, and Popsicles.
- Serve foods at room temperature or chilled; hot foods may contribute to nausea.
- Avoid high-fat and spicy foods if they contribute to nausea. These include fried foods, fatty meats and luncheon meats, whole milk and milk products, butter, margarine, oils, and rich desserts.

Diarrhea

Diarrhea can cause large losses of potassium, sodium, and fluid; it also reduces the time available for absorption of all other nutrients. Severe or chronic diarrhea can lead to nutritional complications including weight loss, hypoproteinemia, metabolic acidosis, and nutrient deficiencies related to decreased transit time.

Common causes of diarrhea include emotional or physical stress; gastrointestinal disorders and malabsorption syndromes (e.g., lactose intolerance); metabolic and endocrine disorders; surgical bowel intervention; bacterial, viral, and parasitic infections; and certain drug therapies. Nutritionally, food allergies and the use of tube feedings may cause diarrhea. Also, coffee or caffeine stimulates peristalsis in some people. Stool frequency may increase from an excessive intake of high-fiber foods or foods with laxative properties such as bran, whole-grain breads and cereals, raw vegetables, fresh fruits, and prunes or prune juice.

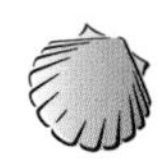

Nutrition therapy varies with the severity and duration of diarrhea. Acute diarrhea lasting 24 to 48 hours usually requires no nutrition intervention other than encouraging a liberal fluid intake to replace losses. For chronic diarrhea, food is withheld for 24 to 48 hours and intravenous fluid and electrolytes are given to maintain hydration. After 1 to 2 days of clear liquids, the diet progresses to a low-fiber diet as tolerated (Box 17.2) to reduce stool bulk and slow gastrointestinal transit time. Small, frequent meals are better tolerated than three large meals. High-potassium foods are encouraged to replace losses.

Until diarrhea completely subsides, it may be prudent to restrict the following:

- Milk because lactose intolerance may be contributing to diarrhea
- Very hot or very cold food and beverages because they stimulate peristalsis
- Coffee, strong tea, some sodas, and chocolate because they contain caffeine
- Prune juice, which is low in fiber but has laxative properties
- Alcohol
- Carbonated beverages because their electrolyte content is low and their osmolality is high, which can promote osmotic diarrhea

A sample low-fiber, milk-free menu appropriate for a patient with diarrhea appears in Box 17.3. Patients with intractable diarrhea that does not respond to traditional medical and nutrition therapy may need bowel rest (total parenteral nutrition, or TPN).

Quick Bite

High potassium foods include

Apricot nectar
Avocado
Banana
Canned apricots and peaches
Cantaloupe
Orange juice
Papaya
Potatoes
Tomato juice
Yogurt

Constipation

Constipation: the difficult or infrequent passage of stools that may be hard and dry.

Constipation can occur secondary to irregular bowel habits, psychogenic factors, lack of activity, chronic laxative use, inadequate intake of fluid and fiber, metabolic and endocrine disorders, and bowel abnormalities (e.g., tumors, hernias, strictures, diverticular disease, irritable colon). Certain medications, such as codeine, aluminum hydroxide, iron supplements, and morphine, cause constipation. Contrary to popular belief, daily bowel movements are not necessary provided the stools are not hard and dry.

A high-fiber diet alleviates constipation. A high-fiber diet is rich in both soluble and insoluble fiber even though only insoluble fiber has been credited with increasing stool bulk and stimulating peristalsis. It is achieved by substituting high-fiber foods for refined, low-fiber foods (Box 17.4). Exactly how much fiber is needed to alleviate constipation varies among individuals. The Adequate Intake set for fiber is 25 g/day for women and 38 g/day for men, approximately double the average American adult intake of approximately 12 to 18 g of fiber per day. Fiber intake is increased gradually to avoid

(*text continues on page 484*)

BOX 17.2 **LOW-FIBER DIET**

Characteristics

This diet restricts insoluble fiber because it increases stool bulk, which decreases transit time and stimulates peristalsis. Soluble fiber has less of an effect on stool bulk and is not restricted.

Indications

- Bowel inflammation as seen in the acute stages of diverticulitis, ulcerative colitis, and regional enteritis
- Esophageal and intestinal stenosis
- Preparation for bowel surgery

Contraindications

- Irritable colon
- Diverticulosis

Guidelines to Achieve a Low-Fiber Diet

Foods recommended:

- Meats: eggs; ground or well-cooked tender meat, fish, and poultry; smooth peanut butter
- Dairy: milk as tolerated, yogurt, pudding, cheeses
- Fruits: juices without pulp except prune juice; most canned or cooked fruit; ripe bananas, peeled apples, citrus sections without membranes
- Vegetables: vegetable juices without pulp; lettuce if tolerated; most well-cooked vegetables without seeds; potatoes without skins
- Breads and cereals: only refined bread and cereal products: white bread, rolls, biscuits, muffins, pancakes, plain pastries; crackers, bagels; melba toast, waffles, refined cereals such as Cream of Wheat, Cream of Rice, and puffed rice; pasta, white rice; quick cooking oatmeal, grits, and farina
- Miscellaneous: plain desserts made with allowed foods such as fruit ices, plain cakes, puddings (rice, bread, plain), and cookies without nuts or coconut; sherbet, ice cream (no nuts or coconut); gelatin; candy such as butterscotch, jelly beans, marshmallows, plain hard candy; honey, molasses, sugar; all fats

Avoid the following foods:

- Protein: tough meats, dried peas and beans, nuts, seeds, lentils, chunky peanut butter
- Dairy: yogurt with seeds or nuts
- Fruits: all other raw, cooked, or dried fruits; prune juice
- Vegetables: most raw vegetables and vegetables with seeds; sauerkraut, winter squash, peas, corn
- Breads and cereals: breads made with whole-grain flour, bran, seeds, nuts, coconut, or dried fruit; corn bread, graham crackers, oatmeal; whole-grain, bran, or granola cereal; cereals containing seeds, nuts, coconut, or dried fruit
- Miscellaneous: nuts, coconut, anything made with nuts or coconut, olives, pickles, seeds, popcorn

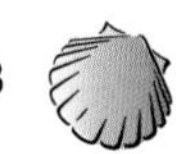

BOX 17.2 (continued)

LOW-FIBER DIET

Sample Menu

Breakfast

Strained orange juice
Cream of rice
Poached egg
White toast with jelly
½ cup milk
Coffee/tea
Salt/pepper/sugar

Lunch

Tomato juice
Sandwich made with white bread, ham, and mustard
Canned peach halves
Sponge cake
½ cup milk
Coffee/tea
Salt/pepper/sugar

Dinner

Roast chicken
White rice
Gelatin made with ripe bananas
½ cup milk
Cooked carrots
Italian bread with olive oil
Coffee/tea
Salt/pepper/sugar

Snack

Saltine crackers
½ cup milk

Potential Problems	Recommended Interventions
Constipation related to low-fiber content of diet: Insufficient fiber intake causes decrease in stool bulk and slowing of intestinal transit time.	Liberalize diet to allow more fiber. This diet is intended to be short-term.
Persistent diarrhea related to poor tolerance of even small amounts of fiber contained in a low-residue diet. Tolerance of fiber varies among patients and conditions.	Further reduce fiber content by eliminating all fruits and vegetables except strained fruit juice.

Patient Teaching

Instruct the patient that

- Fiber is a component of plants and, therefore, is found in fruits, vegetables, grains, and nuts.
- Insoluble fiber, the fiber restricted in this diet, is most abundant in bran, whole wheat breads and cereals, and skins and seeds of fruits and vegetables
- Reducing insoluble fiber slows passage of food through the bowel.
- Diet is intended to be short-term.
- Food preparation techniques to reduce fiber include removing skins, seeds, and membranes of fruits and vegetables that are high in fiber and cooking allowed vegetables until they are very tender.

BOX 17.3

SAMPLE MENU FOR PATIENT WITH DIARRHEA: LOW FIBER, LOW LACTOSE, LOW CAFFEINE

Breakfast

Strained orange juice
Poached egg
2 pancakes with maple syrup
Weak tea with nondairy creamer
Salt/pepper/sugar

Midmorning Snack

6 oz yogurt

Lunch

Tomato juice
Sandwich made with white bread, ham, Swiss cheese, and mustard
Canned peach halves
Weak tea with non-dairy creamer
Salt/pepper/sugar

Midafternoon Snack

Banana
Graham crackers

Dinner

Roast chicken
Cooked carrots
White rice
Italian bread with olive oil
Angel food cake
Weak tea with non-dairy creamer
Salt/pepper/sugar

Snack

Cheddar cheese with saltine crackers

symptoms of intolerance such as increased intestinal gas production, cramping, and diarrhea. If these side effects do occur, they are usually temporary and subside within several days. Long-term studies show that a high-fiber diet, even at levels above current recommendations, is not likely to cause adverse GI symptoms and may actually decrease symptoms of heartburn.

In addition

- Drink at least eight glasses of fluid daily. Hot coffee, tea, or lemon water immediately after waking may help to stimulate peristalsis.
- Encourage the intake of prunes and prune juice, which have laxative effects.
- Encourage regular aerobic exercise, which promotes muscle tone and stimulates bowel activity.

BOX 17.4 **HIGH-FIBER DIET**

Characteristics

- A high-fiber diet is a regular diet that substitutes high-fiber foods for foods low in fiber. Fiber intake should come from eating a wide variety of plant foods rather than from fiber supplements.
- Unprocessed bran may be added as tolerated. At least eight 8-oz glasses of fluid are recommended daily.
- This diet is used to alleviate constipation (a function of insoluble fiber) and to help lower serum cholesterol levels and improve glucose tolerance in diabetes (a function of soluble fiber).

Indications

- For the prevention or treatment of diverticular disease, constipation, irritable bowel syndrome, hypercholesterolemia, and diabetes mellitus
- May aid weight reduction; may help to protect against colon cancer

Contraindications

- Intestinal inflammation or stenosis
- Gastroparesis
- Postgastrectomy or pseudo-obstruction

Guidelines to Achieve a High-Fiber Diet

- Eat 6 to 11 servings from the bread and cereal group daily. Breads and cereals with adequate fiber provide 2 to 5 g of fiber per serving. High-fiber cereals provide 7 to 11 g of fiber per serving. The best choices are whole wheat bread, bran cereals, oatmeal, oat bran, brown rice, wheat germ, and whole wheat pasta.
- Eat 1 serving of dried peas or beans daily.
- Eat 2 to 4 servings of fruit per day. Apples, blackberries, blueberries, figs, dates, kiwifruit, mango, oranges, pears, prunes, strawberries, and raspberries are high in fiber. Eat fruit with the skin on whenever possible.
- Eat 3 to 5 servings of vegetables per day. Cooked asparagus, green beans, broccoli, Brussels sprouts, cabbage, carrots, celery, corn, eggplant, parsnips, peas, snowpeas, Swiss chard, and turnip are good choices.
- Other foods with fiber include popcorn, nuts, sunflower seeds, and sesame seeds.

Sample Menu

Breakfast

Prune juice
Milk
Whole wheat toast with jelly
Orange
Bran cereal
Coffee/tea
Salt/pepper/sugar

Lunch

Split pea soup
Julienne salad made with cheese, egg, Romaine, tomato, carrots, sunflower seeds, and other vegetables as desired
Salad dressing
Date bars
Whole wheat crackers
Apple
Milk
Coffee/tea
Salt/pepper/sugar

(box continues on page 486)

BOX 17.4 (continued)

HIGH-FIBER DIET

Dinner

Roast chicken
Brown rice
Peas
Coleslaw
Bran muffin with margarine
Fresh strawberries over ice cream
Coffee/tea
Salt/pepper/sugar

Snack

Popcorn

Potential Problems	Recommended Interventions
Flatus, distention, cramping, and osmotic diarrhea related to increasing fiber content of the diet too much or too quickly	Initiate a high-fiber diet slowly to develop the patient's tolerance. If symptoms of intolerance persist, reduce fiber content to maximum amount tolerated by the patient.
Possible malabsorption of calcium, zinc, and iron from increased gastrointestinal motility (which allows less time for absorption to occur) or from the binding of these minerals with fiber to form compounds the body cannot absorb	Actual fiber-induced deficiencies are unlikely because the body adapts to a high-fiber diet. However, foods rich in calcium, zinc, and iron should be encouraged.

Patient Teaching

Instruct the patient that

- A high-fiber diet increases stool bulk and speeds passage of food through intestines.
- Fiber intake may be increased by making subtle changes in eating and cooking habits such as eating more fresh fruits and vegetables especially with the skin on.
- Switching to high-fiber breads and cereals can significantly increase fiber intake. The first ingredient on the label should be "whole wheat" or "100% whole wheat," not just "wheat."
- A variety of foods high in fiber should be eaten; numerous forms of fiber exist and each performs a different action in the body (see Chapter 2).
- A meatless main dish made with dried peas and beans is a high-fiber alternative to traditional entrees.
- Fresh or dried fruit make high fiber snacks.
- Although nuts and seeds are high in fiber, they are also high in fat and should be used sparingly.
- Coarse, unprocessed wheat bran is most effective as a laxative. It can be incorporated into the diet by mixing it with juice or milk; by adding it to muffins, quick breads, casseroles, and meat loaves before baking; or by sprinkling it over cereal, applesauce, eggs, or other foods.
- Bran should be added to the diet slowly (up to 3 tbsp/day) to decrease the likelihood of developing flatus and distention.
- Certain foods (in addition to being high in fiber) have laxative effects: prunes and prune juice, figs, and dates.
- At least eight 8-oz glasses of fluid should be consumed daily.

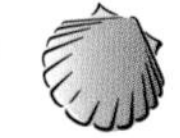

NURSING PROCESS

Ms. Scott is a frail, 79-year-old woman who has been hospitalized for a stroke (cerebrovascular accident, or CVA) for 6 days. Her physical impairments have gradually improved but she continues to have difficulty swallowing and left-sided weakness. On discharge from the hospital she was admitted to a nursing home, where a speech therapist performed a swallowing evaluation. The results indicated that Ms. Scott should be given semisolid foods until her ability to swallow improves. The patient's usual body mass index (BMI) is 19.6. Her current BMI is 18.2.

Assessment

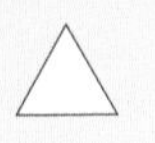

The Following Clinical Data Were Obtained:

Underweight according to BMI with recent weight loss
Status post-CVA with dysphagia
Increased serum sodium, blood urea nitrogen (BUN), and serum osmolality indicate dehydration
Intake and output records indicate poor oral fluid intake

Interviews with Patient and Nursing Staff Revealed:

Patient is fearful of eating and drinking because of frequent choking episodes in the hospital when given liquids.
Patient is anxious about her weight loss.

Nursing Diagnosis

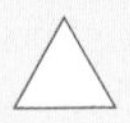

1. Altered Nutrition, Less Than Body Requirements, related to impaired swallowing secondary to CVA.

Planning and Implementation

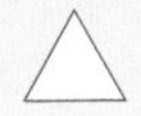

Client Goals

The client will

Swallow food and liquids without aspirating
Return to a regular diet
Consume adequate fluid to correct dehydration
Consume adequate calories and protein to increase BMI to 19.6

Nursing Interventions

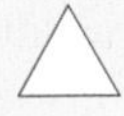

Give mouth care immediately before mealtime to enhance the sense of taste.
Provide a semisolid diet as ordered.
Position the patient in an upright position and tilt her head forward to facilitate swallowing.

(continued)

Feed small amounts at a time and place the food on the right side of the mouth.
Provide encouragement during mealtime.
Offer the patient pudding, custard, and yogurt between meals.
Provide thickened liquids between meals.
Monitor
- Intake and output as well as laboratory values for dehydration
- Swallowing ability, episodes of choking
- For signs and symptoms of aspiration
- Weight and BMI

Evaluation

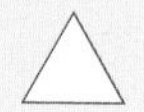

The client

Swallows food and liquids without aspirating
Returns to a regular diet
Consumes adequate fluid to correct dehydration
Consumes adequate calories and protein; increases body mass index to 19.6

DISORDERS OF THE UPPER GI TRACT

The upper GI tract refers to the mouth, esophagus, and stomach. Very little chemical digestion takes place in the upper GI tract; problems here impact nutrition mostly by affecting tolerance to particular foods or textures. Nutrition therapies for dysphagia, gastroesophageal reflux disease, peptic ulcers, and gastritis are discussed below.

Dysphagia

Dysphagia: altered ability to swallow.

Dysphagia can have a profound impact on intake and nutritional status, and it greatly increases the risk of aspiration and its complications of bacterial pneumonia, bronchial obstruction, and chemical pneumonitis. Many conditions cause swallowing impairments. Mechanical causes include obstruction, inflammation, edema, and surgery of the throat. Neurologic causes include amyotrophic lateral sclerosis (ALS), myasthenia gravis, cerebrovascular accident, traumatic brain injury, cerebral palsy, Parkinson's disease, and multiple sclerosis. Refer patients with actual or potential swallowing impairments to the speech pathology department for a thorough swallowing assessment.

Pathophysiology

Swallowing is a complex series of events characterized by four distinct phases.

The *oral preparatory phase* takes place in the mouth, where food (bolus) is chewed in preparation for swallowing. Obviously, liquids need little preparation compared with

 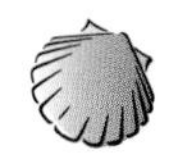

meat and raw vegetables. Patients who have difficulty with this phase may "pocket" food in the cheek, lose food from the lips, or be unable to move food toward the back of the mouth.

In the *oral phase,* the bolus is pushed steadily backward toward the pharynx, which opens to receive the bolus. Impairments in the tongue's muscles or nerves interfere with the oral phase and can cause coughing or choking before the patient swallows. Liquids, because they are difficult to control, are especially problematic.

The *pharyngeal phase* follows. As the food reaches the opening of the pharynx, the swallowing reflex is triggered and the food moves toward and into the esophagus. Food remaining in the throat, prolonged chewing, nasal regurgitation, coughing, choking during or after swallowing, and hoarseness after swallowing are all signs of problems with this phase.

The *esophageal phase* completes the process of swallowing. Peristaltic movements carry the bolus through the esophagus into the stomach. Neurologically impaired patients have less difficulty with this phase than with the other phases. However, obstruction and reduced esophageal peristalsis are concerns. Problems with this phase are less amenable to intervention than problems with the other three phases.

Nutrition Therapy

The goal of nutrition therapy for dysphagia is to modify the texture of foods and/or viscosity of liquids to enable the patient to achieve adequate nutrition and hydration while decreasing the risk of aspiration. Semisolid or medium-consistency foods, such as pudding, custards, scrambled eggs, yogurt, cooked cereals, and thickened liquids, are easiest to swallow and usually safest. As the patient's ability to swallow improves, the variety of food textures may be increased. For instance, patients who master swallowing thick liquids may be introduced to soft foods such as mashed potatoes, plain custards, and smooth cooked cereals. Liberal amounts of melted butter, gravy, and jelly may be used to help moisten foods. Table 17.1 outlines the four different levels of a dysphagia diet based on consistency.

To stimulate the swallowing reflex, food and beverages should be served at optimum temperature—either hot or cold—rather than tepid or room temperature. Tepid foods can be difficult to locate in the mouth and may increase the risk of choking.

Proper feeding techniques are especially important:

- Serve small, frequent meals to help maximize intake.
- Encourage dysphagic patients to rest before mealtime. Postpone meals if the patient is fatigued.
- Give mouth care immediately before meals to enhance the sense of taste.
- Instruct the patient to think of a specific food to stimulate salivation. A lemon slice, lemon hard candy, or dill pickles may also help to trigger salivation. Moderately flavored foods also help to stimulate salivation.
- Reduce or eliminate distractions at mealtime so that the patient can focus his or her attention on swallowing. Limit disruptions, if possible, and do not rush the patient; allow at least 30 minutes for eating.

TABLE 17.1 **DYSPHAGIA DIETS**

Stage/Type of Diet	Description	Foods Allowed
Stage 1: Pureed Diet	Smooth, pudding-like or spoon-thick consistency pureed foods that are homogenous. Eliminates sticky foods such as peanut butter and coarse textured-foods such as nuts and raw fruits and vegetables	Smooth cooked cereals; slurried bread products; milk; yogurt; pudding; applesauce; pureed fruits, vegetables, meats, scrambled eggs, and soups; custard; ice cream; sherbet; liquids thickened as required with commercial thickening agent
Stage 2: Ground Diet	Provides minimum amount of easily chewed foods. Elimi-nates coarse tex-tures, nuts, and raw fruits and vegetables (except banana). Bread is slurried if necessary.	Smooth cooked cereals; bite-sized pasta, rice, and pan-cakes with syrup, if tolerated; slurried bread if necessary; soft poached or scrambled egg; milk and soft milk products; mashed fruit and vegetables without seeds or skins; ground meats or soft casseroles; smooth desserts; liquids thickened as required
Stage 3: Soft, Easy-to-Chew Diet	Similar to mechanical soft diet; consists of soft foods that are not blenderized or pureed. Eliminates tough skins, nuts, dry, crispy, raw, and stringy foods. Meats are minced or diced.	Cooked and ready-to-eat cere-als with milk; poached and scrambled eggs; soft milk products such as yogurt, pudding, cottage cheese, ricotta cheese; rice, pasta, toast without crust if toler-ated; soft fresh or canned fruit without seeds; well cooked or canned vegetables; ground meats or moist, shaved meats with gravy; soft desserts with-out nuts; liquids thickened as required consistency
Stage 4: Modified General Diet	A soft diet that eliminates nuts and deep-fried foods. No foods are chopped or ground.	Foods to avoid include hard bagels, melba toast, hard breadsticks, fruit with skin, hard-to-chew raw vegetables, chewy desserts such as hard marshmallow or caramel, chips, popcorn

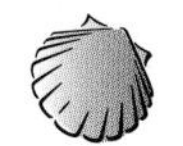

- Place the patient in an upright or high Fowler's position. If the patient has one-sided facial weakness, place the food on the other side of the mouth. Tilt the head forward to facilitate swallowing.
- Use adaptive eating devices such as built-up utensils and mugs with spouts, if indicated. Syringes should never be used to force liquids into the patient's mouth because this can trigger choking or aspiration. Unless otherwise directed, do not allow the patient to use a straw.
- Encourage small bites and thorough chewing.
- Consider tube feedings if the patient is unable to consume an adequate oral diet.

Alcohol interferes with effective swallowing and reduces cough and gag reflexes.

Gastroesophageal Reflux Disease

Gastroesophageal reflux disease (GERD) produces "indigestion" and "heartburn" from the backflow of acidic gastric juices onto the lower esophageal mucosa. The pain may radiate to the neck and throat. It worsens when the person lies down, bends over after eating, or wears tight-fitting clothing. Some people experience regurgitation and over time GERD can lead to esophagitis, dysphagia, and esophageal ulcers and bleeding. However, some people may be relatively asymptomatic, complaining only of a "lump" in their throat.

Pathophysiology

GERD occurs when acidic gastric juices back flow into the esophagus through an incompetent lower esophageal sphincter (LES). GERD is most likely to occur when either the LES or stomach has increased pressure such as in the case of hiatal hernia, the use of alcohol, being overweight, pregnancy, smoking, and delayed gastric emptying.

Nutrition Therapy

Nutrition therapy is one component of a multifactorial approach that includes lifestyle modification, drug therapy, and sometimes surgery. Interventions to reduce or avoid symptoms are to

- Lose weight (if overweight) because weight loss decreases intra-abdominal pressure
- Avoid items that decrease LES pressure, namely
  Alcohol
  Caffeine (coffee, tea, cola)
  Chocolate
  Coffee with or without caffeine
  High-fat foods
  Mint
  Smoking

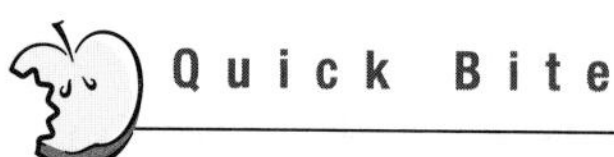

Non-citrus sources of vitamin C

Broccoli
Brussels sprouts
Cantaloupe
Kiwi
Mango
Papaya
Red pepper
Strawberries

- During times of esophagitis, avoid items that may irritate the esophagus such as carbonated beverages, citrus fruits and juices, spicy foods, tomato products, and any other individual intolerances. People who avoid citrus juices and tomato products because of their acidity should be encouraged to eat other sources of vitamin C.
- Avoid large meals to avoid increased gastric pressure.
- Remain upright for 45 to 60 minutes after eating; avoid eating 2 to 3 hours before bedtime; avoid tight-fitting clothing; and elevate the head of the bed 6 to 8 inches while sleeping.

Career Connection

Advertisements for over-the-counter drugs to combat heartburn promise pleasure with impunity by simply popping a pill before or after an eating indiscretion. Although they work well, relying on medications to stave off pain after eating whatever, whenever, and in any amount is foolhardy. All medications have the potential to cause side effects, and pain is a signal that something is wrong. Encourage clients to implement eating and lifestyle changes to see if they alone can prevent symptoms.

Peptic Ulcers

Peptic Ulcer: erosion of the mucosal layer of the stomach (gastric ulcer) or duodenum (duodenal ulcer) caused by an excess secretion of, or decreased mucosal resistance to, hydrochloric acid.

A bacterial infection caused by *Helicobacter pylori* is believed to be the biggest cause of peptic ulcers. *H. pylori,* which occurs in as many as 80% to 90% of patients with peptic ulcers, appears to secrete an enzyme that may deplete gastric mucus, making the mucosal layer more susceptible to erosion. For these patients, destroying the bacteria generally cures the ulcer. The second leading cause of peptic ulcers is the use of nonsteroidal antiinflammatory drugs (NSAIDs) that may damage the stomach lining. Eating spicy food does not cause ulcers.

Compared to the role of antibiotics and drug therapy, nutrition therapy plays a minor, supporting role in the treatment of peptic ulcers. Any foods not tolerated by the individual are eliminated. Although some people benefit psychologically from a strict diet, there is no evidence to support the use of a bland diet to decrease gastric acid secretion or promote healing. Encourage clients to

- Eat a well-balanced diet.
- To prevent increased acid secretion, avoid frequent meals and bedtime snacks.
- Avoid alcohol, cigarette smoking, aspirin, and other NSAIDs.
- Avoid any foods not tolerated especially those that stimulate gastric acid secretion (Box 17.5).

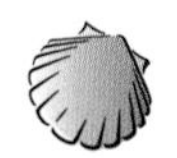

BOX 17.5

FOODS AND SEASONINGS THAT STIMULATE GASTRIC ACID SECRETION

Coffee, regular and decaffeinated
Black pepper
Caffeine
Chili powder
Cloves
Garlic
Peppermint and spearmint oils

Gastritis

Gastritis: inflammation of the gastric mucosa.

Acute gastritis is a temporary inflammation, usually self-limiting, caused by the ingestion of infectious or corrosive substances (e.g., aspirin), food poisoning, radiation therapy, metabolic stress, acute alcoholism, and uremia. Symptoms vary with the source of the irritation and range from mild (heartburn) to severe (vomiting, bleeding, hematemesis). Erosion of the gastric mucosa can lead to massive hemorrhage.

During an attack of acute gastritis, food is withheld for 1 to 2 days and intravenous fluids are provided until symptoms subside. Thereafter, the diet is liberalized according to individual tolerance, but foods known to stimulate gastric acid secretion are avoided (see Box 17.5).

Achlorhydria: lack of hydrochloric acid in the stomach.

Chronic gastritis is marked by progressive and irreversible atrophy of the gastric mucosa related to chronic inflammation. Atrophic gastritis is the most common form of chronic gastritis. Although the exact cause is unknown, chronic atrophic gastritis is associated with *H. pylori* infection and aging. If symptoms occur, they are likely to be

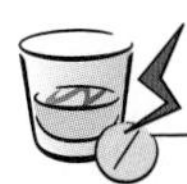

DRUG ALERT

- **Antacids:** Antacids interfere with iron absorption and may cause iron deficiency anemia. They produce other side effects depending on their composition: magnesium may lead to diarrhea, aluminum to constipation, calcium to hypercalcemia, and sodium to fluid retention (sodium-containing antacids are contraindicated for patients who require low-sodium diets).
- **Receptor antagonists:** Histamine H_2 blockers are commonly used in the treatment of peptic ulcers. Cimetidine (Tagamet) decreases gastric secretion, which reduces the absorption of iron, folic acid, and vitamin B_{12}; hyperglycemia and diarrhea may occur. Ranitidine (Zantac) usually produces fewer side effects and interactions than cimetidine but it may cause abdominal discomfort, constipation or diarrhea, and decreased absorption of vitamin B_{12} with long-term use.
- **Antisecretory agents:** The antisecretory drug omeprazole (Prilosec) can cause dry mouth and anorexia.

mild and comparable to those of acute gastritis. The loss of mucosal cell function may lead to achlorhydria, pernicious anemia, and malnutrition. Additional complications include perforation, hemorrhage, and pyloric obstruction related to scar tissue. Early diagnosis and treatment are imperative to prevent irreversible damage.

Gastritis may be treated medically with antacids, antisecretory agents, and antiulcer drugs. A well-balanced diet free of foods that stimulate gastric acid secretion is recommended and individual intolerances are eliminated (see Box 17.5). Clients with pernicious anemia require parenteral injections or nasal sprays of vitamin B_{12}, due to the lack of intrinsic factor necessary for absorption of B_{12}. Achlorhydria may necessitate parenteral iron injections.

DISORDERS OF THE INTESTINES

Steatorrhea: fatty diarrhea that produces loose, foamy, and foul-smelling stools.

Ninety percent to 95% of nutrient absorption occurs in the first half of the small intestine. Impairments in normal small intestine function, for instance, inadequate enzyme levels, rapid transit time, or impaired absorptive surface, can lead to significant malabsorption and malnutrition. Most often, malabsorption affects multiple nutrients. Of greatest concern is the malabsorption of fat (steatorrhea), which causes loss of calories, subsequent weight loss, and numerous secondary nutrient deficiencies such as deficiencies of essential fatty acids, fat-soluble vitamins, and calcium. From those deficiencies, metabolic disturbances may develop (Table 17.2). Compound the problem of decreased absorption with a poor intake and elevated nutritional needs, and malnutrition is almost certainly guaranteed.

The goal of nutrition therapy for malabsorption syndromes is to control steatorrhea, promote normal bowel elimination, restore optimal nutritional status, and promote healing, when applicable:

- A low-fat diet of 35 g or less is indicated if steatorrhea is occurring (Box 17.6). Medium-chain triglycerides (MCT) oil may be used to increase calorie intake (see Chapter 4). MCT oil should be added to the diet gradually to avoid nausea, vomiting, abdominal pain, and distention. The palatability of MCT oil can be improved by substituting it for regular oils in salad dressings and in cooking and baking. However, MCT does not supply essential fatty acids.
- Limit fiber to slow transit time and decrease peristalsis.
- Restrict lactose (milk sugar) even if a lactase deficiency has not been objectively diagnosed. Lactase activity may return to normal after malabsorption has been resolved.
- Increase calories and protein to restore weight and nutritional status. Calorie and protein requirements also increase when healing is required as in the case of regional enteritis, ulcerative colitis and after surgery. Calorie needs may range from 2000 to 3500 cal/day and protein from 1.0 to 1.5 g protein per kilogram.
- Multivitamin, mineral, and water-miscible supplements of fat-soluble vitamins are needed not only to replenish losses but also to facilitate healing and meet increased needs related to the metabolism of a high-calorie, high-protein diet.

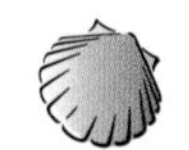

TABLE 17.2 POTENTIAL SECONDARY NUTRIENT DEFICIENCIES AND METABOLIC DISTURBANCES OF MALABSORPTION SYNDROME

Nutrient	Potential Problems
Potential Secondary Nutrient Deficiencies	
Potassium	Muscle weakness
Protein	Hypoalbuminemia, edema, muscle weakness, increased risk of infection, poor wound healing
Iron, folic acid, vitamin B_{12}	Anemia, fatigue, pallor, weakness, palpitations, anorexia, indigestion, sore mouth
Vitamin K	Purpura and easy bleeding
Vitamin A	Roughening of skin, impaired night vision, increased risk of infections
Calcium, magnesium, vitamin D	Osteomalacia and bone pain
Calcium, magnesium	Tetany
B-complex vitamins	Stomatitis, cheilosis, glossitis, and dermatitis
Lactose	Cramping, distention, flatus, and diarrhea after milk ingestion related to secondary lactose deficiency
Potential Metabolic Disturbances	
Impaired absorption of bile salts	Cholesterol gallstone formation (cholesterol from cholesterol-saturated bile may precipitate out into gallstones)
Increased oxalate absorption	Increased risk of oxalate kidney stone formation

- Increase fluid intake to compensate for increased fluid output as necessary (e.g., diarrhea, fistula drainage, blood loss).

A sample low-fat, low-fiber, low lactose menu appears in Box 17.7.

Regardless of the underlying disorder, the diet should be individualized as much as possible to correspond with the patient's likes, dislikes, and intolerances. Small, frequent meals help to maximize intake. Patients who are apprehensive about eating need emotional support and encouragement. If the patient is malnourished, a nasojejunal tube feeding of a hydrolyzed formula or TPN may be used until oral intake is resumed (see Chapter 15). Oral intake should progress to a nutrient-rich diet as soon as possible.

Dumping Syndrome

Dumping syndrome is a complication of gastric surgeries in which the pyloric sphincter is removed, bypassed, or disrupted. Nutritional problems occur until the patient's

(*text continues on page 499*)

BOX 17.6

LOW-FAT DIET

Characteristics

This diet limits the total amount of fat to reduce symptoms of steatorrhea and pain in patients who are intolerant of fat. Foods are baked, broiled, or boiled instead of fried or prepared with added fat. Visible fats on meats are trimmed and poultry skin is removed preferably before cooking. Allowed fats can be used as seasonings or in cooking.

A 50-g fat diet allows

- 6 oz of lean meat or meat substitutes
- Three to five fat equivalents per day
- Moderate portions of all other low-fat and fat-free items

A 25-g fat diet allows

- 4 oz of lean meat or meat substitutes
- One fat equivalent per day
- Moderate portions of all other low-fat and fat-free items

Indications for Use

Malabsorption syndromes such as acquired immunodeficiency syndrome, chronic pancreatitis, Crohn's disease, radiation enteritis, short-bowel syndrome, and chronic cholecystitis, type 1 hyperlipoproteinemia (25 to 35 mg fat)
May also relieve symptoms of GERD

Contraindications

None

Guidelines to Achieve a Low-Fat Diet

Recommended foods

- Meats: lean meat, fish, and skinless poultry; egg whites and low-fat egg substitutes as desired
- Dairy products: milk, yogurt, and puddings that provide less than 1 g fat/serving; low-fat cheese with 3 g fat or less/serving
- Fruits and vegetables: all fruits and vegetables prepared without added fat except avocado and coconut
- Bread and cereals: plain cereals, pasta, macaroni, rice, whole-grain or enriched breads; plain corn or flour tortillas; bagels
- Miscellaneous: sherbet, fruit ices, gelatin, angel food cake, vanilla wafers, graham crackers, nonfat ice cream and frozen yogurt; fruit whips with gelatin; fat-free or skim-milk soups, soft drinks, honey, sugar, seasonings as desired
- Fats: each of the following constitutes one serving (one "equivalent"):
  - 1 tsp butter, margarine, shortening, oil, or mayonnaise
  - 1 tbsp diet margarine, diet mayonnaise, or reduced-calorie cream salad dressing
  - 1 strip crisp bacon
  - 1 tbsp sesame, sunflower, or pumpkin seeds
  - 2 tbsp sour cream, cream cheese, half-and-half, or coffee whitener
  - 1 tbsp heavy cream
  - 2 tsp regular creamy salad dressing
  - 2 tsp peanut butter
  - 2 tsp light cream
  - 6 small nuts
  - 8–10 olives
  - ⅛ medium avocado

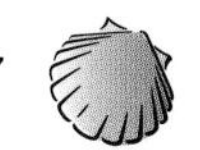

BOX 17.6 (continued)

LOW-FAT DIET

Avoid the following foods:

- Meats: meats with >3 g fat/oz such as fried, fatty, or heavily marbled meats; sausage, lunch meat, spareribs, frankfurters, salt pork, tuna and salmon packed in oil; egg yolks; duck, goose
- Dairy products: 1%, 2%, and whole milk; whole-milk cheeses and yogurt; ice cream
- Fruits and vegetables: any buttered, au gratin, creamed, or fried vegetables; potato chips; chow mein noodles
- Breads and cereals: products made with added fat such as biscuits, muffins, pancakes, doughnuts, waffles, and sweet rolls; breads made with eggs, cheese, or added fat; buttered popcorn; granola-type cereals; popovers; snack crackers with added fat; snack chips; stuffing
- Miscellaneous: cream sauces, gravy; desserts, candy, and anything made with chocolate or nuts; cakes, cookies, pies, pastries

Sample Menu (25 g fat)

Breakfast

Orange juice
Oatmeal
Skim milk
Toast with jelly
Coffee/tea
Salt/pepper/sugar

Lunch

Fat-free vegetable soup
Sandwich: whole-wheat bread, 2 oz skinless chicken breast, lettuce and fat-free mayo
Tossed salad with fat-free dressing
Fruit cocktail
Skim milk
Coffee/tea
Salt/pepper/sugar

Dinner

2 oz broiled fish
Baked potato with salsa
Steamed broccoli
Carrot and celery sticks
Dinner roll with 1 tsp margarine
Fresh strawberries over angel food cake
Skim milk
Coffee/tea
Salt/pepper/sugar

Snack

Unbuttered popcorn
Fruit juice

Potential Problems	Recommended Interventions
Noncompliance related to decreased palatability and satiety from the reduction in fat intake	Encourage the patient to eat a variety of foods and to use nonfat and fat-free versions of familiar foods. Encourage use of butter-flavored sprinkles and sprays to season hot vegetables and potatoes.

(box continues on page 498)

BOX 17.6 (continued)

LOW-FAT DIET

Persistent symptoms of steatorrhea or pain after eating related to fat intolerance	Decrease fat content by eliminating fat equivalents and limiting amount of low-fat meat allowed.
Inadequate intake of iron related to the limited allowance of meat (red meat is the best absorbed source of iron in the diet)	Monitor hemoglobin and hematocrit; recommend iron supplements as needed. Encourage a liberal intake of high-iron foods such as fortified cereals and grains and dried peas and beans. Advise the patient to consume a rich source of vitamin C at each meal to maximize iron absorption.

Patient Teaching

Ensure the patient understands that

- The total amount of dietary fat must be reduced regardless of the source.
- Sources of fat may be visible (e.g., butter, margarine, shortening, fat on meat, salad dressings) or invisible (e.g., marbled meat, whole milk and whole-milk products, egg yolks, nuts).
- Substitutions can be made to individualize the diet.
- Oil-packed tuna and salmon may be used if thoroughly rinsed.
- Fat-free salad dressings may be used as desired.
- Tips for reducing fat content when eating out:
  a. Choose juice or broth-based soup instead of cream soup as an appetizer.
  b. Use lemon, vinegar, low-calorie dressing (if available), or fresh ground pepper on salad or request that the dressing be brought on the side.
  c. Order plain baked or broiled foods.
  d. Avoid warm bread and rolls, which absorb more butter than those at room temperature.
  e. Order fresh fruit, gelatin, or sherbet for dessert.
  f. Request milk for coffee or tea in place of cream and nondairy creamers.

Food preparation techniques to reduce fat content:

- Trim fat from meat and remove skin from chicken before cooking.
- Place meats to be baked or roasted on a rack to allow the fat to drain.
- Bake, broil, steam, or sauté foods in a vegetable cooking spray or allowed fats.
- Cook with bouillon, lemon, vinegar, wine, herbs, and spices instead of adding fat.
- Make fat-free soup stock by preparing the stock a day ahead and refrigerating it overnight. The fat will harden and can easily be removed from the surface. Make fat-free gravies by this method also.
- Purchase "select" grade meats because they are lower in fat than "choice" and "prime" grades.

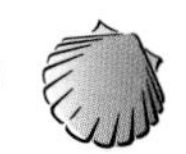

BOX 17.7

SAMPLE MENU FOR PATIENT WITH INFLAMMATORY BOWEL DISEASE: LOW-FAT, LOW-FIBER, LOW LACTOSE, HIGH PROTEIN

Breakfast

Strained orange juice
Scrambled egg substitutes
White toast with jelly
Weak tea
Salt/pepper/sugar

Mid Morning Snack

6 oz nonfat yogurt

Lunch

Apricot nectar
Fat-free chicken noodle soup
Sandwich: white bread, 2 oz skinless chicken breast, and fat-free mayo
Gelatin
Weak tea

Midafternoon Snack

8 oz Boost

Dinner

Tomato juice
2 oz broiled fish
Baked potato with margarine
Green beans
Angel food cake
Weak tea
Salt/pepper/sugar

Snack

8 oz Boost

body adapts to the altered pyloric sphincter. Weight loss after gastric surgery is caused by many factors, including diarrhea, steatorrhea, voluntary restriction of food intake to avoid symptoms, early satiety, and a restrictive diet.

Pathophysiology

Normally, the pyloric sphincter allows controlled amounts of food to move from the stomach into the small bowel. When that sphincter is bypassed or impaired, undigested food is rapidly "dumped" into the duodenum or jejunum. When the duodenum is bypassed, digestive activity that normally occurs there is also bypassed; even when the duodenum is intact, the food moves quickly into the jejunum.

The undigested food in the jejunum is hypertonic, which causes fluid to shift from the plasma and extracellular fluid into the jejunum to dilute the high particle concentration. The large volume of hypertonic fluid in the jejunum causes nausea, distention, crampy pain, and diarrhea within 15 minutes after eating. The fluid shift causes a rapid decrease in circulating blood volume, leading to weakness, dizziness, and a rapid heartbeat.

A secondary reaction, called reactive hypoglycemia, may occur 1 to 2 hours later. The rapid absorption of carbohydrate causes a rapid rise in blood glucose levels. The body compensates by oversecreting insulin, which causes a rapid drop in blood glucose levels and dizziness, perspiration, tachycardia, mental confusion, and syncope.

Maldigestion and malabsorption occur because transit time is rapid and food does not have adequate exposure time with enzymes and bile. Reduced gastric acid secretion may lead to bacterial overgrowth in the stomach or small intestine, causing the malabsorption of fat, fat-soluble vitamins, folate, vitamin B_{12}, and calcium. The excretion of calories and nutrients produces weight loss and increases the risk of malnutrition.

Nutrition Therapy

Strategies to manage dumping syndrome are to (Box 17.8)

- Eat five to six or more small meals daily because the holding capacity of the stomach is reduced. Encourage the client to eat slowly and chew food thoroughly.
- Eliminate simple sugars because they are quickly digested and form a hyperosmolar solution in the jejunum that attracts water. Avoid sugar, gelatin, cookies, soft drinks, undiluted juices, and other high-sugar items.
- Include moderate fat and high protein at each feeding because they are digested more slowly than carbohydrates and do not increase osmolarity as readily.
- Adjust total calorie intake according to weight goals. For instance, weight gain may be indicated for patients undergoing gastric surgery for cancer whereas weight loss is the intended outcome in patients who have gastric bypass surgery to treat obesity.
- Avoid fluids with meals and 1 hour before or after eating. Limit liquid serving sizes to ½ to 1 cup.
- Lie down for 20 to 30 minutes after eating to delay gastric emptying time. (Patients who have reflux should not lie down.)
- Eat foods high in pectin (e.g., apple) and guar gum (e.g., oats), which may help to slow gastric emptying, slow carbohydrate absorption, and blunt the glycemic response. Taking 1 tsp pectin three times daily may be helpful.
- Milk is restricted or eliminated based on tolerance. (Lactose intolerance is common.) Lactose-reduced milk may not be well tolerated because its lactose has been broken down to glucose and galactose, which are simple sugars that may promote dumping.
- Iron, vitamin B_{12}, and folate deficiencies may occur secondary to decreased intake, blood loss, or impaired absorption. Parenteral injections of iron and vitamin B_{12} may be necessary.
- All food and beverages should be served at moderate temperatures; iced or cold beverages may not be tolerated.

BOX 17.8 **ANTI-DUMPING DIET GUIDELINES**

Recommended foods:

- Breads and cereals: whole grain or enriched plain breads, crackers, rolls, unsweetened cereal, rice, pasta
- Vegetables: cooked vegetables, vegetable juice, raw vegetables as tolerated
- Fruit: unsweetened fruit and fruit juices
- Milk and milk products: initially withheld and gradually introduced as tolerated
- Meat and meat alternatives: all allowed
- Fats: all allowed
- Beverages: tea, artificially sweetened soft drinks; diluted fruit juice

Avoid the following foods:

- Sweetened cereals; cereals containing dried fruit; pastries, doughnuts, muffins, coarse cereals; breads containing dried fruit, nuts, or seeds
- Vegetables: any that have sugar added; fried vegetables as tolerated
- Dried fruit, sweetened fruit, sweetened fruit juices
- Milk and milk products (initially)
- Alcohol, coffee, sweetened carbonated beverages, milk-based beverages, fruit drinks and ades
- Cakes, cookies, ice cream, sherbet, frozen yogurt, gelatin, honey, jam, jelly, syrup, sugar

Sample Menu

Breakfast

1 poached egg
1 slice white toast with butter
1 hour later: 6 oz apricot nectar

Midmorning Snack

Firm banana
Butter crackers

Lunch

½ cup cottage cheese with two unsweetened, canned peach halves
Dinner roll with butter
1 hour later: 8 oz artificially sweetened ginger ale

Midafternoon Snack

1 oz cheddar cheese
4 saltine crackers

Dinner

2 oz baked chicken
½ cup white rice with butter
½ cup cooked carrots with butter
1 hour later: hot tea

Bedtime Snack

½ plain bagel with cream cheese

Eventually the diet can be liberalized to include limited amounts of concentrated sweets, larger meal sizes, and some liquid with meals as the remaining portion of the stomach or duodenum hypertrophies to hold more food and allow for more normal digestion.

Lactose Intolerance

Lactose: the disaccharide (double sugar) in milk composed of glucose and galactose.

Lactase is the enzyme responsible for splitting lactose into its component simple sugars, glucose and galactose. For the majority of the world's population, especially Asians, Native Americans, Africans, Hispanics, and people from the Mediterranean, lactase in adults is reduced to only 5% to 10% of the peak levels that occur in infancy.

Pathophysiology

Without adequate lactase, lactose passes through the small intestine undigested. In the colon, lactose ferments, producing short-chain fatty acids and gases. Bloating, cramping, flatulence, and diarrhea are common.

Primary lactose intolerance occurs in "well" people who simply do not secrete adequate lactase. For most of these people, symptoms do not occur at doses less than 4 to 12 g of lactose (e.g., ⅓ to 1 cup of milk) or when lactose is consumed as part of a meal. Individual tolerance varies considerably; simply knowing individual limits (e.g., 8 ounces of milk with dinner is tolerated but 8 ounces of milk between meals is not) is enough to prevent symptoms.

A more problematic lactose intolerance occurs secondary to gastrointestinal disorders that alter the integrity and function of intestinal villi cells, where lactase is secreted. For instance, people with inflammatory bowel disease lose lactase activity when the disease is active and sometimes for a prolonged period afterward. The loss of lactase may also develop secondary to malnutrition because the rapidly growing intestinal cells that produce lactase are reduced in number and function. Secondary lactose intolerance tends to be more severe than primary lactose intolerance. Distention, cramps, flatus, and diarrhea occur within 15 to 30 minutes after lactose ingestion because undigested lactose increases the osmolality of the intestinal contents, resulting in a large fluid shift into the intestines to dilute the particle concentration.

Nutrition Therapy

Nutrition therapy for lactose intolerance is to reduce lactose to the maximum amount tolerated by the individual (Box 17.9). For patients with gastrointestinal disorders, a lactose-restricted diet is indicated at least until the gastrointestinal disorder is resolved and sometimes for a prolonged period thereafter. Because lactose is used as an ingredient in many foods and drugs, it is difficult to eliminate lactose from the diet.

Inflammatory Bowel Disease

Regional enteritis (Crohn's disease) and ulcerative colitis are chronic, inflammatory bowel diseases that produce similar symptoms during periods of exacerbation: diarrhea

BOX 17.9

TEACHING PATIENTS WITH PRIMARY OR SECONDARY LACTOSE INTOLERANCE

Teach the patient to limit lactose (milk sugar) to the level tolerated. Tolerated levels vary among individuals.

The following foods contain high amounts of lactose:

- Milk: whole, 2%, 1%, skim, buttermilk, evaporated, nonfat dry milk, milk solids, sweetened condensed
- Cream; sour cream
- All cheese except aged natural cheeses
- Creamed soups and sauces
- Specialty or flavored instant coffee blends made with creamer
- Cocoa and most chocolate beverages
- Ice cream, sherbet, ice milk, custard
- Puddings, commercial desserts and mixes

Teach the patient to read labels to identify sources of lactose. Products that have milk, butter, margarine, dry milk solids, or whey listed as ingredients contain some lactose. Examples are

- Breads and cereals prepared with milk such as waffles, crepes, and pancakes
- Cookies, cakes, pastries, commercial fruit pie fillings, sherbet
- Cold cuts and hot dogs
- Creamed or breaded meats and vegetables
- Gravy, dried soups, dips, salad dressings
- Commercial French fries, instant potatoes, mashed potatoes
- Butterscotch, caramels, chocolate candy, molasses, peppermints, toffee, chewing gum
- Cordials and liqueurs
- Maraschino cherries
- Powdered soft drinks, hot chocolate mixes, powdered coffee creamer, artificial whipped topping
- Some dietetic and diabetic foods
- Sugar substitutes (Sweet 'N Low and Equal tablets)
- Chocolate; caramels
- Some vitamin and mineral preparations

Other foods with small amounts of lactose include

- Liver, sweetbreads
- Acidophilus milk

Lactate, lactalbumin, and calcium compounds are lactic acid salts and are lactose free. Kosher foods labeled *pareve* are made without milk. Nondairy creamer is also lactose free and may be used in beverages, on cereal, and in cooking if desired. Acidophilus milk or Lactaid milk may be tolerated. Lactaid is available in supermarkets and can be used as a beverage or in cooking. Make sure the patient is aware of the risk for calcium deficiency related to reduction or elimination of milk and dairy products from the diet. Encourage the intake of calcium from nondairy sources such as green leafy vegetables, dates, prunes, canned sardines and salmon with bones, egg yolks, whole grains, nuts, dried peas and beans, and calcium-fortified orange juice. Provide calcium supplements as needed.

Career Connection

Many people self-diagnose lactose intolerance and consequently forsake all milk and dairy products. In fact, milk ranks high on the list of foods that supposedly cause "gas." Yet a double-blind study that gave one glass of milk twice a day to supposedly severely lactose-intolerant people found insignificant symptoms—actually no difference in symptoms—when participants drank milk with or without lactose. Although that study does not exonerate lactose, it clearly shows that for many people "lactose intolerance" is a matter of degree and probably influenced by expectations. These are points lactose-intolerant people may benefit from hearing:

- "Well" people may tolerate milk when it is consumed with food and the serving size is limited to 1 cup or less. Because of its many nutritional attributes (protein, calcium, vitamin D, riboflavin), milk should not be rashly banned from the diet on the assumption of intolerance.
- Milk treated with the enzyme lactase (either LactAid milk or LactAid tablets added to milk by the consumer) has its lactose broken down into glucose and galactose and so is lactose-free.
- Chocolate milk is generally better tolerated than unflavored milk.
- In the production of hard, aged cheese, lactose is converted to lactic acid. If the Nutrition Facts label indicates only 1 or 2 g of sugar/serving (which is lactose in this case), that cheese is probably safe to eat. Processed cheese has more lactose than aged cheese.
- Much of the lactose in yogurt is digested by its bacteria, so it is usually well tolerated. Some brands, however, have milk added.

with possible melena, nausea, vomiting, weight loss, crampy abdominal pain, fever, fatigue, and anorexia.

Pathophysiology

Maldigestion and malabsorption of nutrients may occur from the disease, from surgery to treat the disease, or from medications. As a result, nutritional status is often poor. Patients may avoid specific foods or food types based on experience of pain or diarrhea related to eating. Misconceptions and restrictive diets further limit choices. Malnutrition and anemia are common. Other potential complications with nutritional implications include fistulas and abscesses, hemorrhages, bowel perforations, intestinal obstructions, and dehydration. Inflammatory bowel diseases are characterized by alternating periods of exacerbation and remission.

Nutrition Therapy

The focus of nutrition therapy for acute inflammatory bowel disease is to correct deficiencies by providing nutrients in a form the patient can tolerate. In the acute stage, an elemental tube feeding, possibly one fortified with glutamine, may be indicated to minimize fecal volume. TPN is used for patients who need complete bowel rest or who

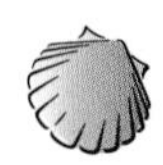

are unable to meet their nutritional requirements through an oral diet or tube feeding. Patients who are fed orally are often reluctant to eat, because they associate eating with pain and diarrhea. Generally, the diet

- Is low in fiber to minimize bowel stimulation. For the same reason, sugar alcohols, caffeine, iced beverages, and carbonated beverages should be avoided.
- Is low in lactose because lactase activity may be reduced or absent. Lactose intolerance may persist for a period after the period of exacerbation has passed.
- Is high in protein and calories to promote healing and restore weight; fat is restricted if the patient has steatorrhea.
- Includes commercial supplements usually needed to meet needs. Appropriate formulas (high-protein, low-fiber, lactose-free, low-fat) may be more numerous and easier to consume than appropriate foods.
- Includes necessary supplemental vitamins and minerals.
- Consists of small, frequent meals that are better tolerated than three large meals and may help to maximize intake.

During remission, a well-balanced diet based on individual tolerance is recommended. Lactose and fiber tolerances vary among individuals. Omega-3 fatty acids, commonly known as "fish oils," may mitigate the inflammatory response.

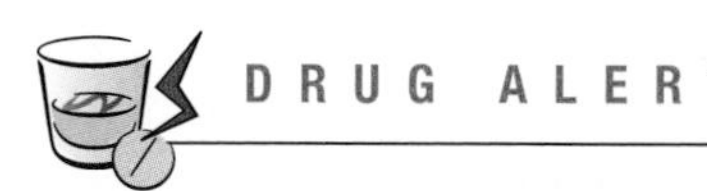

DRUG ALERT

Corticosteroids and Sulfasalazine

Corticosteroids can cause calcium and potassium depletion, sodium retention, and glucose intolerance. Monitor potassium and sodium status. Encourage intake of potassium-rich and calcium-rich foods. Limit sodium if edema or hypertension develops. Monitor serum glucose; long-term use of corticosteroids may necessitate the use of a diabetic diet.

Sulfasalazine interferes with the metabolism and physiologic function of folic acid, leading to folic acid deficiency anemia. Crystalluria and renal stone formation may also occur. Other common side effects include anorexia, nausea, and gastrointestinal upset. Provide folic acid supplements as needed. Encourage a high fluid intake to prevent renal stones. Give with food or milk.

NURSING PROCESS

Mr. Wittmeyer is a 22-year-old man who is admitted to the hospital for suspected Crohn's disease. His chief complaints are crampy abdominal pain, diarrhea, weight loss, fatigue, and anorexia. He has lost 15 pounds since his symptoms began 2 weeks ago. He is prescribed intravenous fluids, sulfasalazine, prednisone, an antidiarrheal medication, and a diet as tolerated.

Assessment

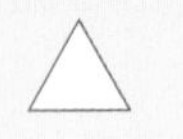

The Following Clinical Data were Obtained:

Recent weight loss of 15 pounds; BMI at 19
Admitted with Crohn's disease; no previous history
Low albumin, hemoglobin, hematocrit showing improvement
Increased serum sodium, BUN, and serum osmolality indicate dehydration

Interview With the Patient Revealed:

Patient is fearful of eating because he relates eating to pain and diarrhea; has been relying mostly on cola for nourishment.
Patient complains of fatigue and anorexia.
Before admission the patient consumed an unrestricted diet with irregular meal schedules and a high intake of milk.

Nursing Diagnosis

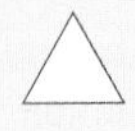

1. Altered Nutrition, Less Than Body Requirements, related to malabsorption secondary to Crohn's disease.

Planning and Implementation

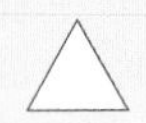

Client Goals

The client will

Experience improvement in symptoms (diarrhea, abdominal pain, fatigue, anorexia).
Restore normal fluid balance.
Consume adequate calories and protein to restore normal weight.
Describe the principles and rationale of nutrition therapy for Crohn's disease and implement the appropriate interventions.

Nursing Interventions

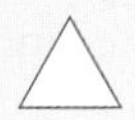

Nursing Therapy

Provide a low-fat, low-fiber, lactose-restricted diet.
Provide lactose-free commercial supplements between meals to enhance protein and calorie intake.
Encourage high fluid intake especially of fluids high in potassium such as tomato juice, apricot nectar, and orange juice.
Monitor
- Intake and output as well as fluid and electrolyte status
- Appetite
- Tolerance to fat (may need to reduce fat level)
- Diarrhea (if patient does not tolerate an oral diet, determine whether an elemental diet or TPN is appropriate)
- Weight changes and BMI

Client Teaching

Instruct the client

On the purpose and rationale of a low-fat, low-fiber, lactose-restricted diet. Advise the patient that he may be able to tolerate fiber and milk after the disease goes into remission.
On the importance of consuming adequate protein, calories, and fluid to promote healing and recovery
To maximize intake by eating small, frequent meals
To avoid colas and other sources of caffeine because they stimulate peristalsis
To eliminate individual intolerances
To chew food thoroughly and avoid swallowing air
On the importance of consuming adequate fluid while taking sulfasalazine
That prednisone should improve his appetite but may cause fluid retention and gastrointestinal upset
To communicate any side effects he experiences from the medications

Evaluation

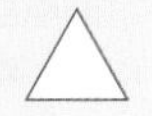

The client

Experiences improvement in symptoms (diarrhea, abdominal pain, fatigue, anorexia)
Attains normal fluid balance
Consumes adequate calories and protein to restore normal weight
Describes the principles and rationale of nutrition therapy for Crohn's disease and implements the appropriate interventions

Celiac Disease (Gluten-Induced Enteropathy, Nontropical Sprue)

Celiac disease is a genetic autoimmune disorder that affects the small intestine when gluten is consumed.

Pathophysiology

Gluten: a general name for the storage proteins gliadin (in wheat), secalin (in rye), and hordein (in barley).

For patients with celiac disease, eating foods that contain gluten (e.g., wheat, rye, barley) causes the intestinal villi to become flattened and atrophied, resulting in a decreased absorptive surface, loss of disaccharidases, and widespread malabsorption of many nutrients including fat, protein, carbohydrate, fat-soluble vitamins, iron, calcium, magnesium, zinc, and some water-soluble vitamins.

Symptoms and their severity vary widely among individuals. Most commonly, celiac disease causes diarrhea, weight loss, muscle wasting, fatigue, and malnutrition. Other common symptoms include iron deficiency anemia, gas, abdominal bloating, edema, and lactose intolerance. Children may display severe irritability, growth stunting, and delayed puberty.

However, many patients with celiac disease eat gluten occasionally or in normal amounts and do not complain of symptoms. Yet even without symptoms, the intestinal mucosa is abnormal in most patients and the risk of cancer, particularly GI lymphoma, is increased. Therefore, the long-term effects of eating even small amounts of gluten are harmful even in asymptomatic patients.

Nutrition Therapy

The only treatment for celiac disease is to completely and permanently eliminate gluten from the diet. A gluten-free diet (Box 17.10) allows the villi to return toward normal, usually within a few weeks, although complete regeneration may never occur. Lactose intolerance secondary to celiac disease may be temporary or permanent.

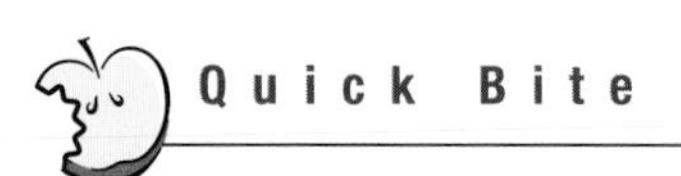

Some alternatives for wheat flour

Cornstarch
Potato flour
White rice flour
Tapioca starch
Quick cooking tapioca
Sweet rice flour
Taro flour
Acorn flour
Almond flour
Brown rice flour
Channa flour (a type of chickpea)

Gluten is found in wheat, rye, and barley—grains that form the foundation of a healthy diet in most cultures. Relatively recently, research has shown that pure oats is gluten free and, therefore, not harmful to people with celiac disease. However, there is worldwide concern that the risk of oats being contaminated with gluten is unacceptably high. Celiac organizations in the United States do not endorse the use of oats.

A gluten-free diet requires a major lifestyle change, so compliance is often a major problem. Gluten-free products (e.g., breads, pastry) made with rice, corn, or potato flour have different textures and tastes than "normal" products and are not well accepted. They are also expensive. Even patients who are willing to comply have difficulty

(*text continues on page 513*)

BOX 17.10

GLUTEN-FREE DIET

Characteristics

This diet eliminates gluten, a protein fraction found in wheat, rye, and barley. Oats are also eliminated due to the high risk of gluten contamination.

Indications

It is used to prevent intestinal villi changes, steatorrhea, and other symptoms characteristic of gluten-sensitive enteropathy, which is also known as celiac disease, celiac sprue, or nontropical sprue. This diet is also used for dermatitis herpetiformis.

Contraindications

None

Guidelines to Achieve a Gluten-Free Diet

Allowed grains and starches include
- Buckwheat
- Rice
- Corn
- Potato
- Tapioca
- Bean
- Sorghum
- Soy
- Arrowroot
- Amaranth
- Quinoa
- Millet
- Tef
- Flours made from nuts

Grains containing gluten that are not allowed
- Wheat including wheat berries, cracked wheat, wheat germ, wheat bran, wheat grass, wheat gluten, wheat nut, wheat starch, farina, bulgar, semolina, durum wheat, graham flour
- Rye
- Barley
- Oats*
- Spelt
- Triticale
- Kamut

Questionable ingredients that should only be used if they can be verified to be made from allowed grains:
- Brown rice syrup (may be made with barley)
- Caramel color
- Dextrin (usually from corn but may be made from wheat)
- Distilled white vinegar
- Emulsifiers

*Pure oats are gluten free, but celiac organizations in the U.S. do not endorse their use due to the high risk of contamination with gluten.

(box continues on page 510)

BOX 17.10 (continued)

GLUTEN-FREE DIET

Flavorings
Flour
Hydrolyzed vegetable protein, hydrolyzed plant protein, or textured vegetable protein
Imported foods labeled "gluten-free" may be made from wheat starch rendered gluten free but still contain small amounts of toxic substances
Ketchup, chili sauce, mustard, bottled meat sauces, horseradish
Malt, malt flavoring (may be made from barley; allowed if made from corn)
Modified food starch or modified starch
Mono- and di-glycerides (in dry products only)
Natural and artificial flavors
Soy sauce or soy sauce solids (many contain wheat)
Other products that often contain gluten:
Breading
Broth
Chip dips
Coating mixes
Communion wafers
Croutons
Imitation bacon
Imitation pepper
Imitation seafood
Licorice
Marinades
Processed meats
Sauces
Self-basting poultry
Soup base
Stuffing
Thickeners

Recommended foods

- Beverages: carbonated drinks, cocoa, coffee, tea, fruit juice, milk, decaffeinated coffee containing no wheat flour, soy milk, wine, rum, vodka derived from grapes or potatoes
- Breads and cereals: products made with arrowroot, cornstarch, cornmeal, potato, rice, soybean, and gluten-free wheat starch flours; pure rice, sago, and tapioca; gluten-free macaroni products; corn bread, muffins, and pone made without wheat flour; corn or rice cereals such as cornflakes, Cream of Rice, hominy, puffed rice, rice flakes, Rice Krispies; grits; rice cakes and wafers; pure corn tortillas; popcorn
- Desserts: cakes, cookies, pastries, and other baked products made with allowed flours; custard, gelatin, homemade cornstarch, tapioca, and rice puddings; ice cream and sherbet prepared without gluten stabilizers
- Fats: butter, corn oil, homemade salad dressings, pure mayonnaise made with allowed vinegar, margarine, other pure vegetable oils
- Fruits: all fruit and fruit juices

BOX 17.10 (continued)

GLUTEN-FREE DIET

- Meat and meat substitutes: all meats, poultry, fish, and shellfish; eggs; dried peas and beans; nuts; peanut butter; aged cheese; soybean and other meat substitutes; tofu; cold cuts, hot dogs, and sausage without fillers.
- Soups: broth, bouillon, clear soups, cream soups thickened with allowed flours
- Vegetables: all plain, fresh, frozen, or canned vegetables except those listed as excluded
- Miscellaneous: pepper; pickles; popcorn; potato chips; sugars and syrups, honey, jelly, jam; hard candy, plain chocolate; pure cocoa; molasses; cider, white, and rice vinegars

Avoid the following foods:

- Beverages: ale, beer, instant coffee containing wheat, Postum, Ovaltine and other cereal beverages, malted milk, instant milk drinks, hot cocoa mixes; nondairy cream substitutes; some herbal teas with barley or barley malt; alcoholic beverages distilled from cereal grains such as gin, whiskey, vodka, beer, ale, malt liquor; some root beers
- Breads and cereals: all products made from wheat, rye, oats, barley, buckwheat, durum, or graham including the following items:

All commercial yeast and quick-bread mixes	Noodles
All-purpose flour	Pancakes
Baking powder biscuits	Pastry flour
Rye flour	Pretzels
Bread crumbs	Bread flour
Self-rising flour	Vermicelli
Crackers and cracker crumbs	Waffles
Kasha	Whole or cracked wheat flours
Matzoh	Zwieback

- Cooked or ready-to-eat cereals containing malt, bran, rye, wheat, oats, barley, wheat germ, bulgur, spelt, cereals made with low-gluten flours
- Desserts: cakes, cookies, pastries, and other baked products made with flours not allowed; prepared mixes, prepared pudding thickened with wheat flour; ice cream cones; ice creams with gluten stabilizers; commercial pie fillings
- Fats: commercial salad dressings that contain gluten stabilizers; homemade salad dressings thickened with flour
- Fruit: any thickened fruits
- Soups: all soups thickened with wheat products or containing barley, noodles, or other wheat, rye, or oat products in any form; bouillon and bouillon cubes with hydrolyzed vegetable protein (HVP)
- Meats prepared with wheat, rye, oats, or barley, or gluten stabilizers or fillers such as some hot dogs, cold cuts, sandwich spreads, sausages, and canned meats; canned pork and beans; turkey basted or injected with HVP or texturized vegetable protein (TVP); breaded fish or meats; tuna canned with HVP
- Sweets: all others not listed previously
- Vegetables: any creamed or breaded vegetables unless allowed ingredients are used; canned baked beans; commercially prepared vegetables with cream sauce or cheese sauce

(box continues on page 512)

BOX 17.10 (continued)

GLUTEN-FREE DIET

Sample Menu

Breakfast

Orange juice
Cornflakes
Skim milk
Coffee
Salt/pepper/sugar

Midmorning Snack

Yogurt
Rice cake

Lunch

Cuban black beans with rice
Pure corn tortilla
Milk
Tapioca pudding
Coffee/tea
Salt/pepper/sugar

Mid-afternoon Snack

Banana

Dinner

Tomato juice
Roast chicken
Baked potato with margarine
Tossed salad with olive oil and cider vinegar dressing
Green beans
Corn bread made without wheat flour
Ice cream made without gluten stabilizers

Bedtime Snack

Apple slices with peanut butter

Additional Considerations

- Patients may be discouraged and overwhelmed when faced with a lifelong restricted diet. Provide support, encouragement, and thorough diet instructions.
- The patient may be temporarily or permanently lactose-intolerant and may require a lactose-restricted diet.
- A celiac crisis may be precipitated by emotional stress.

Potential Problems	Recommended Interventions
Difficulty obtaining a variety of allowed foods from grocery stores related to the highly restrictive nature of the diet.	Encourage the patient to use as many "normal" items as possible such as corn cereals, grits, rice, and rice cereals. They are easy to obtain and less expensive than special products.

BOX 17.10 (continued)

GLUTEN-FREE DIET

Encourage the patient to shop in health-food stores to obtain hard-to-find items such as potato and soybean flours.

Patient Teaching

Instruct the patient on the importance of adhering to the diet even when no symptoms are present. "Cheating" on the diet can damage intestinal villi even if no symptoms develop. To eliminate all wheat, oat, rye, and barley flours and products permanently, the patient should

- Read labels to identify less obvious sources of wheat, rye, oats, and barley used as extenders and fillers. Patients should check with the manufacturer *before* using products of questionable composition.
- Use corn, potato, rice, arrowroot, and soybean flours and their products.
- Use the following as thickening agents: arrowroot starch, cornstarch, tapioca starch, rice starch, sweet rice flour.

The patient should eat an otherwise normal, well-balanced diet adequate in nutrients and calories and should avoid milk and other sources of lactose if not tolerated. Weight gain may be slowly achieved.

Provide the patient with the following aids:

- A detailed list of foods allowed and not allowed
- Information regarding support groups; see websites at the end of this chapter
- Gluten-free recipes

The following companies offer gluten-free products:

- Authentic Foods at authenticfoods.com
- Ener-G Foods, Inc at www.energ.com
- Gluten-Free Pantry at www.Glutenfree.com
- Kingsmill Foods at www.kingsmillfoods.com
- Menu Direct/Dietary Specialties, Inc at www.menudirect.com
- Miss Robens Dietary Foods at www.missroben.com

Ileostomy: a surgically created opening (stoma) on the surface of the abdomen from the ileum.

following the diet because of the pervasiveness of gluten in prepared foods and medications and confusion over identifying sources of gluten on food labels. The diet is very restrictive, requires conscientious label reading, and is difficult to adhere to while eating out.

Ileostomies and Colostomies

Ileostomies and colostomies are performed after part or all the colon, anus, and rectum are removed usually for treatment of severe inflammatory bowel disease, intestinal lesions, obstructions, or colon cancer.

Pathophysiology

Colostomy: a surgically created opening on the surface of the abdomen from the colon.

Effluent: discharged fluid matter.

Potential nutritional problems arise because large amounts of fluid, sodium, and potassium are normally absorbed in the colon. The less colon that remains, the greater the potential for nutritional problems. That is why ileostomies create more problems than colostomies, in which some of the colon is retained. In addition to fluid and electrolyte losses, ileostomies cause a decrease in fat, bile acid, and vitamin B_{12} absorption. Effluent from an ileostomy is liquidy, and fluid and electrolyte losses are considerable. Effluent through a colostomy varies from liquid to formed stools, depending on the length of colon that remains. Over time, adaptation occurs.

Nutrition Therapy

Nutrition therapy for ileostomies and colostomies begins with liquids only. Fruit juices are allowed but are diluted to prevent osmotic diarrhea. The diet is advanced slowly based on individual tolerance. Small frequent meals may be better tolerated. Within 6 to 8 weeks after surgery, the patient should be consuming a near-regular diet. Additional considerations are as follows:

- A high fluid intake (8 to 10 cups daily) is needed to replenish losses. A high fluid intake is especially important for ileostomy patients to maintain a normal urine output and minimize the risk of renal calculi. Many patients inaccurately assume that a high fluid intake contributes to diarrhea. Reassure the patient that excess fluid is excreted through the kidneys, not the stoma.
- Weight loss related to diarrhea or a fear of eating is common. Encourage a high-calorie, high-protein diet to promote healing, replenish losses, and restore normal weight. Encourage patients to verbalize their fears and stress the importance of eating to attain or maintain wellness.
- Fat restriction may be necessary if the patient has steatorrhea or diarrhea from a significant ileal resection. MCT oil is absorbed without bile salts and, therefore, may be used to provide calories.
- Advise the patient regarding what foods cause gas, what foods are likely to cause stomal blockage, what foods help thicken the stool, what foods produce odor, and what foods act as natural intestinal deodorizers (Box 17.11).
- If the patient has a high output, insoluble fiber intake should be minimized because it reduces intestinal transit time. Foods high in soluble fiber, such as oatmeal, applesauce, banana, may help to reduce fluid losses.
- Encourage the patient to eat meals on a schedule to help promote a regular bowel pattern. A small evening meal helps to reduce nighttime stool output.
- Advise the patient to chew food thoroughly because improperly chewed food can cause a stomal blockage.
- Supplemental nutrients may be needed. Because vitamin B_{12} is normally absorbed in the distal ileum, anemia related to vitamin B_{12} malabsorption can occur in patients with ileostomies, necessitating lifelong parenteral injections or

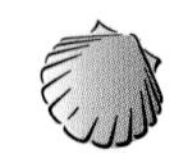

BOX 17.11

OF IMPORTANCE TO PATIENTS WITH AN ILEOSTOMY OR COLOSTOMY

Foods That May Cause Gas

Alcohol and beer
Carbonated beverages
Chewing gum
Chives
Cucumbers
Dried peas, beans and lentils
Eggs
Fried food (some)
Melon
Onions
Peppers
Pickles
Sauerkraut
Vegetables from the cabbage family such as broccoli, Brussels sprouts, cabbage, cauliflower, and turnip

Foods That May Cause Stomal Blockage

Bean sprouts
Cabbage
Carrots (raw)
Celery
Coconut
Corn
Cucumbers
Dried fruit
Green pepper skin
Lettuce
Mushrooms
Nuts
Olives
Peas
Pickles
Pineapple
Popcorn
Seeds
Skins and seeds from fruits and vegetables
Spinach

Foods That May Help To Control Diarrhea

Applesauce
Bananas
Cheese
Creamy peanut butter
Oatmeal or oatbran
Potatoes
Soda crackers
Starchy foods (rice, pasta, barley)
Tapioca
Yogurt

Foods That Produce Odor

Asparagus
Dried peas, beans, and lentils
Eggs
Fish
Garlic
Onions
Some spicy foods
Turnip

Foods That Are Natural Intestinal Deodorizers

Buttermilk
Parsley
Yogurt

nasal sprays of vitamin B_{12}. Additional salt may be needed for patients with ileostomies.

- The patient may experience depression and anxiety related to altered body image, altered body function, and dietary restrictions. Provide emotional support and allow the patient and family to verbalize their feelings. Advise the patient that with time a more normal diet is possible as adaptation occurs. Foods not tolerated initially can be reintroduced in a few months.

Short-Bowel Syndrome

Complications associated with short bowel syndrome, particularly when more than 50% of the bowel has been removed, include malabsorption, maldigestion, dehydration, malnutrition, and metabolic abnormalities related to a decrease in the absorptive area of the intestine.

Pathophysiology

Short-Bowel Syndrome: a complex condition resulting from extensive surgical resection of the intestinal tract usually because of inflammatory bowel disease, cancer, or obstruction.

The actual problems experienced and their severity depend on the amount and location of resected and remaining bowel and if the ileocecal valve was resected. For instance, patients with 150 cm or more of remaining small intestine do not develop short-bowel syndrome, whereas resections of more than 70% of the bowel cause permanent and severe impairments in absorption and metabolic function. Another important factor in the occurrence of symptoms is the amount of time that has elapsed since the resection. Symptoms improve during the first 1 to 2 years after surgery as adaptation takes place.

Short-bowel syndrome is characterized by three postsurgical phases. The first phase lasts for 7 to 10 days after surgery. During this phase, patients experience large fluid and electrolyte losses related to massive diarrhea. The second phase occurs 1 to 3 months after surgery and is the phase during which the majority of adaptation occurs. Diarrhea stabilizes and a positive fluid and electrolyte balance can be achieved with an oral intake. Fat malabsorption continues and deficiencies of calcium and magnesium may become apparent. Some patients reach the third phase of complete adaptation in which nutritional requirements are met through an oral diet.

Nutrition Therapy

Nutrition therapy for short-bowel syndrome is highly individualized, depending on the patient's tolerance. Usually TPN is used as the primary source of nutrition during the first two phases. During the third phase, enteral nutrition is gradually introduced to stimulate the gastrointestinal tract. The complete transition to an oral diet usually occurs when diarrhea is controlled and tolerance to oral feedings improves. Tolerance is enhanced by restricting fat, lactose, fiber, oxalates, and concentrated sweets. Calorie needs may be one and a half to two times above normal in patients who have had 50% or more of their bowel removed. A sample menu appears in Box 17.12. General guidelines to slow the passage of food through the gastrointestinal tract and help reduce diarrhea are to

- Eat six to eight small meals daily.
- Avoid liquids 1 hour before and after each meal.
- Avoid caffeine (coffee, tea, chocolate) and alcohol for the first year after surgery, then use sparingly.
- Reduce fat to a minimum with a goal of less than 8 g per meal if eating six meals per day. It is necessary to read labels to identify hidden sources of fat. MCT oil in doses of 15 mL three to four times a day may be used to supply additional calories.

BOX 17.12

SAMPLE MENU FOR PATIENT WITH SHORT-BOWEL SYNDROME: VERY LOW FAT, LOW LACTOSE, LOW FIBER, LOW SUGAR IN EIGHT SMALL MEALS

Breakfast

Diluted orange juice
Poached egg
White toast with diet jelly

Snack

6 oz artificially sweetened low-fat yogurt

Snack

8 oz Promote (low-fat, lactose-free, high protein oral formula)

Lunch

Fat-free deli turkey on white bread
Banana
Artificially sweetened low-fat yogurt

Snack

8 oz Promote

Snack

Low-fat cheddar cheese on saltines

Dinner

Lean roast beef
Boiled potatoes
Green beans
Unsweetened applesauce

Snack

8 oz Promote

- Use yogurt and aged cheeses, which do not contain lactose and should be well tolerated. Limit lactose to small amounts.
- Avoid foods and medications that contain mannitol and sorbitol (sugar alcohols), because they have a laxative effect.
- Dilute fruit juices and soft drinks to 50% strength by adding water. This lowers their osmolality.
- Avoid acidic foods, such as tomato products and citrus juices, if they cause heartburn.
- Avoid concentrated sweets because they are hyperosmotic and may promote diarrhea.

After a baseline diet is tolerated, restricted categories are reintroduced one at a time. Categories of restricted items should be attempted at 6-month intervals during the first 2 years after surgery. Patients who are unable to adapt need TPN permanently.

Diverticular Disease

Diverticula are caused by increased pressure within the intestinal lumen, which may be related to chronic constipation and long-term low-fiber diets. Studies suggest that the incidence of symptomatic diverticular disease is increased by diets that are low in total dietary fiber and high in total fat or red meat.

Pathophysiology

Diverticula: pouches that protrude outward from the muscular wall of the intestine usually in the sigmoid colon.

Diverticulitis causes cramping, alternating periods of diarrhea and constipation, flatus, abdominal distention, and low-grade fever. Complications include occult blood loss and acute rectal bleeding leading to iron deficiency anemia; abscesses and bowel perforation leading to peritonitis; fistula formation causing bowel obstruction; and bacterial overgrowth (in small bowel diverticula) that leads to malabsorption of fat and vitamin B_{12}.

Nutrition Therapy

Diverticulosis: an asymptomatic condition characterized by diverticula.

Diverticulitis: inflammation and infection that occurs when fecal matter gets trapped in the diverticula.

High-fiber diets appear to decrease the incidence of diverticular disease by producing soft, bulky stools that are easily passed, resulting in decreased pressure within the colon and shortened transit time. However, once the diverticula develop, a high-fiber diet cannot make them disappear. Foods with husks and seeds should be avoided because they can become trapped in diverticula and cause inflammation.

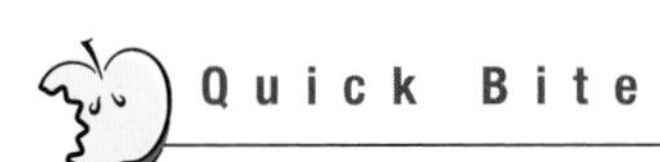

Foods with husks and seeds that may become trapped in diverticula

Corn
Cucumber
Kiwi
Nuts
Popcorn
Raspberries
Strawberries
Tomatoes

A high-fiber diet as tolerated (see Box 17.4) is recommended to prevent and treat diverticulosis. However, a low-fiber diet may be used during an acute phase of diverticulitis or when complications of intestinal bleeding, perforation, or abscess exist. Patients who are treated with a low-fiber diet in the hospital may be reluctant to switch to a high-fiber diet on discharge. Diet compliance depends on the patient's understanding of the rationale and benefits of a high-fiber diet for long-term prevention and treatment of diverticulosis and prevention of diverticulitis.

DISORDERS OF THE ACCESSORY GI ORGANS

The liver, pancreas, and gallbladder are known as accessory organs of the GI tract. Although food does not come in direct contact with these organs, they play vital roles in the digestion of macronutrients. Liver disease, pancreatitis, and gallbladder disease are discussed below.

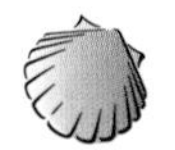

Liver Disease

The liver is a highly active organ involved in the metabolism of almost all nutrients. After absorption, almost all nutrients are transported to the liver, where they are "processed" before being distributed to other tissues. The liver synthesizes plasma proteins, blood clotting factors, and nonessential amino acids and forms urea from the nitrogenous wastes of protein. Triglycerides, phospholipids, and cholesterol are synthesized in the liver, as is bile, an important factor in the digestion of fat. Glucose is synthesized and glycogen is formed, stored, and broken down as needed. Vitamins and minerals are metabolized, and many are stored in the liver. Finally the liver is vital for detoxifying drugs, alcohol, ammonia, and other poisonous substances.

Liver damage can have profound and devastating effects on the metabolism of almost all nutrients. Liver damage can range from mild and reversible (e.g., fatty liver) to severe and terminal (e.g., hepatic coma). Liver failure can occur from chronic liver disease or secondary to critical illnesses.

Pathophysiology

Hepatitis, or inflammation of the liver, is caused by viral infections (types A, B, C, D, and E), alcohol abuse, and hepatotoxic chemicals such as chloroform and carbon tetrachloride. Early symptoms of hepatitis include anorexia, nausea and vomiting, fever, fatigue, headache, and weight loss. Later, dark-colored urine, jaundice, liver tenderness, and possibly liver enlargement may develop. In many cases, liver cell damage that occurs from acute hepatitis is reversible with proper rest and nutrition.

Hepatic Encephalopathy: the central nervous system (CNS) manifestations of advanced liver disease characterized by irritability, short-term memory loss, and impaired ability to concentrate.

Hepatic Coma: unconsciousness caused by severe liver disease.

However, sometimes acute hepatitis advances to chronic hepatitis, which may lead to cirrhosis, liver cancer, and liver failure. Cirrhosis develops when damaged liver cells are replaced by functionless scar tissue, seriously impairing liver function and disrupting normal blood circulation through the liver. Early symptoms include fever, anorexia, weight loss, and fatigue. Glucose intolerance is common. Later, portal hypertension, dyspepsia, diarrhea or constipation, jaundice, esophageal varices, hemorrhoids, ascites, edema, bleeding tendencies, anemia, hepatomegaly, and splenomegaly may develop. Cirrhosis can progress to hepatic encephalopathy and hepatic coma.

The liver "fails" when liver cell loss is extensive. Ominous changes in mental function, such as impaired memory and concentration, slow response time, drowsiness, irritability, flapping tremor, and fecal odor of the breath, signal hepatic encephalopathy, which may progress to hepatic coma. Although the exact cause of these CNS changes are unknown, altered blood amino acid patterns may be involved. The concentration of aromatic amino acids increases because the liver is not able to break them down. Higher-than-normal insulin levels increase the uptake of branched-chain amino acids into muscle cells, so that blood concentrations of these amino acids decrease. The increased ratio of aromatic amino acids to branch-chained amino acids may interfere with the formation of certain neurotransmitters (dopamine and norepinephrine) and cause the formation of substances that may contribute to hepatic coma. However, studies using enteral formulas high in branch-chained amino acids designed for liver failure have yielded inconsistent results regarding their effectiveness.

Increased serum ammonia levels may also be at least partially responsible for CNS manifestations. Ammonia is a CNS toxin produced by the action of gastrointestinal flora on protein (dietary sources, products of muscle catabolism, and protein from gastrointestinal blood loss). Because the malfunctioning liver cannot convert ammonia to urea, serum ammonia levels increase. The drug lactulose prevents the absorption of ammonia in the colon so that it can be excreted in the feces. However, because the degree of increased ammonia in the blood does not correlate with the degree of coma, other nitrogen-containing substances may be involved in the development of hepatic encephalopathy.

Nutrition Therapy

The objectives of nutrition therapy for liver disease are to avoid or minimize permanent liver damage, promote liver cell regeneration, restore optimal nutritional status, alleviate symptoms, and avoid complications. However, depending on the extent of liver damage, regeneration may not be possible.

Malnutrition is common among patients with liver disease and may be related to altered nutrient metabolism, anorexia, nausea, vomiting, maldigestion, and malabsorption. Metabolic rate may be increased or decreased. Glucose intolerance may develop but hyperinsulinism is common. Impaired or reduced bile flow, drug therapy, or alcohol-induced changes in the GI tract may lead to fat intolerance. Fat-soluble vitamins deficiencies may arise secondary to steatorrhea. Meeting nutritional and calorie needs is difficult. A sample menu appears in Box 17.13.

Nutrition therapy guidelines are as follows:

- Increase protein to 1.2 to 1.5 g protein/kg to promote positive nitrogen balance. An adequate protein intake is vital to prevent body protein catabolism and worsening of nutritional status. In a small percentage of patients with cirrhosis, dietary protein can precipitate hepatic encephalopathy. For these patients, a low-protein diet is used and gradually advanced as tolerated. Special formulas high in branched chain amino acids may enable protein intolerant patients to consume more total protein without adverse effects.
- Calorie requirements range from 25 to 35 cal/kg, depending on the stage of the disease (e.g., acute hepatitis vs. stable cirrhosis), history of weight loss, and the presence of additional physiological stressors such as fever and infection.
- Carbohydrates are generally not restricted, even for patients with hyperglycemia, because they are an important source of calories. For patients with either hyper-or hypoglycemia, carbohydrates should be mostly in the form of complex carbohydrates and meal timing should be consistent. Insulin is used to manage elevated glucose levels.
- Fat intake is restricted only if the patient experiences steatorrhea. MCT oil may be used for calories; however, it does not contain the essential fatty acids.
- Eliminate alcohol.
- Limit sodium if ascites is present. Allowances are determined by the accumulation of fluid as measured by sudden weight gain. An allowance of 2000 mg is usually sufficient but more severe restrictions may be necessary (see Chapter 18). High-

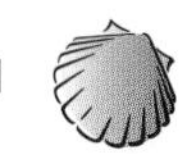

BOX 17.13

SAMPLE MENU FOR PATIENT WITH CIRRHOSIS: HIGH PROTEIN, LIBERAL CARBOHYDRATE, MODERATE FAT, 2 G SODIUM, SOFT DIET

Breakfast

Orange juice
2 poached eggs
2 toast with margarine
Coffee/tea
Salt/pepper/sugar

Snack

8 oz Promote

Lunch

Apricot nectar
Turkey wrap with shredded lettuce and cranberry jelly in tortilla
Steamed asparagus
Angel food cake
Coffee/tea
Salt/pepper/sugar

Snack

Yogurt

Dinner

Apple juice
Lean roast beef
Mashed potatoes with gravy
Cooked carrots
Rice pudding

Snack

8 oz Promote

protein foods are also relatively high in sodium so severe sodium restrictions are difficult to achieve. Low-sodium milk is an option; however, it is unpalatable and most patients find its taste offensive.

- If sodium restriction alone does not effectively control ascites, fluid intake is limited to 1000 to 1500 mL/day as tolerated. Amounts are liberalized as liver function improves. Some patients need a high fluid intake to replace losses caused by fever and vomiting.
- Multivitamin and mineral supplements, especially the B vitamins, vitamin C, and vitamin K, may be necessary to compensate for alterations in metabolism. Impaired liver function increases the risk of vitamin A toxicity; therefore, excess amounts of this vitamin are avoided. Zinc supplements may help to improve appetite.
- Provide small, frequent meals. Malnourished, anorexic patients have difficulty consuming an adequate diet, and nausea may worsen as the day progresses.

High-calorie, high-protein liquid nourishments may be better tolerated than traditional meals. Solicit individual food preferences and work closely with the family.
- A texture-modified diet (i.e., soft, low-fiber, or full liquid) may be needed if a regular diet irritates the esophageal mucosa. Spices, pepper, caffeine, and coarse foods may also irritate esophageal varices. Withhold food if esophageal varices bleed.
- Patients who are unable to consume adequate food or formula orally need enteral or parenteral nutrition. Hepatic formulas have fewer aromatic amino acids and more branch-chained amino acids than routine formulas do.

Liver Transplantation

Liver transplantation is a treatment option for patients with severe and irreversible liver failure. Patients awaiting a transplant usually have long-standing malnutrition; as many as 55% to 100% of people evaluated for a liver transplant are malnourished, and the severity of malnutrition correlates to the degree of liver failure. Moderate to severe malnutrition increases the risk of complications and death after transplantation.

Whenever possible, nutrient deficiencies and imbalances are corrected before the transplantation to promote a positive outcome. Patients waiting for a liver transplant may be given a low-microbial diet to decrease the risk of infection (Box 17.14).

TPN has traditionally been used to deliver nutrition after the surgery. However, early enteral feeding, begun within 12 to 18 hours after transplant, has been shown to be well tolerated and is being used as standard therapy in a growing number of transplant centers. Enteral feedings are discontinued as oral intake increases. Oral nutrition guidelines are as follows:

- Provide 1.2 to 2.0 g protein per kilogram body weight initially. A positive nitrogen balance may be difficult to attain in the first 1 to 2 weeks posttransplant due to the catabolic effects of corticosteroids used to prevent organ rejection.

BOX 17.14

LOW-MICROBIAL DIET

A low-bacteria diet eliminates the following foods:
- Undercooked meats
- Meats and cold cuts from delicatessens; hard-cured salami in natural casing
- All cheese and cheese products including cottage cheese
- Unpasteurized milk and milk products
- All raw vegetables including vegetable garnishes; salads from delicatessens
- Fresh fruit with peels that are eaten such as grapes, cherries, and berries; unpasteurized fruit juices
- Unroasted raw nuts; roasted nuts in the shell
- Fresh salad dressings made from raw eggs
- Unpasteurized honey
- All miso products

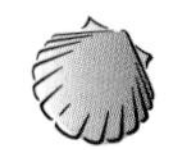

- Calorie needs are estimated at 30 to 35 cal/kg.
- Limit simple sugars if blood glucose levels are elevated.
- Adjust sodium and potassium intakes according to the patient's profile. Sodium allowances range from 2 to 4 g. Patients taking cyclosporine may develop high blood potassium levels.
- Provide supplements of calcium, magnesium, and zinc, which may help to alleviate muscle cramping or impaired sense of taste. Vitamin D supplements of 400 to 800 IU/day are recommended to prevent bone disease.
- After the initial hypermetabolic period, the patient's calorie and protein needs return toward normal. However, long-term complications associated with immunosuppressive therapy, such as excessive weight gain, hypertension, hyperlipidemia, osteopenic bone disease, and diabetes, may require nutrition therapy. Immunosuppressant drugs used to prevent rejection may also cause nausea, vomiting, diarrhea, and mouth sores.

Pancreatitis

Pancreatitis: inflammation of the pancreas.

The pancreas is responsible for secreting enzymes needed to digest dietary carbohydrates, protein, and fat. Until they are needed, those enzymes are held in the pancreas in their inactive form. Inflammation of the pancreas causes digestive enzymes to be retained in the pancreas and converted to their active form so they literally begin to digest the pancreas.

Acute pancreatitis may develop from unknown causes, alcoholism, biliary tract disease, pancreatic cancer; after gastric or biliary tract surgery; or secondary to mumps or a bacterial infection. Chronic pancreatitis, characterized by scarring and tissue calcification, is most often caused by alcohol abuse, although it is also associated with gallstones, hyperparathyroidism, and hyperlipidemia. Symptoms of both acute and chronic pancreatitis include severe abdominal pain, nausea, vomiting, distention, fever, and jaundice. Hyperglycemia, steatorrhea, weight loss, and malnutrition may develop as chronic manifestations.

Acute pancreatitis is treated by reducing pancreatic stimulation. The patient is ordered to have nothing by mouth (NPO) and a nasogastric tube is inserted to suction gastric contents. Appropriate measures are taken to correct fluid and electrolyte imbalance, to control pain, and to treat or prevent symptoms. If the patient is malnourished, a nasojejunal tube feeding (feeding into the jejunum does not stimulate pancreatic secretions) or TPN may be used until oral intake is resumed. As bowel sounds return, serum amylase levels fall; as pain subsides, clear liquids are given. This is progressed to a low-fat diet, then a regular diet as tolerated. Small, frequent meals may be better tolerated initially because they help to reduce the amount of pancreatic stimulation at each meal.

Acute pancreatitis that is not resolved or recurs frequently can permanently damage pancreatic cells, leading to chronic pancreatitis. Because the pancreas normally secretes enzymes in amounts that exceed physiologic need, a decrease in pancreatic enzyme secretion does not necessarily mean that digestion is significantly impaired. However, if the damage is great, digestion is affected, especially fat digestion. If pancreatic enzyme replacements are prescribed, they must be taken with every meal and snack.

The goals of nutrition therapy for chronic pancreatitis are to reduce steatorrhea, to minimize pain, and to avoid acute attacks by

- Limiting fat to the maximum amount that the patient can tolerate without causing steatorrhea or pain—usually 50 g/day or less
- Providing liberal quantities of protein and carbohydrates to replenish calorie and nutrient losses. Patients whose insulin secretion is impaired may need a diabetic diet to help control hyperglycemia.
- Eliminating individual intolerances and gastric acid stimulants (see Box 17.5)
- Providing supplements of vitamin C and the B-complex vitamins as well as water-miscible forms of the fat-soluble vitamins as necessary

Gallbladder Disease

Cholelithiasis: formation of gallstones.

Cholecystitis: inflammation of the gallbladder.

The gallbladder's role in digestion is to store and release bile as needed for the digestion of fat. Bile, which is made in the liver, consists of cholesterol, bile salts, bile pigments, and water. As it is held in the gallbladder, water is slowly removed from bile, making it more concentrated and increasing the likelihood that solids (either cholesterol crystals or pigment material) will precipitate out into clumps known as gallstones. Incomplete emptying of the gallbladder may also be involved in gallstone formation.

A large majority of people with cholelithiasis are asymptomatic, but some experience episodic, upper GI pain that spreads to the chest and shoulders in a manner similar to symptoms of a heart attack. For some people, eating a fatty meal precipitates symptoms; for others, symptoms develop during sleep. Gallstones that obstruct the cystic duct can lead to cholecystitis, causing abdominal pain, nausea and vomiting, jaundice, fever, fat intolerance, and flatulence. Surgical removal of the gallbladder may be used to treat symptomatic gallstones.

No diet modifications are necessary for healthy people with asymptomatic gallstones. Patients with symptomatic gallstones may be told to limit their intake of fat based on the rationale that limiting fat intake reduces stimulation to the gallbladder and minimizes pain. Although some patients' symptoms are aggravated by fat, some studies indicate that fat intolerance is no more common among patients with gallbladder disease than among the general population. Diet modification, therefore, should be individualized according to the patient's tolerance. Foods that are most likely to cause problems are highly seasoned foods, coffee, eggs, broccoli, cauliflower, brussels sprouts, cabbage, onions, legumes, and melons. Coffee, both regular and decaffeinated, has been shown to induce significant increases in plasma cholecystokinin, the hormone released in the upper small bowel that stimulates gallbladder contraction. It is recommended that patients with symptomatic gallstones avoid coffee.

Career Connection

Gallbladder surgery is the most common surgery in the United States. Although the exact cause of gallstones is unknown, they are related to

- Obesity, especially in women. Obese people make more cholesterol, which increases the cholesterol concentration of bile.
- Rapid weight loss, although exactly why this increases the risk of gallstones is unknown. It may be that dieting alters the composition of bile or that fasting or very low calorie diets causes incomplete emptying of the gallbladder, allowing more time for stones to precipitate.
- Increased estrogen, which increases the cholesterol content of bile and may interfere with normal gallbladder contractions. Increased estrogen occurs from the use of birth control pills, hormone replacement therapy, and pregnancy.
- Diabetes, the use of cholesterol-lowering medication, and TPN increase the risk of gallstones, as do surgical resections of the intestines.
- High intakes of simple sugars, alcohol, and animal fat to vegetable fat may increase the risk of gallstones. A diet rich in soluble fiber may lower gallstone risk.

How Do You Respond?

Are fiber pills a good idea for people who can't manage a high-fiber diet? Discourage the use of fiber "pills," which can cause constipation or even intestinal blockages, especially when taken in large amounts and with inadequate fluid. Likewise, over-the-counter laxatives and stool softeners should be used only if recommended by the physician. The easiest way to significantly increase fiber intake is to eat a high-fiber ready-to-eat cereal.

Does a gluten-free diet improve symptoms of autism? Although anecdotal reports claim symptoms of autism improve from a gluten-free diet, there have not been any controlled, double-blind studies published to confirm a connection between gluten and autism.

▲ Focus on Critical Thinking

Respond to the following statements:

1. A bland diet helps to treat ulcers and gastritis.
2. Dumping syndrome is at least partially responsible for the effectiveness of gastric bypass surgery used in the treatment of obesity.
3. Because oats have been determined gluten-free, they should be allowed on a gluten-free diet.

Key Concepts

- Nutrition therapy for gastrointestinal disorders is usually aimed at minimizing or preventing symptoms. For some gastrointestinal disorders, nutrition therapy is the cornerstone of treatment.
- Small, frequent meals may help to maximize intake in patients who are anorexic and avoidance of high-fat foods may lessen the feeling of fullness.
- After nausea and vomiting subside, low-fat carbohydrate foods, such as crackers, toast, oatmeal, and bland fruit, usually are well tolerated. Patients should avoid liquids with meals because liquids can promote the feeling of fullness.
- A low-fiber diet is used to reduce the frequency and volume of fecal output and to slow transit time. It is a short-term diet used for diarrhea, diverticulitis, and malabsorption syndromes, and in preparation for bowel surgery.
- A high-fiber diet increases stool bulk and stimulates peristalsis; it is, therefore, effective against constipation.
- Semisolid foods, such as pudding, yogurt, and cooked cereals, are usually the easiest and safest foods for people with dysphagia. Thin liquids and sticky foods should be avoided.
- People with GERD should lose weight if overweight, avoid large meals and bedtime snacks, eliminate individual intolerances, and avoid items that reduce LES pressure: alcohol, caffeine, chocolate, fatty foods, peppermint and spearmint flavors, and cigarette smoke.
- Patients with ulcers or gastritis should avoid foods that stimulate gastric acid secretion such as pepper, chili powder, alcohol, caffeine, and all coffee.
- Depending on their severity and chronicity, malabsorption syndromes can cause numerous nutritional problems. When steatorrhea occurs, fat is reduced to the maximum amount tolerated. MCT oil may be used to increase calorie intake when fat digestion is impaired.
- Nutrition therapy for dumping syndrome consists of eating small, frequent meals; eating protein and fat at each meal; and avoiding concentrated sugars. Lactose may have to be restricted and liquids should be consumed 1 hour before or after eating instead of with meals.
- Primary lactose intolerance is common in much of the world's adult population; tolerance varies considerably among individuals. Some people tolerate milk with food; others tolerate only lactose-reduced milk. Lactose intolerance that occurs secondary to intestinal disorders is usually more symptomatic than acquired lactose intolerance and requires a more restrictive intake.
- During exacerbation of inflammatory bowel diseases, patients need increased amounts of calories and protein and may not tolerate fiber and lactose. Patients are often reluctant to eat, fearing that food will cause pain and diarrhea. Some patients require enteral or parenteral nutrition for bowel rest. During remission, the diet is liberalized as tolerated.
- A gluten-free diet prevents intestinal villi changes, steatorrhea, and other symptoms in patients with celiac disease. All forms and sources of wheat, oats, rye, and barley must be permanently eliminated from the diet even in patients who are

 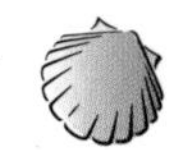

asymptomatic. A gluten-free diet requires major lifestyle changes and is difficult to follow.

- Fluid and electrolytes are of primary concern for patients with ileostomies and colostomies. Low-fiber foods may help to reduce stoma discharge and irritation. Additional calories and protein are needed to promote healing.
- Short-bowel syndrome occurs in patients who have had more than 50% of the small intestine removed. Maldigestion and malabsorption may lead to malnutrition. TPN is usually used until adaptation begins. Calorie and protein requirements increase. Tolerance to fat, lactose, and fiber is impaired.
- A high-fiber diet may prevent diverticulosis and diverticulitis. During acute diverticulitis, however, patients may be given a low-fiber diet to reduce bowel stimulation. Patients are often confused about the apparent inconsistency in nutrition therapy.
- Adequate calories and protein promote liver cell regeneration in patients with hepatitis and cirrhosis. In some people with advanced stage of cirrhosis, a high-protein diet—or a protein intake that is too low—can precipitate a hepatic coma.
- People who have undergone liver transplantation have high protein and calorie needs. Glucose intolerance may occur and sodium and potassium intakes may be restricted depending on the individual's profile. Immunosuppressant drugs may interfere with intake and appetite.
- Chronic pancreatitis is treated with a low-fat diet. Patients who develop glucose intolerance may benefit from a diabetic diet.
- Patients with symptomatic gallstones should avoid coffee (regular and decaffeinated) and eliminate individual intolerances. Overweight patients are encouraged to lose weight gradually.

ANSWER KEY

1. **TRUE** Avoid consuming liquids with meals because they can cause a full, bloated feeling. Encourage a liberal fluid intake between meals with whatever liquids the client tolerates such as clear soup, juice, gelatin, ginger ale, and Popsicles.
2. **TRUE** Carbonated beverages can contribute to diarrhea because their electrolyte content is low and their osmolality is high, possibly leading to osmotic diarrhea.
3. **FALSE** Semisolid or medium-consistency foods, such as pudding, custards, scrambled eggs, yogurt, cooked cereals, and thickened liquids, are easiest to swallow and usually safest.
4. **FALSE** All coffee, both regular and decaffeinated, stimulates gastric acid secretion.
5. **FALSE** MCT oil does provide calories but lacks essential fatty acids, both of which are long-chain (not medium-chain) fatty acids.
6. **TRUE** Hard, aged cheeses like cheddar have most of their lactose converted to lactic acid and, therefore, are generally well tolerated by people with lactose intolerance.
7. **TRUE** Simple sugars are quickly digested and form a hyperosmolar solution in the jejunum that attracts water.
8. **TRUE** For a patient with celiac disease, the long-term effects of eating even small amounts of gluten are harmful even when patients are asymptomatic.

9. **TRUE** Extensive pancreatic damage impairs digestion, especially fat digestion.
10. **FALSE** Most people with gallstones are asymptomatic and do not require any dietary intervention. A low-fat diet may be recommended for symptomatic gallstones to minimize gallbladder stimulation.

WEBSITES

American College of Gastroenterology at **www.acg.gi.org**
American Gastroenterological Association at **www.gastro.org**
Celiac Disease Foundation at **www.celiac.org**
Celiac Sprue Association/USA at **http://csaceliacs.org**
Gluten Intolerance Group at **www.gluten.net**

REFERENCES

Burke, P., Roche-Dudek, M., & Roche-Klemma, K. (2003). *Drug-nutrient resource* (5th ed.). Riverside, IL: Roche Dietitians, LLC.
Celiac Sprue Association. Grains and flours. Available at http://csaceliacs.org/grainsflours.html. Accessed on 1/8/04.
Chicago Dietetic Association and the South Suburban Dietetic Association. (2000). *Manual of clinical dietetics* (6th ed.). Chicago: The American Dietetic Association.
Cunningham, E. (2001). Is there any research to support a gluten- and casein-free diet for a child that is diagnosed with autism? *Journal of the American Dietetic Association, 101,* 222.
Lee, A., & Newman, J. (2003). Celiac diet: Its impact on quality of life. *Journal of the American Dietetic Association, 103,* 1533–1535.
Liebman, B. (2003). GasBusters. *Nutrition Action Health Letter, 30*(4), 1, 3–5.
Mceligot, A., Gilpin, E., Rock, C., et al. (2002). High dietary fiber consumption is not associated with gastrointestinal discomfort in a diet intervention trial. *Journal of the American Dietetic Association, 102,* 549–551.
Thompson, T. (2003). Oats and the gluten-free diet. *Journal of the American Dietetic Association, 103,* 376–379.
Thompson, T. (2001). Wheat starch, gliadin, and the gluten-free diet. *Journal of the American Dietetic Association, 101,* 1456–1459.

For information on the new dietary guidelines 2005 and MyPyramid, visit **http://connection.lww.com/go/dudek**

18

Nutrition for Patients With Cardiovascular Disorders

TRUE	FALSE	
◯	◯	**1** Having a high level of "good" cholesterol lowers the risk of coronary heart disease (CHD).
◯	◯	**2** The optimal level of LDL depends on the number of risk factors a person has.
◯	◯	**3** Homocysteine is an amino acid that, at high levels in the blood, increases the risk of CHD.
◯	◯	**4** Wheat bran and whole wheat grains are the sources of fiber best at lowering LDL.
◯	◯	**5** At high intakes, polyunsaturated fats do not appear to produce any adverse side effects.
◯	◯	**6** People who don't drink alcohol should be encouraged to do so to lower their risk of heart disease.
◯	◯	**7** Stick margarine should be avoided because it is high in saturated fat.
◯	◯	**8** Major sources of saturated fat in the typical American diet—dairy, beef, pork, poultry, and lamb products—also provide substantial amounts of monounsaturated fat.
◯	◯	**9** Weight loss lowers high blood pressure.
◯	◯	**10** The TLC diet is used to lower cholesterol; the DASH diet is used to lower blood pressure.

UPON COMPLETION OF THIS CHAPTER, YOU WILL BE ABLE TO

- Discuss risk factors for CHD.
- Explain how LDL goals are derived.
- Describe the TLC diet and the rationale for the recommended amounts of each particular nutrient.
- Discuss the characteristics of the DASH diet.
- Compare and contrast the TLC and DASH diet.
- Describe other lifestyle modifications that are effective in the prevention and treatment of hypertension.
- Describe teaching points for low-sodium diets.

Coronary Heart Disease: damage to the heart resulting from inadequate supply of blood to the heart.

Cardiovascular diseases are the leading cause of death among Americans. More specifically, coronary heart disease (CHD) is the single leading cause of death and disability in the U.S. An estimated 1.3 million Americans have CHD and approximately 450,000 die from it each year. Intervention trials show that treating modifiable CHD risk factors, such as high blood pressure and high low-density lipoprotein (LDL) cholesterol, decreases fatal and nonfatal cardiovascular events.

This chapter discusses the role of diet in the prevention and treatment of cardiovascular disorders including CHD, hypertension, and congestive heart failure (CHF).

CORONARY HEART DISEASE

Atherosclerosis: the formation of plaques along the smooth inner walls of arteries, which results in progressive narrowing and diminished blood flow to the tissue they supply.

Plaque: deposits of fatty material, cholesterol, calcium, and other blood components that are covered with connective tissue and embedded in the artery wall.

CHD is caused by atherosclerosis, an insidious process characterized by endothelial dysfunction and cholesterol deposition in macrophages and smooth muscle cells in the arterial wall (Fig. 18.1). Initially, fatty streaks form at sites of endothelial injury that may be caused by smoking, high blood pressure, or high blood glucose. Smooth muscle proliferation, inflammation, and calcification cause fatty streaks to harden and enlarge to become plaques. The rupture of unstable plague triggers the formation of a blood clot inside the artery, diminishing or blocking blood flow to tissues. The result can be angina, myocardial infarction (MI), or stroke.

A key factor involved in the development of atherosclerosis is blood pressure. High blood pressure can cause the chronic minimal injury to the endothelial lining that initiates the process of atherosclerosis. Once atherosclerosis develops, plagues cause artery walls to lose their elasticity and become narrowed, resulting in restricted blood flow and increased blood pressure, which further damages artery walls and makes them more susceptible to plaque formation. Thus, the progression of atherosclerosis is self-perpetuating (Fig. 18.2).

Hypercholesterolemia is also crucial in the development of atherosclerosis. CHD is uncommon in societies with mean total cholesterol levels of <180 mg/dL. More specifically, elevated LDL and low HDL are implicated in atherosclerosis.

Risk Assessment

Hypercholesterolemia: generic term to describe high levels of cholesterol in the blood.

Simply put, cholesterol is a major risk factor in the development of CHD. In reality, the relationship between cholesterol and heart disease is complex and influenced by many variables including the amount of "good" and "bad" cholesterol, the concentration of other lipoproteins, genetics, and the presence of independent risk factors. Certain lifestyle habits, such as obesity, inactivity, and diet, play a role, as do other emerging risks such as high homocysteine levels and proinflammatory factors.

"Good" Versus "Bad" Cholesterol

Cholesterol in food is just that: cholesterol—it is not wrapped in a lipoprotein package; it is not good or bad, it just is.

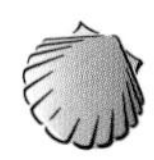

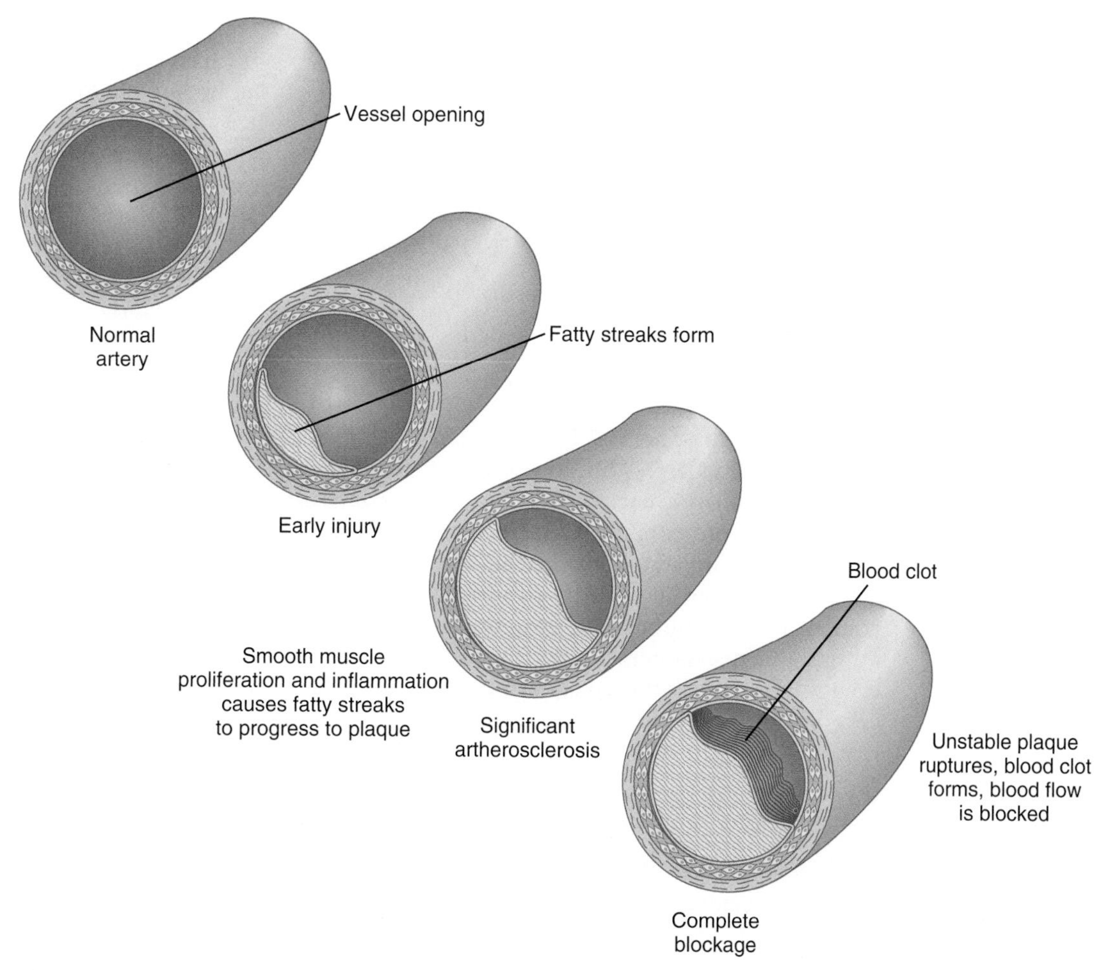

FIGURE 18.1 Schematic of atherosclerosis. The plaque develops by a series of events that begins with microscopic injury to the artery lining. The arteries narrow and the condition is exacerbated by the propensity of clots to form on unstable, ruptured plaques.

In contrast, cholesterol in the blood *is* encased in a lipoprotein package because fat (cholesterol) is insoluble in water (blood). Total cholesterol is a measure of all cholesterol in the blood, 85% to 90% of which is the combined total of high density lipoprotein (HDL) and low density lipoprotein (LDL). Classifications of total, LDL, and HDL cholesterol levels appear in Table 18.1. LDL and HDL perform different functions in the body, which *can* be classified as "good" or "bad."

"Good" Cholesterol. HDL is "good" cholesterol because it acts as a scavenger to take cholesterol out of the serum and transport it to the liver, where it is either recycled or excreted in the bile. As such, HDL is protective against CHD; as HDL goes up, the risk of CHD goes down. Conversely a low HDL is a risk factor for CHD.

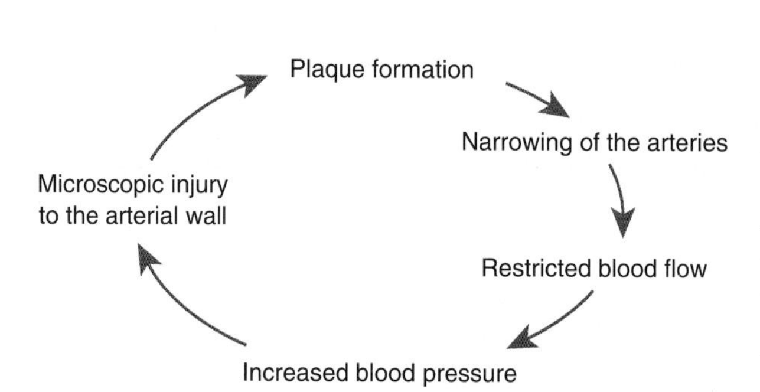

FIGURE 18.2 Perpetuating progression of atherosclerosis.

"Bad" Cholesterol. LDL is the major cholesterol-carrying lipoprotein in the blood. It is "bad" because it transports cholesterol out of the liver into circulation. Animal, laboratory, epidemiologic, and genetic research shows that elevated LDL is a major cause of CHD. Conversely, clinical trials demonstrate that lowering LDL lowers CHD risk, whether initial cholesterol level is high or normal. In addition, recent clinical studies show that even in people with established CHD, LDL-lowering therapy reduces total mortality, coronary mortality, major coronary events, coronary artery procedures, and stroke. As such, both primary and secondary prevention of CHD focuses on lowering LDL. In fact, goals of therapy and parameters for initiating treatment are based on LDL measurements.

Atherogenic: likely to promote atherosclerosis.

However, not all LDL are created equal; LDL particles differ in size, density, and composition. Accumulating evidence indicates that small LDL particles are more atherogenic than larger, less dense particles. In fact, small LDL may increase CHD risk even if LDL concentration is normal. It appears that LDL size and density are influenced by the fatty acid content of the diet.

TABLE 18.1 **ATP III CLASSIFICATION OF LDL, TOTAL, AND HDL CHOLESTEROL (mg/dL)**

LDL Cholesterol	
<100	Optimal
100–129	Near optimal/above optimal
130–159	Borderline high
160–189	High
≥190	Very high
Total Cholesterol	
<200	Desirable
200–239	Borderline high
≥240	High
HDL Cholesterol	
<40	Low
≥60	High

National Cholesterol Education Program, National Heart, Lung, and Blood Institute, National Institutes of Health. (2001). *Third Report of the Expert Panel on Detection, Evaluation, and Treatment of High Blood Cholesterol in Adults. (Adult Treatment Panel III).* (NIH Publication No. 01-3670). Washington, DC: Government Printing Office.

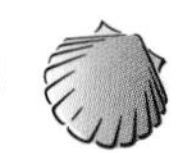

According to The Third Report of the National Cholesterol Education Program (NCEP) Expert Panel on the Detection, Evaluation, and Treatment of High Blood Cholesterol in Adults (Adult Treatment Panel III), a person's healthy or optimal LDL level is determined by the number of major independent risk factors an individual has, with a goal of <100 for the highest risk group and a goal of <160 for the lowest (Table 18.2). A person's risk of developing CHD within 10 years is determined by using the Framingham Point Scores. (To estimate your risk, go to www.nhlbi.nih.gov/guidelines/cholesterol/index.htm and click on 10-year Risk Calculator-online version.) Major independent risk factors are defined as

Cigarette smoking Compelling evidence shows that cigarette smoking increases the risk of CHD. Smoking promotes endothelial damage, increases heart rate, increases blood pressure, lowers HDL, and promotes thrombus formation. The risk of CHD improves with smoking cessation.

Hypertension. Blood pressure ≥140/90 mmHg or the use of antihypertensive medication is an independent risk factor for CHD and stroke. Conversely normalizing blood pressure reduces mortality and morbidity.

Low HDL cholesterol. Low HDL is defined as <40 mg/dL. Conversely, HDL ≥60 mg/dL is considered a negative risk factor and subtracts one risk factor from the total count.

Family history of premature CHD, which is defined as CHD in a first-degree male relative under the age of 55 or in a first-degree female relative under the age of 65.

Age. Age is considered at risk factor for men beginning at age 45; for women, age is a risk beginning at 55.

Other Factors That Impact Risk

In addition to the major independent risk factors outlined above, there are other factors that impact CHD risk. Although they are not factored when setting LDL

TABLE 18.2 **RISK CATEGORIES THAT DEFINE LDL GOAL**

Risk Category	LDL Goal (mg/dL)
Established CHD or CHD equivalent*	<100
2 or more risk factors	<130
0 to 1 risk factor	<160

*Each of the following is considered a CHD equivalent:
clinical heart disease
diabetes
symptomatic carotid artery disease
peripheral arterial disease
abdominal aortic aneurysm

National Cholesterol Education Program, National Heart, Lung, and Blood Institute, National Institutes of Health. (2001). *Third Report of the Expert Panel on Detection, Evaluation, and Treatment of High Blood Cholesterol in Adults. (Adult Treatment Panel III).* (NIH Publication No. 01-3670). Washington, DC: Government Printing Office.

goals, they can be targeted for intervention and their presence may influence treatment decisions.

Metabolic Syndrome

Metabolic syndrome, or syndrome X, is a cluster of metabolic abnormalities that together enhance the risk of CHD at any given LDL level. Cardinal features include abdominal obesity, hypertension, insulin resistance (with or without impaired glucose tolerance), high-serum triglycerides (TG), low HDL, and high concentrations of small, dense LDL. Diagnosis is made when three or more of these risk determinants are present (Table 18.3).

ATP III recognizes metabolic syndrome as a secondary target for risk reduction therapy, right behind the primary target of lowering LDL. All risk factors involved in metabolic syndrome can be improved with weight loss and increased physical activity.

Elevated Triglycerides

Hypertriglyceridemia: generic term to describe high TG levels in the blood.

Studies indicate elevated TG are an independent risk factor for CHD. High TG are related to obesity, physical inactivity, cigarette smoking, excess alcohol intake, and high carbohydrate diets (>60% total calories). Hypertriglyceridemia may also occur secondary to certain diseases (e.g., type 2 diabetes, chronic renal failure), certain drugs (e.g., corticosteroids, estrogens), and genetic disorders. Most often, elevated TG occur as part of metabolic syndrome.

Although the treatment depends on the cause, weight loss and increased activity are recommended when triglycerides are borderline high (150 to 199 mg/dL). Drug therapy may be added when triglycerides are classified as high (200 to 499 mg/dL), and a

TABLE 18.3 **DIAGNOSING METABOLIC SYNDROME**

Metabolic syndrome is confirmed by the presence of three of the following five risks:

Risk Factor	Defining Level
1. Abdominal obesity	
Men	>40 inch waist*
Women	>35 inch waist
2. Triglycerides (mg/dL)	150 or higher
3. HDL (mg/dL)	
Men	<40
Women	<50
4. Blood pressure (mm Hg)	systolic of 130 or higher or diastolic of 85 or higher
5. Fasting blood glucose (mg/dL)	≥110

*Some men can develop multiple metabolic risk factors when waist is 37 to 39 inches.

National Cholesterol Education Program, National Heart, Lung, and Blood Institute, National Institutes of Health. (2001). *Third Report of the Expert Panel on Detection, Evaluation, and Treatment of High Blood Cholesterol in Adults. (Adult Treatment Panel III).* (NIH Publication No. 01-3670). Washington, DC: Government Printing Office.

very low-fat diet ≤15% of total calories is used when triglyceride levels are ≥500 mg/dL. Alcohol should be avoided.

Physical Inactivity

Regular aerobic exercise improves cardiovascular fitness by strengthening the heart and blood vessels and expanding the volume of oxygen the heart can deliver with each beat to reduce overall cardiac workload. Regular exercise reduces the risk of CHD by lowering blood pressure, promoting weight management, increasing HDL, and improving insulin sensitivity. In some people, exercise may also lower LDL. Exercise also appears to reduce inflammation in blood vessels and promotes electrical stability in the heart. Thirty minutes of daily aerobic exercise may provide optimal benefits.

Atherogenic Diet

Dietary fats and cholesterol play a major role in the development of CHD by their impact on blood lipoprotein concentrations. It is well documented that saturated fats and trans fats raise serum cholesterol, particularly LDL. Reducing saturated fat and cholesterol intake, as well as smoking cessation and regular exercise, form the foundation of therapy for the prevention and treatment of CHD. Certainly there are other dietary factors that impact CHD risk.

Other Emerging Risks

The belief that a high-fat diet leads to a high serum cholesterol level that in turn leads to CHD is an oversimplified but frequently held view. Opponents to this hypothesis raise several thought-provoking questions:

- Why do some people eat high-fat diets but have normal cholesterol levels?
- Why do many people with low or normal serum cholesterol levels have CHD but most of those with increased serum cholesterol levels do not have CHD?
- Why does death from cardiovascular disease occur in people with minimal atherosclerosis?
- Conversely, why do so many people with extensive atherosclerosis exhibit no apparent clinical problems?

These questions underscore the fact that although much has been learned about CHD, much has yet to be determined. Genetics certainly play a role. Some other emerging risks include homocysteine and proinflammatory factors.

Homocysteine. Many epidemiologic studies show that a high blood level of the amino acid homocysteine is an independent risk factor for CHD, stroke, peripheral arterial disease, and venous thrombosis. Although the process by which high homocysteine levels cause atherosclerosis is not completely known, an increase in smooth muscle cell growth, arterial damage, and an increased propensity for clot formation are among the suspected mechanisms. High homocysteine levels can occur from a deficiency of folic acid, vitamin B_{12}, and/or vitamin B_6, but a deficiency of folic acid is more likely to cause increased homocysteine levels than deficiencies of the other two vitamins. And although an adequate intake of folic acid, vitamin B_{12}, and vitamin B_6 can lower homocysteine levels, it is not known whether lowering homocysteine through diet lowers CHD risk. Other factors, such as coffee, alcohol, fiber, and exercise, appear to impact homocysteine levels.

Proinflammatory factors. It is now well established that inflammation in the arteries plays a role in the growth of atherosclerotic plaques and promotes blood clot formation. Because of this, there is growing interest in measuring blood levels of C-reactive protein (CRP) to identify low level, asymptomatic inflammation in the body with the ultimate hope that this will be another piece of the puzzle in identifying who is most at risk for CHD. Although studies show that people with high CRP have a higher risk of CHD than similar people with low levels of CRP, it is not known whether lowering CRP lowers CHD risk. Another problem with using CRP is that levels vary as much as 42% when measured repeatedly in the same person without any intervention. If that were true of LDL, the level could vary from 170 (high risk) one week to 99 (low risk) the next without any change in medication, diet, or exercise. At this time, NCEP does not recommend the use of CRP measurement. However, interventions that lower CRP, namely, loss of excess weight, exercise, and smoking cessation, are already advocated for heart health.

Primary and Secondary Prevention and Treatment

Primary Prevention: preventing CHD from developing.

The public health approach for the primary prevention of CHD concentrates on lifestyle changes to lower LDL. These changes include the Therapeutic Lifestyle Change (TLC) diet, along with exercise and weight management. These lifestyle changes along with smoking cessation may also reduce CHD risk by favorably impacting other risk factors such as blood pressure, high triglycerides, and high homocysteine levels. Some people with very high LDL or multiple risk factors may need LDL lowering drugs to achieve their LDL goals (Table 18.4). Remember that LDL goals are based on the number of major independent risk factors an individual has.

Career Connection

The cholesterol-lowering drug Lipitor is currently the best-selling prescription drug in the United States. **While Lipitor and its cousins Zocor, Mevacor, Pravachol, and Lescol can lower cholesterol and CHD risk by as much as one-third, they are not meant to take the place of healthy eating and other lifestyle modifications. Many people mistakenly believe that as long as they are taking medication to control their cholesterol level, they can eat as they wish. In reality, even though these drugs are very powerful, their effectiveness can be undermined by a bad diet. Urge clients to commit to lifestyle changes to give their medication the greatest chance of success.**

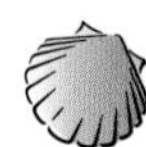

TABLE 18.4

DRUGS AFFECTING LIPOPROTEIN METABOLISM

Drug Class, Agents and Daily Doses	Lipid/Lipoprotein Effects	Side Effects	Contra-indications	Clinical Trial Results
HMG CoA reductase inhibitors (statins)*	LDL ↓ 18–55% HDL ↑ 5–15% TG ↓ 7–30%	Myopathy Increased liver enzymes	Absolute: • Active or chronic liver disease Relative: • Concomitant use of certain drugs†	Reduced major coronary events, CHD deaths, need for coronary procedures, stroke, and total mortality
Bile acid sequestrants‡	LDL ↓ 15–30% HDL ↑ 3–5% TG No change or increase	Gastrointestinal distress Constipation Decreased absorption of other drugs	Absolute: • dysbetalipoproteinemia • TG >400 mg/dL Relative: • TG >200 mg/dL	Reduced major coronary events and CHD deaths
Nicotinic acid¥	LDL ↓ 5–25% HDL ↑ 15–35% TG ↓ 20–50%	Flushing Hyperglycemia Hyperuricemia (or gout) Upper GI distress Hepatotoxicity	Absolute: • Chronic liver disease • Severe gout Relative: • Diabetes • Hyperuricemia • Peptic ulcer disease	Reduced major coronary events, and possibly total mortality
Fibric acids§	LDL ↓ 5–20% *(may be increased in patients with high TG)* HDL ↑ 10–20% TG ↓ 20–50%	Dyspepsia Gallstones Myopathy Unexplained non-CHD deaths in WHO study	Absolute: • Severe renal disease • Severe hepatic disease	Reduced major coronary events

* *Lovastatin (20–80 mg), pravastatin (20–40 mg), simvastatin (20–80 mg), fluvastatin (20–80 mg), atorvastatin (10–80 mg), cerivastatin (0.4–0.8 mg).*

† *Cyclosporine, macrolide antibiotics, various antifungal agents and cytochrome P-450 inhibitors (fibrates and niacin should be used with appropriate caution).*

‡ *Cholestyramine (4–16 g), colestipol (5–20 g), colesevelam (2.6–3.8 g).*

¥ *Immediate release (crystalline) nicotinic acid (1.5–3 g), extended release nicotinic acid (Niaspan®) (1–2 g), sustained release nicotinic acid (1–2 g).*

§ *Gemfibrozil (600 mg BID), fenofibrate (200 mg), clofibrate (1000 mg BID).*

NHLBI, NIH. (2001). *Third Report of the NCEP Expert Panel on Detection, Evaluation, and Treatment of High Blood Cholesterol in Adults. (Adult Treatment Panel III).* (NIH Publication No. 01-3670). Washington, DC: Government Printing Office.

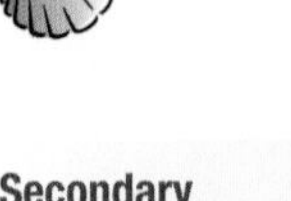

Secondary Prevention: preventing complications from established CHD.

The goal of secondary prevention in people with established CHD or CHD equivalents is to lower LDL to <100 mg/dL. The same lifestyle changes mentioned above are used for all people in this category regardless of initial LDL level because they can lower CHD risk by other means than just LDL lowering. The use of drug therapy is dependent upon LDL level.

Therapeutic Lifestyle Change (TLC) Diet

The TLC diet is low in saturated fat and cholesterol. Table 18.5 compares the recommended nutrient composition in terms of "percentage of total calories" or total quantities per day (e.g., grams, milligrams) with the average American intake. Such terms, however, are meaningless to the general public. How can a person tell if he or she has eaten 200 mg of cholesterol or consumed 7% of his or her calories from saturated fat? Clearly, more user-friendly, positive guidelines focus on what and how much to eat to approximate a healthy intake on a long-term basis. In keeping with the eating style approach as opposed to a therapeutic diet, Figure 18.3 depicts the TLC diet in a MyPyramid format.

Saturated Fat

As saturated fat intake goes up, so do total cholesterol, LDL cholesterol, and the risk of CHD. Conversely, lowering saturated fat intake lowers LDL. The majority of saturated fat in the typical American diet comes from dairy, beef, pork, poultry, and lamb

TABLE 18.5 COMPOSITION OF THE THERAPEUTIC LIFESTYLE CHANGE DIET VERSUS AVERAGE AMERICAN INTAKE

Nutrient	TLC Diet	Average U.S. Diet
Saturated fat (% of calories)	<7	13
Polyunsaturated fat (% of calories)	Up to 10	7
Monounsaturated fat (% of calories)	Up to 20	13
Total fat (% of calories)	25 to 35	34
Carbohydrate (% of calories)	50 to 60	51
Fiber (g/day)	20 to 30	12 to 18
Protein (% of calories)	15	15
Cholesterol (mg/day)	<200	270
Total calories	To maintain desirable body weight/prevent weight gain	

National Cholesterol Education Program, National Heart, Lung, and Blood Institute, National Institutes of Health. (2001). *Third Report of the Expert Panel on Detection, Evaluation, and Treatment of High Blood Cholesterol in Adults. (Adult Treatment Panel III).* (NIH Publication No. 01-3670). Washington, DC: Government Printing Office.

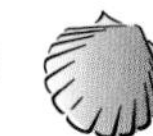

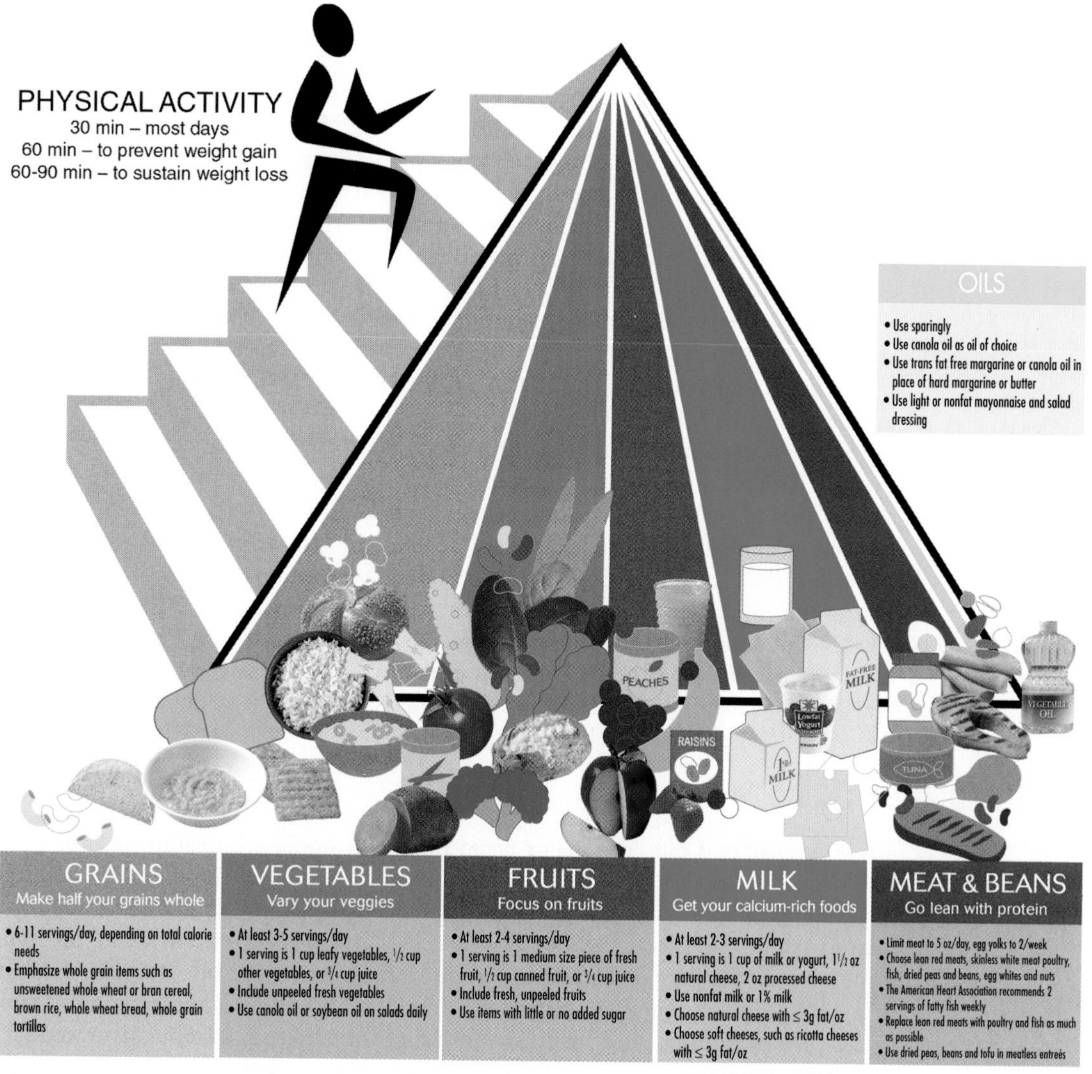

FIGURE 18.3 The Therapeutic Lifestyle Change (TLC) diet in MyPyramid format.

products. Interestingly, these products have substantial amounts of monounsaturated fat. Coconut oil and palm oil are high in saturated fat, but their overall contribution to the diet is relatively small.

Choosing lean meats and trimming away visible fat lower saturated fat intake. Skinless chicken and fish are frequently used in place of red meats. Because even lean meats, poultry, and fish provide saturated fat and cholesterol, portion sizes are limited to 5 oz or less/day. Dry peas and beans and tofu are recommended as substitutes for meat. Low- or nonfat milk, cheese, and yogurt are used in place of full-fat varieties. Butter is replaced with trans fat free margarine.

Polyunsaturated Fats

Polyunsaturated fats are subdivided into omega-6 (n-6) and omega-3 (n-3) fatty acids, although the distinction is not made in the TLC diet. Linoleic acid, the predominate dietary n-6 fatty acid, is an essential fatty acid found in vegetables and vegetable oils such as soybean, corn, sunflower, and safflower. When substituted for saturated fats, linoleic acid lowers LDL and CHD risk but also lowers HDL. In addition, n-6 fatty acids tend to stimulate platelet aggregation, an undesirable side effect.

Omega-3 fatty acids found in fish oils lower triglyceride levels and also CHD risk independently of their effect on lipoproteins. Research indicates that fish oils may reduce the risk of sudden cardiac death, which accounts for almost one-half of all deaths from CHD. Fish oils lower platelet aggregation, decrease inflammatory response mechanisms, and lower blood pressure, all of which lower CHD risk. Fish oils also appear to cause a shift in LDL particle density toward the less dense, less atherogenic type. Although there are no specific recommended levels of fish oil intake in the United States, the American Heart Association recommends at least two servings of fish per week. Plant sources of n-3 fatty acids, such as walnuts, flaxseeds, canola oil, and soybean oil, may also be beneficial. The International Society for the Study of Fatty Acids and Lipids recommends a minimal daily intake of fish oils of 0.65 g/day. Current American intake is about 0.1 to 0.2 g/day.

Monounsaturated Fats

Monounsaturated fats, the major fat in olive oil, canola oil, peanut oil, nuts, seeds, and avocado, lower LDL when they replace saturated fat in the diet. However, they do not appear to lower LDL as much as PUFA do when either is substituted for saturated fat in the diet. The major sources of monounsaturated fat in the typical American diet are those listed for saturated fat plus canola oil. Because they share many sources, the average intake of saturated fat and monounsaturated fat is similar (≈12–13% of calories) and when saturated fat is restricted, monounsaturated fat intake goes down. A decrease in animal fat intake means that olive oil or canola oil intake needs to increase to meet the recommendation that up to 20% of calories be from monounsaturated fat. This tactic is not universally agreed upon, as discussed in the section on total fat (see below).

Trans Fat

Trans fat is a particular type of unsaturated fat that deserves special mention. Like saturated fat, man-made trans fats found in partially hydrogenated fats and foods containing those fats have a positive linear relationship with LDL and so increase the risk of CHD. They also decrease HDL and may be involved in arrhythmias and sudden cardiac death. Although a specific recommendation regarding trans fat intake is not included in the TLC Diet, the Institute of Medicine recommends trans fat intake be as

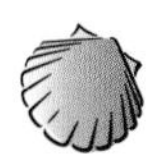

low as possible in the context of a nutritionally adequate diet. That means using "trans fat free" margarines or oils in place of stick margarine and avoiding commercially prepared products containing partially hydrogenated fat such as baked products, processed foods, and shortenings.

Total Fat

The optimal level of total fat intake to prevent CHD is controversial. Does keeping the percentage of calories from fat unchanged, but increasing the amount of monounsaturated fat, offer more protection against CHD than does lowering total fat intake? The controversy stems partly from the observation that low-fat diets lower both LDL and HDL. However, a study in monkeys (which are good predictors of human outcomes) showed that monounsaturated fat, when isocalorically substituted for saturated fat, failed to protect against atherosclerosis even though the ratio of LDL to HDL improved. Also, studies conducted by Dean Ornish show that very low-fat diets do not significantly lower HDL levels most likely because significant weight loss occurs, which raises HDL levels. Ornish's studies show significant improvement or regression of coronary atherosclerosis from a program that combines a strict low-fat, nearly vegetarian diet with exercise, yoga, and meditation.

Another concern regarding increasing monounsaturated fat intake is that dietary sources of monounsaturated fat also provide saturated fat. Adding monounsaturated fat to the diet will counterproductively increase saturated fat intake. Also, adding monounsaturated fat adds calories, which may promote weight gain. Conversely, low-fat diets tend to provide fewer calories because fat is more calorically dense than either carbohydrates or protein. A fat intake of ≤30% of calories combined with regular exercise appears to be important for obesity prevention. Some researchers recommend total fat be limited to 15 to 20% of calories, not the 25 to 35% as recommended in the TLC diet. Still others, such as Dean Ornish and the Pritikin program, recommend fat provide 10% or less of total calories. The best oil to use may be canola because it is low in saturated fat and provides a reasonable balance of n-6 to n-3 fatty acids.

Carbohydrates

When carbohydrates substitute for saturated fat, LDL goes down. Studies show a significant inverse relationship between CHD mortality and the intake of grains, fruit, and vegetables, foods rich in complex carbohydrates. However, a positive relationship has been shown between sugar and syrup intake and CHD mortality, so different types of carbohydrates have different effects on CHD risk. A very high carbohydrate diet is not recommended for people with metabolic syndrome because it may worsen triglyceride level, HDL level, and insulin resistance.

Fiber

High-fiber diets, especially those rich in soluble fiber, lower LDL. As little as 5 to 10 g of soluble fiber can decrease LDL by approximately 3% to 5%. Reductions in LDL are even greater when fiber is added to a high-saturated-fat, high-cholesterol diet. Therefore, a high-fiber intake may provide a cushion against deteriorating compliance, which often occurs over time. Excellent sources of soluble fiber include oats, dried peas and beans, fruit, root vegetables, barley, and flax, although all sources of fiber contain both soluble and insoluble fibers.

Protein

Protein should contribute approximately 15% of total calories. This level is neither restricted nor elevated. Low-saturated-fat sources of protein are recommended, such as lean red meats, skinless white meat poultry, fish, egg whites, dried peas and beans, and nuts.

Cholesterol

Studies show that increasing cholesterol intake increases serum cholesterol levels and is associated with an increased risk of CHD. However, dietary cholesterol has less of an impact on serum cholesterol than saturated fat, but cholesterol may act synergistically with saturated fat to raise serum cholesterol. Although the relationship between dietary cholesterol and serum cholesterol is complex and likely influenced by genetic factors, it is clear that dietary cholesterol should be limited to decrease CHD risk. The sources of cholesterol in the average American diet are egg yolks and the major sources of saturated fat already mentioned. Although individual response varies greatly, a low saturated fat, low cholesterol diet may decrease LDL by ≈15% to 20% compared to the typical American diet.

Career Connection

People with very high LDL (≥ 190 mg/dL) likely have a genetic form of hypercholesterolemia. **For them, diet will not substantially lower LDL to acceptable levels. However, diet, exercise, and weight loss are still important—maybe even more important than for other people—because of the potential beneficial effect on other risks such as blood pressure and insulin sensitivity. It may be a hard sell but diet and medication should not be viewed as mutually exclusive.**

Calories

The recommendation for calories is that they be consumed at a level that will maintain desirable body weight or prevent weight gain. Total calories are determined on an individual basis according to the person's body weight and activity patterns. Weight loss enhances LDL lowering, raises HDL, and improves other risks such as blood pressure and insulin sensitivity.

Other Dietary Components to Cut CHD Risk

Various other dietary components may help to lower CHD risk. Some nutritional supplements purported to prevent or treat cardiovascular problems appears in Box 18.1.

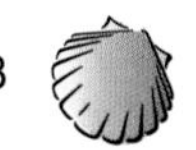

BOX 18.1

NUTRITIONAL SUPPLEMENTS USED TO PREVENT OR TREAT CARDIOVASCULAR PROBLEMS

Tea and green tea extract

A growing body of evidence indicates that regular consumption of tea—either black or green—may reduce the risk of cardiovascular disease. A recent study found that drinking two or more cups of tea per day lowered the risk of fatal heart attacks by 70%. Tea contains a variety of phytochemicals, specifically flavonoids, that may reduce LDL oxidation and/or reduce platelet aggregation. Tea is clearly a healthy choice. But for people who don't want to drink it, standardized green tea extract capsules are available that are purported to be equivalent to four cups of green tea.

Red yeast

The dietary supplement Cholestin is made from red yeast and rice. Its active ingredient is lovastatin, the same active ingredient found in the drug Mevacor. Like Mevacor, red yeast interferes with the liver's ability to synthesize cholesterol. It produces the same therapeutic benefits as lovastatin and also the same side effects, namely gastritis, abdominal discomfort, and increased liver enzyme levels. People who use red yeast are actually self-medicating, a potentially dangerous practice that may circumvent physician-supervised treatment based on the patient's overall CHD risk and actual lipid profile.

Soluble fiber

Fiber supplements may significantly reduce LDL in people with hypercholesterolemia, depending on the type of fiber contained in the supplement. One such supplement is Metamucil, the over-the-counter product approved for sale only as a laxative. Six studies have demonstrated that about 3 tsp of regular flavor Metamucil taken daily for 1.5 to 4 months lowers LDL by 6% to 26% in people with an average initial total cholesterol of 250 mg/dL. As with any source of fiber, an adequate fluid intake is essential. A potential drawback is that some people are allergic to psyllium, the fiber in Metamucil. Possible symptoms of psyllium allergy include wheezing, chest tightness, rashes, and anaphylactic shock in rare instances.

Chromium

Although chromium supplements are advertised to help reduce cholesterol levels, studies have failed to show any beneficial effects.

Hawthorn

An extract of the dried leaves and blossoms of hawthorn is widely used in Europe to treat CHF in its early stages. It reportedly improves the pumping capacity of the heart and reduces susceptibility to cardiac angina by reducing vascular resistance peripherally and in the heart. Hawthorn has a very low incidence of side effects and is considered safe. Even though hawthorn has potential as an important drug for patients with mild CHF, self-treatment of heart disorders is not recommended.

- Do use soft, trans fat free margarine or
- Do choose skim milk and skim-milk products.
- Do fill up on a variety of fruits, vegetables, and whole grains.
- Do use low-fat desserts sparingly.

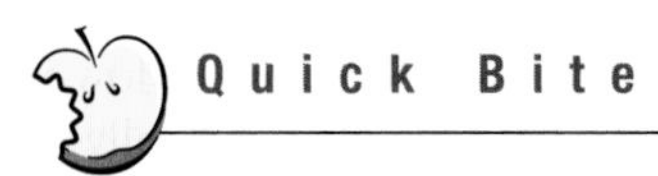

Quick Bite

Low-fat desserts

Low-fat and nonfat frozen yogurt and ice cream
Sherbet
Sorbet
Fruit ice
Popsicles
Angel food cake
Fig bars
Gingersnaps
Other low-fat cakes and cookies

Individualize the message. Instead of making general recommendations that may or may not apply or be doable, it is wise to determine existing positive features of the client's diet and identify where improvement can be made, with "can" defined by the individual. For instance, if a client's "thing" is ice cream, it is unrealistic to believe the client will be able to permanently eliminate ice cream from her diet. Instead, find out if the client is willing to use low-fat ice cream, eat smaller portions, or eat it less frequently. Is the client willing to make more dramatic changes elsewhere, for instance, eat a more vegetarian type diet that would "free up" saturated fat that could be "spent" on ice cream? Work with the individual to find out what foods she is unwilling to give up and what foods have little importance so can be sacrificed. Likewise, offer culturally appropriate interventions (Box 18.2). There is no right or wrong way to achieve the TLC diet guidelines.

Recommend gradual changes. Compliance is more likely to be achieved when small sequential changes are made gradually rather than starting from scratch with a completely new eating style. Encourage the client to set goals he knows he can achieve to create a history of success that will increase the chance of subsequent successes.

Encourage self-monitoring. People who record their total intake for one or more days are more aware of eating and food choices. The written account provides an objective tool for identifying areas that need improvement.

Encourage label reading. Legal definitions of "free," "very low," "low," "reduced," and "less" for fat, saturated fat, cholesterol, and sodium appear in Chapter 8. These descriptions are valid, believable, and useful when comparing different varieties and brands of similar items.

Provide how-to advice. Tips for meal planning and cooking are to

- Eat occasional meatless meals.
- Trim fat from meat before cooking; chicken can be cooked with the skin on but the skin should be removed before eating.
- Use meat more as a condiment than as the main entrée. For example when preparing casseroles, reduce the meat by half and double the complex carbohydrate (rice, potato, pasta).
- Place meats to be baked or roasted on a rack to allow the fat to drain.

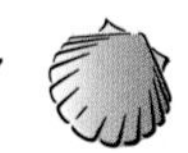

BOX 18.2 **CULTURAL CONSIDERATIONS**

For all cultural groups, emphasize the positive aspects of their eating styles and suggest modifications to lower the fat and sodium content of traditional foods.

African-American Tradition

Traditional soul foods tend to be high in fat, cholesterol, and sodium. On the positive side, there is a heavy emphasis on vegetables and complex carbohydrates.
Changes in cooking techniques can improve fat, cholesterol, and sodium content such as

- Using nonstick skillets sprayed with cooking spray when pan-frying eggs, fish, and vegetables
- Using small amounts of liquid smoke flavoring in place of bacon, salt pork, or ham
- Using more seasonings such as onion, garlic, and pepper, in place of some of the salt
- Substituting fat-free mayonnaise for regular mayonnaise in biscuits
- Using turkey ham or turkey sausage in place of bacon
- Using "lite" or sugar-free syrups
- Using egg substitutes or egg whites in pancakes and biscuits

Mexican-American Tradition

The traditional diet is primarily vegetarian with a heavy emphasis on fruits, vegetables, rice, and dried peas and beans. Processed foods are used infrequently.

Cooking techniques rely on frying and stewing with liberal amounts of oil or lard. High-fat meats and lard are commonly used.

Chinese-American Tradition

Traditional Chinese cooking relies heavily on vegetables and rice with plants providing the majority of calories. Meat is used more as a condiment than an entrée. Cooking techniques tend to preserve nutrients. Sauces add little fat.

Sodium intake is high related to heavy use of soy sauce, MSG, and salted pickles.

Native-American/Alaska Native Traditions

Widely diverse eating styles make useful generalizations difficult.

In general

- Encourage traditional cooking methods such as baking, roasting, boiling, and broiling.
- Encourage the use of traditional meats such as fish, deer, and caribou.
- Remove fat from canned meats.
- Use vegetable oil for frying instead of lard or shortening.

Jewish Tradition

Many traditional foods are high in sodium such as *kosher* meats (salt is used in the koshering process), herring, lox, pickles, canned chicken broth or soups, and delicatessen meats (e.g., corned beef, pickled tongue, pastrami).

Pareve (neutral) nondairy creamers are often used as a dairy substitute at meat meals but they are high in fat. Encourage light and fat-free versions.

(box continues on page 548)

BOX 18.2 (continued)

CULTURAL CONSIDERATIONS

Encourage methods to lower fat in traditional recipes such as

- Baking instead of frying potato pancakes
- Limiting the amount of schmaltz (chicken fat) used in cooking
- Using reduced-fat or fat-free cream cheese on bagels
- Using low-fat or nonfat cottage cheese, sour cream, and yogurt in kugels and blintzes

- Bake, broil, steam, or sauté foods in vegetable cooking spray or allowed oils.
- Prepare foods from "scratch" instead of purchasing convenience foods and mixes, which tend to be high in saturated fat.
- Use recommended oils to season cooked vegetables and in the preparation of salad dressings, marinades, and barbecue sauces.
- Make fat-free soup stock by preparing the stock a day ahead and refrigerating it overnight. The fat will harden and can be removed easily from the surface. Also use this method to make fat-free gravies thickened with cornstarch.
- Use herbs and spices, lemon juice, and flavored vinegars to flavor foods without fat.
- Use these low-fat snack ideas: low-fat yogurt, fresh fruits and vegetables, dried fruit, unbuttered popcorn, unsalted pretzels, bread sticks, melba toast, frozen juice bars, low-fat crackers.

Encourage patience and long-term commitment. It's a lifestyle, not a diet. Whether one-on-one or group counseling, ongoing contact is necessary to provide nutrition education, teach behavior skills, and promote lifestyle modifications.

NURSING PROCESS

Mr. Sanders is a 56-year-old man who recently learned during his routine physical that he has high levels of total cholesterol, LDL, and triglycerides. His HDL is low and his weight is normal. The doctor simply told him to avoid alcohol, exercise, and "watch your diet" but he doesn't know what that means. He comes to you, the corporate nurse, to interpret the doctor's advice.

Assessment

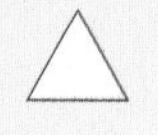

Obtain Clinical Data:

Current weight, height, BMI
Blood pressure

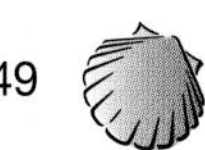

Medical history and comorbidities including diabetes, hypertension, myocardial infarction, alcohol abuse, other CHD risk factors

Abnormal laboratory values especially cholesterol, LDL, HDL, triglycerides, and glucose

Medications that affect nutrition such as diuretics, antihypertensives, antidiabetics, lipid-lowering medications

Interview the Client to Assess:

Understanding the relationship between "diet" and blood cholesterol levels

Motivation to change eating style; previous attempts to modify intake

Usual 24-hour intake including portion sizes, frequency and pattern of eating, method of food preparation, intake of foods high in fat and saturated fat, intake of foods high in soluble fiber

How often meals are eaten out; what and where he eats out

Cultural, religious, and ethnic influences on eating habits

Use of vitamins, minerals, and nutritional supplements: what, how much, and why taken

Psychosocial issues such as living situation and cooking facilities

Usual activity patterns

Use of alcohol, tobacco, and nicotine

Nursing Diagnosis

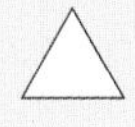

1. Health-Seeking Behaviors, as evidenced by the lack of knowledge of a heart-healthy diet and a desire to learn.

Planning and Implementation

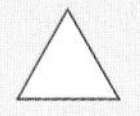

Client Goals

The client will

Experience a decrease in total cholesterol and LDL to the desired level or below (see Table 18.1).

Experience an increase in HDL.

Explain the principles and rationale of nutrition therapy for hypercholesterolemia.

Implement appropriate dietary and lifestyle changes.

Consume a varied and nutritious diet.

Name foods high in saturated fats, polyunsaturated fats, monounsaturated fats, cholesterol, and soluble fiber.

Nursing Interventions

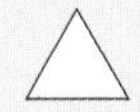

Nutrition Therapy

Recommend changes necessary to achieve the TLC diet

(continued)

Client Teaching

Instruct the client

On the role of the lifestyle changes in managing hypercholesterolemia

On eating plan essentials, including

- Eating up to two egg yolks per week including those used in food preparation.
- Eating up to 5 ounces of lean meat per day emphasizing skinless poultry; lean, well-trimmed cuts of red meat, and fish
- Using canola oils for salads and sautéing
- Eating nuts and seeds in moderation
- Using soft, liquid, or spray trans fat free margarine
- Choosing skim milk and skim-milk products
- Filling up on a variety of fruits, vegetables, and whole grains
- Limiting sugar and sweet intake. Those that are low-fat include low-fat and nonfat yogurt, ice milk, sherbet, sorbet, fruit ice, Popsicles, angel food cake, fig bars, gingersnaps, and other low-fat cakes and cookies
- Increasing soluble fiber intake such as eating more oats and dried peas and beans; drinking at least eight 8-ounce glasses of fluid daily
- Eating two servings of fish per week, if desired
- Avoiding alcohol as advised by the physician

On behavioral matters, including

- How to read labels
- How to order in a restaurant
- The importance of trying new recipes to acclimate to the changes in taste and texture of low-fat dishes
- The importance of regular physical activity

On resources for additional information (see websites at the end of this chapter).

Evaluation

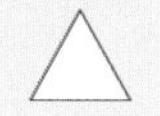

The client

Experiences a decrease in total cholesterol and LDL to the desired level or below

Experiences an increase in HDL

Explains the principles and rationale of nutrition therapy for hypercholesterolemia

Implements appropriate dietary and lifestyle changes

Consumes a varied and nutritious diet

Names foods that are high in saturated fats, polyunsaturated fats, monounsaturated fats, cholesterol, and soluble fiber

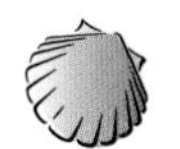

HYPERTENSION

Hypertension is a symptom, not a disease, arbitrarily defined as sustained elevated blood pressure greater than or equal to 140/90 mm Hg. The parameters for "normal" blood pressure have recently been lowered to 119/79 or lower. Blood pressures between normal and high that range from 120/80 to 139/89 have the newly created classification of "prehypertension."

Hypertension is the most common chronic condition in the United States, affecting 50 million American adults. Another 46 million adults have prehypertension. Collectively, this means almost one in two American adults have blood pressure that increases their risk of heart attack or stroke.

Fewer than 5% of cases of hypertension occur secondary to medical problems. In these cases, eliminating the underlying disorder cures the secondary hypertension. In at least 95% of cases, hypertension occurs from unknown causes and is classified as essential, primary, or idiopathic hypertension. Essential hypertension is more common among African-Americans than Caucasians and occurs more frequently among men than women until late middle age. In the United States and other developed countries, the prevalence of hypertension rises progressively with aging, but biologic changes are not the only factor. Age-related increases in blood pressure appear to be related to certain environmental factors, namely, a high salt intake, obesity, physical inactivity, excessive alcohol consumption, and an inadequate intake of potassium and perhaps other minerals. Essential hypertension cannot be cured, but it may be prevented in large numbers of people through lifestyle changes.

Lifestyle changes including nutrition therapy have the potential to be completely effective, produce no adverse side effects, and may preclude the need for drug therapy. As such, they are the focus of primary prevention and the initial treatment of choice for all patients with hypertension. If the patient fails to achieve desired goals, drug therapy (e.g., diuretics, vasodilators, adrenergic blocking agents) may be added. The five lifestyle changes for lowering blood pressure discussed below are remarkably consistent with recommendations to lower LDL.

Lose Weight, If Overweight

Body weight is one of the strongest determinants of blood pressure. Losing weight lowers blood pressure even if ideal weight is not attained and regardless of the degree of overweight. Weight loss may also reduce or eliminate the need for medication and so the potential for toxicity and unpleasant side effects associated with drug therapy. Because weight control has the potential to control hypertension effectively for a large number of people, it is vital for primary prevention and treatment.

The DASH Diet Limited in Sodium

DASH (Dietary Approaches to Stop Hypertension) is a multicenter feeding study funded by the National Heart, Lung and Blood Institute that set out to test if eating

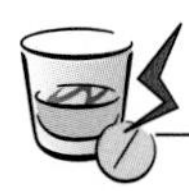

DRUG ALERT

Antihypertensive Drugs

Potassium-wasting diuretics (thiazide and related agents, loop diuretics) can cause constipation, diarrhea, nausea, vomiting, gastrointestinal upset, dry mouth, increased thirst, anorexia, and fluid and electrolyte imbalances. Modify the diet to alleviate unpleasant gastrointestinal side effects, if possible. Often patients who require an increased potassium intake are told to "eat a banana and drink orange juice every day" without any further explanation. Instruct the patient on the many other sources of potassium especially those low in sodium. Advise the client to avoid natural licorice, which tends to cause potassium depletion and sodium retention.

Potassium supplements can lead to nausea, vomiting, gastrointestinal discomfort, and diarrhea and can produce hyperkalemia when used with salt substitutes that contain potassium. Monitor serum potassium levels and observe for signs of hyperkalemia. Advise against the use of potassium-containing salt substitutes.

Because the absorption of **beta-adrenergic blocking agents** (propranolol, metoprolol, atenolol) is enhanced by food, clients should be advised to take them with food.

Elderly patients who are receiving high doses of **captopril** may experience loss of taste.

Some **calcium channel blockers** such as diltiazem (Cardizem, Dilacor) should be taken on an empty stomach because foods that contain fat may decrease their absorption.

whole "real" foods rather than individual nutrients would lower blood pressure as a result of some combination of nutrients, interactions among individual nutrients, or other food factors. The results clearly showed that eating a diet rich in fruit, vegetables, and low-fat dairy products with reduced amounts of fat, red meat, sweets, and sugar-sweetened beverages significantly lowers both systolic and diastolic blood pressures even when sodium is not restricted. It is also clinically proven to lower cholesterol.

A second study, DASH-Sodium, set out to test if limiting sodium on a DASH diet would yield even better results. With both a control and DASH diet, three levels of sodium were tested: 3300 mg (similar to U.S. intake), 2400 mg (the amount used on the Nutrition Facts label), and 1500 mg. The results showed that

- Lowering sodium with either the control diet or DASH diet lowers blood pressure.
- At each sodium level, blood pressure was lower on the DASH diet than on the control diet.
- The greatest reduction in blood pressure occurred at 1500 mg of sodium.
- People with hypertension had the biggest improvement in blood pressure but normotensive people also had large decreases.

The DASH diet is similar to the TLC diet in that it is low in saturated fat and cholesterol and high in fiber. Total fat is also low (unlike the TLC diet) and protein is slightly higher than usual recommendations. What is strikingly different about the DASH diet is that it encourages more fruit, vegetables, and low-fat dairy products and has a separate food group entitled "Nuts, Seeds, and Dried Peas and Beans" from which four to five servings per week are recommended (Table 18.6). The DASH diet provides about two to

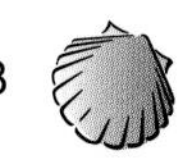

TABLE 18.6

COMPARISON BETWEEN TLC AND DASH DIETS

Food Group	Serving Sizes	Examples and Notes	Daily Servings (except where noted) TLC† Diet	DASH Diet‡	Comments
Grains and grain products	1 slice bread 1 oz dry cereal* ½ cup cooked rice, pasta, or cereal	Whole wheat bread, English muffin, pita bread, bagel, cereals, grits, oatmeal, crackers, unsalted pretzels, and popcorn	6–11	7–8	Both diets recommend whole grain products prepared with little or no added sugar and fat.
Vegetables	1 cup raw leafy vegetable ½ cup cooked vegetable 6 oz vegetable juice	Tomatoes, potatoes, carrots, green peas, squash, broccoli, turnip greens, collards, kale, spinach, artichokes, green beans, lima beans, sweet potatoes	3–5	4–5	
Fruits	6 oz fruit juice 1 medium fruit ¼ cup dried fruit ½ cup fresh, frozen, or canned fruit	Apricots, bananas, dates, grapes, oranges, orange juice, grapefruit, grapefruit juice, mangoes, melons, peaches, pineapples, prunes, raisins, strawberries, tangerines	2–4	4–5	
Low-fat or fat-free dairy foods	8 oz milk 1 cup yogurt 1½ oz cheese	Fat-free (skim) or low-fat (1%) milk, fat-free or low-fat buttermilk, fat-free or low-fat regular or frozen yogurt, low-fat and fat-free cheese	2–3	2–3	Cheese should have $\leq$ 3 g fat/svg.

(table continues on page 554)

TABLE 18.6
(continued)

COMPARISON BETWEEN TLC AND DASH DIETS

Food Group	Serving Sizes	Examples and Notes	Daily Servings (except where noted) TLC[†] Diet	Daily Servings (except where noted) DASH Diet[‡]	Comments
Meats, poultry, and fish	3 oz cooked meats, poultry, or fish	Select only lean; trim away visible fats; broil, roast, or boil, instead of frying; remove skin from poultry	≤ 5 oz/d	≤ 6 oz	TLC diet limits egg yolks to ≤2/week. TLC has dried peas & beans in this group.
Nuts, seeds, and dried peas and beans	⅓ cup or 1½ oz nuts 2 tbsp or ½ oz seeds ½ cup cooked dry beans	Almonds, filberts, mixed nuts, peanuts, walnuts, sunflower seeds, kidney beans, lentils, and peas		4–5 per week	This group is unique to DASH.
Fats and oils	1 tsp soft margarine 1 tbsp low-fat mayonnaise 2 tbsp light salad dressing 1 tsp vegetable oil	Soft margarine, low-fat mayonnaise, light salad dressing, vegetable oils, (e.g., olive, corn, canola, safflower)	≤ 6–8	2–3	TLC diet includes nuts in this group.
Sweets	1 tbsp sugar 1 tbsp jelly or jam ½ oz jelly beans 8 oz lemonade	Maple syrup, sugar, jelly, jam, fruit-flavored gelatin, jelly beans, hard candy, fruit punch, sorbet, ices	Now and then within caloric allowance	5 per week	

*Equals ½–1¼ cups, depending on cereal type.

[†]Calorie level not specified. Low end of each serving range approximates 1600 calories; high end provides approximately 2800 cal

[‡]Amounts appropriate for 2000 calorie diet

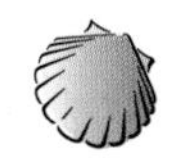

three times the amounts of potassium, magnesium, and calcium most Americans typically consume.

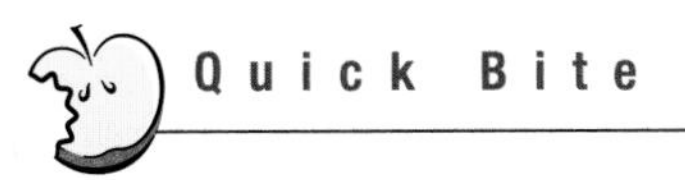

Quick Bite

Sodium content of various ready-to-eat cereals

	Sodium (mg)
Cheerios, 1 cup	280
Rice Chex, 1¼ cup	290
Rice Krispies, 1¼ cup	320
Shredded Wheat, 2 biscuits	0
Grape Nuts, ½ cup	350
Frosted Flakes, ¾ cup	105

Approximately 75% of the 3300 mg of sodium the average American consumes in a day comes from processed or convenience foods (Box 18.3). While 1500 mg sodium may be an optimal intake for blood pressure control, it is not easily achieved, given our grab-and-go style of eating. Tips for lowering sodium intake while eating out appear in Box 18.4. A more reasonable goal is to limit sodium to 2400 mg/day—more than ideal but less than usual. Table 18.7 shows DASH diet menu changes that convert a 2400 mg sodium diet to 1500 mg and 1000 mg of sodium.

Increase Physical Activity

Studies show that increasing activity either alone or as part of a weight-loss program lowers blood pressure. It appears that 30 to 45 minutes of moderate-intensity aerobic exercise may actually be better than a more intense workout. Recommended activities include walking, cycling, dancing, and gardening.

BOX 18.3 **SOURCES OF SODIUM**

The Rule of 7 S's

Soups: canned soups, freeze-dried soup mixes, broth, bouillon (unless salt free)

Sauces: canned gravy, spaghetti sauce, and other cooking sauces; packaged sauce mixes and convenience mixes; ketchup, barbecue sauce, steak sauce, salad dressings

Snacks: processed varieties like corn chips, potato chips, popcorn, pretzels, snack crackers, and salted nuts

Smoked meat and fish: such as bacon, chipped beef, corned beef, cold cuts, ham, hot dogs, sausage, and lox

Sauerkraut: and other foods preserved in brine such as pickles, olives, pickled beets, pickled sausage, pickled herring, and pickled eggs

Seasonings: mustard, horseradish, soy sauce, Worcestershire sauce, meat tenderizer, and monosodium glutamate (MSG)

Sodium-processed cold cuts: bacon, bologna, ham, salami, corned beef

BOX 18.4 **TIPS FOR CONTROLLING SODIUM INTAKE WHILE EATING OUT**

- Request that food not be salted, if possible.
- Choose fruit juice instead of soup for an appetizer.
- Use oil and vinegar or fresh lemon instead of regular salad dressing.
- Choose foods that are grilled, baked, or roasted
- Order plain meat and vegetables without gravy or sauce, or order them "on the side" and use sparingly.
- Choose plain baked potatoes and season sparingly with sour cream, butter, or pepper.
- Select fresh fruit for dessert. If the client is going to splurge, ice cream or sherbet is a better choice than pie, cake, cookies, or other desserts.
- Avoid fast food restaurant meals, which usually are high in sodium. If you have to go, order a child-sized meal.
- Order sandwiches without mayonnaise, sauces, or condiments; load with lettuce, tomato, and onion.

Stop Smoking

Smoking raises blood pressure and is a strong risk factor for CHD.

Limit Alcohol

Consistent and powerful evidence links alcohol consumption (three or more drinks per day) with hypertension. Clients who drink habitually should be advised to limit their consumption to two drinks per day or less. A "drink" is defined as 5 ounces of wine, 12 ounces of beer, or 1.5 ounces of distilled liquor such as rum, bourbon, whiskey, gin, or vodka.

CONGESTIVE HEART FAILURE

CHF is a syndrome characterized by the inability of the heart to maintain adequate blood flow through the circulatory system, which leads to decreased blood flow to the kidneys, excessive sodium and fluid retention, peripheral and pulmonary edema, and finally an overworked and enlarged heart. The severity of CHF can vary from mild to severe. Although the heart and its circulatory efficiency are principally affected initially, the entire circulation is eventually altered.

The treatment of CHF involves treatment of the underlying cause. Physical and mental rest help to decrease cardiac workload. Digitalis may be used to slow the heart rate and strengthen its beat. Diuretic therapy is used to help rid the body of excess fluid. Oxygen therapy may be necessary. Nutrition therapy is used to reduce sodium and fluid retention and to minimize cardiac workload.

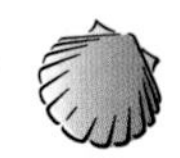

TABLE 18.7

DASH MENU AT THREE DIFFERENT SODIUM LEVELS

2400 mg Sodium Menu	Sodium (mg)	Substitutions to ↓ sodium to 1500 mg	Sodium (mg)	Substitutions to ↓ sodium to 1000 mg	Sodium (mg)
Breakfast		The same as the 2400-mg sodium menu except:		The same as the 1500-mg sodium menu except:	
¾ c wheat flakes cereal	199	2 cups puffed wheat cereal	1		
1 slice whole wheat bread	149				
1 medium banana	1				
1 cup nonfat milk	126				
1 cup orange juice	5				
1 tsp soft margarine	51	1 tsp soft margarine, unsalted	1		
Lunch					
beef sandwich:					
2 oz beef, eye of round	35				
1 Tbsp barbecue sauce	156			1 Tbsp low sodium chili sauce	4
2 slices cheddar cheese, reduced fat	260	2 slices Swiss cheese, natural	109		
1 sesame roll	319			2 slices low sodium bread	14
1 large leaf romaine lettuce	1				
2 slices tomato	22				
1 cup low-fat, low-sodium potato salad	12				
1 medium orange	0				
Dinner					
3 oz cod with lemon juice	90				
½ cup brown rice	5				

TABLE 18.7
(continued)

DASH MENU AT THREE DIFFERENT SODIUM LEVELS

2400 mg Sodium Menu	Sodium (mg)	Substitutions to ↓ Sodium to 1500 mg	Sodium (mg)	Substitutions to ↓ Sodium to 1000 mg	Sodium (mg)
½ c cooked spinach	88			½ cup cooked green beans	6
1 small corn bread muffin	363	1 small dinner roll	146		
1 tsp soft margarine	51	1 tsp soft margarine, unsalted	1		
Snacks					
1 cup fruit yogurt, fat free, no added sugar	107				
¼ cup dried fruit	6				
2 large graham cracker rectangles	156				
1 Tbsp. peanut butter, reduced fat	101	1 Tbsp peanut butter, unsalted	3		
Total Sodium (mg)	1958		1519		979
Approximate Amount					
Calories		2000			
% calories from fat		20			
% calories from saturated fat		6			
Cholesterol		140 mg			
Calcium		1500 mg			
Potassium		4759 mg			
Fiber		30 g			

Nutrition Therapy

Edema related to CHF can be relieved by reducing sodium intake because extracellular fluid retention does not occur in the absence of sodium. Permitted sodium intake may vary from 250 to 2000 mg/day depending on the severity of CHF (Box 18.5). The initial allowance may be progressed as edema subsides. Some clients can tolerate a normal sodium intake after their condition has stabilized.

(*text continues on page 562*)

BOX 18.5

SODIUM-RESTRICTED DIETS

The objective of low-sodium diets is to rid the body of excess sodium and fluid accumulation associated with certain disorders such as liver disease characterized by edema and ascites, CHF, renal disease characterized by edema and hypertension, and adrenocortical therapy. Low-sodium diets also are used in the treatment and possible prevention of hypertension.

Low-sodium diets are contraindicated for clients with sodium-wasting renal diseases such as pyelonephritis, polycystic renal disease, and bilateral hydronephrosis; in pregnancy; for clients with ileostomies; and for those with myxedema.

The characteristics of low-sodium diets vary according to the level of restriction; 500- and 250-mg sodium diets are unpalatable, extremely difficult to follow, and likely to be inadequate in some nutrients. To promote compliance and to allow greater flexibility, exchange lists featuring the sodium content of high- and low-sodium foods may be used.

Levels of Restriction

3000 mg Sodium (130 mEq) Per Day

- Use up to ¼ tsp of salt daily.
- Eliminate high-sodium processed foods and beverages.

2000 mg (87 mEq) Per Day

- Eliminate processed and prepared foods and beverages high in sodium.
- No salt is allowed in cooking or at the table.
- Limit milk and milk products to 16 oz/d.
- Use low-sodium versions of canned and instant products when available.

1000 mg (45 mEq) Per Day

- Follow all 2000-mg sodium restrictions.
- Use only unsalted butter, margarine, and salad dressings.
- Use only low-sodium cheese.
- Limit regular breads to two servings per day; use low-sodium bread, crackers, and other grains.

500 mg (22 mEq) Per Day

- Follow all 1000-mg sodium restrictions.
- Eliminate vegetables naturally high in sodium: beets, beet greens, carrots, kale, spinach, celery, white turnips, rutabagas, mustard greens, chard, peas, and dandelion greens.
- Use only low-sodium bread, no regular bread.
- Eliminate sherbet and flavored gelatin.
- Limit meat to 5 oz/d; one egg may be substituted daily for 1 oz of meat.
- Use distilled water for cooking and drinking if sodium content of water supply is high.

250 mg (11 mEq) Per Day

- Follow all 500-mg sodium restrictions.
- Use low-sodium milk in place of regular milk.

(box continues on page 560)

BOX 18.5 (continued)

SODIUM-RESTRICTED DIETS

Approximate Sodium Content per Food Group

Food Group	mg Sodium/Serving
GRAINS AND GRAIN PRODUCTS	
Unsalted cooked cereal, rice, pasta, ½ cup	0–5
Low sodium bread, 1 slice	5
Ready-to-eat cereal, 1 cup	100–360
Bread, 1 slice	110–175
VEGETABLES	
Fresh or frozen, without salt, ½ cup	1–70
Canned or frozen with sauce, ½ cup	140–460
Tomato juice, canned, ¾ cup	820
FRUIT	
Fresh, frozen, canned, ½ cup	0–5
LOW FAT OR FAT FREE DAIRY PRODUCTS	
Milk, 1 cup	120
Yogurt, 1 cup	160
Natural cheeses, 1½ oz	110–450
Processed cheeses, 1½ oz	600
MEAT, FISH, POULTRY, DRIED PEAS AND BEANS, NUTS	
Beans, cooked from dry, without salt, ½ cup	0–5
Beans, canned, ½ cup	400
Fresh meat, fish, poultry, 3 oz	30–90
Tuna, canned, water pack, 3 oz	250–350
Ham, lean, roasted, 3 oz	1020
FATS	
Margarine, 1 tsp	50–100
Unsalted margarine, 1 tsp	1
Bottled salad dressing, 2 Tbsp	270–400
Oil and vinegar	0

Patient Teaching

(Be more or less specific depending on the level of sodium allowed.)
Provide general information:

- Reducing sodium intake will help the body rid itself of excess fluid and help lower high blood pressure.
- Sodium appears in the diet in the form of salt and to some degree in almost all foods and beverages. Most unprocessed, unsalted foods are low in sodium.
- Approximately 15% of sodium intake comes from salt added during cooking and at the table, 75% comes from processed foods, and 10% is from food and water naturally high in sodium.

BOX 18.5 (continued)

SODIUM-RESTRICTED DIETS

- Sodium-containing compounds are used extensively as preservatives (sodium propionate, sodium sulfite, and sodium benzoate), leavening agents (sodium bicarbonate, baking soda, and baking powder), and flavor enhancers (e.g., salt, MSG) and are found in foods that may not taste salty.
- Many nonprescription drugs (e.g., aspirin, cough medicines, laxatives, antacids), toothpastes, tooth powders, and mouthwashes contain large amounts of sodium and should not be used without a physician's approval.
- Salt substitutes replace sodium with potassium or other minerals. "Low-sodium" salt substitutes are not sodium free and may contain half as much sodium as regular table salt. Use neither type without a physician's approval.
- The preference for salt taste eventually will decrease.
- If the client "cheats" by eating a high-sodium meal or snack, compensate by eating less sodium than normally allowed for the rest of the day.
- Teach the client how to order from a menu while dining out (see Box 18.4).

Teach the client food preparation techniques to minimize sodium intake:

- Foods made from "scratch" generally have less sodium than processed foods and mixes.
- Experiment with sodium-free seasonings such as herbs, spices, lemon juice, vinegar, and wine. Fresh ingredients are more flavorful than dried ones.
- Commercial "salt alternatives" are sodium-free blends of herbs and spices that are not intended to taste like salt but to be used as flavor enhancers.
- If permitted by a physician, salt substitutes may be used although they taste bitter to some people.
- A variety of low-sodium cookbooks are available.

Teach the client how to read labels:

- Salt, MSG, baking soda, and baking powder contain significant amounts of sodium. Other sodium compounds such as sodium nitrite, benzoate of soda, sodium saccharin, and sodium propionate add less sodium to the diet.
- "Sodium free," "low sodium," "very low sodium," and "reduced" or "less" sodium are reliable terms.
- Numerous low- and reduced-sodium products are available: milk, bread and bread products, cereal, crackers, cakes, cookies, pastries, soups and bouillon, canned vegetables, tomato products, meats, entrees, processed meats, hard and soft cheeses, condiments, nuts and peanut butter, butter, margarine, salad dressings, baking powder, and snack foods.
- The difference in taste between some low-sodium products and their high-sodium counterparts is barely noticeable; others taste flat and may need to have herbs or spices added.

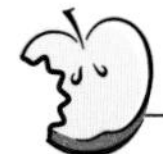
Quick Bite

High-potassium fruits include

Apricots	Melons
Bananas	Raisins
Citrus fruits and their juices	Dried dates
Kiwi	Papaya
Mango	Prune juice
Nectarine	Avocados

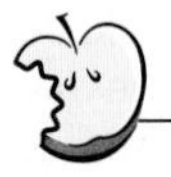
Quick Bite

High-potassium vegetables include

Artichoke
Beets
Brussels sprouts
Mushrooms
Okra
Sweet and white potatoes
Tomatoes and tomato products
Dried peas and beans
Green leafy vegetables
Carrots
Winter squash
Pumpkin
Rutabagas
Parsnips

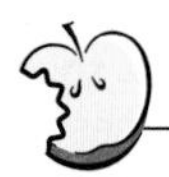
Quick Bite

Potassium-containing salt substitutes

NoSalt
Seasoned NoSalt
Morton Salt Substitute
Morton Lite Salt Mixture
Adolph's Salt Substitute
Adolph's Seasoned Salt
Diamond Crystal
CoSalt

In most cases, sodium restriction used alone or in combination with diuretics (low-sodium diets enhance the sodium-excreting effects of diuretics) effectively reduces fluid volume without the need for fluid restriction. However, fluid restriction may be necessary if edema persists despite a low-sodium diet. Fluid may be limited to 2 L per day or less depending on the client's response to the sodium restriction.

A diet that is low in calories but otherwise nutritionally adequate is indicated for overweight clients. Attaining ideal or slightly underideal weight reduces the cardiac workload. In addition

- Provide five to six small meals per day of nonirritating and non–gas-forming foods to limit gastric distention and pressure on the heart.
- Individualize the diet according to the patient's tolerance. Soft foods reduce the amount of chewing required, an important consideration for fatigued patients.
- Provide adequate potassium based on the type of diuretic prescribed. A high-potassium diet may be indicated for clients who are taking thiazide (potassium-wasting) diuretics or digitalis (Table 18.8). Spironolactone and triamterene are potassium-sparing diuretics that do not warrant the intake or use of additional potassium.
- Initially eliminate caffeine. After the patient's condition has stabilized, coffee intake may be liberalized to four or five cups/day as tolerated.

Malnutrition among CHF patients, known as cardiac cachexia, may occur with poor nutritional intake and long-term use of medication. Nutritional deficiencies can have a severe impact on the heart. Patients with cardiac cachexia need a high-calorie, high-protein, high-nutrient diet within the confines of sodium restriction (1 to 2 g/day). Caloric and nutrient density is important to maximize intake. Often these patients do not tolerate enteral feedings because of access to the thoracic cavity and decreased blood flow to the gastrointestinal tract.

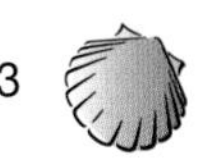

TABLE 18.8 **MEAL PLAN FOR A HIGH-POTASSIUM DIET**

Food Group	Servings/ Day	High-Potassium Choices
Breads and cereal	7	Bran cereals, dark rye and pumpernickel breads
Vegetables	≥ 3	Greens, potatoes, tomatoes, winter squash
Fruit	4	Banana, melon, oranges and orange juice, prune juice
Milk and dairy	2	Malted milk, Ovaltine made with milk
Meat, poultry, fish, dried peas and beans, nuts	≤ 6 oz	Dried peas and beans
Other		Coffee and tea have ≈ 80 mg/cup Pure fats and pure sugars are potassium-free.

NURSING PROCESS

Mrs. Gigante is a 79-year-old widow admitted for CHF. She lives alone. Because she prepares her own meals, she relies heavily on convenience foods such as canned and packaged soups, frozen dinners, canned pasta, and tuna fish sandwiches. She appears thin and has 3+ edema in her lower extremities.

Assessment

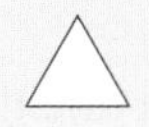

Obtain Clinical Data:

Current weight, height, BMI
Blood pressure
Abdominal girth, presence of edema
Medical history and comorbidities including diabetes, hypertension, myocardial infarction, alcohol abuse, and other CHD risk factors
Abnormal laboratory values, especially cholesterol, lipid profile, triglycerides, blood urea nitrogen, sodium, creatinine, potassium, and glucose
Medications that affect nutrition such as diuretics, antihypertensives, antidiabetics, and lipid-lowering medications
Complaints including activity intolerance, fatigue, and shortness of breath
Urine output

(continued)

Interview the Client to Assess:

Understanding the relationship between sodium, fluid accumulation, and symptoms of CHF
Motivation to change eating style; previous attempts to modify intake
Usual 24-hour intake including portion sizes; frequency and pattern of eating; method of food preparation; problems with anorexia or early satiety; intake of foods high in fat and saturated fat, foods high in sodium, and foods high in potassium
Hydration; input and output
If CHF symptoms impair her abilities to shop, cook, eat, or perform other activities of daily living
Cultural, religious, and ethnic influences on eating habits
Use of vitamins, minerals, and nutritional supplements: what, how much, and why taken
Psychosocial and economic issues such as living situation, cooking facilities, financial status, education, and eligibility for the Meals on Wheels program
Use of alcohol, caffeine, and nicotine
Adherence to prescribed drug therapy

Nursing Diagnosis

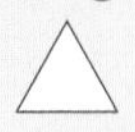

1. Fluid Volume Excess, related to CHF.
2. Decreased Cardiac Output, related to CHF.
3. Health-Seeking Behaviors, as evidenced by the lack of knowledge of a heart-healthy diet and a desire to learn.

Planning and Implementation

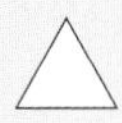

Client Goals

The client will

Attain and maintain normal fluid balance.
Consume a varied and nutritious diet with adequate calories to attain healthy body weight.
Avoid excessive sodium and increase intake of potassium.
Avoid cardiac stimulants.

Nursing Interventions

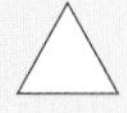

Nutrition Therapy

Provide a 2-g sodium diet as ordered.
Provide five to six small meals to limit gastric distention and pressure on the heart.
Monitor input and output for need for fluid restriction.
Eliminate caffeine until patient has stabilized.

Client Teaching

Instruct the client

On the roles of sodium, fluid, medication, desirable weight, and smoking in managing CHF.

On the availability of the Meals on Wheels program. Explain that Meals on Wheels can provide her with the appropriate diet after discharge to ensure that she gets the proper foods even on days when she feels short of breath or too tired to cook. (Notify the discharge planner that the client may be a candidate for Meals on Wheels.)

On eating plan essentials such as

- Eliminating the use of salt in cooking and at the table
- Using low-sodium canned foods when available
- Avoiding other high-sodium items
- Limiting milk intake to two cups daily
- Restricting caffeine initially
- Increasing intake of high-potassium foods
- Avoiding alcohol
- Adhering to fluid restriction if appropriate

On behavioral matters including

- How to read labels to identify high-sodium foods
- That a gradual reduction in sodium intake may be easier to comply with than an abrupt withdrawal of sodium. Because the preference for salt gradually diminishes when intake is limited, following a low-sodium diet tends to get easier with time.
- Timing meals and snacks to avoid shortness of breath and fatigue
- Physical activity goals if applicable and appropriate

Evaluation

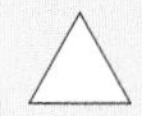

The client

Attains and maintains normal fluid balance

Consumes a varied and nutritious diet with adequate calories to attain healthy body weight; has Meals on Wheels scheduled to provide meals after discharge

Avoids excessive sodium and increases intake of potassium

Avoids cardiac stimulants

How Do You Respond?

What can be done to raise HDL? Low HDL may be related to metabolic syndrome, smoking, very high carbohydrate diets (>60% of calories), and certain drugs. It is not known if raising HDL reduces the risk of CHD, so there are no goals for increasing HDL. The best strategy for people with low HDL is to attain their LDL goal, lose weight if overweight (which may increase HDL by 5 to 20%), and increase their physical activity (which may increase HDL by 5 to 30%). Drug therapy may be considered but drugs do not dramatically increase HDL levels.

Does coffee raise blood pressure? Without doubt, coffee and caffeine cause a transient rise in blood pressure. However, there is no compelling evidence to suggest that drinking coffee significantly increases the risk of developing hypertension. On the other hand, some studies show coffee increases cholesterol and/or CHD risk. Filtered coffee has less of an effect on lipid levels, but both filtered and unfiltered coffee increase homocysteine levels.

▲ Focus on Critical Thinking

Respond to the following statements:

1. A low saturated fat, low cholesterol diet is not necessary if LDL level is normal.
2. It is possible to reverse atherosclerosis through intensive nutrition intervention and other lifestyle changes.
3. The TLC diet and DASH diet can be used interchangeably.

Key Concepts

- The primary focus for the primary and secondary prevention of CHD is to lower LDL. And individual's LDL goal is based on the presence of independent risk factors such as smoking, age, family history, low HDL level, and hypertension.
- Other factors impact CHD risk although they are factored when determining optimal LDL level. Those additional risk factors include metabolic syndrome, high triglycerides, inactivity, an atherogenic diet, elevated homocysteine level, and inflammatory factors.
- Lifestyle modifications recommended to lower total cholesterol and LDL include Therapeutic Lifestyle Change (TLC) Diet, increasing physical activity, and weight loss.
- Saturated fat, trans fat, and cholesterol raise LDL levels. When used in place of saturated fat, complex carbohydrates, polyunsaturated fats, and monounsaturated fat all lower LDL cholesterol as does soluble fiber. Sugars and syrups appear to raise LDL cholesterol. Fish oils protect the heart by means other than LDL lowering.

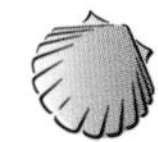

- The optimal percentage of calories from total fat is controversial. The TLC diet guidelines recommend a fat intake of 25 to 35% of total calories whereas many researchers believe a lower fat intake is more effective at lowering CHD risks.
- Changing eating patterns is a lifestyle modification that should be made gradually and sequentially for the greatest chance of long-term success.
- Sterol-rich margarines help to lower LDL but may not be prudent unless the client is at very high risk or already has CHD. Soy products have the potential to lower cholesterol but only with a consistent intake of a large amount. Alcohol reduces the risk of CHD by raising HDL and decreasing platelet aggregation; on the downside, alcohol can raise blood pressure. Sodium restriction helps to prevent hypertension, which in turn helps to prevent CHD.
- Nutrition therapy is the cornerstone of primary prevention and treatment of hypertension. The DASH-sodium diet, which is similar to the TLC diet but has more fruits, more vegetables, and a food group entitled "Nuts, Seeds, and Dried Peas and Beans," is clinically proven to lower blood pressure and cholesterol. Other lifestyle modifications for high blood pressure are to stop smoking, lose excess weight, increase physical activity, and drink alcohol only moderately.
- Usually, a low-sodium diet used with or without diuretics can effectively control fluid balance in clients with CHF without the need for a fluid restriction.

ANSWER KEY

1. **TRUE** A high level of "good" cholesterol (HDL) is protective against CHD.
2. **TRUE** The number of risk factors a person has determines the optimal level of LDL. Major independent risk factors are identified as smoking, hypertension, low HDL, family history of premature CHD, and aging.
3. **TRUE** Although the mechanism is unclear, high levels of homocysteine are considered an independent risk factor for CHD and other atherosclerotic conditions.
4. **FALSE** The sources of fiber best at lowering LDL are the soluble fibers found in oats, dried peas and beans, fruit, root vegetables, barley, and flax. Wheat bran and whole wheat grains are rich sources of insoluble fiber used to promote regularity.
5. **FALSE** Polyunsaturated fats are not considered safe at any level specifically the n-6 fatty acids. They lower HDL and tend to stimulate platelet aggregation. It is recommended that polyunsaturated fat intake be <10% of total calories.
6. **FALSE** Because of the potential health risks and abuse issues, people who do not drink alcohol are not encouraged to do so to lower their risk of heart disease.
7. **FALSE** Stick margarine should be avoided because it contains trans fatty acids that are atherogenic. Trans fat intake should be as low as possible.
8. **TRUE** Major sources of saturated fat in the typical American diet—dairy, beef, pork, poultry, and lamb products—also provide substantial amounts of monounsaturated fat.
9. **TRUE** Weight loss lowers high blood pressure.

10. **TRUE** The TLC diet is used to lower cholesterol and the DASH diet is used to lower blood pressure, but the diets are remarkably similar. In fact, the DASH diet has been clinically proven to lower both blood pressure and cholesterol.

WEBSITES

American Heart Association at **www.americanheart.org**
Heart and Stroke Foundation of Canada at **www.hsf.ca**
National Heart, Lung and Blood Institute at **www.nhlbi.nih.gov**

REFERENCES

American Heart Association. (2004). Journal Report. New stats show heart disease still America's No. 1 killer, stroke No. 3. Available at www.americanheart.org/presenter.jhtml?identifier=3018015. Accessed on 1/15/04.

American Heart Association. (2002). Dietary guidelines. Available at www.americanheart.org/presenter.jhtml?identifier=1330. Accessed on 1/15/04.

Chicago Dietetic Association, South Suburban Dietetic Association, Dietitians of Canada. (2000). *Manual of clinical dietetics.* Chicago: The American Dietetic Association.

Cunningham, E. (2003). How can high-density lipoprotein cholesterol levels be elevated? *Journal of the American Dietetic Association, 103,* 860.

Djousse, L., Folsom, A., Province, M., et al. (2003). Dietary linolenic acid and carotid atherosclerosis: The National Heart, Lung, and Blood Institute Family Heart Study. *American Journal of Clinical Nutrition, 77,* 819–825.

Doherty, J. (Ed.). (2002). Coffee, caffeine and hypertension. *Communicating Food for Health,* June, 72.

Doherty, J. (Ed.). (2002). Coffee or tea? *Communicating Food for Health,* June, 61, 65.

Doherty, J. (Ed.). (2003). CRP and heart attack risk. *Communicating Food for Health,* February, 13, 17.

Fried, S., & Rao, S. (2003). Sugars, hypertriglyceridemia, and cardiovascular disease. *American Journal of Clinical Nutrition, 78*(Suppl.), 873S–880S.

Horn, L., & Ernst, N. (2001). A summary of the science supporting the new National Cholesterol Education Program dietary recommendations: What dietitians should know. *Journal of the American Dietetic Association, 101,* 1148–1154.

Liebman, B. (2003). CRP. Another piece of the heart-disease puzzle? *Nutrition Action Health Letter, 30*(2), 1, 3–7.

Mauger, J., Lichtenstein, A., Ausman, L., et al. (2003). Effect of different forms of dietary hydrogenated fats on LDL particle size. *American Journal of Clinical Nutrition, 78,* 370–375.

McCarron, P. (2002). Dietary approaches to stop hypertension. *Pulse. A Publication for Sports, Cardiovascular, and Wellness Nutritionists, 21*(3), 1–3.

McCarthy, D. (2002). Long-chain omega-3 fatty acids and cardiovascular health. *Pulse. A publication for Sports, Cardiovascular, and Wellness Nutritionists, 21*(1), 1–3.

Mennen, L., Potier de Courcy, G., Guilland, J., et al. (2002). Homocysteine, cardiovascular disease risk factors, and habitual diet in the French supplementation with antioxidant vitamins and minerals study. *American Journal of Clinical Nutrition, 76,* 1279–1289.

National Cholesterol Education Program. (2001). *Third report of the expert panel on detection, evaluation, and treatment of high blood cholesterol in adults (Adult Treatment Panel III). Executive Summary.* (NIH Publication No. 01-3670). Bethesda, MD: U.S. Department of Health and Human Services, Public Health Service, National Institutes of Health.

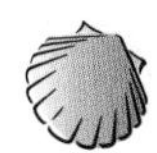

National Heart, Lung, and Blood Institute. Tipsheet. TLC Diet. Daily Food Guide Food Groups. Available at http://nhlbisupport.com/chd1/S2Tipsheets/foodgroup.htm. Accessed on 1/15/04.

National Institutes of Health, National Heart, Lung, and Blood Institute, National High Blood Pressure Program. (2003). *Facts about the DASH Eating Plan*. (NIH Publication No. 03-4082). Bethesda, MD: U.S. Department of Health and Human Services, Public Health Service, NIH, NHLBI.

Rosenberg, I. (Ed.). (2003). The 5 lifestyle steps for lowering blood pressure. *Tufts University Health & Nutrition Letter, 21*(5), 5.

Rosenberg, I. (Ed.). (2003). Was the statin prescription right in the first place? *Tufts University Health & Nutrition Letter, 21*(6), 1, 6.

Rosenberg, I. (Ed.). (2003). At risk for heart disease? Don't expect vitamin E to help. *Tufts University Health & Nutrition Letter, 21*(6), 7.

Schaefer, E. (2002). Lipoproteins, nutrition, and heart disease. *American Journal of Clinical Nutrition, 75*, 191–212.

Simopoulos, A., Leaf, A., & Salem, N. (1999). Essentiality of and recommended dietary intakes for omega-6 and omega-3 fatty acids. *Annals of Nutrition & Metabolism*, 43, 127–130.

For information on the new dietary guidelines 2005 and MyPyramid, visit **http://connection.lww.com/go/dudek**

19

Nutrition for Patients With Diabetes Mellitus

TRUE	FALSE	
⬭	⬭	**1** Carbohydrates impact postprandial glucose levels more than protein or fat.
⬭	⬭	**2** Weight loss lowers the risk of type 2 diabetes only when it is substantial.
⬭	⬭	**3** Increasing physical activity is beneficial even if it does not produce weight loss.
⬭	⬭	**4** Alcohol is more likely to cause hypoglycemia when consumed without food rather than with food.
⬭	⬭	**5** Frequent treatment of hypoglycemia can lead to weight gain.
⬭	⬭	**6** People with diabetes should eat more fiber than the general population should.
⬭	⬭	**7** Foods containing sucrose have a higher glycemic index than starchy foods.
⬭	⬭	**8** All diabetics should be taught how to use exchange lists to plan their meals.
⬭	⬭	**9** Supplemental chromium has been shown to improve glycemic control in people with type 2 diabetes.
⬭	⬭	**10** People with diabetes should limit their intakes of saturated fat and cholesterol.

UPON COMPLETION OF THIS CHAPTER, YOU WILL BE ABLE TO

- List risk factors for type 2 diabetes.
- List goals of nutrition therapy for diabetics.
- Discuss the nutrient recommendations for diabetics.
- Explain how to use exchange lists to implement a meal plan.
- Describe how to convert exchanges into MyPyramid groups to simplify diet counseling.
- Discuss diabetes nutrition therapy in childhood, in pregnancy, and in older adults.

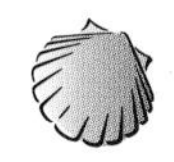

DIABETES

Diabetes Mellitus: a chronic heterogeneous disorder characterized by elevated blood glucose levels (hyperglycemia) related to a relative or absolute deficiency of insulin.

Diabetes is one of the most costly and burdensome chronic diseases of our time and is increasing in epidemic proportions. Approximately 16 million Americans currently have diabetes; that figure is expected to soar to 23 million within the next 10 years. This increase is due almost entirely to an increased prevalence of type 2 diabetes. The prevalence of type 1 diabetes remains relatively stable.

Type 1 Diabetes

Type 1 Diabetes: diabetes characterized by the absence of insulin secretion.

Type 1 diabetes, formerly known as insulin-dependent diabetes mellitus, accounts for only 5% to 10% of all diagnosed cases of diabetes. It is characterized by the absence of insulin, which results from autoimmune response that damages or destroys beta cells, leaving them unable to produce insulin. Although it can occur at any age, it is most often detected before the age of 30 years in people who are normal or slightly below normal weight. All people with type 1 diabetes require exogenous insulin to maintain blood glucose levels.

Type 2 Diabetes

Insulin Resistance: decreased cellular response to insulin.

Impaired Glucose Tolerance: inability to maintain normal glucose levels without excessive amounts of insulin.

Hyperinsulinemia: elevated blood levels of insulin.

Unlike type 1 diabetes in which there is a relatively abrupt end to insulin production, type 2 diabetes is a slowly progressive disease that begins as a problem of insulin resistance. Because cells do not respond to insulin as they should, the pancreas compensates by secreting higher than normal levels of insulin. During this period of impaired glucose tolerance, glucose levels are relatively normal but insulin levels are high. Over time chronic hyperinsulinemia leads to a decrease in the number of insulin receptors on the cells and a further reduction in tissue sensitivity to insulin. Eventually and progressively, insulin sensitivity and insulin secretion deteriorate, and frank type 2 diabetes develops.

The most notable factor involved in the near-epidemic growth of type 2 diabetes is the corresponding increase in the prevalence of obesity and an ever-increasing sedentary American lifestyle. Not all people who are obese and sedentary develop type 2 diabetes, but these are two important risk factors for insulin resistance. Type 2 is most often diagnosed after 40 years of age, but it is being diagnosed in young people in unprecedented numbers because of the increased prevalence of obesity among children and adolescents. Other risk factors for type 2 diabetes appear in Box 19.1.

A multicenter clinical trial called the Diabetes Prevention Program (DPP) found that in a diverse group of overweight people with impaired glucose tolerance, diet and exercise decreased the incidence of diabetes by 58%. Study participants walked at moderate intensity an average of 30 minutes five times per week and decreased their intake of fat and calories. Average weight loss was a modest 5 to 7% of initial weight, or about 15 pounds. This study also found that metformin lowers the incidence of type 2 diabetes by 31%, about one-half as much as the lifestyle interventions. Clearly, millions of

BOX 19.1 **RISK FACTORS FOR TYPE 2 DIABETES**

- ≥45 years of age
- Overweight (BMI ≥ 25 kg/m^2)
- First-degree relative with diabetes
- Chronic physical inactivity
- Member of high-risk ethnic group: African-American, Latino, Native American, Asian-American, Pacific Islander
- Previously identified pre-diabetic condition such as impaired fasting glucose or impaired glucose tolerance
- History of gestational diabetes or giving birth to a baby weighing > 9 pounds
- Hypertensive
- HDL < 35 mg/dL and/or triglyceride level ≥ 250 mg/dL
- Diagnosis of polycystic ovary syndrome
- History of vascular disease

overweight Americans at high risk for type 2 diabetes can delay and possibly prevent the disease with a moderate diet and exercise.

Many people with type 2 diabetes have metabolic syndrome, a cluster of metabolic abnormalities that include insulin resistance, central obesity, low high density lipoprotein cholesterol (HDL), high triglycerides (TG), elevated small low density lipoprotein cholesterol (LDL), and hypertension, all of which contribute to morbidity in type 2 diabetes. Even though nutrition therapy and exercise are capable of controlling glucose levels for the majority of type 2 diabetics, most clients require oral hypoglycemics or insulin because of poor compliance with nutrition and exercise regimens.

Long-Term Complications

Gastroparesis: delayed gastric emptying.

Diabetes significantly increases morbidity and mortality and is the sixth leading cause of death by disease in the United States. Heart disease is the leading cause of death among people with diabetes, and diabetics are 2 to 4 times more likely to die from heart disease compared with age- and sex-matched peers. This increased risk may be partly related to a high incidence of other coronary heart disease risk factors such as hyperlipidemia, obesity, hypertension, and clotting abnormalities. Similarly, the risk of stroke and peripheral vascular disease is significantly higher. Diabetes is the leading cause of new cases of blindness and of end-stage renal disease. Another complication is neuropathy, which can cause gastroparesis, impaired peripheral circulation, and impotence in men. Impaired wound healing can lead to gangrene and amputation. People with diabetes develop complications without being aware that the damage is occurring.

The importance of attaining normal or near normal glycemic control to decrease the incidence and severity of microvascular complications has been confirmed by several large and small trials. Findings suggest that glycemic control also lessens the risk of macrovascular complications, but not to the same extent. Clinical trial data strongly

 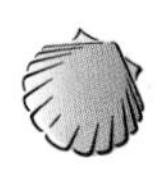

support the importance of treating abnormal lipid levels and hypertension to lower the risk of cardiovascular disease. Nutrition therapy has the potential to delay or prevent diabetes complications by controlling glucose levels, improving blood lipid levels, and controlling hypertension.

DIABETES MANAGEMENT

The overall goals of medical therapy for all people with diabetes are to

- Attain and maintain optimal metabolic controls namely blood glucose levels, blood lipid levels, and blood pressure
- Prevent, delay, or treat complications
- Improve overall health through optimal nutrition and physical activity

These goals are most effectively met through a combination of nutrition therapy, exercise, and drug therapy.

Nutrition Recommendations

Nutrition therapy is an essential component of diabetes management regardless of the client's weight, blood glucose levels, or use of medication. People with diabetes generally have the same nutritional requirements as the general population; therefore, dietary recommendations to promote health and well-being in the general public—lose weight if overweight; eat less saturated fat and cholesterol; eat more fiber and less sodium—are also appropriate for people with diabetes. Because coronary heart disease (CHD) is the leading cause of death among people with diabetes, it makes sense that nutrition recommendations issued by the American Diabetes Association to prevent and treat diabetes are remarkably similar to recommendations put forth by the National Cholesterol Education Program for the primary and secondary prevention of CHD (Chapter 18). Nutrition recommendations for diabetes management are summarized in Table 19.1.

Total Carbohydrate

Glycemic Index: the incremental rise in blood glucose (above baseline) compared to that induced by a standard, usually 50 g glucose or a white bread challenge.

Total carbohydrate intake is the sum of the amount of sugar, starch, and fiber consumed. As a group, carbohydrates have more of an impact on postprandial serum glucose levels than protein or fat does. It is also known that different carbohydrates elicit varying degrees of increase in blood glucose levels. Considering these two facts, obvious assumptions may be that (1) total carbohydrate intake should be restricted and (2) carbohydrates with high glycemic index should be avoided. In reality, neither assumption is correct. Recommendations clearly stress the value in choosing carbohydrates from grains, fruit, and vegetables so that fiber and nutrient needs are met. Although different carbohydrates produce different glycemic responses, there does not appear to be a benefit from a low glycemic index diet compared to a high glycemic

TABLE 19.1 **NUTRIENT RECOMMENDATIONS FOR DIABETES**

Nutrient	Recommendations
Carbohydrates	• Complex carbohydrates in grains, fruits, and vegetables are part of a healthy diet. • Consistency in the amount of total carbohydrate eaten at meals and snacks is more important than the type of carbohydrate consumed. • Together, total carbohydrate and monounsaturated fat should provide ≈60–70% of total calories.
Sweeteners	• Gram for gram, sucrose can replace starch without causing a deleterious affect on glucose levels. • High sugar foods may be high in fat and low in nutrients; they should be used judiciously. • Foods sweetened with fructose should be avoided because they negatively impact serum lipids even though they produce a smaller rise in blood glucose levels compared to other carbohydrates. Natural sources of fructose (fruits, vegetables) do not need to be restricted.
Fiber	• Diabetics may benefit from eating more fiber than they currently do but do not need to eat more fiber than the general public.
Protein	• Protein need may be higher than the RDA but not higher than actual intake. • Current average intake of 15 to 20% of total calories appears adequate and appropriate.
Saturated fat	• Limit to <10% of total calories. If LDL is ≥ 100 mg/dL, limit to <7% of calories.
Polyunsaturated fat	• Should provide up to 10% of total calories. • Omega-3 fats may help to lower triglycerides and other coronary risks without negatively impacting glucose levels.
Monounsaturated fat	• Using more monounsaturated fat and less carbohydrate to make up for the decrease in calories from the decrease in saturated fat does not cause the worsening glucose, insulin, and triglyceride levels seen with a high CHO diet, but monounsaturated fat is higher in calories than CHO and may promote weight gain. • The level of monounsaturated fat should be based on weight and lipid levels.
Trans fat	• Keep as low as possible.
Total fat	• A recommendation for total fat is not made but diets with ≤30% calories from fat may promote modest weight loss.
Cholesterol	• Limit to <300 mg/dl. If LDL is ≥100 mg/dL, lower to <200 mg/dL.

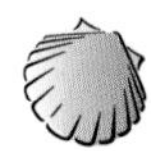

TABLE 19.1 (continued)

NUTRIENT RECOMMENDATIONS FOR DIABETES

Alcohol	• If people choose to drink, alcohol should be limited to 2 drinks/day for men and 1 drink/day for women. • Consume alcohol with food to avoid hypoglycemia.
Vitamin and mineral supplements	• Supplementation is not recommended except for documented deficiencies, folic acid during pregnancy, and calcium to prevent bone disease.
Calories	• Weight loss is a primary goal for type 2 diabetics because it can decrease insulin resistance, improve glucose and lipid levels, and lower blood pressure, even with only modest weight loss. • Lowering calorie intake and increasing physical activity can produce a modest weight loss. • Standard weight loss diets used alone are not likely to produce long-term weight loss.

index diet, in part because many variables affect glycemic index even for a given source of carbohydrate. The bottom line is that the total amount of carbohydrate in meals and snacks is more important than the type or source. A consistent carbohydrate and calorie intake is fundamental to glycemic control.

A recommendation for the optimal amount of carbohydrate has not been made. Rather, the expert consensus is that carbohydrate and monounsaturated fat *together* should provide 60 to 70% of total calories. The optimal contribution of each of these nutrients is based on individual considerations of weight and serum lipid levels. Equivalent LDL lowering is seen when either carbohydrate or monounsaturated fat intake is substituted for saturated fat. However, high-carbohydrate diets increase postprandial glucose and insulin levels, increase serum TG levels, and may decrease HDL compared to isocaloric diets high in monounsaturated fat.

Sweeteners

Isocalorically: of the same calorie level.

Clinical studies demonstrate that when sucrose is isocalorically substituted for starch, there is no difference in glycemic control in either type 1 or type 2 diabetics. Traditional assumptions that sugar causes diabetics' blood glucose levels to rise too high and too quickly no longer hold true. Sucrose and sucrose-containing foods are "allowed" but should be substituted for other carbohydrates in the meal plan, not eaten as "extras." Many long-standing diabetics resist accepting this shift in thinking. Others find the freedom to choose sweetened foods difficult not to abuse. Even though they do not aggravate glycemic control, foods high in sugar are usually nutrient poor and may be high in fat. People with diabetes are advised to consume sucrose judiciously.

The use of fructose as an added sweetener is not recommended because even though it produces a lower postprandial response than other carbohydrates, large amounts of fructose increase LDL and triglycerides in people without diabetes.

However, it is not recommended that diabetics avoid naturally occurring fructose in fruit and vegetables.

Sugar alcohols (sorbitol, mannitol, and xylitol) provide fewer calories and cause a smaller increase in glucose than sucrose and other carbohydrates do. They may cause abdominal gas, discomfort, and osmotic diarrhea when consumed in large amounts.

Nonnutritive sweeteners are safe to use. Saccharin, aspartame, and acesulfame-K, sucralose, and neotame are approved for use by the U.S. Food and Drug Administration (FDA) and may safely be used by diabetics.

Fiber

The recommendations for fiber are the same as for the general population—that is, ≥25 g/day for women and ≈38 g/d for men. Although early studies showed improved glycemic control in diabetics eating large amounts of fiber, later studies have had mixed results. However, foods rich in fiber provide other benefits such as increasing satiety (a plus for weight management); providing vitamins, minerals and phytochemicals; and preventing constipation. People with diabetes are encouraged to eat more fiber than the typical American consumes, but they do not need to eat more than the general population.

Protein

In the typical American diet, including the diets of type 1 and type 2 diabetics, protein provides 15% to 20% of total calories. This level is consistent with the recommendation for protein intake among the general public. Although protein stimulates the secretion of insulin at the same magnitude as carbohydrates, protein does not increase glucose levels. Protein requirement for both type 1 and type 2 diabetics may actually be higher than the normal RDA because of increased protein turnover or increased protein catabolism; estimated protein need does not exceed usual intake, though, because most Americans consume at least 50% more protein than the RDA. Although the current level of intake does not appear to increase the risk of diabetic nephropathy, it is prudent to limit protein intake to ≤20% of total calories.

Fat

A blanket recommendation regarding the optimal level of total fat has not been made because of the leeway allowed in determining monounsaturated fat intake, as previously discussed under the section on Carbohydrates. Specific recommendations have been made for saturated fat, polyunsaturated fat, cholesterol, and trans fat.

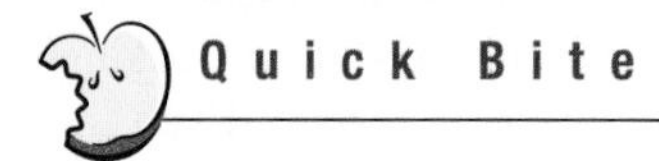

Lowering saturated fat intake means

Choosing nonfat or low-fat milk, cheese, and yogurt
Choosing only lean meats and limiting portions to ≈ 5 oz/day

 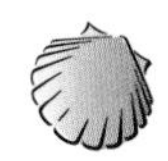

Saturated Fat

Consistent with recommendations made for the primary and secondary prevention of coronary heart disease, people with diabetes are urged to limit their intake of saturated fat. There is strong evidence in populations with type 2 diabetes and among people without diabetes that saturated fat worsens insulin resistance, raises LDL, and, therefore, increases the risk of CHD. The recommendation to limit saturated fat to <10% of total calories or to <7% of calories if LDL level is ≥100 mg/dL is a prudent measure.

Polyunsaturated Fat

Polyunsaturated fats have not been well studied in diabetics. Consistent with the TLC diet, polyunsaturated fat should contribute up to 10% of total calories. Omega-3 fatty acids have a positive effect on lowering triglyceride levels and do not appear to adversely affect glucose levels if intake is ≤3 g/day.

Trans Fat

Trans fat raises LDL cholesterol, lowers HDL cholesterol, and, therefore, increases CHD risk. Several studies suggest trans fats also have a negative impact on insulin sensitivity. Like the recommendation made to the general public, trans fat intake should be minimized.

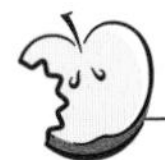

Quick Bite

Limit trans fat by

Using a soft, trans fat free spread in place of margarine
Avoiding processed foods such as frozen French fries, frozen chicken fingers, potato chips
Avoiding fried fast food
Avoiding commercially baked products such as cakes, cookies, crackers, and doughnuts

Total Fat

What is the optimal level of total fat for people with diabetes? The answer is not clear. An individual's weight and lipid levels must be considered.

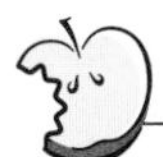

Quick Bite

Total fat is lowered by choosing

Only lean meats and in limited amounts
Foods baked, broiled, boiled, or roasted instead of fried
Only low-fat or nonfat dairy products
Low fat or nonfat versions of salad dressings, margarines, snack foods, and desserts

- Lowering fat to <30% of calories may help to promote weight loss. Many experts believe weight loss is better achieved with an even lower fat intake such as 20% to 25% of calories. However, lowering the percentage of calories from fat inherently means that the percentage of calories from carbohydrates increases. This may have deleterious affects on postprandial glucose levels, triglyceride levels, and HDL level. On the other hand, if lower fat means greater weight loss, these outcomes may be negated because weight loss improves glucose tolerance and HDL levels. The question is: will lowering fat intake help the individual client to lose weight?

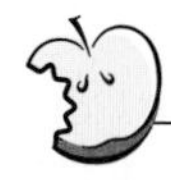

Quick Bite

Increasing monounsaturated fat with lower carbohydrates means

Using olive oil in place of butter, margarine, or other salad dressings
Using nuts in place of meat occasionally
Cutting starch by one or two servings each meal

- Diabetics with a high level of triglycerides may see a greater improvement in their lipid, glucose, and insulin levels by consuming a fat intake higher than 30% (and correspondingly fewer carbohydrate calories) *with the increase in fat coming from monounsaturated fat*. But a higher-fat diet may undermine weight loss. The question is: will the individual client be able to achieve a negative calorie balance if fat intake is high?

Cholesterol

The recommendation is to limit cholesterol to 300 mg or less to decrease the risk of cardiovascular disease. However, the new dietary guidelines for primary and secondary prevention of CHD suggests cholesterol be limited to <200 mg/day. People with diabetes appear more sensitive to dietary cholesterol than the general population.

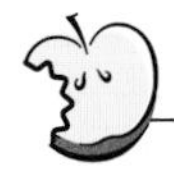

Quick Bite

To cut cholesterol

Limit egg yolks to two/week.
Limit foods high in saturated fat (full fat dairy products, beef, pork, lamb).
Avoid organ meats.

Calories

Weight loss has traditionally been the focus of nutritional intervention for type 2 diabetics. A negative calorie balance quickly lowers high glucose and triglyceride concentrations even before weight loss occurs. Conversely, a positive calorie balance increases glucose and triglyceride concentrations and increases the risk of weight gain. A high-

 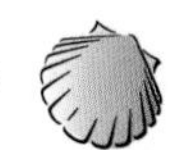

calorie diet, whether or not it is high in carbohydrate, directly promotes insulin resistance. Even though long-term weight loss is seldom achieved, losing weight is a primary goal.

There is no one proven strategy that can be uniformly recommended to promote weight loss in all clients. For instance, although standard weight loss diets that provide 500 to 1000 fewer calories than usual daily intake do promote weight loss, long-term outcomes are poor without other interventions such as exercise and behavior modification. Very-low-calorie diets (≤800 calories/day) produce substantial weight loss and rapid improvements in blood glucose and lipid levels in people with type 2 diabetes, but weight gain is common after the diet stops. Drug therapy to treat obesity may be useful but (1) the effect is modest, (2) the drugs only work as long as they are taken, and (3) optimal benefits are achieved when drugs are combined with diet, exercise, and behavior modification. Bariatric surgery can lead to substantial weight loss and remission of type 2 diabetes, but it is considered an unproven option.

Vitamin and Mineral Supplements

The vitamin and mineral requirements of diabetics are not different from those of the general population. Deficiencies of potassium and magnesium may aggravate glucose intolerance; they can be easily detected with a blood test and corrected with supplements. Chromium deficiency may also impair glucose tolerance in diabetics, but benefit from supplementation has not been conclusively proven. Supplements provide no proven benefit in managing diabetes unless underlying nutrient deficiencies exist. Exceptions include folic acid to prevent birth defects and calcium to prevent osteoporosis.

Alcohol

Moderate use of alcohol in well-controlled diabetics does not affect blood glucose levels. However, alcohol intake should be limited to two or fewer drinks daily. Alcohol should be consumed with food but not between meals because it can cause hypoglycemia. In addition, type 1 diabetics should not reduce their food intake to compensate for alcohol calories. Alcohol should be avoided during pregnancy and lactation and by people who have a history of alcohol abuse.

Additional Considerations for Type 1 Diabetes

Additional considerations for type 1 diabetes revolve around insulin:

- In type 1 diabetes, the most effective approach to controlling postprandial hyperglycemia is adjusting premeal doses of insulin based on amount of carbohydrate to be consumed.
- For people receiving fixed insulin regimens, carbohydrate intake should be consistent each day at breakfast, each day at lunch, and each day at dinner as well as snacks. Note that the amount of carbohydrate *at each meal* in a given day is not necessarily equal: for instance, the carbohydrate content every day at breakfast may be less than at lunch.
- Good glycemic control is associated with weight gain, which adversely affects blood glucose and lipid levels, blood pressure, and overall health. To prevent weight gain, keep total calories to weight maintenance levels.

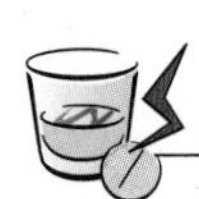

DRUG ALERT: MEDICATIONS USED TO CONTROL BLOOD GLUCOSE LEVELS

Insulin

Different kinds of insulin differ in their onset, peak time, and duration. Meal timing should match insulin action for maximum effectiveness. Exogenous insulin increases the risk of hypoglycemia; in people with type 2 diabetes, it stimulates appetite, promotes weight gain, and aggravates insulin resistance, leading to an even greater need for insulin.

Oral Agents

The type of drug prescribed depends on the patient's fasting and postprandial glucose levels, body weight, and response to therapy. Because each class of oral agents works by a different mechanism to help reduce blood glucose levels, combinations of oral agents are often prescribed. They vary in duration of action, dose response, and side effects. Sometimes after a few months or years of use, a previously effective drug will fail to work.

Alpha-glycosidase inhibitors marketed in the United States are acarbose (Precose) and miglitol (Glyset). Because they work by delaying the digestion of carbohydrates, they should be taken with the first bite of each meal. Poor compliance is a concern. Gas and diarrhea are common side effects. Although they do not cause hypoglycemia, they may be used in conjunction with other drugs that do. If hypoglycemia develops in this case, it should be treated with pure glucose because glucose is absorbed without undergoing digestion.

The biguanide metformin (brand name Glucophage, Glucophage XR) works by inhibiting hepatic glucose production and increases sensitivity of peripheral tissues to insulin. GI side effects are uncommon but it may cause diarrhea or a metallic aftertaste.

The meglitinide repaglinide (brand name Prandin) stimulates the release of insulin from pancreatic beta cells and thus has the potential to cause hypoglycemia. Unlike other oral agents, repaglinide works very quickly. It is taken with each meal or up to 30 minutes before mealtime. Because it is gone from the bloodstream in 3 to 4 hours, it does not raise insulin levels over a long period.

Sulfonylureas stimulate pancreatic beta cells to produce more insulin. Because insulin is increased, weight gain, hypoglycemia, and hyperinsulinemia are risks. Sulfonylureas may be used as monotherapy or in combination with other drugs. Brand names in this class include Diabinese, Amaryl, Glucotrol, Glucotrol XL, DiaBeta, Micronase, Glynase PresTab, Tolinase, and Orinase. Although they all have a similar effect on blood glucose levels, they differ in their side effects and in how often they need to be taken. For instance, Glucotrol appears to be more effective when taken ½ hour before meals and Orinase is the shortest acting so the risk from hypoglycemia is lessened.

Thiazolidinediones increase tissue sensitivity to insulin. They are taken once or twice daily with food and may cause weight gain. Troglitazone (brand name Rezulin), the first drug in this class approved for use in the United States, was removed from the market in

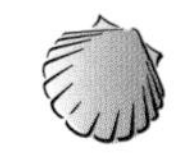

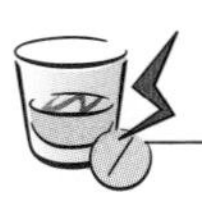

DRUG ALERT: MEDICATIONS USED TO CONTROL BLOOD GLUCOSE LEVELS
(continued)

March 2000 at the request of the FDA after confirmed reports of severe liver failure and death related to its use. Two other drugs in this class, rosiglitazone (Avandia) and pioglitazone (Actos), are purported to be less toxic than troglitazone. Regular monitoring of liver function is recommended.

Combination Drugs

Combination drugs include Glucovance (metformin + glyburide), Avandamet (metformin + rosiglitazone) and Metaglip (metformin + glipizide). See information above for each constituent drug.

Additional Considerations for Type 2 Diabetes

Weight loss and increased activity can prevent type 2 diabetes. Once type 2 diabetes is diagnosed, weight loss and increased activity can normalize blood glucose levels and prevent or delay complications, so efforts to promote weight loss and increased activity are high priority. In addition

- Control of blood glucose improves when meals and snacks are relatively consistent in number, timing, and carbohydrate content every day.
- Eating meals 4 to 5 hours apart may help postprandial glucose levels to return to baseline.
- Drug therapy is used to help manage type 2 diabetes when exercise and nutrition therapy fail to achieve glycemic control. Drugs are used in addition to, not in place of, diet and exercise. Drug therapy begins with oral agents. Thirty percent to 40% of type 2 diabetics eventually use insulin to help control their blood glucose levels.

Transforming Recommendations into Meals

Knowing the recommended proportion of nutrients people with diabetes should consume provides the backdrop to converting percentages of calories into actual foods, serving sizes, meals, and food. Calorie requirements are determined, approximate grams are calculated, and servings are decided upon. The complete process is shown in Box 19.2. The actual blueprint for eating may be implemented by a variety of approaches such as the diabetic exchange lists, carbohydrate counting, or a basic MyPyramid.

Exchange Lists for Meal Planning

Devised by the American Diabetic Association and the American Dietetic Association, the *Exchange Lists for Meal Planning* is a framework for choosing a healthy diet that is relatively consistent in total calories and the amounts of carbohydrate, protein, and fat eaten daily. Its three major categories are Carbohydrates, Meat and Meat Substitutes,

BOX 19.2

THE PROCESS OF CALCULATING A DIABETIC DIET

Example: A 30-year-old woman, who is 5 feet 6 inches tall, weighs 169 pounds. She agrees a ½ pound/week weight loss is a realistic goal.

The Process (numbers are rounded):

1. Calculate weight in kilograms.

   169 pounds divided by 2.2 pounds/kg = 77 kg

2. Calculate total calorie requirements using the standard figure of 30 cal/kg.

   77 kg × 30 cal/kg = 2310 cal

3. Subtract 500 to promote ½ pound weight loss/week. (1 # = 3500 cal divided by 7 days/week = 500 calorie deficit).

   2310 cal − 500 cal = 1800 cal

4. Within the general parameters, choose the percentage of calories from carbohydrates, protein, and fat.

   Choose 55% cal from CHO
   20% cal from protein
   25% cal from fat
   100% total cal

5. Convert percentage of total calories into calories.

   1800 cal × 55% CHO = 990 CHO cal
   × 20% pro = 360 pro cal
   × 25% fat = 450 fat cal
   1800 total cal

6. Convert calories into grams.

   900 CHO cal divided by 4 cal/g = 248 g CHO
   360 pro cal divided by 4 cal/g = 90 g pro
   450 fat cal divided by 9 cal/g = 50 g fat

7. Convert grams into servings, utilizing the values given in the exchange lists. The number of servings of fruit, vegetables, and milk are based on individual preference. The servings from the remaining lists are determined mathematically.

		Goals:	**248 g**	**90 g**	**50 g**
List	**Per Serving**	**Number of Servings**	**CHO (g)**	**Pro (g)**	**Fat (g)**
Fruit	15 g CHO	3	45	-	-
Nonstarchy vegetables	5 g CHO, 2 g pro	3	15	6	-
Milk, nonfat	12 g CHO, 8 g pro	3	36	24	-
			96		

a. 248 g CHO goal
   − 96 g already accounted for
   152 g remaining divided by 15 g CHO/svg starch = 10 svg starch to meet total CHO goal

Starch		10	150	30	-
			246 g CHO	60	

BOX 19.2 (continued)

THE PROCESS OF CALCULATING A DIABETIC DIET

	Number of Servings	CHO (g)	Pro (g)	Fat (g)
b. 90 g pro goal – 60 g already accounted for 30 g remaining divided by 7 g pro/oz of meat = 4 oz of meat to meet total protein goal				
Meat, lean (1 svg = 7 g pro, 3 g fat)	4 oz	0	28 88 g pro	12
c. 50 g fat goal – 12 g already accounted for 38 g remaining divided by 5 g fat/svg of fat = 7 svg fat to meet total fat goal				
Fat (1 svg = 5 g fat)	7	0	0	35 47 g fat

8. Devise a meal plan considering individual preference (see Box 19.3).

and Fats. Within each major category are subgroups that form the exchange lists (Fig. 19.1). Portion sizes are specified so that each serving within a list contains approximately the same amount of carbohydrates, protein, fat, and calories.

Exchange lists simplify meal planning, eliminate the need for daily calculations, provide flexibility and variety, ensure a relatively consistent intake, and emphasize important nutrition principles such as limiting and modifying fat and controlling sodium intake. However, the exchange lists may not be appropriate or acceptable for all age, ethnic, and cultural groups; individual adjustments may be vital for compliance. Characteristics of the exchange lists are as follows:

- The Carbohydrate category contains five exchange lists: starch, fruit, milk, other carbohydrates, and vegetables. With the exception of the vegetables list, all other lists within the carbohydrate group contain approximately the same amount of carbohydrate and can generally be substituted for one another.
- The Meat and meat substitute category is divided into four groups based on fat content. All four groups provide the same amount of protein and no carbohydrates.
- The Fat category supplies only fat. It is divided into three sublists based on the predominate type of fat: monounsaturated fats, polyunsaturated fats, and saturated fats.
- With the exception of the starch, fruit, milk, and other carbohydrates exchanges, items from one list cannot be exchanged for items in a different exchange list (e.g., 1 cup of milk can be exchanged for 1 serving of fruit but not for 1 serving of meat or fat).
- Portion sizes are important because consistency can only be achieved if the portions consumed are of the appropriate size. Food should be weighed or measured until portion sizes can be estimated accurately.
- The number of servings allowed from each exchange list depends on the calorie content and composition of the diet and corresponds as closely as possible to the client's preferences and food habits.

Carbohydrate Group

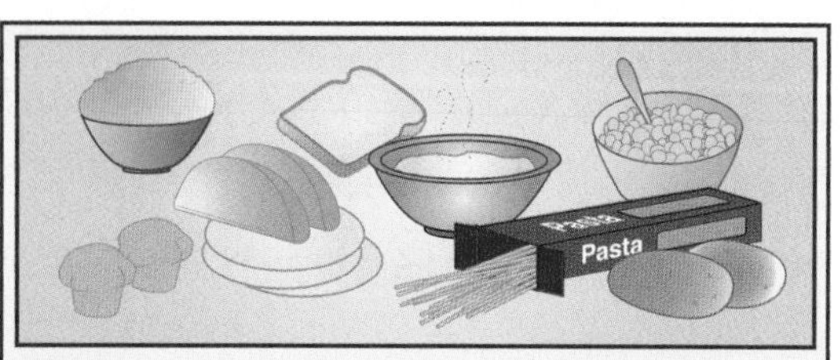

Starch

1 exchange equals:
- 15g carbohydrate
- 3g protein
- 80 calories

Examples of an exchange:
- 1 slice bread
- 3/4 c ready-to-eat cereal
- 1/2 c cooked cereal
- 1/3 c cooked rice or pasta
- 1/2 c cooked beans, peas or lentils
- 1/2 c corn, yams, or potatoes
- 1/2 bagel, English muffin, or bun
- 1 tortilla, waffle, roll, taco, or matzoh
- 3 cups microwave popcorn

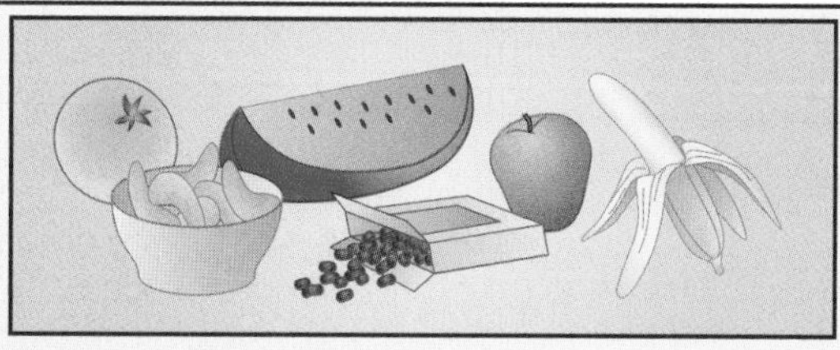

Fruits

1 exchange equals:
- 15g carbohydrate
- 60 calories

Examples of an exchange:
- 1 small orange, apple, banana, or nectarine
- 1/2 c canned sweet cherries, fruit cocktail, or pears
- 1 1/4 c strawberries or watermelon cubes
- 1/2 large grapefruit
- 2 Tbsp raisins

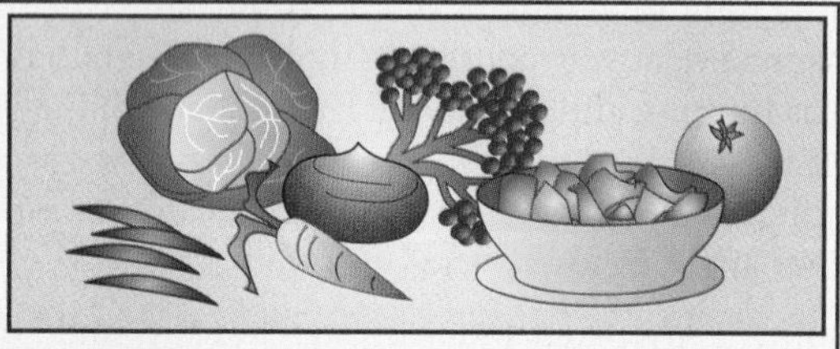

Vegetables

1 exchange equals:
- 5g carbohydrate
- 2g protein
- 25 calories

Examples of an exchange:
- 1/2 c cooked carrots, greens, green beans, brussel sprouts, beets, broccoli, cauliflower, or spinach
- 1 c raw carrots, radishes, or salad greens
- 1 large tomato

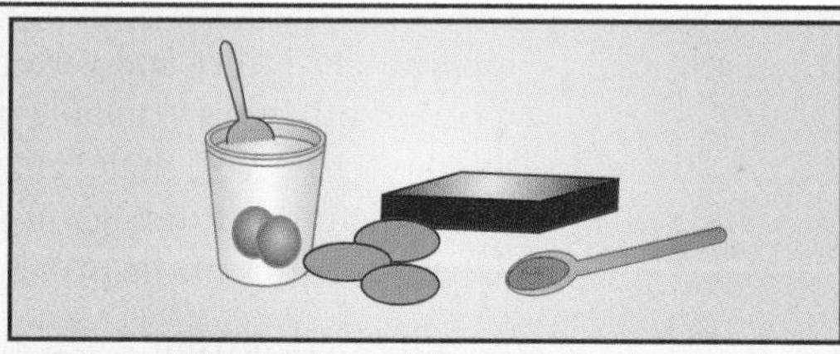

Other carbohydrates

1 exchange equals:
- 15g carbohydrate or 1 starch or 1 fruit or 1 milk calories vary with fat content; portion sizes are small

Examples of an exchange:
- 3 gingersnaps
- 1 Tbsp regular jam or jelly
- 1/2 c frozen yogurt or regular gelatin
- 1 small unfrosted brownie
- 1 chewy fruit snack roll

FIGURE 19.1 Exchange lists.

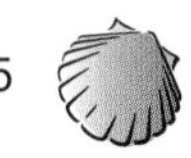

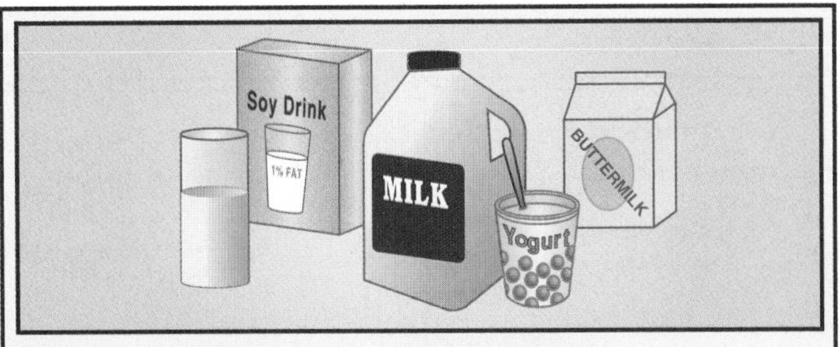

Milk (3 sublists based on fat content)

1 exchange equals:
12g carbohydrate
8g protein
0 to 8g fat
calories vary with fat content

Examples of a fat-free exchange (0 to 3g fat, 90 cal):
1 c fat-free or 1% milk
1 c fat-free or lowfat buttermilk
3/4 c fat-free plain yogurt

Examples of a reduced-fat exchange (5g fat, 120 cal):
1 c 2% milk
3/4 c plain lowfat yogurt
1 c soy milk

Examples of a whole fat exchange (8g fat, 150 cal):
1 c whole milk
3/4 c plain whole milk yogurt
1 c kefir

FIGURE 19.1 (Continued)

- Meal patterns specify the number of servings from each exchange list allowed for each meal and snack (Box 19.3). Glycemic control is improved when exchanges are not "saved" from one meal to use at another, especially for clients who are taking insulin or oral agents.
- Certain foods and beverages are considered "free" because they provide less than 5 g of carbohydrate or less than 20 cal per serving. Some of these items have serving sizes specified; those choices should be limited to three servings per day, preferably over the course of the day. Items without a portion size, such as sugar substitutes, may be used as desired.
- A combination foods list gives examples of how mixed dishes can be calculated into a meal plan; components are identified, then classified according to their representative exchange lists. For instance, one-fourth of a 12-inch thin-crust cheese

Meat and Meat Substitute Group

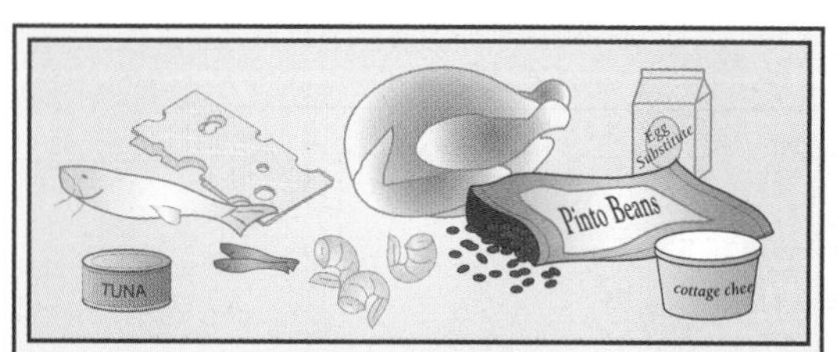

Meat and substitutes (very lean)

1 exchange equals:
7g protein
0 to1g fat
35 calories

Examples of an exchange:
- 1 oz chicken or turkey (white meat, no skin)
- 1 oz cod, flounder, or haddock
- 1 oz tuna (canned in water)
- 1 oz clams, crab, lobster, scallops, shrimp, or imitation seafood
- 1 oz fat-free cheese
- 1/2 c cooked beans, peas, or lentils* counts as 1 very lean meat plus 1 starch exchange
- 1/4 c fat-free or low-fat cottage cheese
- 2 egg whites (or 1/4 c egg substitute)

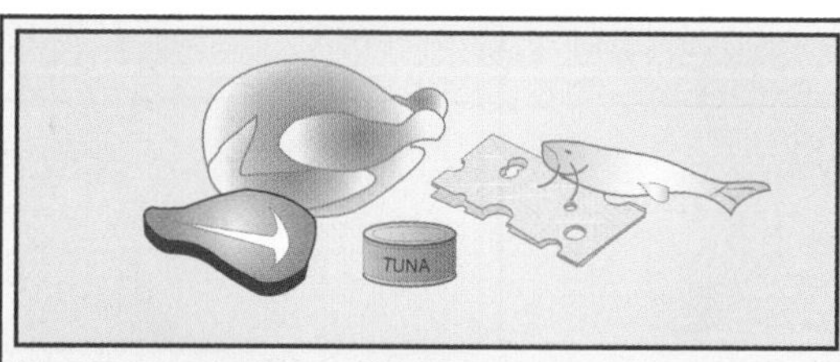

Meat and substitutes (lean)

1 exchange equals:
7g protein
3g fat
55 calories

Examples of an exchange:
- 1 oz beef or pork tenderloin
- 1 oz chicken or turkey (dark meat, no skin)
- 1 oz salmon or catfish
- 1 oz tuna (canned in oil, drained)
- 1 oz low-fat cheese or luncheon meats

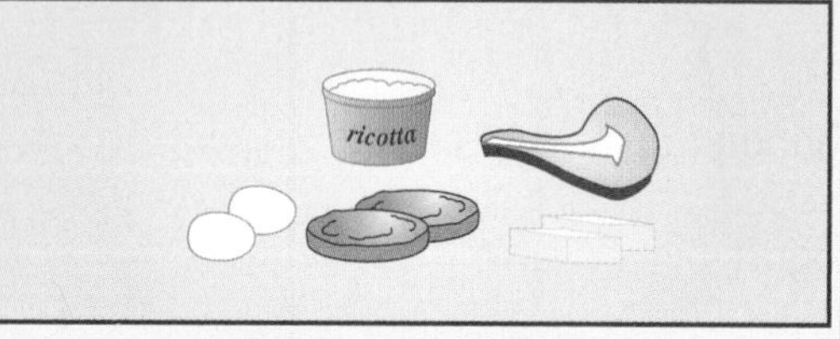

Meat and substitutes (medium-fat)

1 exchange equals:
7g protein
5g fat
75 calories

Examples of an exchange:
- 1 oz ground beef
- 1 oz pork chop
- 1 egg
- 1/4 c ricotta
- 4 oz tofu
- 1 oz chicken (dark meat, with skin)
- 1 oz any fried fish product

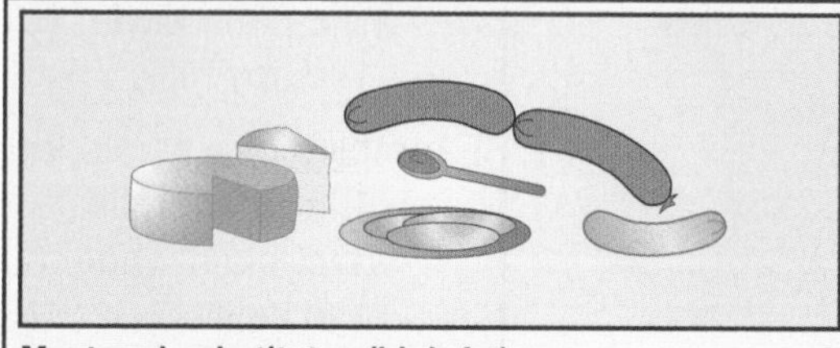

Meat and substitutes (high-fat)

1 exchange equals:
7g protein
8g fat
100 calories

Examples of an exchange:
- 1 oz pork sausage, spareribs, or ground pork
- 1 oz luncheon meat (such as bologna)
- 1 oz regular cheese (such as cheddar or American)
- 1 small hot dog (turkey or chicken)
- 1 tbs peanut butter

FIGURE 19.1 (Continued)

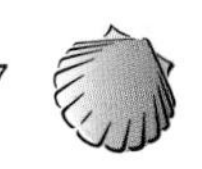

Fat Group

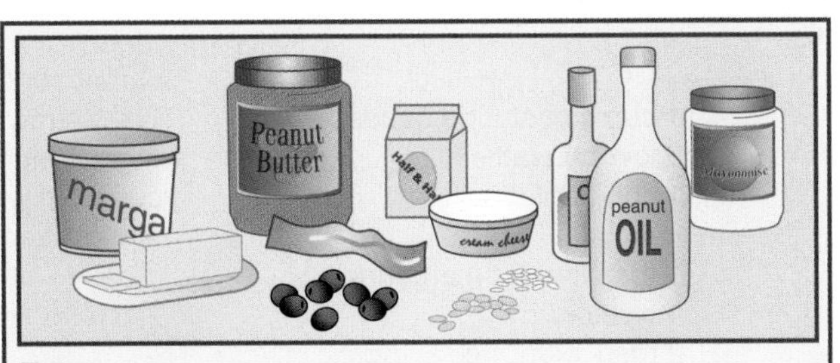

Fats

1 exchange equals:
- 5g fat
- 45 calories

Examples of monounsaturated fat exchanges:
- 1 tsp olive, canola, or peanut oil
- 8 large black olives
- 1/2 tbsp peanut butter
- 2 tsp tahini

Examples of polyunsaturated fat exchanges:
- 1 tsp stick, tub, or squeeze margarine
- 1 tsp regular mayonnaise
- 1 tbsp reduced fat mayonnaise
- 1 tsp corn, safflower, or soybean oil
- 4 English walnut halves
- 1 tbsp pumpkin or sunflower seeds

Examples of saturated fat exchanges:
- 1 slice cooked bacon
- 1 tsp butter
- 2 tbsp shredded coconut
- 1 T regular cream cheese
- 2 T regular sour cream
- 2 T half and half

FIGURE 19.1 (Continued)

pizza counts 2 starch exchanges (the crust), 2 medium-fat meat exchanges (the cheese), and 1 fat exchange (oil in and on the crust).

- Fast foods are also calculated into a meal plan according to their composition. For instance, one 6-inch submarine sandwich is listed as 3 starch exchanges (the roll), 1 vegetable exchange (lettuce, tomato, onion), 2 medium-fat meat exchanges (2 ounces of luncheon meats), and 1 fat exchange (oil or mayonnaise).

BOX 19.3 **SAMPLE 1800-CALORIE MEAL PLAN AND MENUS**

Meal plan	Sample menu 1	Sample menu 2
Breakfast		
		A parfait consisting of
1 fruit	1 cup cantaloupe cubes	1¼ cup strawberries
2 starch	2 low-fat waffles	½ cup low-fat granola
1 milk	1 cup nonfat milk	⅔ cup plain whole fat yogurt (also counts as 2 fat exchanges)
2 fat	1 tbsp low-fat margarine 4 walnuts	
"Free"	2 tbsp sugar free syrup Coffee	Tea
Lunch		
3 starch 2 meat, lean 2 fat 1 vegetable	1 6 inch submarine (counts as 3 starch, 2 meat, 1 vegetable, and 2 fat because medium fat meat is used)	Beef burrito (counts as 3 starch, 1 meat, 2 fats because medium fat meat is used)
1 milk, nonfat	1 cup nonfat milk	1 cup nonfat milk
1 fruit	1 small apple	1 small banana
Dinner		
3 starch	2 taco shells	1 cup spaghetti
2 meat	2 oz taco meat	2 1 oz meatballs
2 vegetables	1 cup combined lettuce, tomato, onion 1 cup combined carrot and celery sticks	1 cup tomato sauce
2 fat	(used in higher fat taco meat)	(used in higher fat meatballs)
1 milk	1 cup nonfat milk	1 cup nonfat milk
1 fruit	1 cup papaya cubes	¾ cup blueberries
Bedtime snack		
2 starch	1 cup nonfat milk (exchanged for 1 starch) 5 vanilla wafers	2 plain rice cakes
1 fat	(count as 1 starch + 1 fat)	½ tbsp peanut butter

- The exchange list approach is best suited to people who want or need structured meal-planning guidance and are able to understand complex details. Some clients progress from using the exchange lists to carbohydrate counting.

Carbohydrate Counting

Carbohydrate counting is a relatively new meal planning approach available at a basic or advanced level that offers an alternative to the use of traditional exchange lists. Resulting

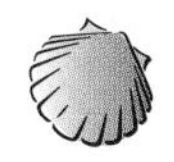

from advances in diabetes management, carbohydrate counting is based on the concepts that a carbohydrate is a carbohydrate is a carbohydrate and that carbohydrates are what affect postprandial glucose levels. Emphasis is on consuming a consistent quantity of total carbohydrate without restricting the type. Although carbohydrate counting has the advantage of focusing on a single nutrient (carbohydrates) rather than all the energy-yielding nutrients, protein and fat cannot be disregarded, especially if weight is a concern.

Because of its greater flexibility, this method allows the client to feel more in control and offers the potential for improved glucose control. On the minus side, carbohydrate counting requires clients to keep food records initially and periodically, and they must also record blood glucose levels before and after eating. Some clients may see weighing and measuring foods as a disadvantage. In addition, the goals of weight control and healthful eating may be forgotten or forsaken when the emphasis is placed solely on carbohydrate.

MyPyramid

On the other hand, people who cannot master the details of the exchange lists or carbohydrate counting may benefit from using MyPyramid as a tool. Although it is less than ideal, consistency in the amount of servings from various food groups may be achieved, even if the quality of food choices is not considered (e.g., fat, sodium). To compensate for intricate details that may be lost in the translation, such as "lean" meat and "nonfat" milk, it may be prudent to recommend fewer fat servings than the exchange calculations. For instance, in the meal plan outlined in Box 19.3, each exchange except for the fat group could be loosely converted to the corresponding food guide group in approximately the same number of servings. Assuming that not all choices from the grains, milk, and meat group will be low-fat or nonfat, a reasonable adaptation is to suggest the client limit fat servings to one per meal.

Changing Behaviors

Career Connection

The diagnosis of diabetes often triggers anxiety and uncertainty. **People often see "diet" as the most difficult part of treatment. Even people with healthy eating styles may need to make changes in their intake to improve glycemic control. Giving someone a preprinted list of do's and don'ts can add to a resentful client's frustration. Take time to listen.**

- **What do you want from nutrition counseling?**
- **What behaviors do you want to change?**
- **What changes can you make in your present lifestyle?**
- **What obstacles may prevent you from making changes?**
- **What changes are you willing to make right now?**
- **What changes would be difficult for you to make?**

Mastering the intricacies of eating for diabetes—what, how, when, and why—occurs over a continuum from learning basic facts to assimilating and implementing information. Individuals differ in how much information they want or need to know and in

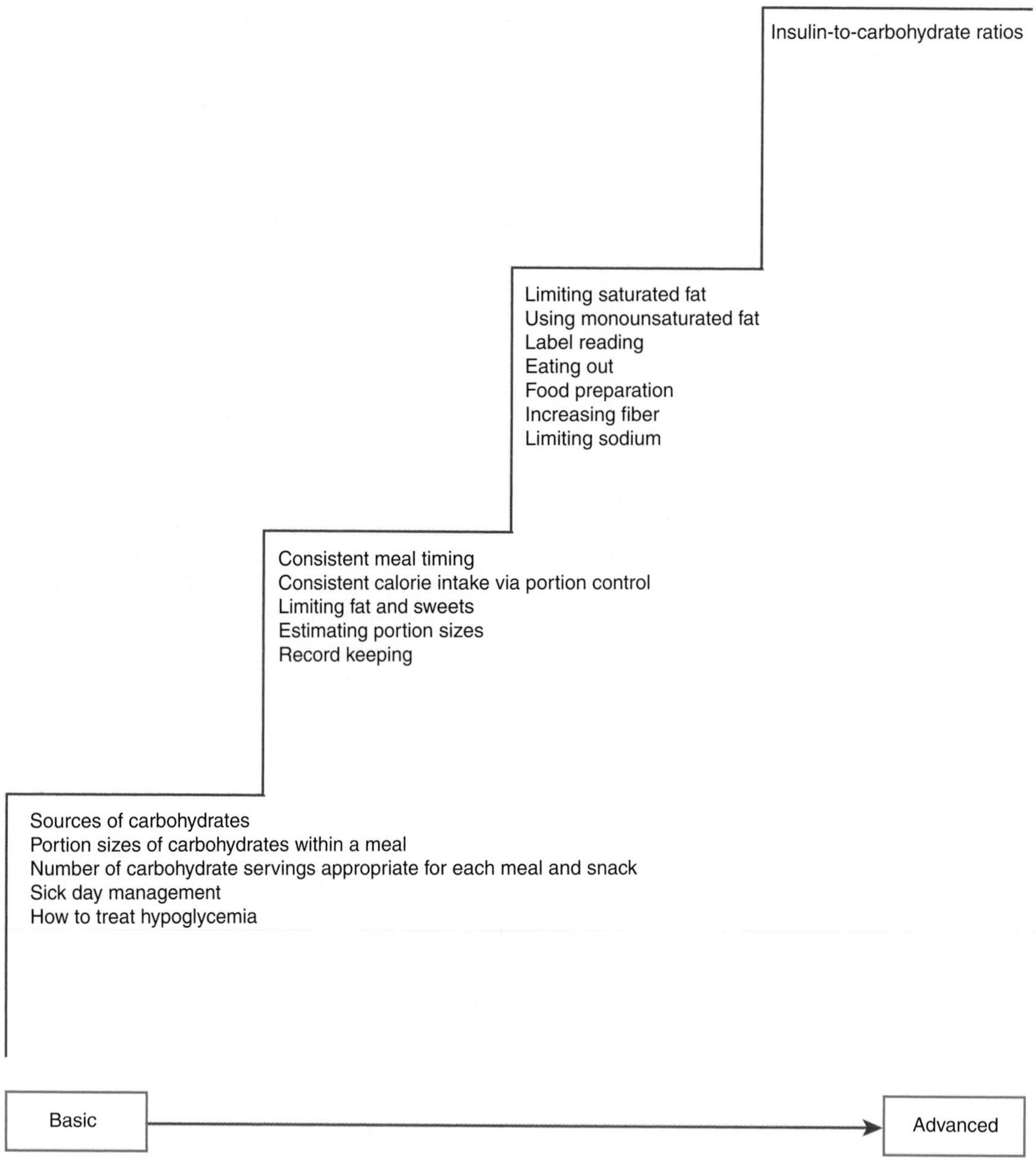

FIGURE 19.2 An illustration of knowledge and skills attained in step-wise fashion. Actual progression and concepts learned vary among individuals.

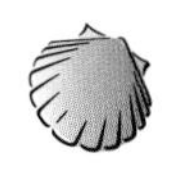

how motivated they are to improve their eating behaviors. Ideally, positive changes occur progressively over time in step-wise fashion (Fig. 19.2) with the client actively involved in goal setting, self-monitoring, and record keeping. In reality, motivation to follow a meal plan may be initially high, but commitment and diligence may dwindle when clients realize that "cheating" does not cause immediate illness. Periodic and ongoing follow-up may improve compliance. Arming the client with behavior skills, such as tips for eating out and tips for food purchasing and label reading (Box 19.4), provides them with the tools to make better choices.

Exercise

Exercise is an important aspect of treatment for both types of diabetes regardless of weight status unless it is contraindicated for other medical reasons.

For people with type 1 diabetes who engage in planned exercise, reducing insulin may be the best way to prevent hypoglycemia. The other alternative to prevent hypoglycemia is to eat more food, which over time is counterproductive to weight management. However, if exercise is unplanned, an additional 10 to 15 g carbohydrate per hour of moderate activity is recommended. More intense exercise requires more carbohydrate.

Exercise has not been shown to improve glycemic control among people with type 1 diabetes, but it imparts other important benefits such as improving cardiovascular fitness, promoting bone strength, and enhancing the sense of well-being. However, when diabetes is poorly controlled, exercise may worsen hyperglycemia; without adequate insulin, the muscle cannot adequately use glucose, so the liver compensates by producing or releasing stored glucose.

Because exercise lowers the blood glucose level, the optimal time for insulin-dependent diabetics to exercise is within 2 hours after eating; exercise beyond that time is more likely to cause hypoglycemia. Clients should test their blood glucose level before exercising and eat a carbohydrate snack if the level is lower than 100 mg/dL. After exercise, the risk of hypoglycemia continues for up to 24 to 36 hours because exercise increases insulin sensitivity in muscle.

Among people with type 2 diabetes, exercise offers substantial benefits. Regular exercise improves blood glucose control independent of weight loss. It also reduces insulin resistance, improves blood lipid levels, improves blood pressure, and enhances sense of well-being and quality of life. Exercise helps to maintain long-term weight reduction. Type 2 diabetics who are treated with oral hypoglycemic agents or insulin may experience exercise-induced hypoglycemia; they should monitor their blood glucose levels, exercise within 2 hours after eating, and stop activity if signs and symptoms of hypoglycemia develop.

Managing Acute Complications

Clients who effectively manage their blood glucose levels may avoid acute complications. Ideally, food intake, activity patterns, and medications work in concert to keep fasting and postprandial glucose levels within acceptable ranges. In reality, blood glucose levels

BOX 19.4

BEHAVIOR SKILLS

Tips for Eating Out

- Eat the same size portion you would at home. Order only what you need and want.
- Select a restaurant with a variety of choices.
- Eat slowly.
- Choose tomato juice, unsweetened fruit juice, clear broth, bouillon, consommé, or shrimp cocktail as an appetizer instead of sweetened juices, fried vegetables, or creamed or thick soups.
- Choose fresh vegetable salads and use oil and vinegar or fresh lemon instead of regular salad dressings, or request that the dressing be put on the side. Avoid coleslaw and other salads with the dressing already added.
- Order plain (without gravy or sauce) roasted, baked, or broiled meat, fish, and poultry instead of fried, sautéed, or breaded entrées. Avoid stews and casseroles. Request a doggie bag if the portion exceeds the meal plan allowance.
- Order steamed, boiled, or broiled vegetables.
- Choose plain, baked, mashed, boiled, or steamed potatoes, rice, or noodles.
- Select fresh fruit for dessert.
- Request a sugar substitute for coffee or tea, if desired.

Tips on Food Purchasing and Label Reading

Studies show that women use nutrition information on food labels when deciding what foods to buy. The more confident they are in their ability to read food labels, the greater the chance that they will make appropriate food purchases. Therefore, it is important to teach people, especially women, about how to read food labels.

A big area of confusion is the claims on food labels such as "low fat" and "good source of fiber." Clients need assurance that these claims are defined by labeling laws and are reliable. Another misconception regards the sugar content listed on the Nutrition Facts label. Clients need to know that the value listed includes both natural and added sugars. For instance, milk, which has 12 g of sugar per 8-oz serving, appears to be a "high sugar" food but the "sugar" is naturally present lactose, not added sucrose. Clients also need to know that

- Fresh, frozen (without sugar), and water-packed canned fruits are preferable, but sweetened canned fruit is acceptable if it is rinsed under running water for at least 1 minute to remove the sugary syrup.
- Sugar goes by many names on the ingredient list such as high-fructose corn syrup, invert sugar, sorghum, dextrose, and maltose.
- Sugar alcohols, such as sorbitol and xylitol, can cause diarrhea in large amounts.
- Dietetic products are not necessarily calorie-free or specifically intended for diabetics. Foods that are labeled "dietetic" may be made without sugar, without salt, with a particular type of fat, or for special food allergies. Read the ingredient label and check with a diet counselor before adding a dietetic food to the diet—or avoid dietetic foods altogether because they are expensive and usually do not taste as good as the foods they are intended to replace.
- Ingredients are listed in descending order by weight. Therefore, foods that list sugar near the beginning of the ingredient list may be high in sugar (the exception is when foods contain few ingredients).

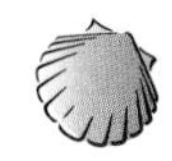

may be out of normal range due to factors that may or may not be under the individual's control, leading to acute complications.

Routine Hyperglycemia

Persistent hyperglycemia detected through routine monitoring means that there is an imbalance among food, medication, and activity. Strategies to correct hyperglycemia that occurs at a particular time of day include reducing carbohydrate content of the previous meal, eliminating or reducing the size of the previous snack, changing the time of the previous meal or snack, increasing activity in the hours before the hyperglycemia is detected, adjusting the previous insulin dose, or a combination of these strategies. The actual intervention used depends on the client's needs, lifestyle, and preferences.

Hyperglycemia Related to Acute Illness

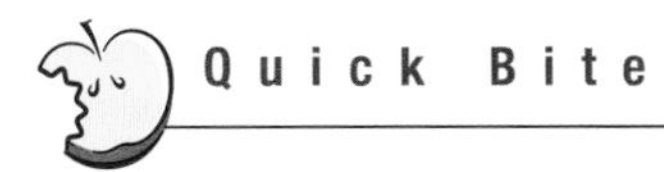

Quick Bite

Each of the following has approximately 15 g of carbohydrate and may be acceptable during illness

6 ounces regular ginger ale
½ cup ice cream
½ cup apple juice
1 frozen juice bar
½ cup sherbet
½ cup regular gelatin
½ cup orange juice
1 cup creamed soup.

Acute illnesses, even mild ones such as a cold or flu, can significantly raise blood glucose levels. Unless otherwise instructed by the physician, clients should maintain their normal medication schedule while monitoring their blood glucose levels and testing their urine for ketones every 3 to 4 hours. Clients should eat the usual amount of carbohydrate, divided into smaller meals and snacks if necessary. Clients whose blood glucose levels are higher than 250 mg/dL do not need to consume all their usual carbohydrate intake. If a normal diet is not tolerated, clients should rely on liquids to prevent hypoglycemia and to replenish losses that may occur from vomiting or diarrhea. Generally, 15 g of carbohydrate (i.e., one starch, fruit, milk, or other carbohydrate exchange) should be eaten every 30 minutes and 1½ cups of fluid should be taken every hour.

Hypoglycemia

Hypoglycemia is often referred to as insulin reaction. It occurs from taking too much insulin (or sulfonylureas, but less frequently), inadequate food intake, delayed or skipped meals, extra physical activity, or consumption of alcohol without food.

Blood glucose levels of 70 mg/dL or less require immediate action. Clients should be advised to carry a readily absorbable source of carbohydrate with them at all times to treat hypoglycemia. See Box 19.5 for suggested treatment of hypoglycemia. Frequent treatment of hypoglycemia can lead to weight gain. Frequent bouts of hypoglycemia also means that the care plan needs to be revised or the client needs to be counseled to ensure better adherence.

Patients with long-standing diabetes may develop hypoglycemic unawareness. This occurs because the body no longer signals hypoglycemia. Consistent monitoring of blood glucose is especially important for people who are not cognizant of hypoglycemic symptoms.

BOX 19.5 **SUGGESTED TREATMENT FOR HYPOGLYCEMIA**

1. Consume 15 g of readily absorbable carbohydrate. This amount should raise blood glucose levels by 50 to 100 mg/dL in 15 to 30 minutes. Any of the following will work:
   4 to 6 ounces or regular soft drink
   4 ounces of orange juice
   2 or 3 glucose tablets (5 g each)
   1 tablespoon of honey
   1 tablespoon of brown sugar
   4 or 5 Life Savers
   5 or 6 large jelly beans
2. Retest blood glucose in 15 minutes. If glucose is at or below 50 to 80 mg/dL, consume another 15 g of carbohydrate.
3. Retest blood glucose in 15 minutes. If glucose is within normal range (80 to 120 mg/dL) and it is still 1 hour or longer until the next meal or snack, consume another 15 g of carbohydrate.
4. Retest blood glucose and monitor symptoms.

Life Cycle Considerations

Diabetes nutrition therapy can influence growth and development in children and adolescents, the outcome of pregnancy, and the quality of life in older adults. Special considerations for each group are presented here.

Children and Adolescents

Children's and adolescents' increased nutritional needs related to growth, irregular eating patterns, and erratic activity levels complicate management of their diabetes. Children

Career Connection

Nutrition therapy for children with diabetes is impacted by the stage of growth and development. **Age-based assumptions may not be reliable or valid due to variability in the rate of physical and emotional development. Consider the following:**

- **Is the child responsible for any or all of his or her diabetes management?**
- **Does the child feed himself or herself?**
- **Do the child's routine and activity expenditure differ on weekdays and on the weekend?**
- **What is the child's school schedule?**
- **What is the child's social life?**
- **Are school lunches eaten?**
- **Does the child have food jags or use food to manipulate parents?**
- **If the child does not attend school, who is the primary caretaker during the day?**

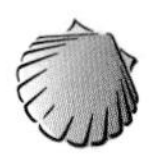

with diabetes appear to have the same nutrient needs as their age-matched peers. Nutrition recommendations for children are the same for adults, but children require more frequent adjustments in insulin and food intake to compensate for growth and activity needs. Failure to provide adequate calories and nutrients results in poor growth, as does poor glycemic control and inadequate insulin administration. Conversely, excessive weight gain occurs from excessive calorie intake, overtreatment of hypoglycemia, or excess insulin administration. Neither withholding food nor having a child eat when not hungry is an appropriate strategy to manage glucose levels. Rather, individualized meal plans and intensive insulin regimens can provide flexibility for erratic eating, activity, and growth.

Pregnancy

Pregnant women with preexisting type 1 or type 2 diabetes are at increased risk of spontaneous abortion and pregnancy-induced hypertension. Women with diabetes tend to have bigger babies (macrosomia), probably as a result of high glucose levels. After about 13 weeks' gestation, babies produce their own insulin: high glucose levels in the mother lead to increased fetal insulin secretion, which acts as a growth hormone to stimulate fat deposition. Hyperglycemia also increases the risk of birth defects, especially during the first few weeks of pregnancy. Other risks to the infant include life-threatening hypoglycemia and respiratory distress syndrome.

Preconception counseling, early prenatal care, and ongoing counseling throughout pregnancy are needed to help maintain glycemic control. The nutritional needs during pregnancy are similar for women with and without diabetes. Women of healthy weight (BMI of 20 to 26) need approximately 30 cal/kg of weight, whereas women who are obese prior to pregnancy should limit their calorie intake to 24 cal/kg. Consistent timing and carbohydrate composition of meals and snacks are important to avoid hypoglycemia. A bedtime snack, preferably one that provides carbohydrate, protein, and fat, is usually necessary to sustain blood glucose levels throughout the night. Some women may need a snack during the night, such as a glass of milk, to prevent morning hypoglycemia.

Gestational diabetes is diabetes that occurs only during pregnancy and is usually resolved after delivery. However, many women with gestational diabetes develop type 2 diabetes later in life. Women with gestational diabetes should avoid excessive weight gain during pregnancy and should maintain a reasonable weight thereafter. For some women with gestational diabetes, modest energy and carbohydrate restrictions may be appropriate. A regular eating pattern of three meals with two to three snacks, including a bedtime snack, should be established. Blood glucose monitoring is important to evaluate the effectiveness of nutrition therapy and to identify the need for drug therapy. If insulin is used, maintaining carbohydrate consistency at meals and snacks is a priority. If midmorning hyperglycemia is a problem, carbohydrate intake at breakfast should be limited to less than 20% of the day's total (Box 19.6).

Diabetes in Later Life

There are unique considerations related to aging that affect glycemic control. First, blood glucose levels rise with age for reasons that are unclear. Treatment may not be instituted for glucose elevations that are considered "high" in younger populations but

BOX 19.6

EXAMPLE OF LIMITING CARBOHYDRATES EATEN AT BREAKFAST TO <20% OF TOTAL CARBOHYDRATE INTAKE

In a 2100-calorie diet

→ If carbohydrate provides 45% of total calories, the grams of total carbohydrate/day are 945.

2100 cal × 45% = 945 carbohydrate calories

→ Converting calories into grams yields 236 g carbohydrate/day

945 carbohydrate calories divided by 4 cal/kg = 236 g/day

→ 236 g CHO/day × 20% = 47 g at breakfast

→ 47 g divided by 15 g carbohydrate/carbohydrate group = 3 carbohydrate servings for breakfast

→ 3 carbohydrate group servings is then implemented as per the client's preference such as

- 2 pieces of toast and 1 cup of milk
- ¾ of a 4 oz bagel
- 3 pancakes
- ¼ of a 12 inch thin crust cheese pizza

Career Connection

When counseling older adults

- **Keep teaching sessions short.**
- **Relay only as much information as necessary.**
- **Go slowly and summarize frequently.**
- **Minimize distractions.**
- **Include a spouse or family member.**
- **Speak clearly; face clients who have a hearing impairment.**
- **Use appropriate written materials; do not overload the client with information that is nice to know but not essential.**
- **Ask the clients to write down skills or procedures (e.g., insulin injection, home glucose monitoring) in their own words.**

may be "normal" for the elderly. Cognitive impairments, such as memory loss, impaired concentration, dementia, and depression, may preclude self-management. Physical impairments may impede exercise. Sensory impairments, such as decreased hearing, poor eyesight, and decreased senses of taste and smell, may complicate teaching and self-management. For instance, older clients who could clinically benefit from insulin may be treated instead with oral agents if poor eyesight or decreased manual dexterity precludes self-injection. Older adults may be at greater nutritional risk for a variety of reasons including poor dentition, physical impairments that make shopping or cooking difficult, poor appetite related to lack of socialization, and an inadequate food budget. For many, a strict calorie-controlled diet is more harmful than beneficial.

Because older adults are more susceptible to severe hypoglycemia, a fasting target level of 120 to 150 mg/dL may be considered appropriate.

Diabetic Diets in the Hospital

Career Connection

When people with diabetes are hospitalized

- Patients given clear or full liquid diets should receive approximately 200 g of carbohydrate per day in equally divided amounts at meals and snacks. Sugar-free liquids should not be used. Adjustments in diabetes medications may be needed to achieve glycemic control.
- Food intake should be progressed as soon as possible after surgery with the goal of providing adequate carbohydrates and calories.
- Continuous monitoring is needed during catabolic illnesses to ensure that nutritional needs are met and hyperglycemia is prevented. Overfeeding exacerbates hyperglycemia.
- For tube feedings, standard enteral formulas (≈ 50% carbohydrate) or a lower-carbohydrate content formula (33 to 40% carbohydrate) may be used. Both types require glucose monitoring so that adjustments can be made in glucose-lowering medications as needed.

Traditionally. standardized calorie-level meal plans based on the exchange lists have been used to provide "diabetic" diets to hospitalized diabetics. The physician would order a specific-calorie-level "ADA diet" that was composed of specific percentages of carbohydrate, protein, and fat. Because the ADA (American Diabetes Association) no longer endorses any single meal plan or specified nutrient composition, it is recommended that this term and approach no longer be used.

Also considered obsolete are "no concentrated sweets," "no sugar added," "low sugar," and "liberal diabetic" diets. They do not reflect the diabetes nutrient recommendations and unnecessarily restrict sugar. These diets may give patients the false impression that glycemic control is achieved by limiting sugar.

A suggested alternative to the traditional "ADA diet" is a consistent-carbohydrate meal plan. In this approach, calories are not specified but carbohydrate intake is consistent; that is, breakfast supplies approximately the same amount of carbohydrate each day, lunch is likewise consistent from day to day, and so are dinner and snacks. A typical day's intake from meals and snacks may range from 1500 to 2000 cal, with adjustments made for individual patients as needed. Appropriate modifications in fat intake are made, and consistent timing of meals and snacks is stressed. However, just as there is no longer one diabetic diet, neither is there one correct way to provide nutrition therapy to hospitalized diabetics.

Diabetics are no longer admitted to the hospital for diabetes management and education. Hospital stays are shorter and patients tend to be sicker. For these reasons, diabetes self-management education, including nutrition therapy counseling, is usually best provided in an outpatient or home setting. Acute care settings have neither the time nor the resources to completely teach diabetes management.

NURSING PROCESS

Mrs. Wilson is a 69-year-old woman referred to a home health agency for a home visit to provide nutrition/diabetes education. When she was diagnosed with diabetes 5 years ago, the doctor told her to avoid sugar and take DiaBeta twice a day. She is 5 feet 2 inches tall and weighs 185 pounds.

Assessment

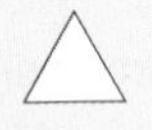

Obtain Clinical Data:

Current BMI; recent weight history

Medical history and comorbidities including hyperlipidemia, hypertension, cardiovascular disease, renal impairments, neuropathy, and gastrointestinal complaints

Abnormal laboratory values especially fasting blood glucose, glycosylated hemoglobin, total cholesterol, LDL-C, HDL-C, triglycerides, and albumin

Record of blood glucose monitoring

Blood pressure measurement

Medications taken that affect nutrition such as insulin, other oral agents, lipid-lowering medications, cardiac drugs, antihypertensives, and anticoagulants

Interview the Client to Assess:

Understanding of the relationship between food, exercise, and blood glucose levels

Ability to understand attitude toward health and nutrition, and readiness to learn

Motivation to change eating style; how she implemented the “avoid sugar” advice. For instance, did she simply not use sugar in her tea or did she also know that cakes, cookies, pies, and candy are sources of sugar?

Usual 24-hour intake including portion sizes, frequency and pattern of eating, method of food preparation, intake of high-fat foods, intake of high-sugar foods, use of salt and salty foods. Determine whether mealtimes are relatively consistent or variable from day to day.

Appropriateness of usual calorie intake and overall nutritional adequacy. Assess types of carbohydrate, protein, and fat usually consumed. Assess usual intake of foods high in fiber especially soluble fiber such as oats, oat bran, and dried peas and beans.

Cultural, religious, and ethnic influences on eating habits

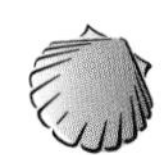

Psychosocial and economic issues such as the living situation, cooking facilities, adequacy of food budget, education, need for food assistance, and level of family and social support
Usual activity patterns; willingness and ability to increase activity
Use of vitamins, minerals, and nutritional supplements: what, how much, and why they are taken
Use of alcohol

Nursing Diagnosis

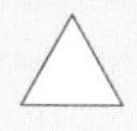

1. Altered Health Maintenance, related to the lack of knowledge of diet management of diabetes mellitus.

Planning and Implementation

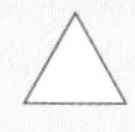

Client Goals

The client will
Short-term

- State three signs/symptoms of hypoglycemia.
- Eat three meals plus a bedtime snack at approximately the same times every day.
- Use artificially sweetened soft drinks and use sugar substitute in her tea.
- Use fruit for dessert every day instead of the usual cake or cookie.
- Monitor her blood glucose level daily.
- State three emergency foods to use during hypoglycemic episodes.
- Walk 10 minutes three times a day at least 3 days per week.

Long-term

- Lose 10 pounds in 6 months.
- Consistently maintain preprandial blood glucose levels less than 120 mg/dL.
- Avoid hypoglycemia.
- Improve lipid profile.
- Prevent or delay chronic complications.
- Eat a nutritionally adequate, varied, and balanced diet.
- Increase physical activity to 30 minutes daily five times a week.

Nursing Interventions

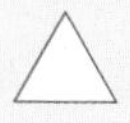

Nutrition Therapy

Introduce basic concepts: which foods contain carbohydrates, appropriate serving sizes for carbohydrates in a meal, and how many carbohydrate servings are appropriate for each meal and snack. Allow the client to verbalize her feelings and thoughts about diabetes and nutrition therapy.

(continued)

Client Teaching

Instruct the client

On the role of nutrition therapy in managing blood glucose levels, including

- That nutrition therapy is essential and that nutrition is important even when no symptoms are apparent
- That medication is used in addition to nutrition therapy not as a substitute

On eating plan essentials, including the importance of

- Eating meals and snacks at regular times every day
- Eating approximately the same amount of food every day especially the same amount of carbohydrates
- Reducing portion sizes for gradual weight loss
- Eating enough high-fiber foods such as oats, oat bran, and dried peas and beans
- Using less fat, sugar, and salt

On behavioral matters, including

- How to read labels to identify foods that are low in fat and low in saturated fat
- Reducing high-sugar and high-fat foods to help promote weight loss
- Not skipping meals or the bedtime snack
- Physical activity goals

Where to get additional information

Evaluation

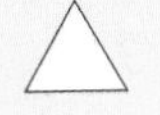

The client

Short-term

- States three signs/symptoms of hypoglycemia
- Eats three meals plus a bedtime snack at approximately the same times every day
- Uses artificially sweetened soft drinks and uses sugar substitute in her tea
- Uses fruit for dessert every day instead of the usual cake or cookie
- Monitors her blood glucose level daily
- States three emergency foods to be used during hypoglycemic episodes
- Walks 10 minutes three times a day at least three times per week

Long-term

- Loses 10 pounds in 6 months
- Consistently maintains preprandial blood glucose levels below 120 mg/dL
- Avoids hypoglycemia
- Improves lipid profile
- Prevents chronic complications
- Eats a nutritionally adequate, varied, and balanced diet
- Increases physical activity to 30 minutes daily five times a week

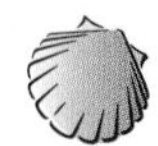

How Do You Respond?

How can I follow a diabetic diet with my relentless "sweet tooth"? Small amounts of sweet foods are permitted, especially if weight is not a problem, as long as they are counted as part of the meal plan, not added as "extras." Diabetic cookbooks are helpful in incorporating sweet foods into the eating pattern. Calorie-free foods sweetened with nonnutritive sweeteners (e.g., saccharin, aspartame) add sweetness and interest without calories. Encourage the client to use artificially sweetened soft drinks, gelatin, and hard candy.

What is "functional" hypoglycemia? Functional hypoglycemia (hyperinsulinism) is a disorder characterized by an excessive insulin secretion in response to carbohydrate-rich foods that causes blood glucose levels to fall to 40 mg/dL or less. Symptoms of hypoglycemia, such as weakness, hunger, nervousness, trembling, sweating, and faintness, usually develop 2 to 4 hours after eating. In severe cases, convulsions and loss of consciousness may occur. Approximately 15% of cases lead to diabetes. The goal of nutrition therapy is to avoid stimulating insulin secretion. The diabetic exchange lists may be used to implement the following strategies:

- Limit total carbohydrate intake to 100 to 125 g/day.
- Use only small amounts of simple sugars.
- Eat small, frequent meals, each containing protein and/or fat, to help slow the rate of carbohydrate absorption, decrease the rise in blood glucose levels, and reduce insulin secretion. A liberal protein intake is encouraged.
- Encourage fiber intake, especially soluble fiber.
- Lose weight, if overweight.
- Avoid alcohol.

▲ Focus on Critical Thinking

Respond to the following statements:

1. Glycemic index is an important consideration in choosing carbohydrates.
2. Telling people with type 2 diabetes that they may be able to delay or prevent long-term complications by losing weight and exercising should be enough motivation to change their behavior.
3. A high carbohydrate, low-fat diet is the optimal diet for all diabetics.

Key Concepts

- Type 1 diabetes is characterized by the lack of insulin secretion. It is usually diagnosed before the age of 30 years in people who are of normal or below normal weight.

- Ninety percent to 95% of diabetes cases are type 2 diabetes. It is characterized by hyperinsulinemia and insulin resistance. Hyperglycemia provides constant stimulation for insulin secretion, further aggravating hyperinsulinemia.
- Tight glycemic control delays or prevents the onset of long-term microvascular complications and probably macrovascular complications as well.
- Nutrition therapy is the cornerstone of treatment for all diabetics, regardless of weight status, use of medication, blood glucose levels, and presence or absence of symptoms. The goals of nutrition therapy are to achieve optimal blood glucose and lipid levels, attain or maintain reasonable weight, and avoid acute and chronic complications.
- Nutrient needs of people with diabetes are not different than the general population. Dietary recommendations to promote health and well-being are also appropriate for people with diabetes. Because they are at high risk, people with diabetes should consume a diet consistent with the TLC Diet for the primary and secondary prevention of CHD.
- The American Diabetes Association recommends that people with diabetes consume approximately 10% of total calories from saturated fat, 10% from polyunsaturated fat, and 10% to 20% from protein. The remaining calories are to be divided between carbohydrates and monounsaturated fats depending on the client's lipid levels, usual dietary pattern, and weight status.
- Sucrose ("sugar") is no longer considered detrimental to glucose control so long as it is eaten as part of the meal plan and not as an "extra." However, if weight loss is a goal, high-sugar foods should be limited.
- Diets for diabetics are not "one size fits all." Dietary changes should be made sequentially and restrictions kept to a minimum to maximize compliance.
- Clients who want or need only basic nutrition therapy information may benefit from using MyPyramid as a tool or single-topic resources geared to the client's interests.
- Exchange lists and carbohydrate counting are two approaches to meal planning that allow flexibility while promoting day-to-day consistency in the amount of carbohydrate consumed.
- Children and adolescents have a greater variation in their daily calorie needs than do adults because of their nutritional needs for growth and their more erratic activity and eating patterns.
- Pregnant diabetics need to closely monitor their blood glucose levels and eat three meals and two to three snacks daily. The bedtime snack is especially important to avoid morning hypoglycemia.
- Elderly diabetics may need to be treated more conservatively than younger diabetics because they are more susceptible to severe hypoglycemia, are at greater nutritional risk, and may have physical or sensory impairments that complicate self-management.
- Diabetic diets in the hospital were traditionally identified as "ADA diets." Because there is no one diabetic diet recommended for all people with diabetes, this term should be discontinued.

ANSWER KEY

1. **TRUE** Carbohydrates impact postprandial glucose levels more than protein or fat.
2. **FALSE** Modest weight loss, such as 5% to 7%, has been shown to dramatically reduce the risk of type 2 diabetes.
3. **TRUE** Even if it does not produce weight loss, increasing physical activity improves glucose control, reduces insulin resistance, improves blood lipid levels, improves blood pressure, and enhances sense of well-being and quality of life.
4. **TRUE** Alcohol is more likely to cause hypoglycemia when consumed without food rather than with food.
5. **TRUE** Frequent treatment of hypoglycemia, meaning eating extra carbohydrates, can lead to weight gain.
6. **FALSE** People with diabetes should eat more fiber than the average American but do not need more than the general population.
7. **FALSE** Foods containing sucrose may have a higher glycemic index than starchy foods, but generalizations may not be accurate because many variables affect glycemic index. For instance, a baked potato has a higher glycemic index than does chocolate milk.
8. **FALSE** The exchange lists may be too complicated for some people to implement successfully. MyPyramid can be used as a suitable teaching tool as long as specific information about carbohydrates is provided.
9. **FALSE** Supplemental chromium improves glycemic control in people with type 2 diabetes only if they are deficient in chromium.
10. **TRUE** People with diabetes should limit their intake of saturated fat and cholesterol because their risk of CHD is very high.

WEBSITES

American Diabetes Association at **www.diabetes.org**
Joslin Diabetes Center at **www.joslin.org**
National Institute of Diabetes and Digestive and Kidney Diseases at **www.niddk.nih.gov**

REFERENCES

American Diabetes Association. (2004). Nutrition principles and recommendations in diabetes. *Diabetes Care, 27,* (Suppl. 1), S36–S46.

American Diabetes Association. (2004). Physical activity/exercise and diabetes. *Diabetes Care, 27,* (Suppl. 1), S58–S62.

American Diabetes Association. (2004). Diabetes nutrition recommendations for health care institutions. *Diabetes Care, 27,* (Suppl. 1), S55–S57.

American Diabetes Association, American Dietetic Association. (2003). *Exchange lists for meal planning.* Alexandria, VA: American Diabetes Association; Chicago: American Dietetic Association.

American Diabetes Association and National Institute of Diabetes and Digestive and Kidney Diseases. (2004). Prevention or delay of type 2 diabetes. *Diabetes Care, 27,* (Suppl. 1), S47–S54.

Brekke, H., Jansson, P., Mansson, J., & Lenner, R. (2003). Lifestyle changes can be achieved through counseling and follow-up in first-degree relatives of patients with type 2 diabetes. *Journal of the American Dietetic Association, 103,* 835–843.

Daly, A., Franz, M., Holzmeister, L, et al. (2003). New diabetes nutrition resources. *Journal of the American Dietetic Association, 103,* 832–834.

Kelley, D. (2003). Sugars and starch in the nutritional management of diabetes mellitus. *American Journal of Clinical Nutrition, 78*(Suppl.), 858S–864S.

National Institute of Diabetes and Digestive and Kidney Diseases. (2003). *National Diabetes Statistics fat sheet: General information and national estimates on diabetes in the United States.* NIH Publication No. 04-3892. Bethesda, MD: U.S. Dept. Health and Human Services, National Institutes of Health.

Pastors, J., Franz, M., Warshaw, H., et al. (2003). How effective is medical nutrition therapy in diabetes care? *Journal of the American Dietetic Association, 103,* 827–831.

U.S. Department of Health and Human Services. (2002). Diet and exercise delay diabetes and normalize blood glucose. Available at www.nih.gov/news/pr/feb2002/hhs-06.htm. Accessed on 1/22/04.

Wing, R., Goldstein, M., Acton, K., et al. (2001). Behavioral science research in diabetes. *Diabetes Care, 24,* 117–123.

Woods, T. (2003). Diet and exercise: Preemptive strikes on type 2 diabetes. *Journal of the American Dietetic Association, 103,* 843.

Yeh, G., Eisenberg, D., Kaptchuk, T., & Phillips, R. (2003). Systematic review of herbs and dietary supplements for glycemic control in diabetes. *Diabetes Care, 26,* 1277–1294.

For information on the new dietary guidelines 2005 and MyPyramid, visit **http://connection.lww.com/go/dudek**

20

Nutrition for Patients With Renal Disorders

TRUE	FALSE	
○	○	**1** Early in the course of chronic renal disease, limiting protein may help to preserve kidney function.
○	○	**2** Foods high in protein tend to be high in phosphorus.
○	○	**3** Milk is an excellent source of high biologic value protein for people with pre-end stage renal disease.
○	○	**4** All people with renal impairments need to limit their sodium intake.
○	○	**5** People with chronic renal disease tend to have accelerated atherosclerosis and may benefit from eating more monounsaturated fat.
○	○	**6** Dialysis causes protein requirements to increase about 50% above normal.
○	○	**7** People receiving peritoneal dialysis absorb calories from the dialysate.
○	○	**8** People who have gained more than 2 pounds between dialysis treatments have eaten too many calories.
○	○	**9** People with calcium oxalate renal stones should avoid calcium.
○	○	**10** The most effective nutritional intervention for renal stones is to increase fluid intake.

UPON COMPLETION OF THIS CHAPTER, YOU WILL BE ABLE TO

- Discuss the nutrient recommendations for pre-end stage renal disease (ESRD), ESRD, acute renal failure, and nephrotic syndrome.
- Describe what those nutrient recommendations mean in terms of teaching clients what to eat.
- List ways to promote dietary compliance.
- Describe nutritional interventions for renal stones.

Nitrogenous Wastes: wastes produced from nitrogen, namely ammonia, urea, uric acid, and creatinine.

Rennin: an enzyme secreted by the kidneys in response to a reduced blood flow that stimulates the release of aldosterone.

The kidneys perform many vital endocrine and exocrine functions. They maintain normal blood volume and composition by reabsorbing needed nutrients and excreting wastes through the urine. Urinary excretion is the primary method by which the body rids itself of excess water, nitrogenous wastes, electrolytes, sulfates, organic acids, toxic substances, and drugs. The kidneys help to regulate acid–base balance by secreting hydrogen ions to increase pH and excreting bicarbonate to lower pH. The kidneys are involved in blood pressure regulation through the action of rennin and in red blood cell production through the action of erythropoietin. Because vitamin D is converted to its active form in the kidneys, they have an important role in maintaining normal metabolism of calcium and phosphorus.

This chapter discusses nutrient recommendations for pre-end stage renal disease (ESRD), ESRD, posttransplant, acute renal failure (ARF), and nephrotic syndrome. Nutrition recommendations for preventing and treating kidney stones are presented.

RENAL DISEASE

Erythropoietin: a hormone secreted by the kidneys that stimulates the bone marrow to produce red blood cells.

Active Form of Vitamin D: 1,25-dihydroxycholecalciferol.

Renal damage and subsequent loss of renal function profoundly affect metabolism, nutritional requirements, and nutritional status. As urine output decreases, fluid and electrolytes accumulate in the blood. The retention of nitrogenous wastes leads to uremic syndrome. Acidosis occurs because the kidneys are unable to excrete excess acid produced through normal metabolic processes. Reabsorption of some nutrients is impaired, which causes them to be lost in the urine. GI absorption of some minerals, such as calcium and iron, is impaired. Impaired synthesis of renin, erythropoietin, and vitamin D can lead to high blood pressure, anemia, and bone demineralization, respectively. Certain peptide hormones, such as insulin, parathyroid hormone, and glucagon, are not adequately inactivated, which contributes to altered metabolism. Accelerated atherosclerosis increases the risk of congestive heart failure, myocardial infarction, and further renal damage. Poor intake related to dietary restrictions, anorexia, alterations in taste, nausea, vomiting, stomatitis, depression, or anxiety is common. In addition, nutrients may be lost secondary to drug therapy, dialysis, or renal transplantation. In short, the disruption to homeostasis is profound.

Renal damage can occur secondary to kidney disorders such as glomerulonephritis, polycystic kidney disease, obstructive kidney stones, or congenital kidney malformations. Diabetes is the leading cause of renal failure in the United States. Hypertension and hypercholesterolemia also increase the risk of renal disease. Some people diagnosed with early renal disease may never progress to irreversible late stage disease. Lifestyle changes, including diet, can slow the progress of the disease when initiated early.

Nutrition Therapy

Nutrition therapy has an integral role in the management of renal disease. Its lofty goals are to:

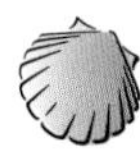

Uremic Syndrome: a cluster of symptoms related to the retention of nitrogenous substances in the blood such as fatigue, decreased mental acuity, muscle twitches, cramps, anorexia, unpleasant nausea, vomiting, diarrhea, itchy skin, gastritis, and GI bleeding.

- Reduce renal workload to delay or prevent further kidney damage
- Restore or maintain optimal nutritional status
- Control the accumulation of uremic toxins such as urea, phosphorus, sodium, and sometimes potassium

The optimal interventions needed to meet these objectives vary among individuals and according to the nature, severity, and stage of the disease. Generally, diet modifications are made in response to symptoms and laboratory values and, therefore, require frequent monitoring and adjustment. Alterations in the intake of protein, calories, sodium, fluid, potassium, phosphorus, calcium, and other vitamins and minerals are necessary initially or eventually. The diet is both complex and dynamic. Table 20.1 summarizes the nutrient recommendations in chronic renal disease discussed here.

Pre–End Stage Renal Disease

Pre-ESRD, a predialysis condition, is characterized by an increase in serum creatinine levels secondary to a decline in renal function. The goals of nutrition therapy are to (1) help preserve remaining renal function; therefore, the focus is on limiting the intake of protein and phosphorus; and (2) control risk factors such as blood glucose levels and hypertension as appropriate. Potassium is usually not a concern until urine output is less than 1 L/day. A sample menu appears in Box 20.1.

Protein

Pre-end Stage Renal Disease: the period of renal failure when renal function is impaired but not to the degree where dialysis or transplant is required. Also known as renal insufficiency.

Protein restriction is the cornerstone of nutrition therapy for pre-ESRD. Studies show that protein restriction can slow the progression of renal disease, although the optimal level of dietary protein has not been determined. In theory, less protein intake generates less urea, so BUN levels decrease and symptoms of uremia, such as nausea and vomiting, improve.

A narrow margin of error exists with regard to protein intake. Whereas too much protein increases BUN levels and the symptoms of uremia, too little protein results in body protein catabolism (which increases serum potassium and BUN levels) and protein malnutrition as evidenced by low serum albumin levels. Low serum albumin is a strong predictor of mortality in patients starting dialysis.

For pre-ESRD, the recommended daily protein intake is 0.6 to 1.0 g/kg of ideal or adjusted body weight, a range that extends from slightly below the normal RDA for protein (0.8 g/kg) to slightly above. Protein allowance may begin at 1.0 g/kg and be adjusted downward as the disease progresses. Limiting protein to 0.6 g/kg can be difficult to implement because most Americans generally consume almost twice this level.

There is some evidence to suggest that some animal proteins, such as red meat, are more damaging to the kidneys than are vegetable proteins such as soy. Because restricting protein is so difficult, a compromise may be to substitute vegetable protein for some animal protein.

TABLE 20.1

NUTRIENT RECOMMENDATIONS FOR CHRONIC RENAL DISEASE

Nutrient	Pre-End Stage Renal Disease	Hemodialysis	Peritoneal Dialysis
Protein	0.6–1.0 cal/kg; >50% HBV sources	1.1–1.4 g/kg; >50% HBV sources	1.2–1.5 g/kg; >50% HBV sources
Calories	35 cal/kg ideal or adjusted weight (<60 years old) 30–35 cal/kg ideal or adjusted weight (>60 years old)	35 cal/kg ideal or adjusted weight (<60 years old) 30–35 cal/kg ideal or adjusted weight (>60 years old)	35 cal/kg ideal or adjusted weight (<60 years old) 30–35 cal/kg ideal or adjusted weight (>60 years old) Subtract calories absorbed from dialysate
Sodium	Individualized or 1–3 g/day	Individualized or 2–3 g/day	Individualized or 2–4 g/day
Potassium	Individualized per lab values	Individualized per lab values or 40 mg/kg ideal or adjusted weight	Individualized per lab values
Phosphorus	Individualized or 8–12 mg/kg ideal or adjusted weight	Individualized or <17 mg/kg ideal or adjusted weight	Individualized or <17 mg/kg ideal or adjusted weight
Calcium	Individualized per calcium, phosphorus, PTH lab values	Individualized per lab values; approximately 1000 mg/day	Individualized per lab values; approximately 1000 mg/day
Fluid	Individualized	500–750 mL + urine output/day	Individualized
Vitamin and mineral supplement	Individualized	Individualized	Individualized

Renal Practice Group of the American Dietetic Association. (2002). *National renal diet: Professional guide* (2nd ed.). Chicago: American Dietetic Association.

BOX 20.1

SAMPLE RENAL MENUS: PRE-ESRD DIET VERSUS ESRD DIET

Sample Pre-ESRD Diet: 42 g Protein, at least 2300 Calories	**Sample ESRD Diet: 90 g Protein Diet, 2600 cal, 2g K, 3g Na, 1200 mg P**
Breakfast	
½ cup orange juice	1 medium canned plum
1 English muffin	1 English muffin
At least 1 tbsp margarine	1 tbsp margarine
	2 eggs fried in margarine
Jelly	Jelly
Coffee	1 cup coffee
Sugar	Sugar
Nondairy creamer	Nondairy creamer
Lunch	
Sandwich made with	
1 oz turkey	2 oz turkey
2 slices white bread	2 slices white bread
At least 2 tbsp mayonnaise	2 tbsp mayonnaise
lettuce	lettuce
1 slice tomato	1 slice tomato
1 small apple	1 small apple
Ginger ale	1 cup milk
Snack	
2 fruit rollups	4 sugar cookies
Dinner	
2 oz roast beef	4 oz toast beef
low sodium gravy	low sodium gravy
½ cup unsalted noodles with 2 tbsp margarine	½ cup unsalted noodles with 2 tbsp margarine
½ cup carrots with margarine	½ cup carrots
Lettuce, onions, cucumbers, green pepper salad with olive oil and vinegar dressing	Lettuce, onions, cucumbers, gr pepper salad with olive oil and vinegar dressing
⅛ blueberry pie	⅛ blueberry pie
Ginger ale	1 cup ginger ale
Snacks	
Carbonated beverages*	
Marshmallows, gum drops, hard candy	Marshmallows, gum drops, hard candy

*As allowed, depending on fluid needs.

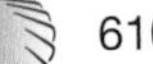

Career Connection

Even though highly motivated clients can successfully lower their protein intake, maintaining a consistently low protein intake is extremely difficult. Consider that a client who weighs 70 kg (154 pounds) whose level of renal function allows only 0.6 g protein/kg would be allowed to eat only 42 g of protein/day. Look how quickly protein adds up even before meats are considered.

A reasonable core diet may be

6 servings from the grain group × 3 g protein/average serving	= 18 g pro
3 servings of vegetables × 2 g protein/average serving	= 6 g pro
½ cup milk (limited because of the phosphorus)	= 4 g pro
Total before meat:	28 g pro

42 g total −28 g used so far = 14 g left for meat, fish, and poultry. At 7 g protein/ounce, the client is "allowed" only 2 oz of meat/day plus the amounts of foods listed above. Fruit is virtually protein-free but may not be eaten freely because of its potassium content. The only other source of protein-free calories available: pure sugars and pure fats.

Strategies that may help promote dietary adherence are to

- Encourage clients to weigh and measure foods for accuracy.
- Provide positive messages about what to eat rather than emphasizing food restrictions.
- Encourage social support from family and friends.
- Foster the client's perception as successfully adhering to the plan. People who are more confident in their ability to adhere to the eating plan make better choices.
- Provide feedback on self-monitoring and biochemistry data. Correlation of records with laboratory data enables the client to see cause-and-effect, reinforces the importance of nutrition therapy, and opens the door for problem solving.
- Encourage the client to try low protein breads, cereals, cookies, gelatin, and pastas. Acceptability varies greatly among low protein products, so if a client does not like one brand, it does not mean he won't like another.

Calories

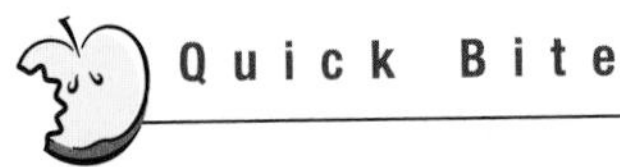

Renal formulas designed for pre-end stage renal disease that provide calories with limited amounts of protein, fluid, and electrolytes are

Renalcal Diet
Suplena

Adequate calories are needed to prevent weight loss and spare body protein from catabolism. Taking in too few calories can have the same effect as eating too much protein: BUN levels rise because body proteins are broken down for energy.

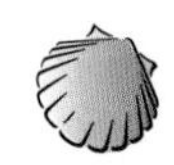

Calorie recommendations are 35 cal/kg for adults under 60 years of age and 30 to 35 cal/kg for those who are older. In contrast to healthy eating messages for the general population, clients who must limit their intake of protein are advised to increase their intake of pure sugars and pure fats to meet their calorie requirements while keeping protein low. Pure sugars and pure fats are protein-free even though they are not considered "nutritious" foods by normal standards (Box 20.2). In this population in whom diabetes and hyperlipidemia are common, an increased intake of pure sugars and pure fats is seemingly contraindicated. The best protein-free calorie option is to choose fats rich in monounsaturated fats such as canola oil, olive oil, and trans fat–free margarines.

BOX 20.2

SOURCES OF PROTEIN-FREE CALORIES AND SEASONINGS

Protein-Free Calories

Beverages*
- Alcoholic
- Carbonated (colas may be restricted due to their relatively high phosphorus content)
- Cranberry juice cocktail
- Fruit drinks and punches
- Kool-Aid
- Lemonade, limeade
- Tang

Candies
- Buttermints
- Candy corn, fondant
- Chewy fruit snacks
- Cotton candy
- Fruit chews, fruit rollups
- Gum
- Gumdrops
- Jelly beans
- Life Savers
- Lollipops
- Marshmallows
- Mints

Desserts
- Fruit ice*
- Juice bar
- Popsicle*
- Sorbet

Fats
- Butter and margarine (unsalted)
- Coconut
- Mayonnaise, oils
- Powdered coffee whitener
- Shortening
- Tartar sauce

Sweeteners
- Corn syrup
- Honey
- Jams
- Jellies
- Maple syrup
- Marmalade
- Sugar: confectioners, white, brown

Protein-Free Seasonings

Flavoring extracts
Herbs
Spices
Vinegar

*As allowed by fluid restriction.

Phosphorus

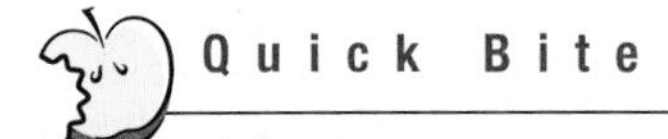

Quick Bite

High-phosphorus foods include

Beer	Dairy products
Bran	Dried peas and beans
Bran cereal	Meat
Cheese	Nuts
Chocolate	Peanut butter
Cola	

Like protein restriction, low-phosphorus diets have been shown to delay the progression of renal disease. A high phosphorus intake contributes to hyperphosphatemia, which stimulates parathyroid hormone PTH secretion, which in turn promotes loss of bone mass and increases the risk that damaging deposits of calcium and phosphorus will form in the kidneys and other soft tissues. Restricting phosphorus is appropriate for all stages of renal disease. On the plus side, low-protein diets are usually low in phosphorus and may effectively control hyperphosphatemia in pre-ESRD.

Controlling Blood Glucose Levels

Studies clearly show that controlling blood glucose levels can prevent renal damage and reverse early kidney hyperfiltration. Consistent meal timing and consistent carbohydrate intake, as well as increased physical activity and weight loss, help to control blood glucose levels. See Chapter 19 for nutrition therapy for diabetes.

Controlling Hypertension

Controlling high blood pressure reduces the risk of renal disease. In people diagnosed with renal disease, controlling blood pressure reduces the rate of kidney function decline, reduces the likelihood that dialysis or transplant will be required, and decreases mortality. Weight loss, limiting alcohol consumption, and healthy eating can significantly lower blood pressure. Studies confirm that a diet rich in fruits and vegetables and low in fat, saturated fat, and sodium can lower blood pressure. See the DASH diet in Chapter 18.

Food Guidance for Pre-ESRD

In terms of food, nutrition recommendations for pre-ESRD can be summarized as follows:

- Limit meat intake to <5 to 6 oz/day for most men and <4 oz/day for most women. Protein intakes less than this may actually worsen symptoms and cause weight loss with increased risk of malnutrition. However, as renal function deteriorates, more drastic cuts in protein intake may be necessary, including limiting regular breads and cereals.
- Limit dairy products including milk, yogurt, ice cream, and frozen yogurt, to ½ cup/day. Nondairy creamers are a low-phosphorus alternative, but they can be high in saturated fat.

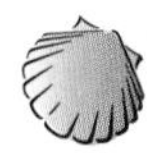

- Limit cheese to 1 oz hard cheese/day or ⅓ cup cottage cheese/day.
- Limit high-phosphorus foods to 1 serving or less/day. High-phosphorus foods include beer, chocolate, cola, nuts, peanut butter, dried peas and beans, bran, bran cereals, and some whole grains.
- Lowering sodium intake can help to maintain normal blood pressure or lower high blood pressure.
- A consistent intake of carbohydrate with regularly timed meals is important for people with diabetes.
- Because loss of renal function changes vitamin and mineral requirements, caution clients against using any vitamin, mineral, or nutritional supplement without prior approval from their physician.

End Stage Renal Disease: a severe stage of chronic renal failure that requires life-sustaining treatment with either dialysis or a kidney transplant. BUN may be as high as 150 to 250 mg/dL.

End Stage Renal Disease

Glomerular Filtration Rate (GFR): the rate at which the kidneys form filtrate as determined by the amount of creatinine excreted per 24 hours. Normal GRF is about 120 to 130 ml/min.

End-stage renal disease occurs when glomerular filtration rate falls to <25 ml/min; serum creatinine levels steadily increase, overt symptoms are apparent, and dialysis or transplantation are required. Malnutrition is common in people with ESRD and is associated with increased morbidity and mortality. A high-protein, low-phosphorus, low-potassium, low-sodium, fluid-restricted diet is used to help maintain acceptable blood chemistries, blood pressure, and fluid status between dialysis treatments. Saturated fat and cholesterol may also be restricted because of hyperlipidemia. Other nutrients of concern include calcium, vitamin D, vitamins, and trace minerals. A sample menu appears in Box 20.1.

Protein

Once dialysis is initiated, the need for protein increases to greater than normal levels to compensate for the loss of serum proteins and amino acids in the dialysate. However, most people receiving dialysis consume less than the recommended 1.2 g/kg/d. Achieving this level of intake within the confines of other restrictions is difficult.

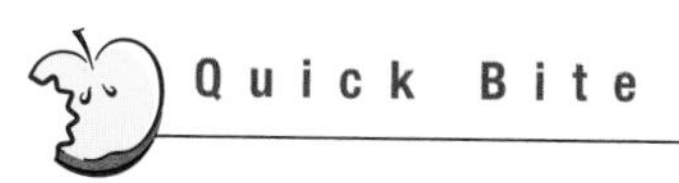

Quick Bite

Sources of high biologic protein are

Eggs	Meat
Milk products	Fish
Soy	Poultry

It is recommended that at least 50% of protein intake be from high biologic sources. The rationale for using high biologic proteins, which provide adequate amounts of all the essential amino acids, is that they promote reuse of circulating nonessential amino acids for protein synthesis and by doing so minimize urea production.

Calories

Daily consumption of 35 cal/kg of ideal or adjusted weight is recommended for adults under 60 years of age. Clients over 60 years old may need 30 to 35 cal/kg. The protein-sparing effect of sufficient calories enables dietary protein to be used

Dialysate: the dialysis solution used to extract wastes and fluid from the blood.

Career Connection

Calorie requirements are typically based on an amount per kilogram of weight. But which weight? Ideal? Actual? Usual? Adjusted? Currently nutrient guidelines are based on ideal body weight, but ideal may not be appropriate for all clients. For clients who are significantly underweight, using ideal can lead to overfeeding and the risk of refeeding syndrome. For clients who are obese, using ideal weight ignores the increase in muscle mass. A common practice is to calculate an adjusted body weight for clients who are obese, based on the premise that an obese person has a greater percentage of body fat, which is much less metabolically active than muscle tissue and requires fewer calories.

Adjusted weight = [(actual weight–ideal weight) × FFM factor] + ideal weight

FFM (fat free mass) factor = 0.22–0.33 for women
0.19–0.38 for men

Example: For a 200 (91 kg) pound woman whose ideal weight is 100 pounds (45 kg):
[(200 pounds – 100 pounds) × .28 (middle of the FFM factor range for women)] + 100 pounds
100 pounds × .28 = 28 pounds + 100 pounds = 128 pounds adjusted weight
128 is then divided by 2.2 to get adjusted weight in kilograms, which is approximately 58 kg

Compare using different weights:

Actual wt	Ideal wt	Adjusted wt
91 kg	45 kg	58 kg
× 35 cal/kg	× 35 cal/kg	× 35 cal/kg
3185 total cal	1575 total cal	2030 total cal

The bottom line is that there is currently no validated method for calculating calorie and protein needs in obese people. Nutrient recommendations should be viewed as starting points that are refined over time, based on the individual's lab values and other factors. The same holds true for people who are significantly underweight.

to replenish the protein lost through the dialysate and maintain normal body proteins.

Because hyperlipidemia is common, a low–saturated fat, low-cholesterol diet is prudent. Lean meats, nonfat milk (allowed only in limited amounts because of the phosphorus content), and egg whites are the best choices of animal protein. Canola oil, olive oil, and trans fat-free soft margarines are recommended sources of fat.

Clients receiving peritoneal dialysis need to decrease their calorie intake to compensate for the glucose calories absorbed from the dialysate (approximately 340 to 680 cal/day). Likewise, sedentary clients and post-transplantation clients who are taking immunosuppressive steroids may require fewer calories to avoid excess weight gain.

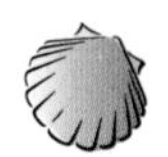

Phosphorus

A low phosphorus intake continues to be important: Vitamin D deficiency, which occurs as the kidneys fail to convert the vitamin to its active form, alters the metabolism of calcium, phosphorus, and magnesium, resulting in hyperphosphatemia, bone demineralization, bone pain, and possible calcification of the soft tissues (e.g., eyes, skin, heart, lungs, blood vessels, and kidneys).

A low phosphorus intake is relatively easy to achieve when protein intake is restricted as in the case of pre-ESRD. However, when dialysis begins and protein allowance increases, phosphorus intake correspondingly increases. Phosphate binders in addition to dietary restriction are necessary to control serum phosphorus levels for the majority of patients. Phosphate binders must be taken with all meals and snacks. Table 20.2 lists the calcium, phosphorus, and protein contents of selected foods.

Potassium

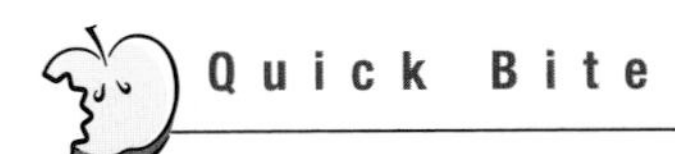

Low-potassium vegetables include

Beans, wax and green	Escarole
Bean sprouts	Green pepper
Cabbage	Lettuce
Cucumber	Water chestnuts
Endive	Watercress

Potassium allowance is based on the individual's lab values. A general recommendation for people undergoing hemodialysis is to allow 40 gm/kg of ideal or adjusted weight, but again, lab values dictate dietary allowance. Clients receiving continuous ambulatory peritoneal dialysis, as well as those taking potassium-wasting diuretics or those experiencing vomiting or diarrhea, are at risk of hypokalemia. GI bleeding, acidosis, catabolism, and hyperglycemia increase the risk of hyperkalemia. Individual needs vary widely.

Sodium and Fluid

The client's blood pressure, weight, serum electrolyte levels, and urine output determine the amount of sodium and fluid allowed. Most renal diets contain a moderate amount of sodium (2 to 4 g/day), but some clients with advanced renal failure are unable to conserve sodium and a sodium deficit may occur if sodium intake is restricted. If the client does not have edema, hypertension, or signs of heart failure, increasing the sodium intake as tolerated may slightly improve GFR. Actual sodium allowance is determined on an individual basis.

Fluid allowance is determined by urine output. Generally, daily fluid allowance exceeds urine output by 500 mL to 750 mL to account for the amount of insensible losses through skin, lungs, and perspiration. Sodium and fluid allowances are set at levels that control weight gain between treatments to 1 to 2 pounds, although much larger gains are common.

TABLE 20.2

CALCIUM, PHOSPHORUS, AND PROTEIN CONTENT OF SELECTED FOODS

Item	Amount	Calcium (mg)	Phosphorus (mg)	Protein (g)
Bread, Cereal, Rice, and Pasta Group				
White bread	1 slice	27	24	2
Whole wheat bread	1 slice	20	64	3
Long-grain rice	½ cup	10	81	3
Corn tortilla	1 med	44	79	1
Vegetable Group				
Artichoke, boiled	1 med	135	258	3
Cassava, raw	3.5 oz	91	70	3
Kale, frozen, boiled	½ cup	90	18	2
Okra, boiled	½ cup	77	37	2
Spinach, boiled	½ cup	122	50	3
Turnip greens, boiled	½ cup	99	21	1
Fruit Group				
Orange juice, calcium-fortified	¾ cup	200	25	0
Avocado, raw	1 med	13	45	2
Cypres, dried	10	43	67	2
Mango, raw	1 med	21	23	1
Strawberries, raw	½ cup	10	14	0
Milk, Yogurt, and Cheese Group				
Skim	1 cup	302	247	8
1%	1 cup	300	235	8
2%	1 cup	297	232	8
Whole	1 cup	291	228	8
Goat milk	1 cup	326	270	9
Chocolate milk (with 1% milk)	1 cup	287	256	8
Plain low-fat yogurt with nonfat dry milk	1 cup	415	326	12
Plain whole-milk yogurt	1 cup	274	215	8
Low-fat fruit-flavored yogurt	1 cup	314	247	8
Cheddar	1 oz	214	145	7
Cottage cheese, 1% fat	½ cup	78	170	12
Mozzarella, part skim	1 oz	147	105	7
Ricotta, part skim	½ cup	337	226	8
Swiss	1 oz	272	171	8
Ice cream, vanilla soft serve	½ cup	138	106	4

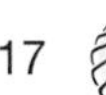

TABLE 20.2
(continued)

CALCIUM, PHOSPHORUS, AND PROTEIN CONTENT OF SELECTED FOODS

Item	Amount	Calcium (mg)	Phosphorus (mg)	Protein (g)
Meat, Poultry, Fish, Dry Beans, Eggs, and Nuts Group				
Ground beef, broiled	3½ oz	12	191	27
Ham, cured, roasted	3½ oz	6	224	19
Veal, ground, broiled	3½ oz	17	217	24
Beef liver, braised	3½ oz	7	404	24
Chicken breast, roasted	½	13	196	27
Salmon, chinook	3 oz	24	316	22
Tuna, white, canned	3 oz	12	185	20
Refried beans, canned	½ cup	45	109	7
Great northern beans, canned	½ cup	70	178	7
Egg, poached	1	25	89	6
Almonds, blanched	1 oz	73	150	6
Peanut butter	2 tbsp	13	101	7
Sunflower seeds, dry roasted	1 oz	20	327	6
Fats, Oils, and Sweets				
Sour cream	2 tbsp	28	20	1
Cola	12 oz	11	44	0
Milk chocolate bar	1.55 oz	84	95	3
Orange sherbet	½ cup	52	38	1

Career Connection

For many clients on dialysis, limiting fluid intake is the biggest challenge. Teaching clients *why* the fluid restriction is important is only half the battle; teaching them *how* to control their intake and thirst is vital. Strategies to relieve thirst include

- Use ice or popsicles within the fluid allowance—very cold things are better at relieving thirst.
- Suck on hard candy or mints.
- Chew gum.
- Frequent mouth rinsing with refrigerated water.
- Suck on a lemon wedge.
- Bread with applesauce or jelly may relieve dry mouth.
- Control blood glucose levels, as appropriate.
- Try frozen grapes.
- Use small glasses instead of large ones.
- Apply petroleum jelly to the lips.

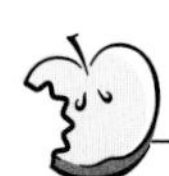

Quick Bite

Sources of fluid in addition to beverages consumed include

Gelatin	Liquid medication
Gravy	Popsicles
Ice (melts to 9/10 initial volume)	Sauces
Ice cream (melts to ½ initial volume)	Sherbet
Ice milk (melts to ½ initial volume)	Soup

Calcium

Hypocalcemia in ESRD is related to altered vitamin D metabolism, impaired intestinal absorption of calcium, and hyperphosphatemia. Foods high in calcium, namely dairy products, are also high in phosphorus and so are not allowed freely. It is not likely that calcium requirement can be met through food alone when dairy products are restricted. Calcium carbonate taken between meals acts like a calcium supplement; taken with meals, it functions as a phosphorus binder so the amount of calcium absorbed is diminished. Calcium supplements are adjusted according to the individual's calcium, phosphorus, and PTH lab values.

Vitamin D

Supplements of the active form of vitamin D promote calcium absorption to help maintain blood calcium levels and prevent bone disease. Doses are individualized to maintain desirable serum calcium levels (see Drug Alert).

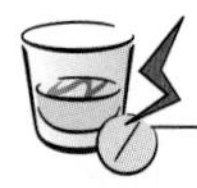

DRUG ALERT

Drugs Used During Chronic Renal Disease

Epoetin alfa (Procrit, Epogen) is recombinant human erythropoietin, which stimulates bone marrow production of red blood cells. It is used to treat anemia of chronic renal failure in which there is an erythropoietin deficiency.

Possible side effects include worsening hypertension, edema, fatigue, nausea, vomiting, and diarrhea.

Because deficiencies of iron, vitamin B_{12}, and folic acid can cause a poor response, it is important to identify and prevent nutritional deficiencies.

Calcitriol (Calcijex, Rocaltrol) is the active form of vitamin D (1-25-dihydroxycholecalciferol). It is used to manage hypocalcemia in patients receiving chronic renal dialysis. Vitamin D raises serum calcium levels and decreases parathyroid hormone levels. An adequate intake of calcium and fluids is important. The risk of hypermagnesemia is increased when calcitriol is used with magnesium-containing antacids.

Vitamins

Alterations in vitamin metabolism, intake, or requirements occur secondary to renal disease and dialysis. Deficiencies of water-soluble vitamins occur frequently in clients with renal failure and may be caused by inadequate intake related to anorexia or dietary restrictions; altered metabolism related to uremia or medications; or increased losses related to dialysis. For instance, amounts greater than the RDA of folic acid and vitamin B_6 are recommended to promote red blood cell production. Conversely, less than normal amounts of vitamin C are recommended for people with ESRD because vitamin C increases the risk of oxalate stones and many people with renal failure have high blood oxalate levels.

Fat-soluble vitamins tend not to be removed by dialysis; however, except for vitamin D mentioned previously, supplements of fat-soluble vitamins usually are not necessary. In fact, vitamin A supplementation is contraindicated in clients with ESRD because of reported toxicity.

Specially formulated vitamin supplements are available with the appropriate levels of essential vitamins for people with renal disease. Regular multivitamin preparations may provide too much of some vitamins (e.g., Vit A) and too little of others (e.g., folic acid).

Trace Minerals

Renal failure can cause toxic accumulations of aluminum and magnesium; products containing either of these minerals, such as antacids or supplements, should be avoided. Clients who are undergoing dialysis may develop a deficiency of zinc, which could contribute to anorexia and taste alterations. Supplements are recommended if a zinc deficiency is identified. Zinc supplements and iron supplements should not be taken at the same time, nor should zinc supplements be taken within 1 hour before meals or within 2 hours after eating.

Iron supplements plus human erythropoietin are used to treat anemia of ESRD. Iron supplements may cause gastrointestinal upset and constipation, and they should not be taken with calcium or zinc supplements. Potential side effects of recombinant human erythropoietin appear in the accompanying Drug Alert.

Meal Planning

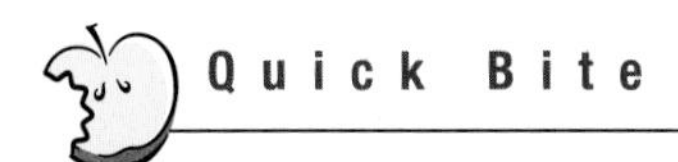

Low-potassium fruits include

Applesauce	Lemon
Blueberries	Papaya nectar
Cranberries	Peach nectar
Cranberry juice cocktail	Pears, canned
Grape juice	Pear nectar

Unlike the relatively simple food guidance offered for pre-ESRD, the "diet" for ESRD is complex and seemingly unrealistic. How can a high protein intake be achieved if phosphorus is restricted? How can adequate calories be consumed if fat and saturated fat are problems? And with so many restrictions, what is left to eat anyway?

Designing a "diet" to provide enough of what the individual needs, but not so much as to worsen symptoms of uremia and fluid retention, is a complex task. An even greater challenge is converting grams, milligrams, and calories into servings of particular foods and acceptable menus. Yet the biggest hurdle is getting the client to make permanent changes in eating habits and food choices. Nutritional success stories seem to be scarce.

The National Renal Diet, developed by the Renal Dietitians Dietetic Practice Group of the American Dietetic Association, simplifies meal planning through the use of food lists (referred to as "choices," rather than "exchanges," to eliminate confusion with diabetic exchanges). For pre-dialysis renal disease, choices include protein, fruit, calorie and flavorings. For people on dialysis, the choices are identified as protein; fruit and vegetable; dairy and phosphorus; bread, cereal and grain; fluid; and calorie and flavoring. Foods are grouped into lists based on their protein, sodium, potassium, and/or phosphorus content; calories are also addressed, and fluids may be considered. For instance, the Fruit Choice list is divided into three groups based on the potassium content, and the Bread, Cereal, and Grain Choices is split into two lists, one of which has higher levels of sodium, potassium, and/or phosphorus. Portion sizes are specified so that relative consistency in nutrient intake can be achieved. Items within a list may be substituted for each other; substitutions from one list to another are not appropriate.

An individualized meal pattern specifies the number of choices permitted from each list; actual allowances are based on laboratory data and clinical symptoms and correspond as closely as possible to the client's food preferences and habits. The composition, complexity, and number of choice lists used in the treatment of renal failure vary considerably among institutions. Despite the use of "choice" lists, trying to adhere to a renal diet is extremely challenging. The diet is complex; modifications are numerous, extensive, and lifelong; and changes are frequent.

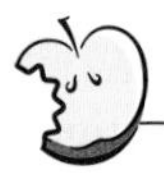

Quick Bite

Renal formulas designed for clients undergoing dialysis that provide calories and protein in a limited volume and low electrolytes are

Magnacal Renal
Nephro
Novasource Renal
NutriRenal

Additional meal planning considerations are as follows:

- Clients with uremia may experience a deterioration of appetite as the day progresses. Encourage a good breakfast.
- Highly seasoned or strongly flavored foods may be preferred because of changes in the sense of taste attributed to uremia.
- Clients should initially weigh or measure portion sizes and, thereafter, periodically spot-check portion sizes for accuracy because either too little or too much

 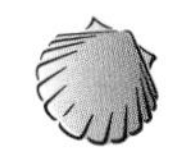

protein in the diet can cause BUN levels to increase and uremic symptoms to return.

- Protein allowance should be spread over the whole day instead of saving it all for one meal.
- Renal formulas may be necessary to achieve adequate protein and calorie intake within the context of other dietary restrictions.
- Foods high in potassium include fruit (especially bananas, citrus fruits and juices, melons, raisins), potatoes, tomatoes, dried peas and beans, whole grains, milk, and fresh meat. The potassium content of vegetables and potatoes can be reduced by cutting them into small pieces, soaking them overnight, and boiling them in fresh water.

Kidney Transplantation

Kidney transplantation is a treatment option for people with ESRD. As with any surgery, the immediate postoperative diet is high in protein and calories to promote healing; nutrient needs gradually decrease after the initial postoperative period (Table 20.3).

TABLE 20.3 **POST-TRANSPLANT NUTRIENT RECOMMENDATIONS FOR ADULTS**

Nutrient	Acute Post-Transplant Recommendations	Maintenance Post-Transplant Recommendations
Protein	1.3–2.0 g/kg wt or adjusted for obesity	0.8–1.0 g/kg
Calories	30–35 cal/kg wt or adjusted weight	25–30 cal/kg or adequate to maintain desirable weight
Fat	30–50% non protein calories	<7% saturated fat, <200 mg cholesterol/day
Sodium	4 g/day or unrestricted if HTN/edema are absent	2–4 g/day based on blood pressure and presence of edema
Fluid	High volume given to stimulate urine output; 500 mL + urine output	Generally not restricted
Vitamin and mineral supplements	Not indicated if oral intake is adequate and balanced	Not mandatory; multivitamin is acceptable. 1000–1500 mg calcium with vitamin D may be appropriate.

Dietitians in Nutrition Support Dietetic Practice Group. (Hasse, J. & Blue, L. [Ed.]) (2002). *Comprehensive guide to transplant nutrition.* Chicago: American Dietetic Association.

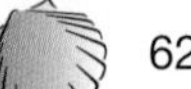
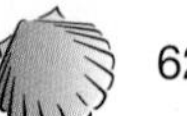

Patients usually begin with liquids within 24 hours after surgery and quickly progress to solid foods. Patients with persistent hyperglycemia may benefit from a carbohydrate-controlled diet. Pretransplant dietary restrictions may be necessary until the new kidney functions normally. Nutritional supplements may be necessary but tube feedings are rarely needed. General guidelines are as follows:

- During the immediate post-transplant period, protein needs may be as high as 1.3 to 2.0 g/kg due to surgical stress, high-dose corticosteroid therapy, muscle catabolism, and preexisting malnutrition. If the grafted kidney fails to work immediately, dialysis rather than dietary protein restriction is used to control uremia.
- Provide calories to maintain reasonable weight and spare protein. Corticosteroids may contribute to obesity, but other drugs may promote weight loss related to anorexia, nausea, vomiting, and diarrhea.

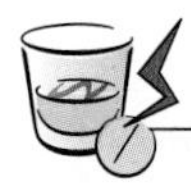

DRUG ALERT

Drugs Used After Renal Transplantation

Corticosteroids (e.g., prednisone) cause protein catabolism, negative nitrogen balance, glucose intolerance, sodium and fluid retention, potassium excretion, and impaired calcium absorption. Gastrointestinal upset may occur. Possible diet modifications include increasing protein and potassium and limiting sodium. Small, frequent meals may help to minimize gastrointestinal distress. A diabetic diet may be indicated for hyperglycemia.

Cyclosporine (Neoral, Sandimmune) commonly causes GI distress, nausea, vomiting, and diarrhea. Other potential side effects include hypertension, hyperlipidemia, and hyperkalemia. Sodium and potassium intakes may be restricted; because cyclosporine is nephrotoxic, a renal diet may be used. Dietary fat decreases drug absorption.

Immunosuppressants (muromonab-CD3, Orthoclone, antithymocyte globulin) are less toxic than cyclosporine but may cause nausea, vomiting, diarrhea, and anorexia. Fever and stomatitis may occur.

Azathioprine (Imuran) may cause esophageal sores, vomiting, diarrhea, and macrocytic anemia. A liquid or soft diet may be needed.

- Limit fat to less than 30% of total calories, saturated fat to <7% of calories, and cholesterol to <200 mg/day because blood lipid levels are often elevated. Elevated low density lipoprotein cholesterol has been associated with chronic rejection in renal transplant recipients.
- Limit sodium to 4 g/day. No restriction is necessary in the absence of hypertension and edema.
- Adjust potassium intake according to diuretic therapy.
- Supplements of phosphorus and magnesium may be necessary.

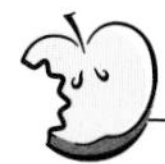

Quick Bite

A 4-g sodium diet is very liberal with few restrictions. The client may simply be told to not use salt in cooking or at the table and to avoid obviously salty foods such as

Cold cuts
Convenience foods such as frozen dinners and dried soup mixes
Fast foods
Pickled vegetables
Salted snack foods
Salty condiments such as soy sauce, dill pickles, mustard, ketchup
Smoked, salted, and kosher meats
Regular canned soup, vegetables, meat, and sauces

NURSING PROCESS

Allen Parker is 34 years old and has had type 1 diabetes for 27 years. He has a history of mild hypertension and mild anemia and complains of sudden weight gain and "swelling." His BUN and creatinine have been steadily increasing over the last several years. During his last appointment, the doctor told Allen to watch his protein intake and avoid salt. His diabetes is fairly well controlled with diet and multiple insulin injections. The doctor has diagnosed renal insufficiency and asked you to talk to Allen about his diet.

Assessment

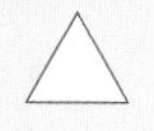

Obtain Clinical Data:

Current height, weight, BMI, recent weight history
Medical history including cardiovascular disease, hypertension, diabetes, and history of renal disease
Abnormal laboratory values, especially BUN, creatinine, lipid levels, glucose, albumin, electrolytes, phosphorus, calcium, hemoglobin, and hematocrit
Urine specific gravity
Blood pressure
Medications that affect nutrition such as diuretics, insulin, and lipid-lowering medications

Interview Client to Assess:

Understanding of the relationship between diet and renal function, specifically the role of protein, calories, sodium, potassium, phosphorus, calcium, and fluid

(continued)

Motivation to change eating style; how successful he was at avoiding salt
Usual 24-hour intake, portion sizes, frequency and pattern of eating. Assess usual quantity and quality of protein consumed and whether most of the protein is of high biologic value (usually animal sources) or of low biologic value (gelatin and plant sources). Assess the use of salt and intake of high-sodium foods: cold cuts, bacon, frankfurters, smoked meats, sausage, canned meats, chipped or corned beef, buttermilk, cheese, crackers, canned soups and vegetables, convenience products, pickles, and condiments. Determine if a salt substitute is used and, if so, its chemical composition. Assess intake of calories, potassium, calcium, and fluid.
Cultural, religious, and ethnic influence on eating habits
Psychosocial and economic issues such as living situation, cooking facilities, financial status, employment, and education
Use of vitamins, minerals, and nutritional supplements: what, how much, and why taken
Use of alcohol and nicotine
Physical complaints such as fatigue, taste changes, anorexia, nausea, vomiting, diarrhea, muscular twitches, and muscle cramps

Nursing Diagnosis

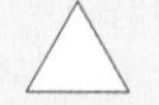

1. Fluid Volume Excess, related to impaired renal function

Planning and Implementation

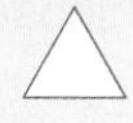

Client Goals

The client will

Maintain normal urinary output.
Achieve and maintain normal blood pressure.
Achieve normal or near-normal electrolyte levels.
Maintain adequate glucose control.
Consume adequate calories to minimize tissue catabolism.
Attain and maintain adequate nutritional status.
Describe the rationale and principles of nutrition therapy for renal insufficiency and implement appropriate dietary changes.
Practice self-management strategies especially self-monitoring protein intake.

Nursing Interventions

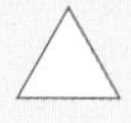

Nutrition Therapy

The doctor has prescribed a 50-g protein, 2-g sodium diet in addition to the patient's normal 2400-cal diabetic diet.

Client Teaching

Instruct the client

On the role of nutrition therapy in the treatment of renal insufficiency

On eating plan essentials, including

- Limiting protein, emphasizing high-quality proteins, spreading protein allowance over the whole day
- Consuming adequate calories
- Limiting high-sodium foods, not adding salt during cooking or at the table

On behavioral matters including

- How to weigh and measure foods to ensure accurate portion sizes
- To self-monitor protein intake
- To weigh himself at approximately the same time every day with the same scale while wearing the same amount of clothing. Unexpected weight gain or loss should be reported to the physician.
- That renal diet cookbooks are available to increase variety

On attitudinal adjustment. Learn to view the diet as an integral component of treatment and a means of life support. Strict adherence to the diet can improve the quality of life and decrease the workload on the kidneys.

Evaluation

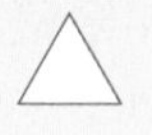

The client

Maintains normal urinary output
Achieves and maintains normal blood pressure
Achieves normal or near-normal electrolyte levels
Consumes adequate calories to minimize tissue catabolism
Attains and maintains adequate nutritional status
Describes the rationale and principles in nutrition therapy of renal insufficiency and implements the appropriate dietary changes
Practices self-management strategies, especially self-monitoring protein intake

Acute Renal Failure

Acute renal failure (ARF) is the sudden but often reversible loss of renal function characterized by rising blood levels of urea and other nitrogenous wastes and oliguria or anuria. During the initial anuric phase, aggressive treatment with dialysis is required. Even though urine output begins to increase in the next phase (oliguric phase), dialysis is typically used. As the diuretic phase begins, dehydration is a risk as urine output rises as high as 1½ to 2 times normal. Optimally, the convalescent phase follows as normal renal function is restored.

Complications of ARF include infection, which is the leading cause of death in these clients. Hyperkalemia may result in cardiac arrest, metabolic acidosis, hypercatabolism, circulatory overload (dyspnea, orthopnea, pulmonary congestion, pulmonary edema), hypertension, hypertensive crisis, convulsions, and neurologic abnormalities. ARF may progress to CRF; at least 5% of clients with acute tubular necrosis require long-term hemodialysis. ARF is fatal in 50% of cases.

The primary focus of treatment is to correct the underlying disorder so as to prevent permanent renal damage. Dialysis is used to keep BUN levels lower than 100 mg/dL and creatinine levels lower than 8 mg/dL. Diuretics and other measures to restore fluid and electrolyte balance are used. Symptomatic anemia is treated with transfusions of packed red blood cells. Nutrition therapy may help to lessen the workload of the kidneys and restore optimal nutritional status.

The optimal diet for clients with ARF is more elusive than the optimal diet for CRF. Although the exact nutritional requirements are not known, it is evident that needs vary among individuals and according to the phase of ARF and that diet restrictions are liberalized once dialysis is instituted.

Protein

Protein recommendations are based on the degree of renal function, the level of underlying stress, and whether dialysis therapy is used. Clients under mild stress and not receiving dialysis therapy may be limited to 0.6 g protein per kilogram body weight. As GFR returns to normal or dialysis begins, the protein allowance is increased to promote nitrogen balance and tissue healing. Depending on the type of dialysis used and levels of underlying stress, protein intake may increase to as high as 1.5 to 2.0 g/kg.

Calories

Calorie requirements depend on the rate of catabolism and metabolism and range from 30 to 45 cal/kg. Carbohydrate modules, pure fats, refined sugars, and low-protein starches are used liberally.

Fluid

For both the oliguric and diuretic phases of ARF, fluid intake should equal total fluid output per 24 hours plus an additional 500 mL, depending on the client's hydration status. Up to 3 L of fluid may be needed daily to prevent dehydration during the diuretic phase.

Potassium

Life-threatening hyperkalemia that occurs during the oliguric phase of ARF is related to potassium retention and tissue catabolism, which causes potassium to leave the cells and enter the serum. Diets that are low in potassium (2 g/day or less) and exchange resins such as Kayexalate may be used during the oliguric phase to reduce serum potassium levels. Once diuresis begins, large amounts of potas-

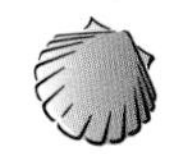

sium are excreted and potassium supplements may be necessary to avoid hypokalemia.

Sodium

Sodium intake is adjusted according to urine output, serum sodium level, symptoms of sodium imbalance, and concurrent use of dialysis. Typically, 2 to 3 g/day is recommended, although sodium may be restricted to < 2 g/day during the anuric phase. As with potassium, sodium requirements increase during the diuretic phase to replace increased losses.

Method of Feeding

Clients who are unable to eat because of critical illness or impaired gastrointestinal function secondary to ARF may need enteral or parenteral nutrition. Special enteral and parenteral renal formulas are available. Fluid restrictions may complicate either type of feeding.

Nephrotic Syndrome

Nephrotic Syndrome: a collection of symptoms that occurs when increased capillary permeability in the glomeruli allow serum proteins to leak into the urine.

Nephrotic syndrome may be caused by diabetes, hypertension, infection, immunological and hereditary conditions, and certain chemicals. Symptoms include hypoalbuminemia, massive edema, hyperlipidemia, and blood hypercoagulation. Loss of proteins in the urine, such as albumin, immunoglobulins, transferrin, and vitamin D-binding protein, may lead to protein malnutrition, anemia, vitamin D deficiency, and increased risk of infection. Accelerated atherosclerosis is a distinguishing feature that increases not only the risk of cardiovascular disease, but also the risk of progressive renal damage. In some cases, treating the underlying disorder corrects nephrotic syndrome. In others, especially diabetes, nephrotic syndrome may be a sign of progressive renal deterioration.

The goals of nutrition therapy are to minimize edema, replace nutrients lost in the urine, and reduce the risk of progressive renal damage. Nutrients of primary concern are protein and sodium. Additional modifications in fat, cholesterol, and calorie intake may be indicated.

Protein

Protein intake should be sufficient to meet protein needs but not excessive so as to accelerate renal deterioration and increase urinary protein losses. An intake of 0.7 to 1.0 g/kg/day, a level close to the RDA, is recommended. Consuming a soy-based vegetarian diet appears to decrease urinary protein losses and lower serum lipid levels.

Sodium and Fluid

A low-sodium diet, in conjunction with drug therapy, is needed to control edema and hypertension. Generally, a 2-g sodium diet is recommended, but a more severe restriction may be necessary depending on the client's response to diuretics. A fluid restriction is generally not necessary. Daily weights are used to assess fluid status.

Fat and Cholesterol

The Total Lifestyle Change (TLC) Diet discussed in Chapter 18 for the primary and secondary prevention of coronary heart disease is recommended to control elevated lipid levels seen in nephrotic syndrome. Drug therapy may be combined with the low saturated fat (<7% of calories), low cholesterol (<200 mg/day) diet for maximum effectiveness. Studies have shown that in high-risk clients with IgA nephropathy, early and prolonged treatment with fish oil supplements slows disease progression.

Calories

A calorie intake of 35 cal/kg is recommended to spare protein. However, gradual weight loss in overweight clients improves serum lipid levels and blood pressure.

Kidney Stones

Struvite: magnesium ammonium phosphate crystals formed by the action of bacterial enzymes.

Kidney stones are one of the most common and painful urologic disorders. Precipitation of insoluble crystals in the urine leads to formation of stones that vary in size from sand-like "gravel" to large, branching stones. Although they form most often in the kidney, they can occur anywhere in the urinary system.

Approximately 80% of stones contain calcium, and most of these are composed of calcium oxalate; fewer calcium stones are composed of calcium phosphate. Approximately 10% of stones are composed of uric acid and 10% are struvite. Cystine (an amino acid) stones are rare and occur only in people with cystinuria, an autosomal recessive disorder.

The likelihood of kidney stones increases when urine volume is low, which favors the precipitation of stones. For instance, people who lose large amounts of fluid through ileostomies have low urine output and an increased risk of kidney stones. Certain occupational circumstances that limit fluid intake (e.g., in delivery people and salespeople) may also increase risk, as does living in the southeastern United States (the "stone belt"). It has been suggested that the increased risk is related to low urine volume secondary to increased perspiration caused by high environmental temperatures or to increased absorption of calcium secondary to vitamin D activation from greater sunlight exposure.

Excessive intakes of protein, sodium, calcium, and oxalate may increase the risk of stone formation in susceptible people.

Protein. High intakes of protein increase urinary excretion of calcium, oxalate, and uric acid and reduce urinary pH. These factors increase the risk for forming uric acid and/or calcium oxalate stones.

Sodium. Because the body rids itself of excess sodium through the urine, the greater the sodium intake, the greater the level of urinary sodium. High urinary sodium increases urinary excretion of calcium and uric acid.

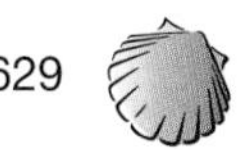

Oxalates. Endogenous oxalate production provides more urinary oxalate than dietary intake does. Although certain foods are rich sources of oxalate and are well absorbed, such as spinach, rhubarb, beets, nuts, chocolate, tea, wheat bran, and strawberries, the bioavailability of oxalate in other foods, such as Swiss chard and collards, is low. Unfortunately, studies on bioavailability are lacking, so conservative advice is that people with calcium oxalate stones should avoid all foods high in oxalate (Box 20.3.)

BOX 20.3 **FOODS HIGH IN OXALATE**

Foods Known to Increase Urinary Oxalate

Spinach
Rhubarb
Beets
Nuts
Chocolate
Tea
Wheat bran
Strawberries

Other High-Oxalate Foods That May or May Not Increase Urinary Oxalate

Beer
Instant coffee
Grits
Wheat germ
Whole wheat flour
Fruitcake
Berries: blackberries, gooseberries, black raspberries
Concord grapes
Red currants
Damson plums
Tangerine
Baked beans with tomato sauce
Peanut butter
Tofu
Sweet potatoes
Beans (wax or legumes)
Celery
Dark leafy greens
Eggplant
Leeks
Summer squash
Cocoa
Carob
Vitamin C intake in excess of RDA

Calcium. Hypercalciuria, an inherited condition, is the cause of stones in more than half of all clients. Although it would seem that limiting calcium intake would be beneficial, people who follow a low-calcium diet excrete more calcium in their urine than they consume, indicating that calcium is being lost from bone. Therefore, most adults with hypercalciuria are urged to consume 800 mg calcium/day, preferably from food. That translates to two 1-cup servings of milk or yogurt with the remaining calcium coming from less significant, nondairy sources. Dietary calcium may favorably bind with dietary oxalate in the intestines, forming an insoluble compound that the body cannot absorb. The decrease in urinary oxalate that occurs with increased dietary calcium is proportionally more significant than the accompanying rise in urinary calcium levels. However, consuming the RDA for calcium from supplements or antacids appears to increase the risk of calcium stones. In cases where hypercalciuria is not caused by excessive GI absorption of calcium, 1000 mg of calcium/day is recommended.

Nutrition Therapy

The most effective nutritional intervention for the treatment and prevention of all renal calculi is to increase fluids and thereby dilute the urine. It is also the intervention that clients are most apt to comply with. A high urine output not only helps the client to pass an existing stone, but also decreases the likelihood that another stone will precipitate out of the urine. A daily fluid intake of 3 L is recommended with at least 50% from water. Coffee (regular and decaffeinated), tea, and wine may lower the risk of kidney stone formation while grapefruit juice may increase the risk. Fluid intake should increase when perspiration increases such as with hot weather and exercise. At least 8 to 12 ounces of fluid, preferably water, should be consumed before bedtime because urine normally becomes more concentrated at night.

Additional recommendations for clients with calcium stones are as follows:

- Avoid high intakes of protein and sodium.
- People at risk for oxalate stones should avoid megadoses of vitamin C because the body can synthesize oxalate from vitamin C.
- Maintain adequate calcium intake. Restricting calcium intake has not been shown to decrease stone formation and may worsen osteoporosis.
- Avoid high-oxalate foods (see Box 20.3).

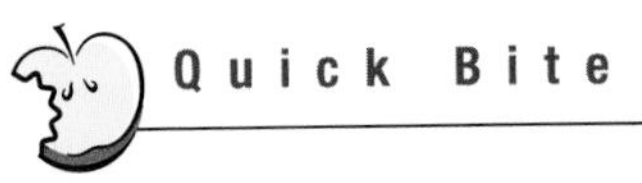

High-purine foods include

Red meats, especially organ meats
Anchovies
Sardines
Scallops

Recommendations for clients with uric acid stones are as follows:

- Low-purine diets are sometimes used in conjunction with medication but their benefits are unproven.
- Consume protein in moderation because high protein intakes acidify the urine. However, drugs are much more effective and consistent at lowering urinary pH.
- Limit alcohol.

How Do You Respond?

Does cranberry juice prevent urinary tract infections? Although conclusive evidence is lacking, it appears that cranberry juice is effective against urinary tract infections because it contains an ingredient that may prevent bacteria from adhering to the lining of the urinary tract, thereby promoting their excretion. However, not all bacteria are sensitive to the juice, and protection lasts only as long as the juice is consumed regularly. Clients who are prone to urinary tract infections and like cranberry juice should be encouraged to consume it regularly just in case. The only other dietary recommendation for urinary tract infections is to increase fluid intake to flush bacteria.

Are omega-3 fish oil supplements beneficial for people on hemodialysis? In addition to their cardioprotective effects, supplements of omega-3 fats have been shown to improve uremic pruritus, decrease vascular access graft thrombosis, and decrease the dose of erythropoietin needed to maintain hemoglobin level within the goal range for people on hemodialysis. The American Heart Association recommends people with or at risk of heart disease consume 1 g of EPA and DHA per day, but people on dialysis may need as much as 2 g daily. Future research may show that omega-3 from fish are equally effective as those from supplements. In the meantime, advise clients who want to use an omega-3 supplement, instead of increasing fish consumption, to first talk to their physician to determine the best dose for the individual. Caution them against using brands made from halibut and/or shark liver oils because they may contain toxic levels of vitamin A. Fish oil supplements should be stored in the refrigerator to avoid rancidity.

▲ Focus on Critical Thinking

Respond to the following statements:

1. For someone with ESRD, it is necessary to eat enough protein even if this means exceeding the phosphorus allowance.
2. For clients with pre-ESRD, it is better to eat too little protein than too much.
3. People with calcium kidney stones should limit calcium intake.

Key Concepts

- Loss of renal function profoundly affects metabolism, nutritional status, and nutritional requirements. The nutrients most affected are protein, calcium, phosphorus, vitamin D, fluid, sodium, and potassium.
- Diet modifications for renal disease are complex, unpalatable, and frequently adjusted according to the client's laboratory values and symptoms.

- Protein restriction remains the cornerstone of dietary treatment for pre-ESRD because limiting protein has the potential to lessen renal workload and slow disease progression.
- There is a narrow margin of error regarding protein intake: too little protein results in body protein catabolism, which has the same effect as eating too much protein, namely, an increase in BUN levels.
- A high-calorie diet is indicated whenever protein intake is restricted to ensure that the protein consumed will be used for specific protein functions, not for energy requirements.
- Usually clients with pre-ESRD need to limit phosphorus and, if blood pressure is a problem, sodium. Potassium is usually not restricted.
- Fluid allowance is based on urine output plus an additional 500 mL to 750 mL to account for insensible losses.
- Calcium metabolism is impaired because of faulty vitamin D metabolism, impaired intestinal absorption, and hyperphosphatemia as a result of loss of renal function. A high calcium intake from food is not achievable when phosphorus is restricted.
- When dialysis is instituted, dietary restrictions are liberalized; a high protein intake is recommended to compensate for protein lost through the dialysate.
- ARF represents an even greater nutritional challenge than CRF. Protein, sodium, potassium, phosphorus, and fluid are adjusted according to lab data, use of dialysis, renal function, and drug therapy.
- Clients who experience renal transplantation may need to alter their diets to lessen the side effects of immunosuppressant therapy. Steroids cause hyperglycemia, sodium retention, weight gain, potassium depletion, loss of calcium from the bones, and gastrointestinal upsets.
- A fluid intake of 3 L/day or more is the most effective nutritional intervention for the prevention of renal calculi.

ANSWER KEY

1. **TRUE** Early in the course of chronic renal disease, limiting protein may help to preserve kidney function but there are no guarantees and the optimal level of protein intake is not known.
2. **TRUE** Foods high in protein tend to be high in phosphorus. Other high-phosphorus foods include cola, chocolate, beer, bran, and bran cereal.
3. **FALSE** Although milk is an excellent source of high biologic value protein, it is high in phosphorus and so it can only be consumed in limited amounts (½ cup/day).
4. **FALSE** Some people with advanced renal failure are unable to conserve sodium, and a sodium deficit may occur if sodium intake is restricted.
5. **TRUE** People with chronic renal disease tend to have accelerated atherosclerosis and may benefit from eating more monounsaturated fat while restricting their intakes of saturated fat and cholesterol.
6. **TRUE** Dialysis causes protein requirements to increase about 50% above normal because proteins and amino acids are lost in the dialysis.

7. **TRUE** People receiving peritoneal dialysis may absorb 100 to 200 g of glucose from the dialysate, which is 340 to 680 calories.
8. **FALSE** Weight gain between dialysis treatments reflects fluid retention. Excessive weight gain between dialysis treatments means the intake of sodium and fluid are too high, not that calorie intake is too high.
9. **FALSE** Most people with hypercalciuria should consume 800 mg calcium/day. Restricting calcium intake does not decrease the risk of calcium stones because high calcium levels are maintained at the expense of bone. Dietary calcium may bind with oxalate in the GI tract to promote its excretion.
10. **TRUE** The most effective nutritional intervention to treat or prevent all types of renal stones is to increase fluid intake to dilute the urine. It also is the intervention clients are most likely to comply with.

WEBSITES

American Association of Kidney Patients at **www.aakp.org**
American Kidney Fund at **www.kidneyfund.org**
Kidney Information Clearinghouse at **www.renalnet.org**
National Institute of Diabetes and Digestive and Kidney Diseases at **www.niddk.nih.gov**
National Kidney Foundation at **www.kidney.org**
Nephron Information Center at **www.nephron.com**
www.ikidney.com

REFERENCES

American Kidney Fund. (2002). Public Information Series: Facts about kidney diseases and their treatment. Available at www.kidneyfund.org. Accessed on 1/28/04.
Chicago Dietetic Association, The South Suburban Dietetic Association, Dietitians of Canada. (2000). *Manual of clinical dietetics* (6th ed.). Chicago: American Dietetic Association.
Harum, P. (2002). Diet therapy goals. Is a low protein diet good for the management of nondialyzed chronic renal failure patients? Available at www.ikidney.com/iKidney/InfoCenter/NephrologyIncite/Archive. Accessed on 1/30/04.
Hasse, J., & Blue, L. (2002). *Comprehensive guide to transplant nutrition*. Chicago: American Dietetic Association.
Karalis, M. (2001). Everything you need to know about fluids . . . but were afraid to ask. Available at www.ikidney.com/iKidney/Lifestyles/NutritionalTipsHelpfulHints. Accessed on 1/30/04.
Karalis, M. (2000). Understanding the psychology of living on a renal diet. Available at www.ikidney.com/iKidney/Community/pro2Pro/Dietitians. Accessed on 1/30/04.
O'Connell, B. (2002). Eating right for healthy kidneys. Available at www.ikidney.com/iKidney/Lifestyles/NutritionalTips/JustDiagnosed. Accessed on 1/30/04.
Renal Dietitians Dietetic Practice Group of the American Dietetic Association. (2002). *National renal diet: Professional guide* (2nd ed.). Chicago: American Dietetic Association.
Vergili-Nelsen, J. (2003). Benefits of fish oil supplementation for hemodialysis patients. *Journal of the American Dietetic Association, 103,* 1174–1177.

For information on the new dietary guidelines 2005 and MyPyramid, visit **http://connection.lww.com/go/dudek**

21

Nutrition for Patients With Cancer or HIV/AIDS

TRUE	FALSE	
○	○	**1** Nutrition problems are not likely to develop until cancer metastasizes.
○	○	**2** Clients who are adequately nourished may be better able to withstand the effects of cancer treatment.
○	○	**3** Cachexia is directly related to the amount of calories consumed.
○	○	**4** The appetite of clients with anorexia tends to improve as the day progresses.
○	○	**5** The risk of nausea may be lessened by not eating 1 to 2 hours before chemotherapy and radiation.
○	○	**6** A cheese sandwich may be a better option than hot roast beef for someone with taste alterations.
○	○	**7** Lipodystrophy can be prevented with a low-fat diet.
○	○	**8** You can identify clients with HIV who are experiencing malabsorption because they have diarrhea.
○	○	**9** Clients with HIV/AIDS have problems with appetite and intake similar to those of cancer clients.
○	○	**10** Nutritional counseling of clients with HIV/AIDS should include how to avoid foodborne illnesses.

UPON COMPLETION OF THIS CHAPTER, YOU WILL BE ABLE TO

- Discuss how cancer and cancer therapies affect nutritional status.
- Describe nutritional interventions to minimize the following side effects: anorexia, nausea and vomiting, taste alterations, and sore mouth.
- Discuss three ways to increase a client's calorie and protein intake.
- Explain how HIV/AIDS affects nutritional status.
- Discuss nutrition therapy goals and interventions for clients with HIV/AIDS.

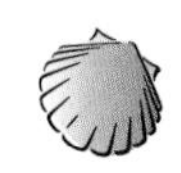

This chapter is devoted to cancer and acquired immunodeficiency syndrome (AIDS), two diseases characterized by body wasting and malnutrition. Although nutrition therapy cannot cure either disease, it has the potential to maximize the effectiveness of drug therapy, minimize side effects of the disease and its treatments, and improve overall quality of life.

NUTRITION AND CANCER

The relationships among diet, nutritional status, and cancer are complex and multifaceted. As discussed in Chapter 8, approximately 35% of all cancer deaths are related to dietary factors. Some components of food may promote cancer and others may help to prevent cancer promotion. For people who have cancer and are being aggressively treated, nutrition intervention can help to maintain weight and nutritional status and, therefore, has the potential to reduce the risk of side effects, optimize the chance for successful cancer treatment, and decrease morbidity and mortality. Conversely, poor nutrition can lead to malnutrition, which may increase the severity of side effects and decreases the chance of survival. For the terminally ill, palliative nutrition may improve quality of life and enhance the client's sense of well-being.

Effect of Cancer on Nutritional Status

Cancer and its treatments can have profound and devastating effects on nutritional status, leading to protein–calorie malnutrition, the most common secondary diagnosis in cancer patients. Protein–calorie malnutrition is a major cause of morbidity and mortality. Moreover, cancer patients identify nutrition problems as the most important factor affecting their sense of well-being, more important than sexuality or continued employment.

Local Effects

Local tumor effects produce many nutritional problems. Most notably, growing tumors of the gastrointestinal tract can cause obstruction, nausea, vomiting, impaired digestion, delayed transit, and malabsorption. Ascites related to ovarian and genitourinary cancers may lead to early satiety, progressive protein malnutrition, and fluid and electrolyte imbalances. Pain related to tumor bulk or location may cause severe anorexia and poor oral intake. Tumors of the central nervous system that cause confusion or somnolence may lead to poor intake related to poor attention. Other potential problems vary with the cancer location (Table 21.1).

Systemic Effects

Cancer causes systemic nutritional problems by altering body metabolism. Although metastatic cancers may produce more pronounced changes, even localized cancers can

TABLE 21.1 **POTENTIAL LOCAL EFFECTS OF CANCER ON NUTRITION**

Cancer Location	Potential Impact on Nutrition
Head and neck	Difficulty chewing and swallowing
Esophagus	Dysphagia related to obstruction GERD
Stomach	Fluid and electrolyte imbalance related to vomiting Early satiety
Small bowel	Maldigestion and malabsorption Protein-losing enteropathy related to lymphatic obstruction within the intestinal villi Bowel obstruction
Colon	Malabsorption Bowel obstruction
Liver	Watery diarrhea related to an increase in serotonin, histamines, and other substances
Pancreatic cancer	Maldigestion and malabsorption Diabetes
CNS	Dysphagia

produce generalized effects. Metabolic alterations include increased energy expenditure, increased protein catabolism and whole-body protein turnover (reuse of amino acids that are generated by protein metabolism), increased lipolysis, and preferential use of fat as an energy source. In addition, tumors can produce hormone-like substances that alter nutrient absorption and metabolism. Other substances produced by cancer cells may alter sense of taste, promote anorexia, or contribute to cancer cachexia.

Cancer Cachexia

Cachexia: a wasting syndrome marked by weakness and progressive loss of body weight, fat, and muscle.

Cachexia is estimated to cause 20% to 40% of cancer deaths. It is characterized by early satiety, anorexia, anemia, loss of immunocompetence, and severe weight loss, which is defined as an unintentional loss of 10% or more of body weight within 6 months. Cachexia diminishes quality of life, impairs wound healing, increases the risk of infection, and increases the risk of mortality.

The etiology of cachexia is not completely understood. It does not appear to be directly related to tumor size, type, or extent, although people with GI cancers are at particular risk for cachexia. Also, cachexia is not simply a matter of inadequate intake: it can develop in people who appear to be consuming adequate calories and protein, but because of the disease, are malabsorbing nutrients. Unlike simple starvation, to which the body adapts by lowering metabolic rate, the metabolic rate in cachexia is not adaptive and may increase, decrease, or be normal. Altered metabolism and factors produced by the tumor are among the several factors suspected of contributing to the development of cachexia (Fig. 21.1). Because factors other than inadequate intake are involved, aggressive nutritional intervention does not ensure a cure. Because cachexia

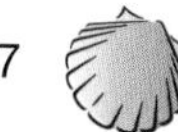

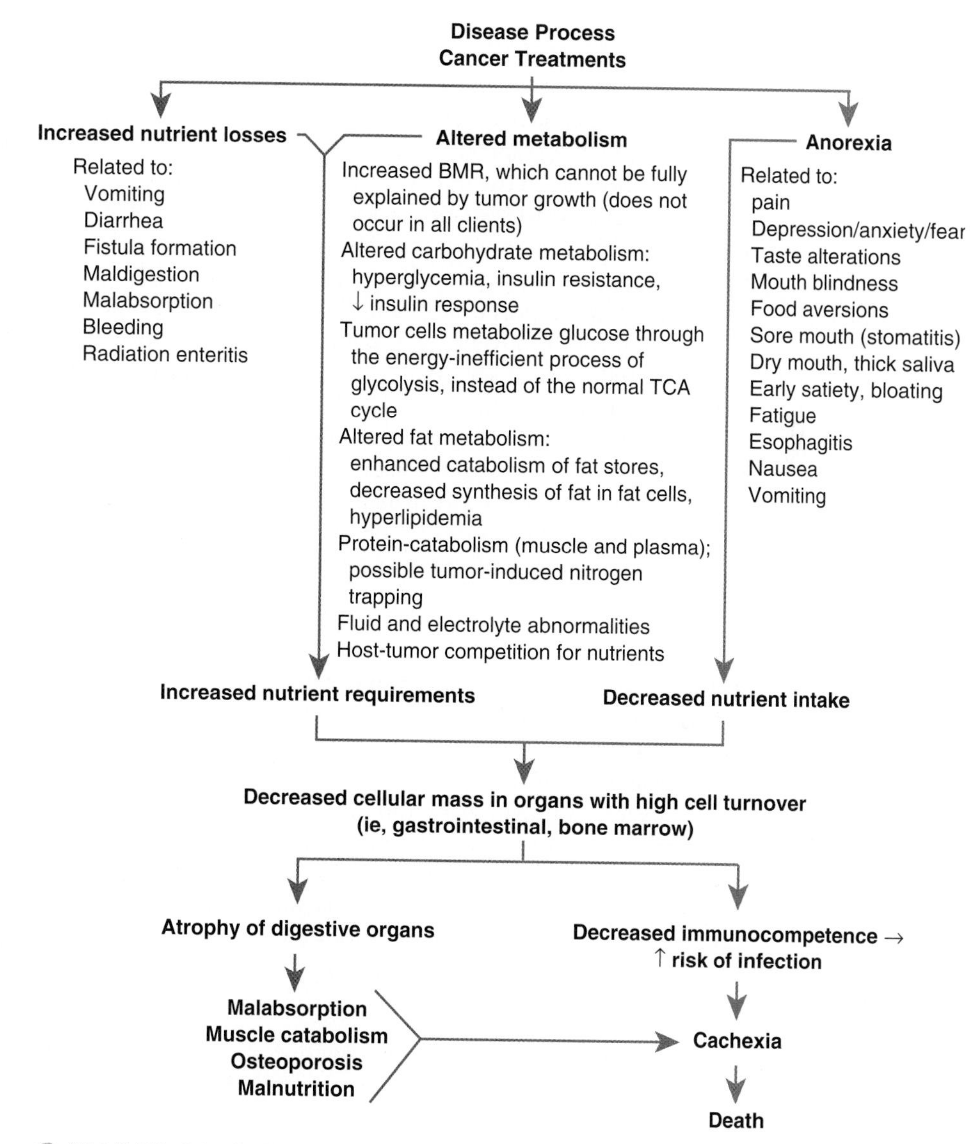

FIGURE 21.1 Factors contributing to cachexia.

is easier to prevent than to treat, nutritional support should be initiated before the downward spiral of malnutrition develops.

Effect of Cancer Therapies on Nutritional Status

Cancer may be treated with surgery, chemotherapy, radiation, immunotherapy, or a combination of therapies. Some hematologic cancers are treated by bone marrow transplantation. Each treatment modality can contribute to progressive nutritional deterioration related to systemic or localized side effects that interfere with intake, increase nutrient losses, or alter metabolism. Actual response to each therapy depends on the individual and the type and extent of treatment.

Nutritional support used as an adjuvant to effective cancer therapy helps to sustain the client through adverse side effects and may reduce morbidity and mortality. Nutrition therapy can reverse weight loss, restore or maintain immunocompetence, help to restore normal metabolism, enhance tolerance for antineoplastic therapy, maintain body composition during nutritional repletion, and reduce postoperative morbidity. However, for nutritional support to improve the results of cancer therapy, the therapy itself must have a reasonable chance of success. Evidence suggests that aggressive nutritional support may be of little value or even detrimental when it is used in conjunction with ineffective cancer treatment.

Surgery

Surgery is often the primary treatment for cancer; approximately 60% of people diagnosed with cancer undergo some type of cancer-related surgery. People who are malnourished prior to surgery are at higher risk of morbidity and mortality. If time allows, nutritional deficiencies are corrected prior to surgery.

Postsurgical nutritional requirements increase for protein, calories, vitamin C, B vitamins, and iron to replenish losses and promote healing. Physiological or mechanical barriers to good nutrition can occur depending on the type of surgery, with the greatest likelihood of complications arising from GI surgeries. Table 21.2 outlines potential side effects and complications incurred for various types of surgery.

Chemotherapy

More than 90 different chemotherapy drugs are approved for use in the U.S. Given alone or in combination, chemotherapy drugs damage the reproductive ability of both malignant and normal cells, especially rapidly dividing cells such as well-nourished cancer cells and normal cells of the gastrointestinal tract, respiratory system, bone marrow, skin, and gonadal tissue. Cyclic administration of multiple drugs is given in maximum tolerated doses. See the Supplement Alert later in the chapter for a list of herbal products that may interfere with the metabolism of drugs.

The side effects of chemotherapy vary with the type of drug or combination of drugs used, dose, rate of excretion, duration of treatment, and individual tolerance. Chemotherapy side effects are systemic and, therefore, potentially more numerous than

 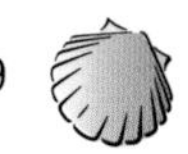

TABLE 21.2 POTENTIAL COMPLICATIONS OF SURGERY

Type	Potential Complications
Head and neck resection	Difficulty chewing and swallowing Tube feeding dependency
Esophagectomy or esophageal resection	Early satiety Regurgitation Fistula formation Stenosis Vagotomy →decreased stomach motility, decreased gastric acid production, diarrhea, steatorrhea
Gastric resection	"Dumping syndrome": crampy diarrhea that develops quickly after eating; accompanied by flushing, dizziness, weakness, pain, distention, and vomiting Hypoglycemia Esophagitis Decreased gastric motility Fat malabsorption and diarrhea Deficiencies in iron, calcium, and fat-soluble vitamins Vitamin B_{12} malabsorption related to lack of intrinsic factor
Intestinal resection	Malnutrition related to generalized malabsorption Fluid and electrolyte imbalance Diarrhea Increased risk of renal oxalate stone formation and increased excretion of calcium Metabolic acidosis
Massive bowel resection	Steatorrhea Malnutrition related to severe generalized malabsorption Metabolic acidosis Dehydration
Ileostomy or colostomy	Fluid and electrolyte imbalance
Pancreatic resection	Generalized malabsorption Diabetes mellitus

the localized effects seen with surgery or radiation. The most commonly experienced nutrition-related side effects are anorexia, fatigue, nausea and vomiting, taste alterations or aversions, sore mouth or throat, diarrhea, early satiety, and constipation. Side effects increase the risk of malnutrition and weight loss, which may prolong recovery time between treatments. When subsequent chemotherapy treatments are delayed, successful treatment outcome is potentially threatened.

Radiation

Radiation causes cell death; particles of radioactive energy break chemical bonds, disrupting reproductive ability. Although radiation injures all rapidly dividing cells, it is most lethal for the poorly differentiated and rapidly proliferating cells of cancer tissue. Recovery from sublethal doses of radiation occurs in the interval between the first dose and subsequent doses. Normal tissue appears to recover more quickly from radiation damage than cancerous tissue does.

Side effects are specific for the area irradiated, usually develop around the second or third week of treatment, then diminish 2 or 3 weeks after radiation therapy is completed.

The type and intensity of radiation side effects depend on the type of radiation used, the site, the volume of tissue irradiated, the dose of radiation, the duration of therapy, and individual tolerance. Patients most at risk for nutrition-related side effects are those who have cancers of the head and neck, lungs, esophagus, cervix, uterus, colon, rectum, and pancreas. Potential complications of radiation are shown in Table 21.3. Nutrition intervention is directed toward alleviating symptoms. Patients who are well nourished are better able to withstand the side effects of treatment.

TABLE 21.3 **POTENTIAL COMPLICATIONS OF RADIATION**

Area	Potential Complications
Head and neck	Altered or loss of taste ("mouth blindness") Xerostomia (dry mouth) Thick salivary secretions Difficulty swallowing and chewing Loss of teeth Mucositis Stomatitis
Lower neck and midchest	Acute: esophagitis with dysphagia Delayed: fibrosis, esophageal stricture, dysphagia Nausea Edema
Abdomen and pelvis	Extensive radiation to upper or middle abdomen may → nausea and vomiting Acute or chronic bowel damage → cramps, steatorrhea, malabsorption, disaccharidase deficiency, protein-losing enteropathy, bowel constriction, obstruction, or fistula formation Chronic blood loss from intestine and bladder Pelvic radiation → increased urinary frequency, urgency, and dysuria
CNS	Nausea Dysgeusia

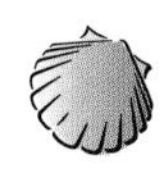

Immunotherapy

Immunotherapy seeks to enhance the body's immune system to help control cancer. Potential adverse effects include fever, which increases protein and calorie requirements, and nausea, vomiting, and diarrhea. Impaired intake can lead to malnutrition, which can interfere with healing and recovery.

Bone Marrow Transplantation

Bone marrow transplantation is used primarily to treat hematologic cancers. Bone marrow transplantation is preceded by high-dose chemotherapy and possibly total-body irradiation to suppress immune function and destroy cancer cells. Nutritional side effects arise from high-dose chemotherapy, total body irradiation, and immunosuppressants, which are given before and after the procedure. Anorexia, taste alterations, nausea, vomiting, oral dryness, thick saliva, constipation, mucositis, stomatitis, esophagitis, and intestinal damage that causes severe diarrhea and malabsorption are reported. Neutropenia leaves the patient susceptible to infection, so precautionary measures must be taken to prevent foodborne illness (Box 21.1). Total parenteral nutrition (TPN) may be needed for 1 to 2 months after bone marrow transplantation.

Nutrition Therapy in Cancer Treatment

The needs of cancer clients change as they move along the continuum of recovery. For instance, clients in the first phase, the initial period after diagnosis that may include surgery, may not need specific information about what to eat. They may not have experienced any side effects of cancer that interfere with intake or nutritional status. Advice that may or may not be needed in 6 months is inappropriate for a client who

BOX 21.1

STRATEGIES TO REDUCE THE RISK OF FOODBORNE ILLNESS

- Wash hands before and after handling food and eating and after using the restroom.
- Cook all meat, fish, and poultry to the well-done stage.
- Do not eat raw or uncooked eggs such as soft boiled eggs, "over easy" eggs, or Caesar salads with raw eggs in the dressing.
- Do not eat sushi, raw seafood, raw meats, or unpasteurized milk or dairy products.
- Do not drink water unless it is known to be safe.
- Refrigerate foods immediately after purchase.
- Wash fruits and vegetables thoroughly in clean water.
- Refrigerate leftovers immediately after eating; thoroughly reheat before eating.
- Discard leftovers after 3 days.
- Avoid cross-contamination by using separate cutting boards and work surfaces for raw meats and poultry; keep work surfaces clean.
- Keep hot foods >140°F and cold food <40°F.
- Use expiration dates on food packaging to discard foods that may be unsafe to eat.

feels overwhelmed by the task of coming to terms with a cancer diagnosis. Side effects appear in the next phase as the client undergoes treatment. During this phase, some clients believe there is nothing food or nutrition therapy can do to help them feel better. At the other end of the spectrum are clients who believe dietary changes can cure, arrest, or treat their disease. The goal is to get clients to the middle ground, where they feel empowered with the sense that they can take an active role in their own recovery. Finally, the long-term recovery phase begins as the client resumes a normal intake. Acute care needs transition into long-term goals of optimal nutrition for health and well-being and secondary cancer prevention.

Nutrition Goals

Career Connection

Loss of dignity and control, change in sexuality and body image, and loss of appetite can create a frustrating, seemingly hopeless situation for the client; food may be used to express anger and resentment. Think beyond the nutritional value of food:

- **Allow the client and family to verbalize feelings; emphasize a positive, supportive, team-effort approach.**
- **Although the client may need the encouragement and support of family and friends, putting them in a position of "force-feeding" the client may add tension to an already stressful situation.**
- **Encourage the client to be an active participant in his/her nutritional care. For instance,the client and the health care team may "contract" for an acceptable amount of weight loss. As long as the client does not lose more weight than was agreed on, the client is in charge of his or her own nutritional care.**

Regardless of whether or not the patient is undergoing active therapy, recovering from therapy, or in remission, the benefits of consuming adequate calories and nutrients are well documented. Used as an adjunct to cancer treatment, the goals of aggressive nutrition intervention are to

- Prevent or correct nutrient deficiencies
- Preserve lean body mass
- Optimize tolerance to treatment
- Minimize nutrition-related side effects
- Maintain strength and energy
- Improve immunocompetence
- Promote wound healing
- Maximize quality of life

In cases where nutrition therapy cannot achieve weight gain, nutrition therapy may help to

- Lessen side effects
- Reduce risk of infection

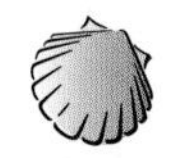

- Reduce asthenia
- Improve sense of well-being

For people with terminal cancer, the focus of nutrition is comfort and relief of side effects.

Nutrient Needs

A "typical" cancer client does not exist. Whereas some clients present with weight loss and malnutrition at the time of cancer diagnosis, others are well nourished and asymptomatic. The course of treatment may be aggressive or palliative; it may include surgery, chemotherapy, radiation or a combination of treatments. The effect on nutritional status and intake may be mild or dramatic. As such, a standard "cancer" diet does not exist; nutrient needs are highly individualized and are not static. Factors to consider when determining the client's nutritional needs are

- Client's age
- Actual weight, recent weight changes
- Current intake
- Pre-existing medical conditions
- Presence and severity of side effects
- Client's ability to perform activities of daily living and participate in physical activity
- Physical signs of malnutrition such as loss of subcutaneous fat and wasting
- Laboratory values that may indicate protein malnutrition such as albumin, prealbumin, and serum transferrin
- Serum electrolyte and mineral levels such as sodium, potassium, magnesium, and calcium

A regular diet is used as a starting point and individualized as needed, such as increasing protein and calories, instituting interventions to alleviate side effects, and changing the method of feeding.

Increasing Protein and Calories

Usually, a high-protein diet of 1.5 to 2.0 g/kg is prescribed to prevent body protein catabolism or replenish lean tissue. Calorie needs range from 25 to 35 cal/kg for weight maintenance to 40 to 50 cal/kg to replenish body stores. Although it is commonly assumed that all cancer clients develop anorexia and cachexia, weight gain is a common side effect of chemotherapy for breast cancer. Calories and protein are adjusted to meet the individual's needs.

An increase in protein and calories can be achieved by having the client

- Eat more food, which is not a realistic option for most people experiencing side effects of cancer or cancer treatments.
- Eat food that has been modified to be more protein- and calorie-dense. This approach can be effective if the client or caregiver understands how to modify a variety of foods, but may not be consistently achieved. Suggestions for increasing protein and calorie density appear in Box 21.2.

BOX 21.2

WAYS TO INCREASE THE PROTEIN AND CALORIE DENSITY OF FOODS

To Increase Protein and Calories

- Add skim milk powder to milk to make double-strength milk; chill well before serving.
- Use double-strength milk on hot or cold cereals and in scrambled eggs, soups, gravies, casseroles, milk shakes, and milk-based desserts.
- Substitute whole milk for water in recipes.
- Add grated cheese to soups, casseroles, vegetable dishes, rice, and noodles.
- Use peanut butter as a spread on slices of apple, banana, pear, crackers, or waffles; use as a filling for celery.
- Add finely chopped, hard-cooked eggs to sauces, soups, and casseroles.
- Choose desserts made with eggs or milk such as sponge cake, angel food cake, custard, and puddings.
- Dip meat, poultry, and fish in eggs or milk and coat with bread or cereal crumbs before baking, broiling, or pan frying.
- Use yogurt as a topping for fruit, plain cakes, or other desserts; use in gravies and dips.

To Increase Calories

- Mix cream cheese with butter and spread on hot bread and rolls.
- Whenever possible, add butter to hot foods: breads, pancakes, waffles, soups, vegetables, potatoes, cooked cereal, rice, and pasta.
- Substitute mayonnaise for salad dressing in salads, eggs, casseroles, and sandwiches.
- Add dried fruit, nuts, or granola to desserts and cereal.
- Use whipped cream on pies, fruit, pudding, gelatin, ice cream, and other desserts and in coffee, tea, and hot chocolate.
- Use marshmallows in hot chocolate, on fruit, and in desserts.
- Top baked potatoes, vegetables, and fruits with sour cream.
- Snack frequently on nuts, dried fruit, candy, buttered popcorn, cheese, granola, and ice cream.
- Use honey on toast, cereal, and fruit and in coffee and tea.

- Consume high-protein, high-calorie nutritional supplements. This strategy is the easiest and most consistent way to achieve a high-calorie, high-protein intake. Supplements may be consumed between meals and as meal replacements if necessary. Products like Ensure and Boost come in high-protein and high-calorie versions and in a variety of flavors to help reduce taste fatigue. Serving them over ice may improve acceptance. Promote is a high-protein, bland-tasting option for clients who dislike the sweetness of other products. Instant breakfast mix is a less expensive option for at-home use for clients who are not lactose intolerant. Because taste varies considerably among products, encourage clients to try a variety.

Minimizing Side Effects

Alleviating eating problems is paramount to promoting an adequate intake. Modifications in texture, temperature, and eating schedule, as well as administering medications to control side effects, may optimize intake.

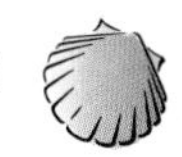

Anorexia

Anorexia, which may be continuous or sporadic, is among the most common symptoms in people with cancer. Appetite is often best in the morning and deteriorates gradually throughout the day. A major cause of anorexia is food odor. To limit the client's exposure to food odors in the hospital, remove the tray cover before the tray is placed in front of the client so that food odors can dissipate. The following tips may help to manage anorexia:

- Overeat during "good" days.
- Eat a high-protein, high-calorie, nutrient-dense breakfast if appetite is best in the morning.
- Eat small, frequent meals (e.g., every 2 hours by the clock).
- Limit low-calorie and empty-calorie items such as carbonated beverages.
- Increase the nutrient density of foods by adding butter, skim milk powder, peanut butter, cheese, honey, or brown sugar.
- Limit liquids with meals to avoid early satiety and bloating at mealtime.
- Use liquid supplements (instant breakfast mixes, milk shakes, commercial supplements) in place of meals when appetite deteriorates or the client is too tired to eat.
- Enhance appetite with light exercise, a glass of wine or beer if not contraindicated, and the use of appetite stimulants.
- Make eating a pleasant experience by eating in a bright, cheerful environment, playing soft music, and enjoying the company of friends or family.
- Experiment with recipes, flavorings, spices, and the consistency of food. Preferences may change daily.
- Avoid strong food odors if they contribute to anorexia. Cook outdoors on a grill, serve cold foods rather than hot foods, or use takeout meals that do not need to be prepared at home.
- Use appropriate medications to control pain, nausea, and depression.

Nausea and Vomiting

Nausea and vomiting occur as a result of cancer and cancer therapies especially chemotherapy. Acute nausea and vomiting can develop within 2 hours after drug administration and may last up to 24 hours. Some drugs can produce delayed nausea and vomiting beyond the day of chemotherapy, which may last for 3 to 5 days or even up to 3 weeks. Rarely, nausea and vomiting persist from one cycle of chemotherapy to the next. Clients who have poor control of emesis may experience anticipatory nausea and vomiting. Nausea may persist even after vomiting is controlled, and it can have a more devastating impact on quality of life. Long-term survival may be affected if the client refuses or postpones chemotherapy treatments because of nausea and vomiting.

Anticipatory Nausea and Vomiting: nausea and vomiting that occur before or during chemotherapy, at a time when symptoms normally would not be expected.

The following tips may help to manage nausea:

- Eat foods served cold or at room temperature because hot foods may contribute to nausea.
- Eat high-carbohydrate, low-fat foods such as toast, crackers, yogurt, sherbet, cooked cereal, soft or canned fruits, watermelon, bananas, fruit juices, and angel food cake.
- Avoid fatty, greasy, fried, or strongly seasoned foods.

- Keep track of and avoid foods that cause nausea.
- To decrease the likelihood of nausea, avoid eating 1 to 2 hours before chemotherapy or radiotherapy.
- Take antiemetics as prescribed even when symptoms are absent.

Fatigue

Fatigue is one of the most distressing side effects of both chemotherapy and radiation. It differs from fatigue in healthy people in that it is more intense, persists longer, and it is not relieved by sleep. It tends to peak within a few days after chemotherapy, then declines until the next treatment, when the cycle repeats itself. Fatigue significantly impairs quality of life by decreasing mental activity, work capacity, and activities of daily living. Recognizing their decline in function, clients may feel hopelessness and despair. Clients are often too tired to eat, and food purchasing and preparation may be exhausting. Fatigue impairs intake, and poor intake exacerbates fatigue.

The following tips may help to manage fatigue:

- Encourage a good breakfast because fatigue may worsen as the day progresses.
- Engage in regular exercise if possible.
- Consume easy-to-eat foods that can be prepared with a minimal amount of effort.
- Drink oral supplements between meals or as a meal replacement as necessary.
- Use convenience foods and labor-saving appliances (e.g., blender, Crock-Pot, toaster oven, microwave oven, dishwasher).
- Drink adequate fluids because chronic dehydration contributes to fatigue.
- Assistance may be available from Meals On Wheels or other community services.

Taste Changes

Taste changes may result from cancer or cancer treatments. Radiation-induced taste alterations usually develop by the third week of therapy and return to normal within 1 year.

Clients who experience taste changes are more likely to lose weight. Conversely, clients who lose weight may be more likely to develop taste alterations. Elemental zinc has been shown to correct taste abnormalities. If prescribed, zinc should be taken with food or milk to decrease the risk of gastrointestinal irritation. The most common taste changes are a decreased threshold for urea (bitter) and an increased threshold for sucrose (sweet). The following tips may help to manage taste changes:

- Suck on hard candy during therapy if chemotherapy causes a bitter or metallic taste.
- Use plastic utensils and dishes.
- Encourage drinking fluids with meals to reduce unpleasant tastes.
- Tart foods such as citrus juices, cranberry juice, pickles, or relishes may help to overcome metallic taste.
- Practice good oral hygiene before eating to eliminate unpleasant tastes.
- Experiment with a variety of seasonings especially if the oral mucosa is not impaired.
- Avoid anything that tastes unpleasant.
- Meats may be better tolerated if served cold or at room temperature or if highly flavored with strong seasonings, sweet marinades, or sauces such as cranberry sauce, jelly, or applesauce.

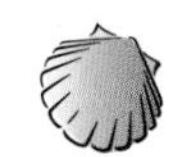

- If red meats (beef and pork) have a "bad," "rotten," or "fecal" taste, eat other high-protein foods such as eggs, cheese, mild fish, nuts, and dried peas and beans. If those sources are not tolerated, milk shakes, eggnogs, puddings, ice cream, and commercial supplements can provide sufficient protein and calories.
- Add the juice from half of a freshly squeezed lemon to commercial supplements to lessen excessive sweetness and bitter aftertaste that affects people with cancer.
- Add a pinch of salt to decrease the sweetness of sugary foods.
- Serve attractively presented food in a bright, cheerful environment.

Food Aversions

Food aversions may be intermittent or may worsen as the day progresses. To avoid learned aversions, instruct the client to avoid his or her favorite foods or fast completely before receiving radiation or chemotherapy. If nausea and vomiting tend to occur at about the same time each day, withholding food beforehand may help to avoid learned aversions.

Sore Mouth (Stomatitis)

Stomatitis may produce taste alterations, mouth blindness, or the association between eating and pain. Analgesics (as prescribed) before meals reduce pain associated with eating. Stomatitis also increases susceptibility to *Candida albicans* infections, which may cause ulcerated white or yellow patches on the oral mucosa and further diminish taste sensation. The following tips may help to manage stomatitis:

- Practice good oral hygiene (thorough cleaning with a soft-bristle toothbrush or cotton swabs plus frequent mouth rinses with normal saline and water or baking soda and water). Commercial mouthwashes containing alcohol may irritate and burn the oral mucosa.
- Cut food into small portions.
- Avoid spices, acidic foods, coarse foods, salty foods, alcohol, and smoking that can aggravate an already irritated oral mucosa.
- Eat a soft or liquid bland diet, drink plenty of fluids, and avoid hot foods and beverages. Try mashed potatoes, macaroni and cheese, scrambled eggs, and cooked cereals.
- Cold items may help to numb the oral mucosa. Try frozen bananas, applesauce, canned fruit, watermelon, cottage cheese, yogurt, ice cream, puddings, custards, and instant breakfast mixes.
- Straws may ease swallowing.
- Avoid wearing ill-fitting dentures.

Dry Mouth or Thick Saliva

Clients with decreased saliva production are susceptible to dental caries. Encourage good oral hygiene, frequent mouth rinsing, and the avoidance of concentrated sweets. Provide mouth care immediately before mealtime for added moisture. The following tips may help to manage dry mouth:

- Take small bites and chew food thoroughly.
- Avoid dry, coarse foods.
- Eat soft or moist foods (e.g., foods with gravies or sauces).

- Avoid foods that stick to the roof of the mouth such as peanut butter.
- Drink high-calorie, high-protein liquids between meals.
- Sugar-free fluids containing citric acid such as lemonade, frozen juice bars, and sherbet, may help to stimulate secretions.
- Use ice chips and sugar-free hard candies and gum between meals to relieve dryness.
- Artificial saliva and the use of straws may facilitate swallowing. Petroleum jelly applied to the lips may help to prevent drying.

Diarrhea

Diarrhea may occur secondary to radiation, chemotherapy, GI surgery, or emotional distress. Complications include dehydration, hyponatremia, and hypokalemia. Antidiarrheals should be used shortly before a meal. The following tips may help to manage diarrhea:

- Replace fluid and electrolytes with broth, soups, sports drinks, and canned fruit.
- Limit caffeine, hot or cold liquids, and high-fat foods because they aggravate diarrhea.
- Avoid gassy foods and liquids such as dried peas and beans, cruciferous vegetables, carbonated beverages, and chewing gum.
- Foods high in pectin and other soluble fibers such as oatmeal, cooked carrots, bananas, peeled apples, and applesauce, may help to slow transit time.
- Avoid artificially sweetened candy or gum containing sorbitol.
- Drink fluid throughout the day and at least 1 cup after each loose bowel movement.
- Unless tolerance to lactose has been confirmed, limit or avoid milk.

Method of Feeding

For both physiologic and psychological reasons, an oral diet is preferred whenever possible. When oral intake is inadequate or contraindicated, enteral or parenteral nutrition can be a safe and effective way to nourish critically ill cancer patients who cannot consume an adequate oral intake. A client may be a candidate for nutrition support if one or more of the following criteria are met:

- Weight of <80% of ideal or a recent unintentional weight loss of >10% of usual weight
- Malabsorption of nutrients related to disease, short bowel syndrome, or cancer treatments
- Fistulas or draining abscesses
- Inability to eat or drink for > 5 days
- Moderate or high nutritional risk as determined by nutritional screening or assessment
- Client or caregiver demonstrate competency in nutrition support for discharge planning

Nutritional support can improve nutritional status and quality of life and therefore may prevent disruptions in treatment schedule that could potentially impact treatment out-

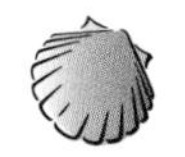

come. What is not known is whether or not nutritional support improves survival; the debate regarding the effect of nutrition support on tumor growth continues. The advantages and disadvantages of nutritional support, as well as individual considerations that include diagnosis, prognosis, degree of malnutrition, and GI function, must be thoroughly evaluated. Table 21.4 summarizes benefits, indications, and contraindications of nutrition support for cancer patients. For more on enteral and parenteral nutrition, see Chapter 15.

TABLE 21.4 **BENEFITS, INDICATIONS, AND CONTRAINDICATIONS WITH ENTERAL AND PARENTERAL NUTRITION SUPPORT**

	Enteral Nutrition Support	Parenteral Nutrition Support
Benefits	Uses gut Fewer complications Easier to administer than parenteral nutrition Less costly than parenteral nutrition	Can provide adequate nutrition when oral and enteral modes are contraindicated or inadequate
Indications	GI cancers Severe complications that jeopardize treatment in an already malnourished patient	Nonfunctional GI tract Severe diarrhea/ malabsorption Severe mucositis or esophagitis High-output GI fistulas that cannot be bypassed by enteral intubation Severe preoperative malnutrition
Contraindications	Nonfunctional GI tract Malabsorption disorders Mechanical obstructions Severe bleeding Severe diarrhea Intractable vomiting GI fistulas that preclude tube placement Prolonged ileus Prognosis not consistent with aggressive nutrition therapy	Functional GI tract Need for support for <5 days Inability to obtain IV access Poor prognosis not consistent with aggressive nutrition therapy Additional relative contraindications are that the patient does not want parenteral nutrition, the patient is hemodynamically unstable, profound metabolic and/or electrolyte abnormalities exist, and/or the patient is anuric without dialysis.

Career Connection

Supportive measures for palliative nutrition therapy include

- Controlling unpleasant side effects, such as pain, constipation, nausea, vomiting, and heartburn, with medication
- Respecting the client's wishes regarding the level of nutritional support desired
- Providing adequate mouth care to control dryness and thirst
- Respecting the client's personal tastes and preferences
- Ensuring a pleasant eating environment and serving attractive food
- Serving food of appropriate textures
- Using a team approach that includes physician, dietitian, and nurse

Palliative Nutrition Therapy

For clients whose prognosis is terminal, the value of nutritional support is a controversial ethical issue. No benefit is derived from aggressively feeding a client whose cancer is not being treated because both body weight gain and tumor growth are stimulated. Instead, nutrition should be maintained as an integral component of palliative care, with the goals of providing comfort and improving the quality of life. Eating should be encouraged as a source of pleasure, not as an adjunct to treatment. The client's requests and preferences are more important than the nutritional quality of the diet.

Nutritional Supplements

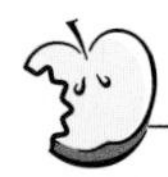

Quick Bite

Legitimate clinical trials are underway to test the effectiveness of nutritional supplements as an adjunct to traditional cancer treatments, such as

Shark cartilage in patients receiving chemotherapy and radiation therapy who have non-small cell lung cancer that cannot be surgically removed
Mistletoe extract with chemotherapy for the treatment of solid tumors
Fish oils to enhance the ability of radiation to kill cancer cells while reducing side effects
Milk thistle to reduce liver damage in children receiving chemotherapy for acute lymphoblastic leukemia

People faced with a cancer diagnosis are desperate to do whatever it takes to eradicate the disease. Nutritional supplements, such as vitamins and herbs, are often perceived to be a potentially beneficial, non-risky option that may improve quality of life, enhance immune system functioning, relieve symptoms, or even cure the dis-

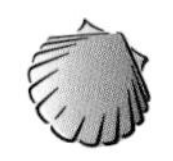

ease. It is estimated that approximately 63% of people with cancer use nutritional supplements.

At this time, few clinical studies have been conducted to confirm the benefits or dangers of using supplements as part of cancer treatment or prevention. For instance, although there is growing evidence that plants may help to protect against cancer, exactly which compounds are beneficial and in what amounts are not known. A case in point is that although populations with a high intake of beta-carotene rich foods have lower rates of lung cancer, a clinical study testing beta-carotene supplements in smokers had to be halted because the supplements actually *increased* the rate of lung cancer. Supplements can alter liver enzyme activity and so influence the metabolism of drugs, including chemotherapy drugs (see Supplement Alert). Supplements should not be assumed to be safe or beneficial simply because they are "natural," and clients should be encouraged to discuss supplements with their physician before using them.

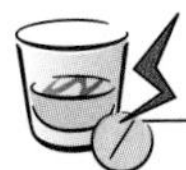

SUPPLEMENT ALERT

Some herbs alter the metabolism of drugs. When herbs increase the metabolism of drugs, blood concentration is less than anticipated and effectiveness is reduced. When drug metabolism is decreased, an increase in blood concentration can lead to toxicity or increased side effects.

The following herbs may cause increased blood levels of certain drugs:
- Siberian Ginseng
- Goldenseal
- Turmeric
- Milk thistle

The following herbs may render certain drugs less effective:
- Garlic
- St. John's Wort

Prevention of Secondary Cancers

After successful treatment of cancer, the focus of nutrition shifts from "getting enough" to establishing healthy eating practices consistent with dietary recommendations designed to reduce the risk of cancer in the general public. Prevention strategies recommended by the American Cancer Society are to

- Eat a variety of healthy foods with an emphasis on plant sources.
- Eat five or more servings of a variety of fruits and vegetables daily.
- Choose whole grains over processed, refined grains and sugars.
- Limit consumption of red meats, especially processed meats and high fat meat.

- Choose foods to help maintain a healthy weight.
- Drink alcohol only in moderation, if at all.

The American Institute of Cancer Research has issued similar recommendations but advocates 5 to 10 daily servings of fruits and vegetables. Additional recommendations are to chose foods low in salt and to prepare and store food safely. Although following these recommendations may reduce the risk of cancer, it does not guarantee cancer prevention. See Chapter 8 for the role of nutrition in cancer prevention.

NURSING PROCESS

Karen is a 59-year-old reformed smoker who now calls herself a "health nut." She was recently diagnosed with lung cancer. She had surgery to remove her right lung and is now receiving chemotherapy for cancerous "spots" on the left lung and stomach. She has lost 28 pounds and complains of nausea, vomiting, and a bad taste in her mouth. Because she has followed an "anticancer" diet for years, she is reluctant to now change her eating habits and eat more protein, fat, and calories. She eats mostly fruit, sherbet, and skim milk.

Assessment

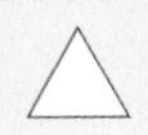

Obtain Clinical Data:

Height, current weight, body mass index (BMI), usual weight, rate of weight loss

Medical history such as diabetes, heart disease, or hypertension

Types of drugs the client is receiving through chemotherapy; other prescribed medications that affect nutrition

Physician's goals and plan of treatment

Laboratory data: serum albumin, serum transferrin, thyroxine-bound prealbumin, retinol-binding protein, serum electrolytes, and other abnormal values. Nitrogen balance study, if available.

Fluid intake and output

Interview the Client to Assess:

Usual 24-hour intake, portion sizes, frequency and pattern of eating, food aversions, daily fluid intake

Pattern of nausea and vomiting. Determine how the client has coped with nausea, vomiting, and taste changes.

Understanding of increased nutritional needs related to cancer and cancer therapies

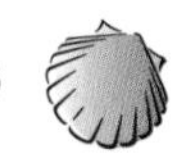

Willingness to change her attitudes toward food and nutrition
Cultural, religious, and ethnic influences on eating habits
Psychosocial and economic issues such as financial status, employment, and outside support system
Usual activity patterns
Use of vitamins, minerals, and nutritional supplements. Determine what, how much, and why the client is using each.
Use of alcohol and nicotine

Nursing Diagnosis

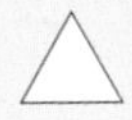

1. Altered Nutrition: Less Than Body Requirements, related to nausea, vomiting, and taste changes secondary to cancer/cancer therapy.

Planning and Implementation

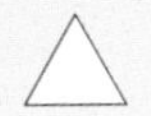

Client Goals

The client will

Eat six to eight times daily.
Verbalize the importance of consuming adequate protein and calories and the role of fat in providing required calories.
Switch from skim milk to 2% milk.
Drink at least 16 ounces of a high calorie, high protein supplement daily.
Practice ways to increase protein and calorie density of foods consumed.
Maintain present weight until chemotherapy is completed.
List interventions she will try at home to help relieve nausea and taste alterations.

Nursing Interventions

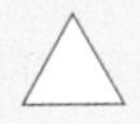

Nutrition Therapy

Provide a high-protein house diet as ordered.
Provide 8 ounces of Boost Plus three times daily between meals.

Client Teaching

Instruct the client

That an adequate nutritional status reduces the side effects of treatment, may make cancer cells more receptive to treatment, improves quality of life, and may increase survival rate. Poor nutritional status may potentiate chemotherapeutic drug toxicity.
That a preventative eating style is no longer appropriate. Consuming adequate protein and calories (even fat calories) is the major priority.

(continued)

On eating plan essentials, including

- Protein sources the client may tolerate despite nausea and taste changes such as eggs, cheese, mild fish, nuts, dried peas and beans, milk shakes, eggnogs, puddings, ice cream, instant breakfast mixes, and commercial supplements
- How to increase the protein and calorie density of foods eaten
- To eat small, frequent "meals" to help maximize intake but to avoid eating 12 hours before chemotherapy
- To drink ample fluids 1 to 2 days before and after chemotherapy to enhance excretion of the drugs and to decrease the risk of renal toxicity

On interventions to minimize nausea such as

- Eating foods served cold or at room temperature
- Eating high-carbohydrate, low-fat foods such as toast, crackers, yogurt, sherbet, cooked cereal, soft or canned fruits, watermelon, bananas, fruit juices, and angel food cake
- Avoiding fatty, greasy, fried, and strongly seasoned foods

On behavior to help maximize intake, including

- Viewing food as a medicine, rather than a social pleasure, that must be "taken" even when the desire to eat is lacking
- Keeping track of and avoiding foods that cause nausea
- Taking antiemetics as prescribed even when symptoms are absent
- Sucking on hard candy during chemotherapy and using plastic utensils and dishes to mitigate the "bad taste" in her mouth
- Avoiding anything that tastes unpleasant

Evaluation

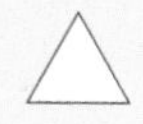

The client

Eats six to eight times daily
Verbalizes the importance of consuming adequate protein and calories and the role of fat in providing required calories
Switches from skim milk to 2% milk
Drinks at least 16 ounces of a high-calorie, high-protein supplement daily
Practices ways to increase protein and calorie density of foods consumed
Maintains present weight until chemotherapy is completed
Lists interventions she will try at home to help relieve nausea and taste alterations

NUTRITION AND IMMUNODEFICIENCY

Nutritional status and immunity are interrelated. The inflammatory and immune response to infection increases nutrient requirements and the risk for malnutrition. Conversely, nutrient deficiencies and sometimes excesses can impair immune system

 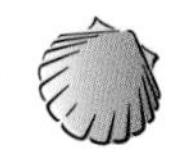

function and the ability to fight infection. Specifically, chronic malnutrition decreases the number of T lymphocytes, slows natural killer cell activity and interleukin-2 production, reduces B cell function, alters cytokine activity, and reduces the ability of neutrophils to phagocytose and kill bacteria. For clients with HIV, optimum nutrition may delay disease progression and improves quality of life.

Effect of HIV Nutritional Status

People with HIV are at increased nutritional risk. HIV infection, secondary infection, malignancies, and drug therapies can cause symptoms or side effects that impair intake, alter nutrient metabolism, decrease nutrient availability, or increase nutritional requirements. Despite more effective antiretroviral drugs, weight loss, malnutrition, and wasting are common problems in HIV. Why this is true is not completely understood. It may be that even after drug treatment, there is enough of the virus left to cause a chronic inflammatory response that compromises nutrition.

Wasting: Although many definitions exist, wasting is generally described as an unintentional loss of 10% of body weight.

Wasting is an AIDS-defining condition characterized by unintentional weight loss of 10% in the presence of diarrhea or chronic weakness and documented fever for at least 30 days that is not attributable to a concurrent condition other than HIV infection itself. Although both lean body mass and fat tissue are lost, the loss of lean body mass is much greater. Wasting exacerbates illness and is associated with significant morbidity such as fatigue, weakness, and reduced quality of life. Numerous prospective and retrospective studies demonstrate a significant relationship between weight loss and mortality, disease progression, or both.

Like cancer cachexia, the cause of wasting in AIDS is multifactorial and varies among individuals. Changes in metabolism, GI abnormalities, cytokine production, and poor intake may be contributing factors.

Changes in Metabolism

Accelerated metabolism, and thus the need for additional calories and nutrients, may occur from infection, fever, cancer, and/or drug-induced reactions. Although increased *resting* energy expenditure is common among patients with HIV, it is not a universal finding. In addition, *total* energy expenditure may be less due to a decrease in physical activity. Studies show that reversing wasting is not contingent on reversing elevated resting energy expenditure.

Although there are a variety of other metabolic alterations related to HIV infection, such as altered rates of protein turnover, decreased rates of muscle protein synthesis, and increased rates of hepatic lipogenesis, it is not known to what extent they contribute to wasting.

GI Abnormalities

Diarrhea and malabsorption are common among people infected with HIV and may occur secondary to intestinal infections, drug therapy, low serum albumin, gastrointestinal malignancies, and AIDS enteropathy. Because malabsorption can occur in the absence of diarrhea, malabsorption should not be excluded on the basis of normal bowel patterns alone. Uncorrected, malabsorption can lead to malnutrition, wasting, and impaired quality of life. Whereas rapid weight loss (>4 kg in <4 months) is associated with periods of acute infection, more gradual weight loss (>4 kg in >4 months) tends to be related to GI complications.

Cytokine Production

Excessive production of cytokines has been implicated in the metabolic abnormalities, anorexia, and wasting that accompanies HIV infection. However, it is not known if the elevated cytokine levels are a cause or an effect of progressing HIV disease.

Poor Intake

Cytokines: proteins secreted by various cell types that regulate the intensity and duration of immune responses.

Inadequate calorie intake, whether from poor intake and/or increased requirements, is an important factor contributing to wasting. Intake may be poor because of anorexia, infection, fatigue, mouth ulcers, depression, anxiety, nausea, vomiting, diarrhea, impaired swallowing, impaired taste, esophageal ulcerations, and/or shortness of breath. In addition, the opportunity to eat may be restricted if specific eating schedules are necessary to avoid food and drug interactions. Studies show that low intakes of thiamin, riboflavin, niacin, vitamin B_6, vitamin E, and iron are associated with more rapid disease progression.

Nutrition Therapy

The goals of nutrition therapy are to

- Forestall or reverse wasting
- Treat or minimize symptoms/side effects of HIV disease and antiretroviral therapies
- Enhance the effectiveness of drug therapy
- Prevent food-borne illness

Nutrition therapy begins with an individualized assessment that determines the client's level of risk based on weight, weight change, changes in body composition, biochemical markers of malnutrition, clinical signs of malnutrition, adequacy of intake, and symptoms of HIV or side effects of treatment that impact intake or nutritional status. An individualized plan of care is designed that takes into account the client's socioeconomic, cultural, and ethnic background. Nutrition counseling deals with how, what, why, and when to eat to optimize health and quality of life. Ideally, nutrition therapy begins before the client exhibits any symptoms of HIV disease even if intake appears adequate, because the effectiveness of nutrition therapy may be limited once the client is ill enough to need hospital care.

Forestall or Reverse Wasting

Although it is recognized that weight loss and disease progression are related, the relationship between calorie intake and weight loss is unclear. Some studies show no as-

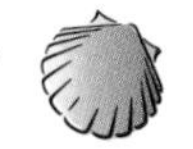

Career Connection

Nurses are in an ideal position to provide nutrition counseling when appropriate and to recommend referrals to the dietitian as needed. Counseling may include

- **How to cope with side effects such as anorexia, nausea, and vomiting.**
- **Guidelines for evaluating nutritional supplements and products. Remind clients that there are no supplements or diets that cure HIV/AIDS and that some therapies are potentially harmful. Advise clients to be skeptical when they hear the words "breakthrough," "magical cure," and "new discovery." Likewise, "detoxify," "purify," and "energize" are nonscientific jargon, not medical terms.**
- **The benefits of using high protein supplements. Products such as Boost High Protein, Boost Plus, Ensure HN, and Ensure Plus provide quick and easy protein and calories.**
- **The benefits of comfort foods. Clients with HIV disease may experience anger, depression, and anxiety. Comfort foods may provide some consolation and may be appealing when other foods are not. Even if the nutritional value of comfort foods is small, their emotional value is important.**
- **Information on food and drug interactions.**
- **Information about home-delivered meals that may be available from a local AIDS service provider.**

sociation between calorie intake and weight loss; others show there is a correlation. Although optimal calorie and nutrient intake cannot guarantee weight maintenance, it can improve quality of life.

Calories

Exact calorie and nutrient requirements for patients with HIV/AIDS have not yet been established, so there are no universally accepted standards. A reasonable starting range to estimate baseline calorie needs may be 35 to 45 cal/kg, which can be adjusted as needed. (The standard for a healthy adult is generally approximately 30 cal/kg.) Individual requirements are likely to vary more among people with HIV than among the general population, and opportunistic infections and malignancies elevate calorie needs.

HIV Research of the Nutrition Infection Unit at Tufts University School of Medicine specifies calorie recommendations according to the client's clinical status:

- 37 cal/kg if the client's weight is stable and there are no secondary infections
- 45 cal/kg if the client has an opportunistic infection
- 55 cal/kg if the client is losing weight

Protein

A high-protein diet may be prescribed, especially for clients with serum protein depletion and loss of lean body tissue. A protein intake of 1.2 to 2.0 g/kg is frequently recommended, although there are no data to support this recommendation. This recommendation translates to a rule-of-thumb guideline of 100 to 150 g/day for men and 80 to 100 g/day for women.

Vitamins and Minerals

Decreased serum levels of vitamins and minerals, a frequent finding in HIV-infected clients, are most likely related to poor intake. Although low serum levels of some vitamins and minerals are associated with increased rates of disease progression and mortality, there have been no controlled studies showing vitamin or mineral supplementation reverses wasting, delays disease progression, or improves survival. Unless a specific nutrient deficiency is diagnosed, one or two multivitamin and mineral tablets (without extra iron) that supply 100% of the RDA are generally recommended.

Method of Feeding

Clients who are unable to consume an adequate oral intake may require tube feeding for supplemental or complete nutrition. Because many formulas have the potential to cause diarrhea, the client's tolerance should be closely monitored. Advera and Impact are commercial formulas designed for clients with impaired immune function.

Clients with intractable vomiting, severe secretory diarrhea, or bowel obstruction may be candidates for TPN. However, the use of TPN is controversial because it may not be able to stop progressive wasting in clients who have systemic infections. Some studies have found that TPN increases body fat without increasing body cell mass. The client should be counseled on the potential risks and benefits of both enteral and parenteral nutrition.

Other Interventions for Wasting

Combined with nutrition therapy, exercise can help to prevent or treat wasting. Exercise can improve fitness level, restore lean body mass, improve insulin sensitivity, improve lipoprotein profiles, and enhance sense of well-being. Studies show that moderate exercise does not cause deleterious effects on immune function or viral load in people with HIV. Clients should be encouraged to engage in both aerobic and resistance exercise as tolerated.

One or more drugs may be used to combat wasting, depending on the contributing factors. Those used most frequently include appetite stimulants, testosterone replacement, growth hormone, or anabolic steroids. Their benefits and disadvantages are presented in Table 21.5.

Treat or Minimize Symptoms

Clients with HIV/AIDS may experience problems with appetite and intake similar to those of cancer clients. Nutrition therapy recommendations made earlier in this chapter for anorexia, nausea and vomiting, fatigue, taste changes, food aversions, stomatitis, dry mouth, and diarrhea are appropriate for HIV-infected clients as well as for people with cancer. As in the case of cancer, liquid commercial supplements are frequently used because they tend to leave the stomach quickly, are easy to consume, and provide significant quantities of calories and protein. Small frequent feedings (e.g., six to nine times daily) are encouraged even when appetite is lacking. Two complications not previously addressed under cancer are malabsorption and metabolic alterations associated with lipodystrophy.

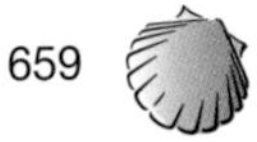

TABLE 21.5 DRUGS USED TO COMBAT WASTING

Drug	Benefits	Disadvantages
Appetite Stimulants		
Megestrol acetate (Megace)	Potent appetite stimulant Promotes weight gain Increases sense of well-being	Majority of weight gain is fat Potential side effects include deep vein thrombosis, hypogonadism, adrenal suppression
Dronabinol (Marinol)	Subjectively stimulates appetite; in controlled studies, was not proven to increase appetite Weight gain not consistently increased	May cause heartburn, nausea, dry mouth, drowsiness
Testosterone (given to men with low levels of testosterone)	Increases lean body mass and muscle strength without negatively affecting CD4 cell counts, especially when clients do resistance exercises while taking the drug	Reduces HDL cholesterol Exacerbates liver disease
Recombinant Human Growth Hormone	Promotes weight gain Increases lean body mass	Expensive Generally must be given every day Potential side effects include joint stiffness, joint swelling, and diarrhea May cause hyperglycemia Contraindicated during critical illness

Lipodystrophy (also known as fat redistribution syndrome): a condition characterized by changes in body shape such as loss of peripheral fat (e.g., in face, buttocks, arms, and legs) and central fat deposition (in abdomen and back of the neck). Weight may not change. Glucose intolerance, elevated triglycerides, and elevated cholesterol may also occur.

Malabsorption

Controlling diarrhea and malabsorption can substantially improve quality of life. Although diarrhea may seem to be triggered by eating, clients need to understand that limiting food intake to control diarrhea only exacerbates wasting. Interventions listed for diarrhea may be appropriate. For malabsorption with or without diarrhea, a low-fat diet is recommended. Supplemental medium-chain triglyceride (MCT) oil may be needed for additional calories. MCT oil does not require pancreatic lipase or bile for digestion and absorption and therefore can be absorbed easily by people with impaired digestion or absorption.

Metabolic Alterations of Lipodystrophy

Lipodystrophy is not life threatening, but emotional distress caused by the significant changes in body shape and social stigmatization may cause clients to decrease or stop their antiretroviral therapies. Although nutrition therapy cannot reverse the changes in body shape, it may help to improve the metabolic abnormalities of glucose intolerance, hypertriglyceridemia, and hypercholesterolemia. Specifically, a Mediterranean diet low in saturated fat and refined sugar, relatively high in monounsaturated fat, and high in fiber-rich whole grains, fruits, and vegetables may help to improve lipoprotein profiles and glucose tolerance. See Chapter 4 for more on the Mediterranean diet.

Enhance Effectiveness of Drug Therapy

Due to food/drug interactions, medication schedules and food restrictions are both complex and strict. Some clients stop antiretroviral therapies because they are convinced that the drugs' side effects and complicated regimens are not worth the effort. Maximum effectiveness of drug therapy is dependent on compliance with the medication schedule and food restrictions. Table 21.6 lists drugs that should be taken on an empty stomach and those that need to be taken with food.

Prevent Foodborne Illness

Because people with HIV/AIDS have compromised immune systems, steps should be taken to reduce the risk of foodborne illness (see Box 21.1). See Chapter 9 for more on foodborne illness.

How Do You Respond?

Should people with cancer take antioxidant supplements? Nutrition experts recommend that people with or without cancer consume a wide variety of at least five servings of fruits and vegetables daily to obtain antioxidants and other substances that may protect against cancer. On the other hand, supplements provide only a few selected ingredients, not the whole package of potentially beneficial compounds. Also, high doses of antioxidant supplements, namely vitamins A, C, and E, beta-carotene, and selenium, may actually interfere with the effectiveness of chemotherapy: these antioxidants may destroy beneficial free radicals that would otherwise kill cancer cells. High doses of antioxidants may prevent apoptosis (programmed cell death) of tumor cells. Animal research is underway to determine if depleting antioxidants in the diet may enhance apoptosis of cancer cells and thereby slow tumor growth. Until more is known, clients undergoing chemotherapy should eat normal amounts of fruits and vegetables and avoid taking antioxidant supplements.

Doesn't canola oil cause cancer? The rumors that canola oil causes cancer stems from the fact that canola is derived from rapeseed. Rapeseed is naturally high in erucic acid, a fatty acid shown to be harmful to animals. However, in the 1970s, traditional plant breeding methods led to the creation of a low–erucic acid rapeseed, which is used to make canola oil. Numerous studies have shown no human health risks associated with canola oil.

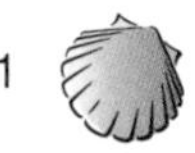

TABLE 21.6

HIV MEDICATIONS AND TIMING OF FOOD INTAKE

Drug Class	Take With Food	Take on Empty Stomach	Take Without Regard to Food
Nucleoside reverse transcriptase inhibitors (NRTI)	**Tenofovir (Viread)**	**Zidovudine (Retrovir-AZT-ZDV)** If it must be taken with food to decrease GI side effects, a low-fat meal is recommended **Zidovudine-lamivudine (Combivir, AZT-3TC)** If it must be taken with food to decrease GI side effects, a low-fat meal is recommended **Zidovudine-lamivudine–abacavir (Trizivir, AZT-3TC-ABC)** If it must be taken with food to decrease GI side effects, a low-fat meal is recommended **Didanosine (Videx EC-ddl)** Take at least 30 min before or 2 h after a meal. Take only with water.	**Lamivudine (epivir-3TC)** Fewer side effects if taken with meals **Abacavir (Ziagen-ABC)** **Stavudine (zerit-d4T)** **Zalcitabine (Hivid-ddC)**
Nonnucleoside reverse transcriptase inhibitors (NNRTI)			**Delavirdine (Rescriptor-DLV)** **Efavirenz (Sustiva-EFV)** Avoid high-fat meal. **Nevirapine (Viramune-NVP)**
Protease Inhibitors	**Sequinavir (soft-gel capsule) (Fortovase-SQVsgc)** Take with or up to 2 h after a full meal. **Sequinavir (hard-gel capsule) (Invirase-SQV)** Take with or up to 2 h after a full meal with high calories and high-fat foods for better absorption. **Lopinavir-ritonavir (Kaletra, LPV-RTV)** Better with high-fat meal. **Ritonavir (Novir-RTV)** Mix oral solution with chocolate milk or supplements to improve taste. **Nelfinavir (Viracept-NLF)** Take with meal or snack that includes a high protein food to increase absorption and decrease GI side effects.	**Indinavir (Crixivan-IDV)** Take at least 1 h before or 2 h after a meal or with a low- or non-fat meal.	**Amprenavir (Agenerase-APV)** Avoid high-fat meal.

▲ Focus on Critical Thinking

Respond to the following statements:

1. People undergoing treatment for cancer should limit their intake of fat because it may increase the risk of some types of cancer.
2. If TPN is not going to prolong a client's life, it should not be used.
3. It is easier to prevent malnutrition and weight loss in clients with cancer or HIV than it is to treat it.

Key Concepts

- Without early and aggressive nutritional interventions, cancer and HIV/AIDS can have profound and devastating effects on nutritional status, often resulting in wasting and malnutrition.
- Cancer alters metabolism by increasing energy expenditure, increasing protein catabolism, increasing fat catabolism, and increasing the use of fat for energy.
- Neither the incidence nor the severity of cachexia can be related directly to calorie intake or tumor weight.
- Nutrition therapy cannot cure cancer or HIV/AIDS, but it may improve tolerance to therapies and promote quality of life.
- In general, the nutrition therapy for cancer and for HIV/AIDS is similar: minimize side effects that interfere with nutrient intake and use and increase protein and calorie intake.
- For most people undergoing chemotherapy, fatigue and nausea and vomiting are among the most distressing side effects.
- Increasing the calorie and protein densities of the diet is generally more acceptable than increasing the volume of food served.
- No benefit is derived from force-feeding a client whose cancer is not being aggressively treated.
- Malnutrition may speed the progression from HIV disease to AIDS.
- Nutrient requirements for people with HIV/AIDS have not been determined, but it appears that calorie and protein needs are increased.
- Clients with cancer or HIV/AIDS are susceptible to nutritional "cures" and may use unorthodox diets or supplements that may be detrimental to their health.

ANSWER KEY

1. **FALSE** Even cancers that have not metastasized can cause generalized nutritional effects.
2. **TRUE** Clients who are adequately nourished are better able to withstand the effects of cancer treatments.
3. **FALSE** Although anorexia can contribute to the development of cachexia, neither the incidence nor the severity of cachexia can be related directly to calorie intake.

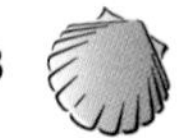

4. **FALSE** The cancer patient's appetite is generally better in the morning and tends to deteriorate as the day progresses.
5. **TRUE** The cancer patient should avoid eating 1 to 2 hours before chemotherapy or radiation therapy to decrease the likelihood of nausea.
6. **TRUE** Taste alteration may be caused by cancer treatment; if roast beef has a "bad" or "rotten" taste, a cheese sandwich is a high-protein alternative.
7. **FALSE** A low-fat diet cannot prevent lipodystrophy, but clients who develop lipodystrophy with hypercholesterolemia may benefit from a low–saturated fat diet to help lower serum cholesterol.
8. **FALSE** Diarrhea does not necessarily accompany malabsorption caused by HIV infection. Malabsorption cannot be ruled out on the basis of bowel movements alone.
9. **TRUE** Patients with HIV/AIDS may well experience problems related to appetite and intake similar to those of cancer patients.
10. **TRUE** The risk of foodborne infections in patients with HIV/AIDS can be reduced by educating them on food and water safety such as the importance of refrigerating foods, washing fruit and vegetables, and cooking meats thoroughly.

WEBSITES RELATED TO CANCER

American Botanical Council at **www.herbalgram.org**
American Cancer Society at **www.cancer.org**
American Institute for Cancer Research at **www.aicr.org**
American Society for Clinical Oncology at **www.asco.org**
National Cancer Institute at **www.cancer.gov**
National Center for Complementary and Alternative Medicine (NCCAM) at **www.nccam.nih.gov**
Oncology Nursing Society at **www.ons.org**

WEBSITES RELATED TO HIV/AIDS

AIDS Education Global Information System (AEGIS) at **www.aegis.com**
Association of Nutrition Services Agencies at **www.aidsnutrition.org**
AIDSinfo (A Service of the U.S. Department of Health and Human Services) at **www.aidsinfo.nih.gov**
HIV Research of the Nutrition Infection Unit at Tufts University School of Medicine at **www.tufts.edu/med/nutrition-infection/hiv/**
Center for HIV Information from the University of California San Francisco School of Medicine at **www.hivinsite.org**
Centers for Disease Control, Division of HIV/AIDS Prevention (DHAP) **http://www.cdc.gov/hiv/dhap.htm**
Community Programs For Clinical Research on AIDS, CPCRA (Government-funded research) at **http://www.cpcra.org/**
Food and Drug Administration HIV/AIDS Page at **http://www.fda.gov/oashi/aids/hiv.html**
Health Resources and Services Administration (HRSA) HIV/AIDS Services at **http://hab.hrsa.gov**
National Institute of Allergy & Infectious Diseases (NIAID), Division of Acquired Immunodeficiency Syndrome (DAIDS) at **http://www.niaid.nih.gov/daids/default.htm**

National Institutes of Health, National Center for Complementary and Alternative Therapies at **http://nccam.nih.gov**
National Institutes of Health Office of AIDS Research at **http://www.nih.gov/od/oar/**

REFERENCES

American Cancer Society. (2002). The complete guide—nutrition and physical activity. Available at www.cancer.org. Accessed on 12/17/03.
American Institute of Cancer Research. (2002). Should cancer patients taken antioxidant supplements? *AICR ScienceNow, 1,* 2–3.
Chicago Dietetic Association, the South Suburban Dietetic Association, and Dietitians of Canada. (2000). *Manual of clinical dietetics* (6th ed.). Chicago: American Dietetic Association.
Gentry, M. (Ed.) (2003). Diet as medicine for cancer patients. *American Institute for Cancer Research Newsletter on Diet, Nutrition and Cancer Prevention, 79,* 8.
Gerrior J., Kantaros, J., Coakley, E., et al. (2001). The fat redistribution syndrome in patients infected with HIV: Measurements of body shape abnormalities. *Journal of the American Dietetic Association, 101,* 1175–1180.
Memorial Sloan-Kettering Cancer Institute. (2003). About herbs, botanicals, and other products. Frequently asked questions. Available at www.mskcc.org. Accessed on 2/10/04.
Mulligan, K., & Schambelan, M. (2003). HIV-associated wasting. Available at www.hivinsite.org/InSite?page=kb-04-01-08. Accessed on 2/9/04.
National Cancer Institute. (2003). Nutrition in cancer care (PDQ): Supportive care. Available at www.nci.nih.gov. Accessed on 2/9/04.
National Center for Complementary and Alternative Medicine. (2003). Complementary and alternative medicine in cancer treatment: Questions and answers. Available at www.cis.nci.nih.gov/fat/9_14.htm. Accessed on 2/10/04.
Nerad, J., Romeyn, M., Silverman, E., et al. (2003). General nutrition management in patients infected with Human Immunodeficiency Virus. *Clinical Infections Diseases, 36*(Suppl. 2), S52–62.
Shattuck, D. (2001). Complexities beyond simple survival: Challenges in providing care for HIV patients. *Journal of the American Dietetic Association, 101,* 13–15.
Wood, M., Potts, E., & Connors, J. (2003). HIV nutrition and health. Building a high-quality diet. Available at www.tufts.edu/med/nutrition-infection/hiv/health_high quality_diet.html. Accessed on 2/13/04.
Woods, M., Spiegelman, D., Knox, T., et al. (2002). Nutrient intake and body weight in a large HIV cohort that includes women and minorities. *Journal of the American Dietetic Association, 102,* 203–211.

For information on the new dietary guidelines 2005 and MyPyramid, visit **http://connection.lww.com/go/dudek**

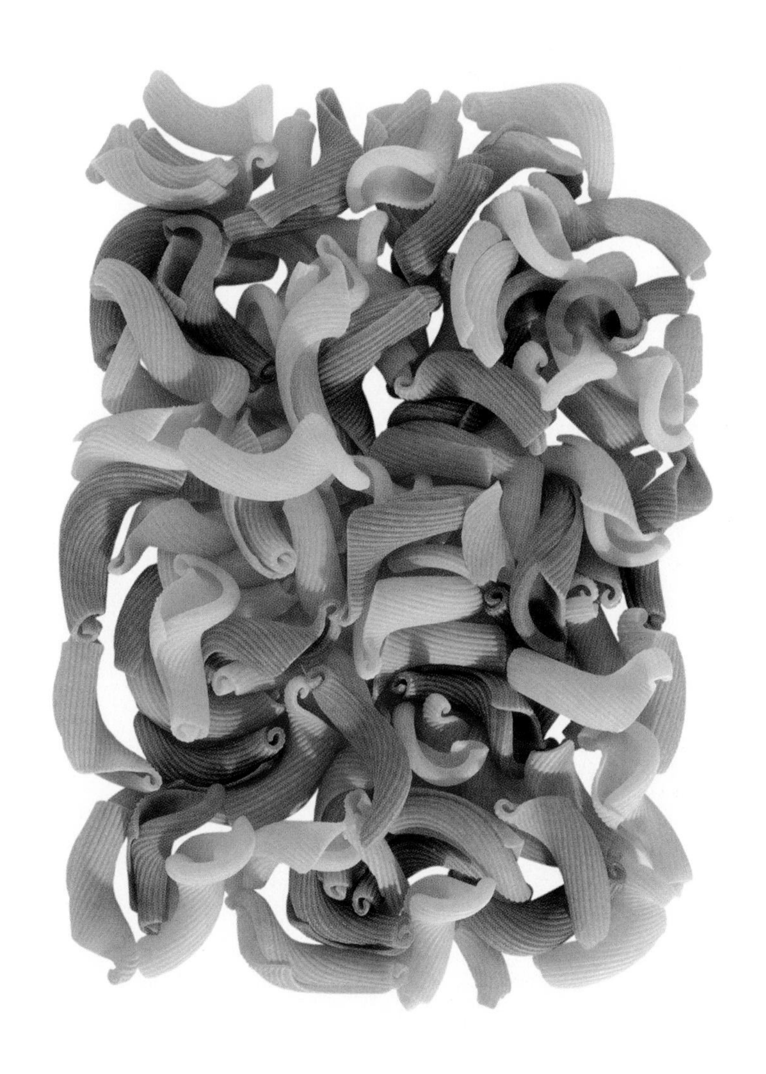

APPENDICES

1

Dietary Reference Intakes (DRIs): Recommended Intakes for Individuals, Vitamins (Food and Nutrition Board, Institute of Medicine, National Academies)

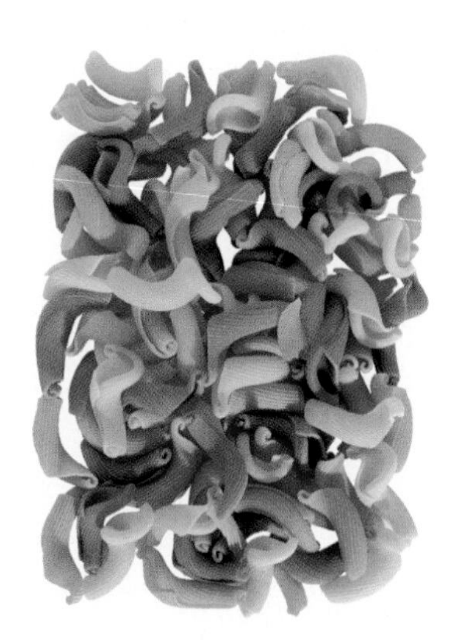

Life Stage Group	Vitamin A (µg/d)[a]	Vitamin C (mg/d)	Vitamin D (µg/d)[b,c]	Vitamin E (mg/d)[d]	Vitamin K (µg/d)	Thiamin (mg/d)
Infants						
0–6 mo	400*	40*	5*	4*	2.0*	0.2*
7–12 mo	500*	50*	5*	5*	2.5*	0.3*
Children						
1–3 y	**300**	**15**	5*	**6**	30*	**0.5**
4–8 y	**400**	**25**	5*	**7**	55*	**0.6**
Males						
9–13 y	**600**	**45**	5*	**11**	60*	**0.9**
14–18 y	**900**	**75**	5*	**15**	75*	**1.2**
19–30 y	**900**	**90**	5*	**15**	120*	**1.2**
31–50 y	**900**	**90**	5*	**15**	120*	**1.2**
51–70 y	**900**	**90**	10*	**15**	120*	**1.2**
>70 y	**900**	**90**	15*	**15**	120*	**1.2**
Females						
9–13 y	**600**	**45**	5*	**11**	60*	**0.9**
14–18 y	**700**	**65**	5*	**15**	75*	**1.0**
19–30 y	**700**	**75**	5*	**15**	90*	**1.1**
31–50 y	**700**	**75**	5*	**15**	90*	**1.1**
51–70 y	**700**	**75**	10*	**15**	90*	**1.1**
>70 y	**700**	**75**	15*	**15**	90*	**1.1**
Pregnancy						
≤18 y	**750**	**80**	5*	**15**	75*	**1.4**
19–30 y	**770**	**85**	5*	**15**	90*	**1.4**
31–50 y	**770**	**85**	5*	**15**	90*	**1.4**
Lactation						
≤18 y	**1,200**	**115**	5*	**19**	75*	**1.4**
19–30 y	**1,300**	**120**	5*	**19**	90*	**1.4**
31–50 y	**1,300**	**120**	5*	**19**	90*	**1.4**

NOTE: This table (taken from the DRI reports, see www.nap.edu) presents Recommended Dietary Allowances (RDAs) in **bold type** and Adequate Intakes (AIs) in ordinary type followed by an asterisk (*). RDAs and AIs may both be used as goals for individual intake. RDAs are set to meet the needs of almost all (97 to 98 percent) individuals in a group. For healthy breastfed infants, the AI is the mean intake. The AI for other life stage and gender groups is believed to cover needs of all individuals in the group, but lack of data or uncertainty in the data prevent being able to specify with confidence the percentage of individuals covered by this intake.

[a] As retinol activity equivalents (RAEs). 1 RAE = 1 µg retinol, 12 µg β-carotene, 24 µg α-carotene, or 24 µg β-cryptoxanthin. The RAE for dietary provitamin A carotenoids is two-fold greater than retinol equivalents (RE), whereas the RAE for preformed vitamin A is the same as RE.

[b] Cholecalciferol. 1 µg cholecalciferol = 40 IU vitamin D.

[c] In the absence of adequate exposure to sunlight.

[d] As α-tocopherol. α-Tocopherol includes RRR-α-tocopherol, the only form of α-tocopherol that occurs naturally in foods, and the 2R-stereoisomeric forms of α-tocopherol (RRR-, RSR-, RRS-, and RSS-α-tocopherol) that occur in fortified foods and supplements. It does not include the 2*S*-stereoisomeric forms of α-tocopherol (SRR-, SSR-, SRS-, and SSS-α-tocopherol), also found in fortified foods and supplements.

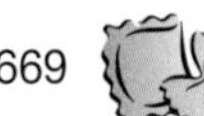

Riboflavin (mg/d)	Niacin (mg/d)[e]	Vitamin B_6 (mg/d)	Folate (μg/d)[f]	Vitamin B_{12} (μg/d)	Pantothenic Acid (mg/d)	Biotin (μg/d)	Choline[g] (mg/d)
0.3*	2*	0.1*	65*	0.4*	1.7*	5*	125*
0.4*	4*	0.3*	80*	0.5*	1.8*	6*	150*
0.5	6	0.5	150	0.9	2*	8*	200*
0.6	8	0.6	200	1.2	3*	12*	250*
0.9	12	1.0	300	1.8	4*	20*	375*
1.3	16	1.3	400	2.4	5*	25*	550*
1.3	16	1.3	400	2.4	5*	30*	550*
1.3	16	1.3	400	2.4	5*	30*	550*
1.3	16	1.7	400	2.4[h]	5*	30*	550*
1.3	16	1.7	400	2.4[h]	5*	30*	550*
0.9	12	1.0	300	1.8	4*	20*	375*
1.0	14	1.2	400[i]	2.4	5*	25*	400*
1.1	14	1.3	400[i]	2.4	5*	30*	425*
1.1	14	1.3	400[i]	2.4	5*	30*	425*
1.1	14	1.5	400	2.4[h]	5*	30*	425*
1.1	14	1.5	400	2.4[h]	5*	30*	425*
1.4	18	1.9	600[j]	2.6	6*	30*	450*
1.4	18	1.9	600[j]	2.6	6*	30*	450*
1.4	18	1.9	600[j]	2.6	6*	30*	450*
1.6	17	2.0	500	2.8	7*	35*	550*
1.6	17	2.0	500	2.8	7*	35*	550*
1.6	17	2.0	500	2.8	7*	35*	550*

[e] As niacin equivalents (NE). 1 mg of niacin = 60 mg of tryptophan; 0–6 months = preformed niacin (not NE).

[f] As dietary folate equivalents (DFE). 1 DFE = 1 μg food folate = 0.6 μg of folic acid from fortified food or as a supplement consumed with food = 0.5 μg of a supplement taken on an empty stomach.

[g] Although AIs have been set for choline, there are few data to assess whether a dietary supply of choline is needed at all stages of the life cycle, and it may be that the choline requirement can be met by endogenous synthesis at some of these stages.

[h] Because 10 to 30 percent of older people may malabsorb food-bound B_{12}, it is advisable for those older than 50 years to meet their RDA mainly by consuming foods fortified with B_{12} or a supplement containing B_{12}.

[i] In view of evidence linking folate intake with neural tube defects in the fetus, it is recommended that all women capable of becoming pregnant consume 400 μg from supplements or fortified foods in addition to intake of food folate from a varied diet.

[j] It is assumed that women will continue consuming 400 μg from supplements or fortified food until their pregnancy is confirmed and they enter prenatal care, which ordinarily occurs after the end of the periconceptional period—the critical time for formation of the neural tube.

2

Dietary Reference Intakes (DRIs): Recommended Intakes for Individuals, Elements (Food and Nutrition Board, Institute of Medicine, National Academies)

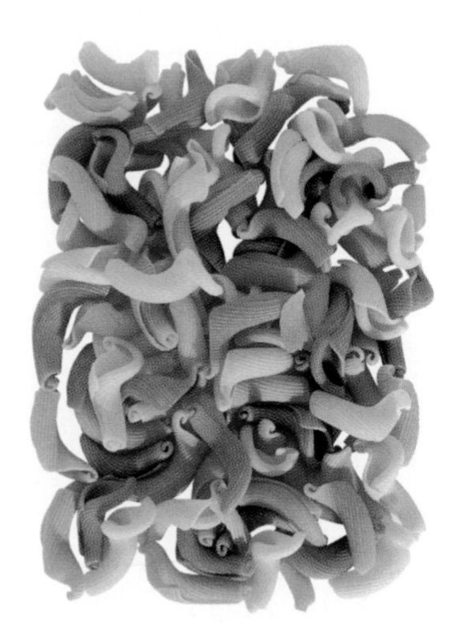

Life Stage Group	Calcium (mg/d)	Chromium (μg/d)	Copper (μg/d)	Fluoride (mg/d)	Iodine (μg/d)	Iron (mg/d)	Magnesium (mg/d)	Manganese (mg/d)	Molybdenum (μg/d)	Phosphorus (mg/d)	Selenium (μg/d)	Zinc (mg/d)
Infants												
0–6 mo	210*	0.2*	200*	0.01*	110*	0.27*	30*	0.003*	2*	100*	15*	2*
7–12 mo	270*	5.5*	220*	0.5*	130*	**11**	75*	0.6*	3*	275*	20*	**3**
Children												
1–3 y	500*	11*	**340**	0.7*	**90**	**7**	**80**	1.2*	**17**	**460**	**20**	3
4–8 y	800*	15*	**440**	1*	**90**	**10**	**130**	1.5*	**22**	**500**	**30**	5
Males												
9–13 y	1,300*	25*	**700**	2*	**120**	**8**	**240**	1.5*	**34**	**1,250**	**40**	**8**
14–18 y	1,300*	35*	**890**	3*	**150**	**11**	**410**	2.3*	**43**	**1,250**	**55**	**11**
19–30 y	1,000*	35*	**900**	4*	**150**	**8**	**400**	2.3*	**45**	**700**	**55**	**11**
31–50 y	1,000*	35*	**900**	4*	**150**	**8**	**420**	2.3*	**45**	**700**	**55**	**11**
51–70 y	1,200*	30*	**900**	4*	**150**	**8**	**420**	2.3*	**45**	**700**	**55**	**11**
>70 y	1,200*	30*	**900**	4*	**150**	**8**	**420**	2.3*	**45**	**700**	**55**	**11**
Females												
9–13 y	1,300*	21*	**700**	2*	**120**	**8**	**240**	1.6*	**34**	**1,250**	**40**	**8**
14–18 y	1,300*	24*	**890**	3*	**150**	**15**	**360**	1.6*	**43**	**1,250**	**55**	**9**
19–30 y	1,000*	25*	**900**	3*	**150**	**18**	**310**	1.8*	**45**	**700**	**55**	**8**
31–50 y	1,000*	25*	**900**	3*	**150**	**18**	**320**	1.8*	**45**	**700**	**55**	**8**
51–70 y	1,200*	20*	**900**	3*	**150**	**8**	**320**	1.8*	**45**	**700**	**55**	**8**
>70 y	1,200*	20*	**900**	3*	**150**	**8**	**320**	1.8*	**45**	**700**	**55**	**8**
Pregnancy												
≤18 y	1,300*	29*	**1,000**	3*	**220**	**27**	**400**	2.0*	**50**	**1,250**	**60**	**12**
19–30 y	1,000*	30*	**1,000**	3*	**220**	**27**	**350**	2.0*	**50**	**700**	**60**	**11**
31–50 y	1,000*	30*	**1,000**	3*	**220**	**27**	**360**	2.0*	**50**	**700**	**60**	**11**
Lactation												
≤18 y	1,300*	44*	**1,300**	3*	**290**	**10**	**360**	2.6*	**50**	**1,250**	**70**	**13**
19–30 y	1,000*	45*	**1,300**	3*	**290**	**9**	**310**	2.6*	**50**	**700**	**70**	**12**
31–50 y	1,000*	45*	**1,300**	3*	**290**	**9**	**320**	2.6*	**50**	**700**	**70**	**12**

NOTE: This table presents Recommended Dietary Allowances (RDAs) in **bold type** and Adequate Intakes (AIs) in ordinary type followed by an asterisk (*). RDAs and AIs may both be used as goals for individual intake. RDAs are set to meet the needs of almost all (97 to 98 percent) individuals in a group. For healthy breastfed infants, the AI is the mean intake. The AI for other life stage and gender groups is believed to cover needs of all individuals in the group, but lack of data or uncertainty in the data prevent being able to specify with confidence the percentage of individuals covered by this intake.

SOURCES: Dietary Reference Intakes for Calcium, Phosphorus, Magnesium, Vitamin D, and Fluoride (1997); Dietary Reference Intakes for Thiamin, Riboflavin, Niacin, Vitamin B_6, Folate, Vitamin B_{12}, Pantothenic Acid, Biotin, and Choline (1998); Dietary Reference Intakes for Vitamin C, Vitamin E, Selenium, and Carotenoids (2000); and Dietary Reference Intakes for Vitamin A, Vitamin K, Arsenic, Boron, Chromium, Copper, Iodine, Iron, Manganese, Molybdenum, Nickel, Silicon, Vanadium, and Zinc (2001). These reports may be accessed via www.nap.edu.

3

Dietary Reference Intakes (DRIs): Recommended Intakes for Individuals, Macronutrients (Food and Nutrition Board, Institute of Medicine, National Academies)

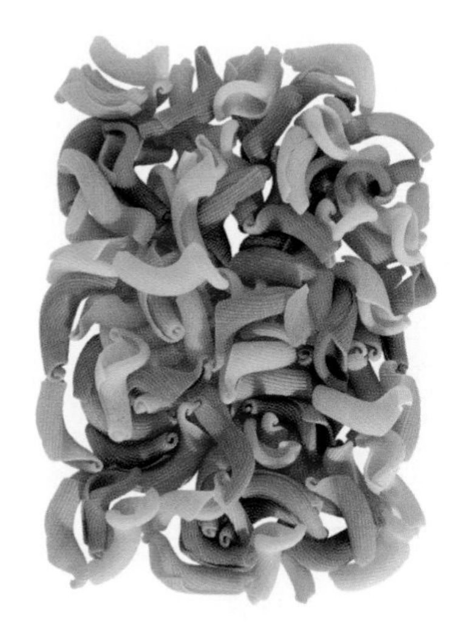

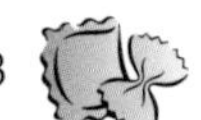

Life Stage Group	Carbohydrate (g/d)	Total Fiber (g/d)	Fat (g/d)	Linoleic Acid (g/d)	α-Linolenic Acid (g/d)	Protein[a] (g/d)
Infants						
0–6 mo	60*	ND	31*	4.4*	0.5*	9.1*
7–12 mo	95*	ND	30*	4.6*	0.5*	**13.5**
Children						
1–3 y	**130**	19*	ND	7*	0.7*	**13**
4–8 y	**130**	25*	ND	10*	0.9*	**19**
Males						
9–13 y	**130**	31*	ND	12*	1.2*	**34**
14–18 y	**130**	38*	ND	16*	1.6*	**52**
19–30 y	**130**	38*	ND	17*	1.6*	**56**
31–50 y	**130**	38*	ND	17*	1.6*	**56**
51–70 y	**130**	30*	ND	14*	1.6*	**56**
>70 y	**130**	30*	ND	14*	1.6*	**56**
Females						
9–13 y	**130**	26*	ND	10*	1.0*	**34**
14–18 y	**130**	26*	ND	11*	1.1*	**46**
19–30 y	**130**	25*	ND	12*	1.1*	**46**
31–50 y	**130**	25*	ND	12*	1.1*	**46**
51–70 y	**130**	21*	ND	11*	1.1*	**46**
>70 y	**130**	21*	ND	11*	1.1*	**46**
Pregnancy						
14–18 y	**175**	28*	ND	13*	1.4*	**71**
19–30 y	**175**	28*	ND	13*	1.4*	**71**
31–50 y	**175**	28*	ND	13*	1.4*	**71**
Lactation						
14–18 y	**210**	29*	ND	13*	1.3*	**71**
19–30 y	**210**	29*	ND	13*	1.3*	**71**
31–50 y	**210**	29*	ND	13*	1.3*	**71**

NOTE: This table presents Recommended Dietary Allowances (RDAs) in **bold type** and Adequate Intakes (AIs) in ordinary type followed by an asterisk (*). RDAs and AIs may both be used as goals for individual intake. RDAs are set to meet the needs of almost all (97 to 98 percent) individuals in a group. For healthy breastfed infants, the AI is the mean intake. The AI for other life stage and gender groups is believed to cover needs of all individuals in the group, but lack of data or uncertainty in the data prevent being able to specify with confidence the percentage of individuals covered by this intake.

[a] Based on 0.8 g protein/kg body weight for reference body weight.

SOURCE: Dietary Reference Intakes for Energy, Carbohydrate, Fiber, Fat, Fatty Acids, Cholesterol, Protein, and Amino Acids (2002). This report may be accessed via www.nap.edu.

4

Acceptable Macronutrient Distribution Ranges

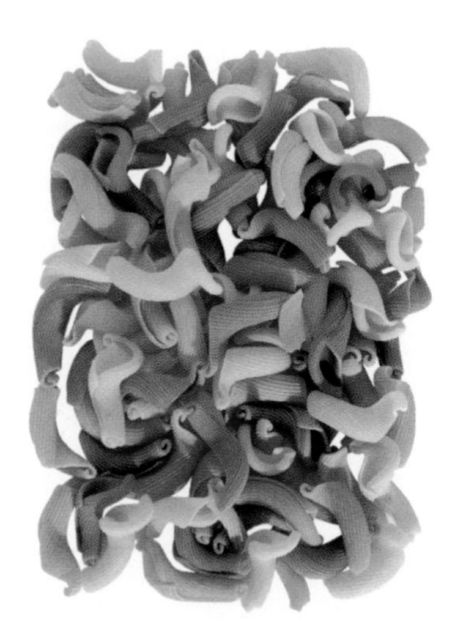

	Range (percent of energy)		
Macronutrient	Children, 1–3 y	Children, 4–18 y	Adults
Fat	30–40	25–35	20–35
n-6 polyunsaturated fatty acids* (linoleic acid)	5–10	5–10	5–10
n-3 polyunsaturated fatty acids* (α-linolenic acid)	0.6–1.2	0.6–1.2	0.6–1.2
Carbohydrate	45–65	45–65	45–65
Protein	5–20	10–30	10–35

*Approximately 10% of the total can come from longer-chain n-3 or n-6 fatty acids.

SOURCE: Dietary Reference Intakes for Energy, Carbohydrate, Fiber, Fat, Fatty Acids, Cholesterol, Protein, and Amino Acids (2002). This report may be accessed via www.nap.edu.

5

Growth Charts

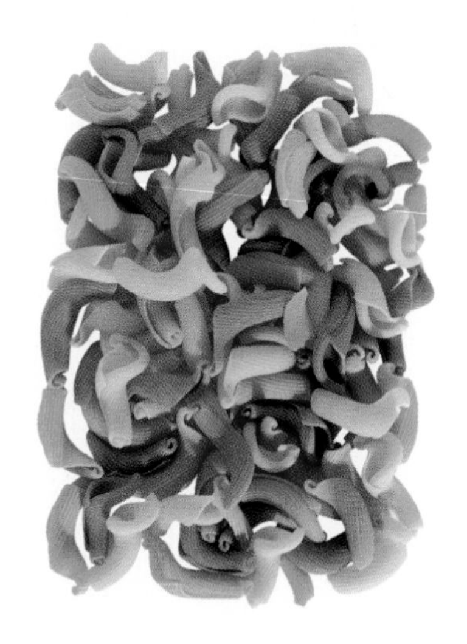

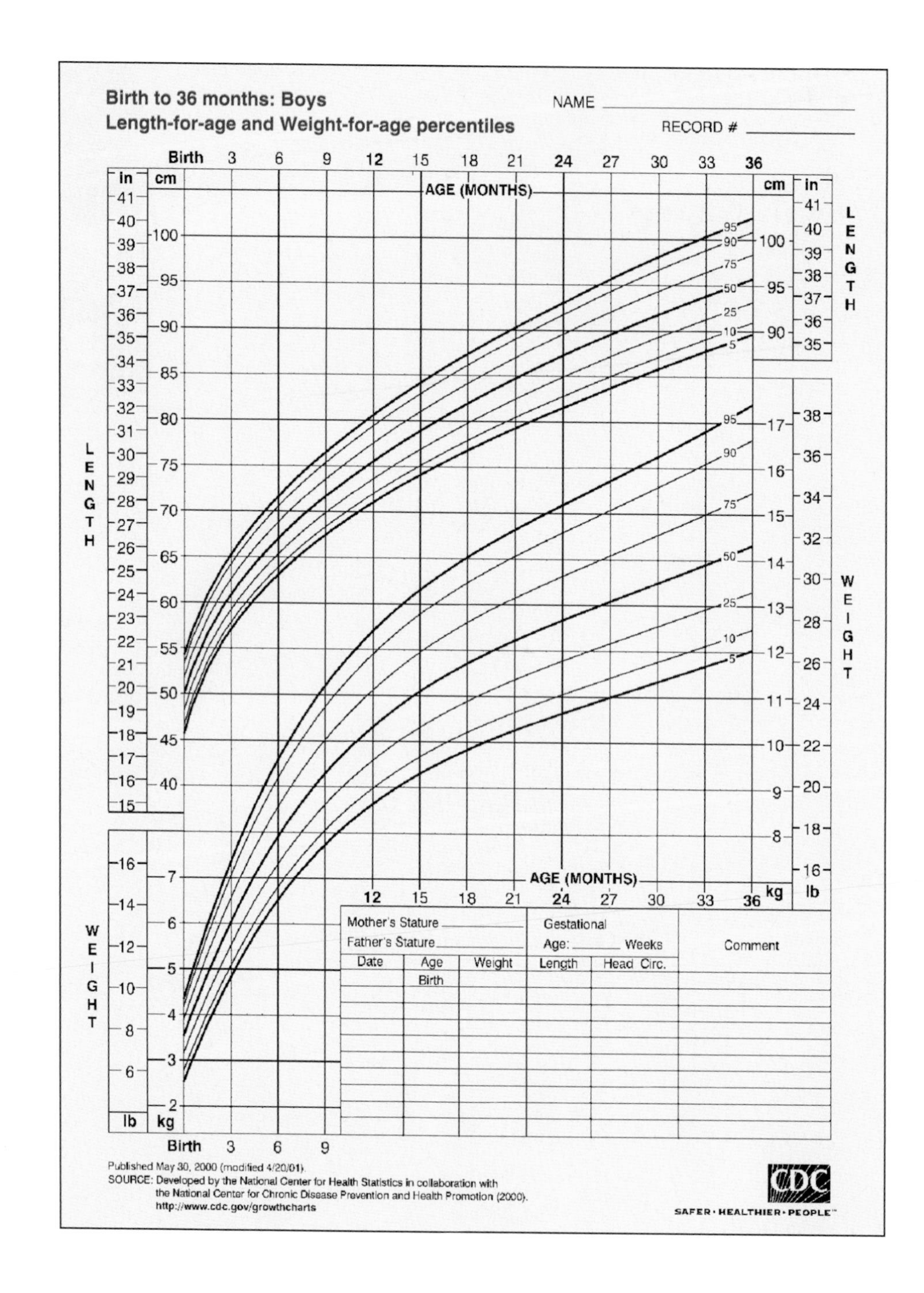
Birth to 36 months: Boys
Length-for-age and Weight-for-age percentiles
NAME
RECORD #
AGE (MONTHS)
LENGTH
WEIGHT
Mother's Stature
Father's Stature
Gestational
Age: Weeks
Comment
Date
Age
Weight
Length
Head Circ.
Birth
Published May 30, 2000 (modified 4/20/01).
SOURCE: Developed by the National Center for Health Statistics in collaboration with
the National Center for Chronic Disease Prevention and Health Promotion (2000).
http://www.cdc.gov/growthcharts
CDC
SAFER · HEALTHIER · PEOPLE

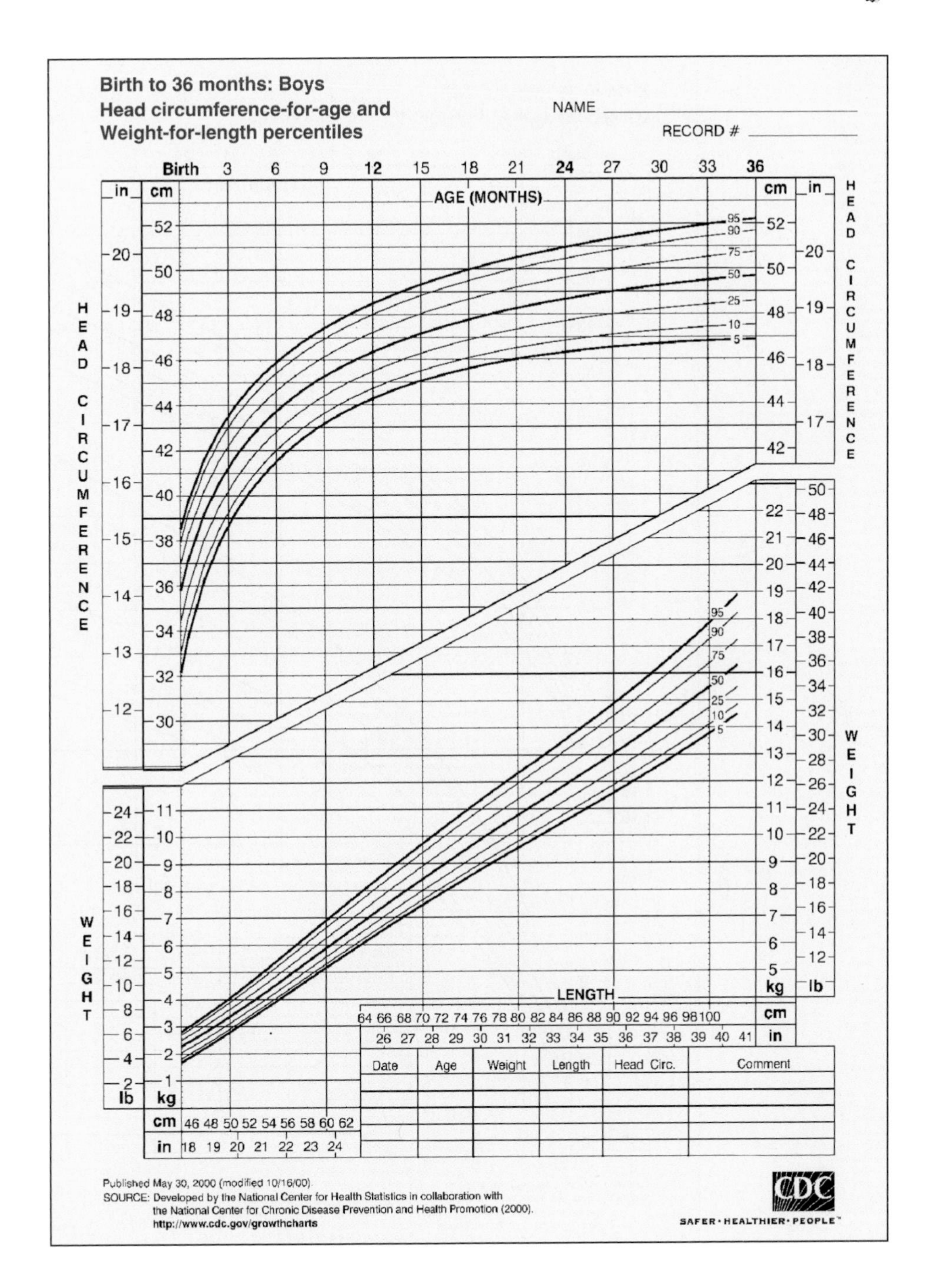

Birth to 36 months: Boys
Head circumference-for-age and
Weight-for-length percentiles
NAME
RECORD #
Birth 3 6 9 12 15 18 21 24 27 30 33 36
AGE (MONTHS)
HEAD CIRCUMFERENCE
WEIGHT
LENGTH
Date
Age
Weight
Length
Head Circ.
Comment
Published May 30, 2000 (modified 10/16/00).
SOURCE: Developed by the National Center for Health Statistics in collaboration with
the National Center for Chronic Disease Prevention and Health Promotion (2000).
http://www.cdc.gov/growthcharts
CDC
SAFER · HEALTHIER · PEOPLE

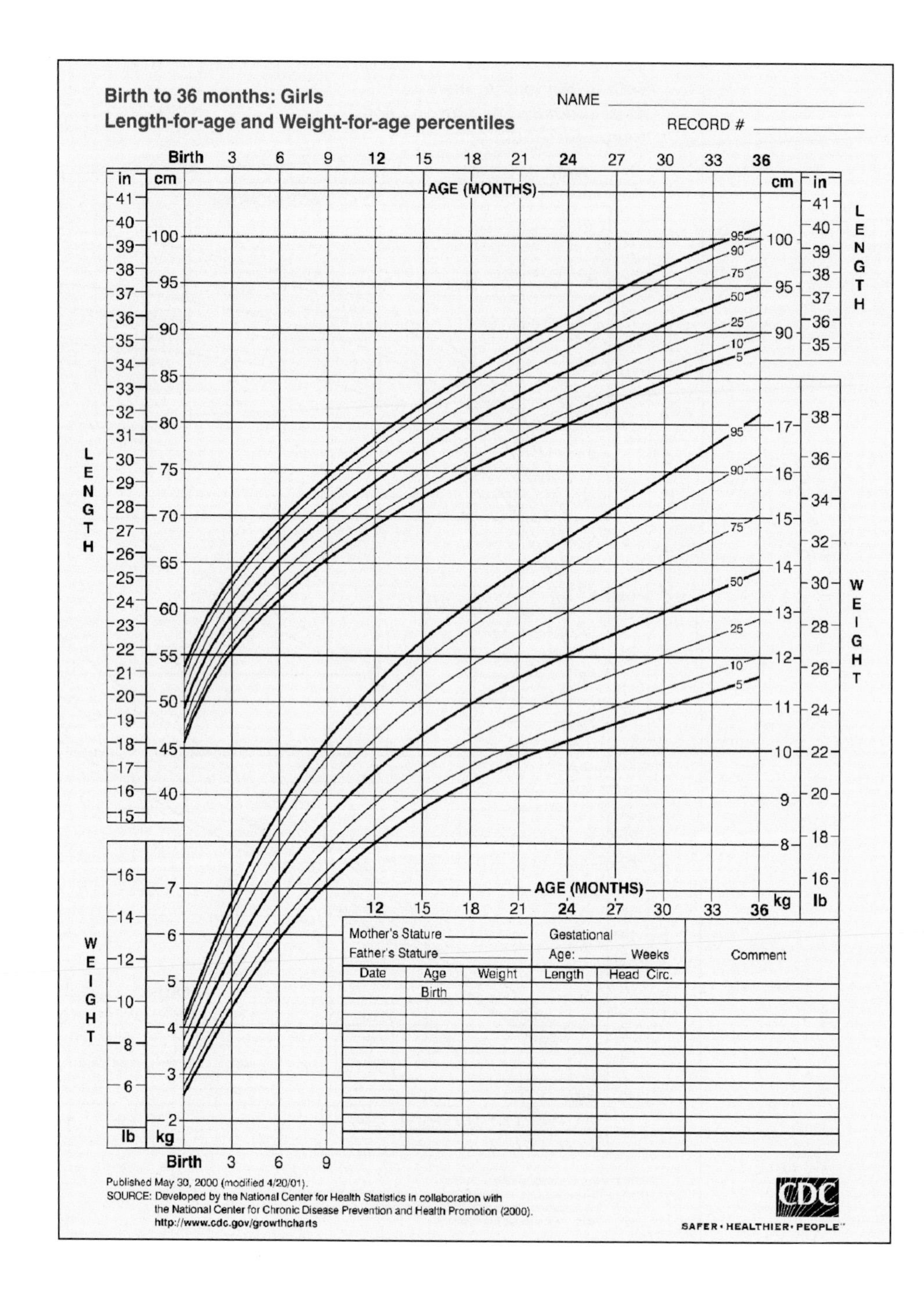
Birth to 36 months: Girls
Length-for-age and Weight-for-age percentiles
NAME
RECORD #
Birth 3 6 9 12 15 18 21 24 27 30 33 36
AGE (MONTHS)
in
cm
LENGTH
WEIGHT
kg
lb
95
90
75
50
25
10
5
Mother's Stature
Father's Stature
Gestational
Age: Weeks
Comment
Date
Age
Weight
Length
Head Circ.
Birth
Published May 30, 2000 (modified 4/20/01).
SOURCE: Developed by the National Center for Health Statistics in collaboration with the National Center for Chronic Disease Prevention and Health Promotion (2000).
http://www.cdc.gov/growthcharts
CDC
SAFER · HEALTHIER · PEOPLE™

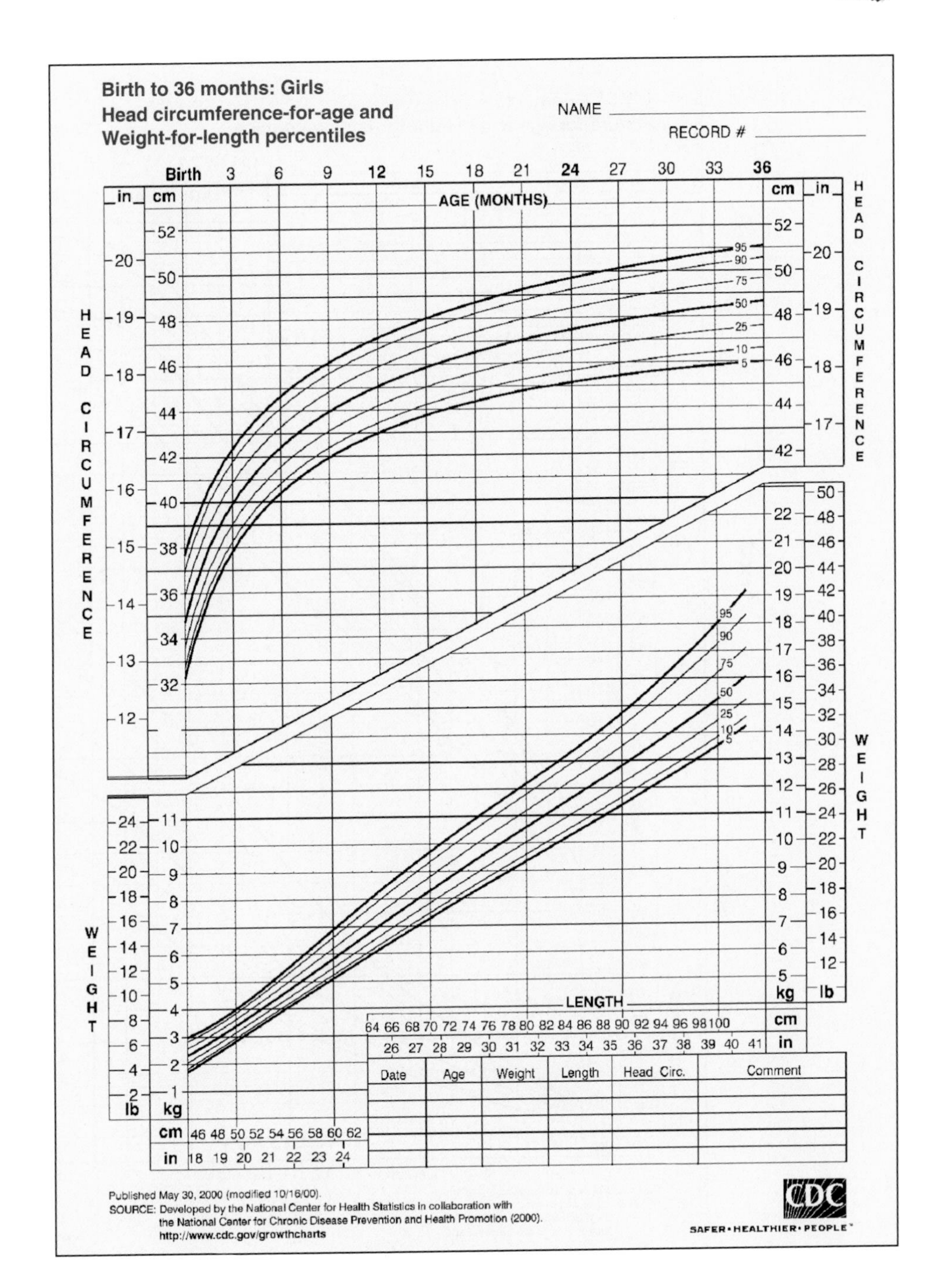
Birth to 36 months: Girls
Head circumference-for-age and
Weight-for-length percentiles
NAME
RECORD #
Birth 3 6 9 12 15 18 21 24 27 30 33 36
AGE (MONTHS)
HEAD CIRCUMFERENCE
WEIGHT
LENGTH
in cm
kg lb
95 90 75 50 25 10 5
Date Age Weight Length Head Circ. Comment
Published May 30, 2000 (modified 10/16/00).
SOURCE: Developed by the National Center for Health Statistics in collaboration with the National Center for Chronic Disease Prevention and Health Promotion (2000).
http://www.cdc.gov/growthcharts
CDC
SAFER • HEALTHIER • PEOPLE

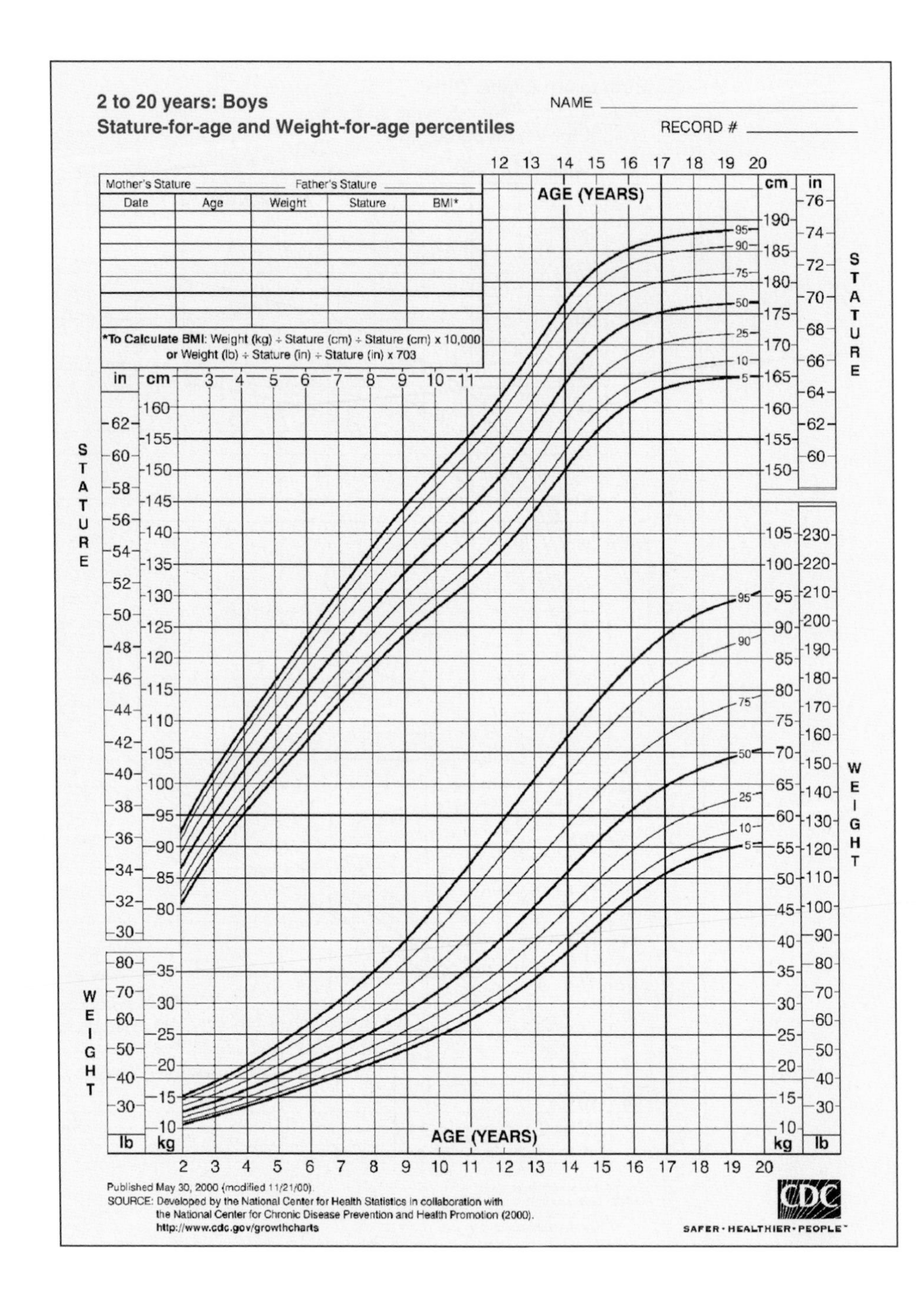
2 to 20 years: Boys
Stature-for-age and Weight-for-age percentiles
NAME
RECORD #
Mother's Stature
Father's Stature
Date
Age
Weight
Stature
BMI*
*To Calculate BMI: Weight (kg) ÷ Stature (cm) ÷ Stature (cm) x 10,000
or Weight (lb) ÷ Stature (in) ÷ Stature (in) x 703
AGE (YEARS)
STATURE
WEIGHT
in
cm
kg
lb
95
90
75
50
25
10
5
Published May 30, 2000 (modified 11/21/00).
SOURCE: Developed by the National Center for Health Statistics in collaboration with
the National Center for Chronic Disease Prevention and Health Promotion (2000).
http://www.cdc.gov/growthcharts
CDC
SAFER · HEALTHIER · PEOPLE™

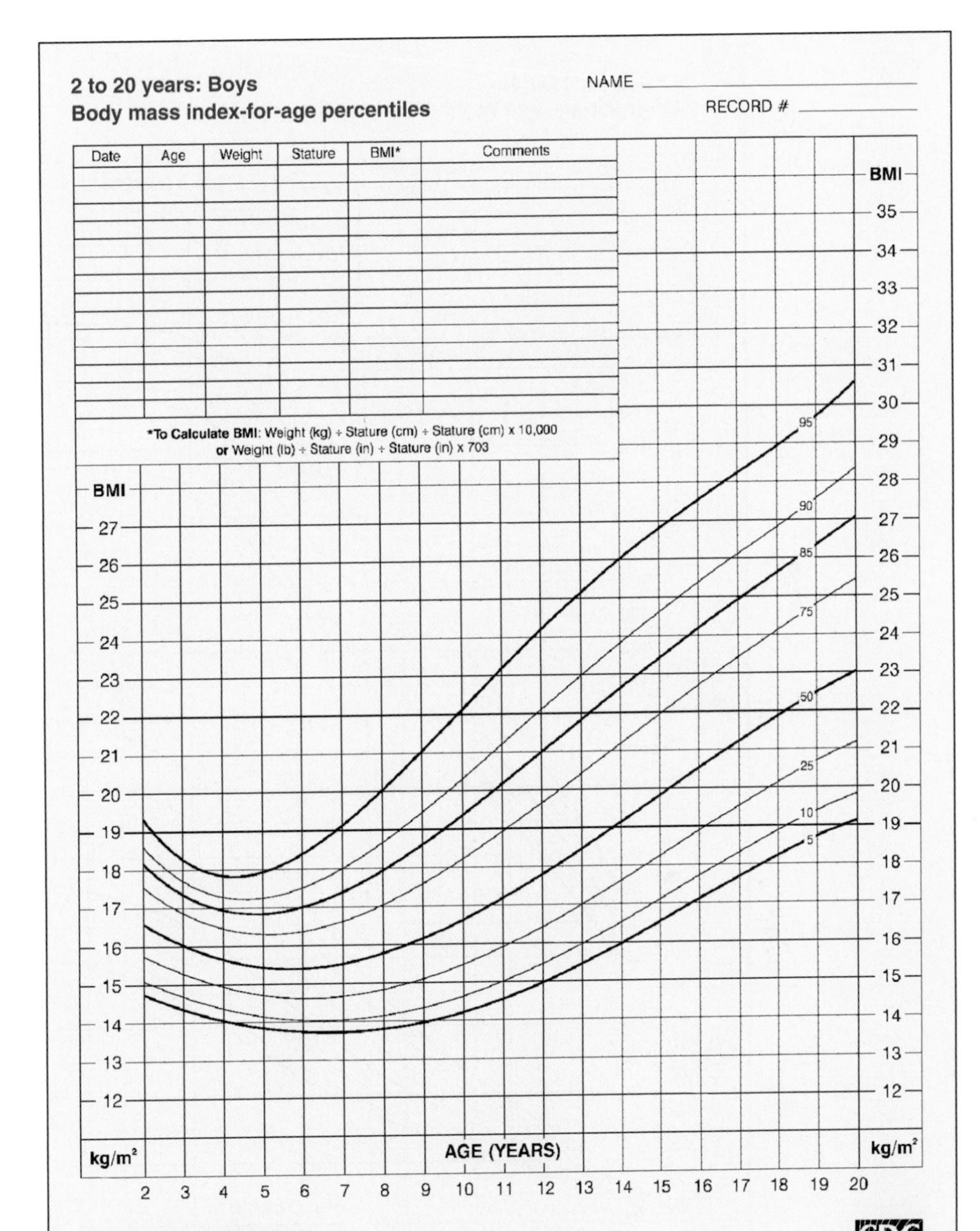

Published May 30, 2000 (modified 10/16/00).
SOURCE: Developed by the National Center for Health Statistics in collaboration with the National Center for Chronic Disease Prevention and Health Promotion (2000).
http://www.cdc.gov/growthcharts

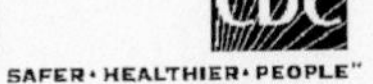

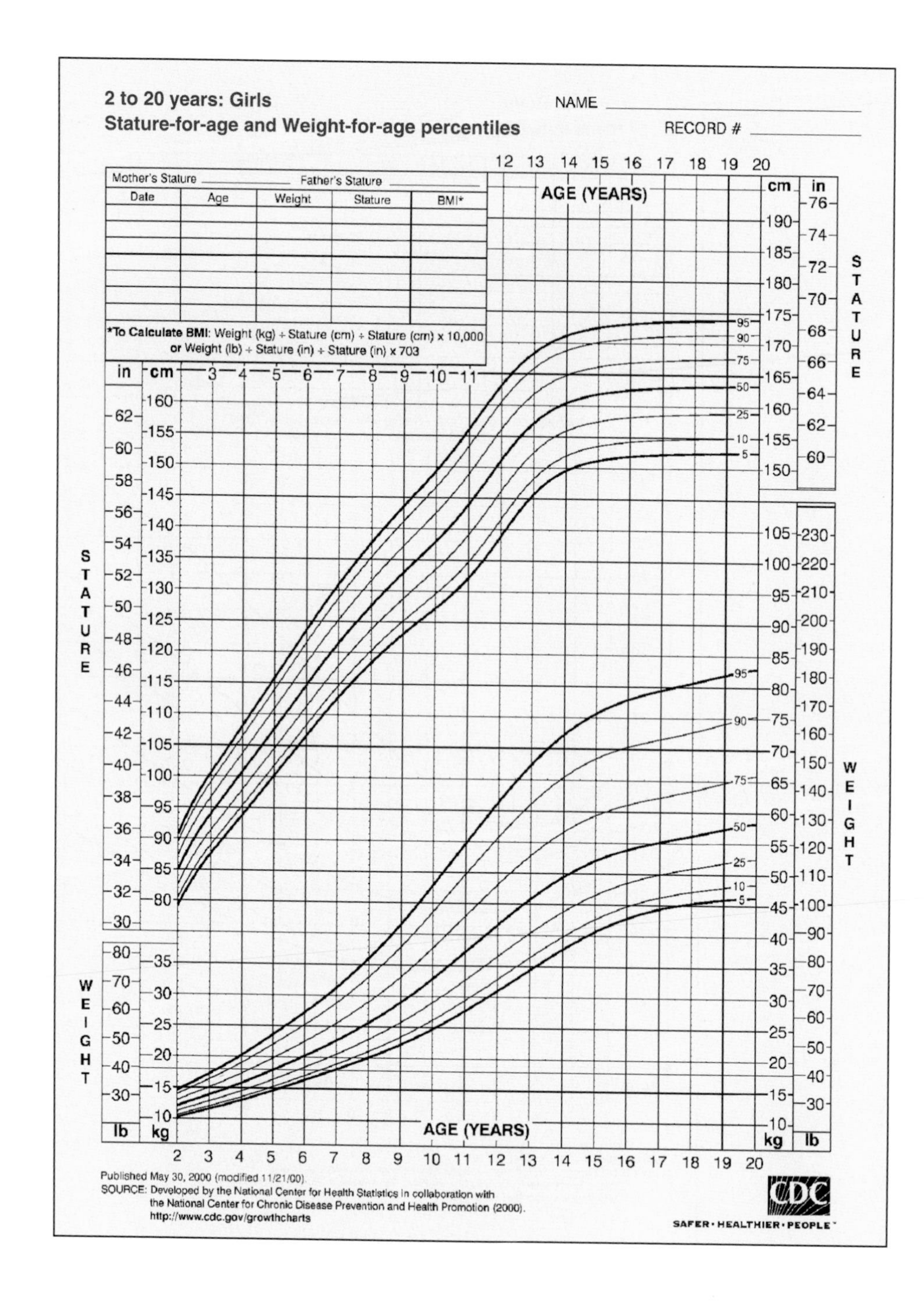

2 to 20 years: Girls
Stature-for-age and Weight-for-age percentiles
NAME
RECORD #
Mother's Stature
Father's Stature
Date
Age
Weight
Stature
BMI*
*To Calculate BMI: Weight (kg) ÷ Stature (cm) ÷ Stature (cm) x 10,000
or Weight (lb) ÷ Stature (in) ÷ Stature (in) x 703
AGE (YEARS)
STATURE
WEIGHT
Published May 30, 2000 (modified 11/21/00).
SOURCE: Developed by the National Center for Health Statistics in collaboration with
the National Center for Chronic Disease Prevention and Health Promotion (2000).
http://www.cdc.gov/growthcharts
CDC
SAFER • HEALTHIER • PEOPLE

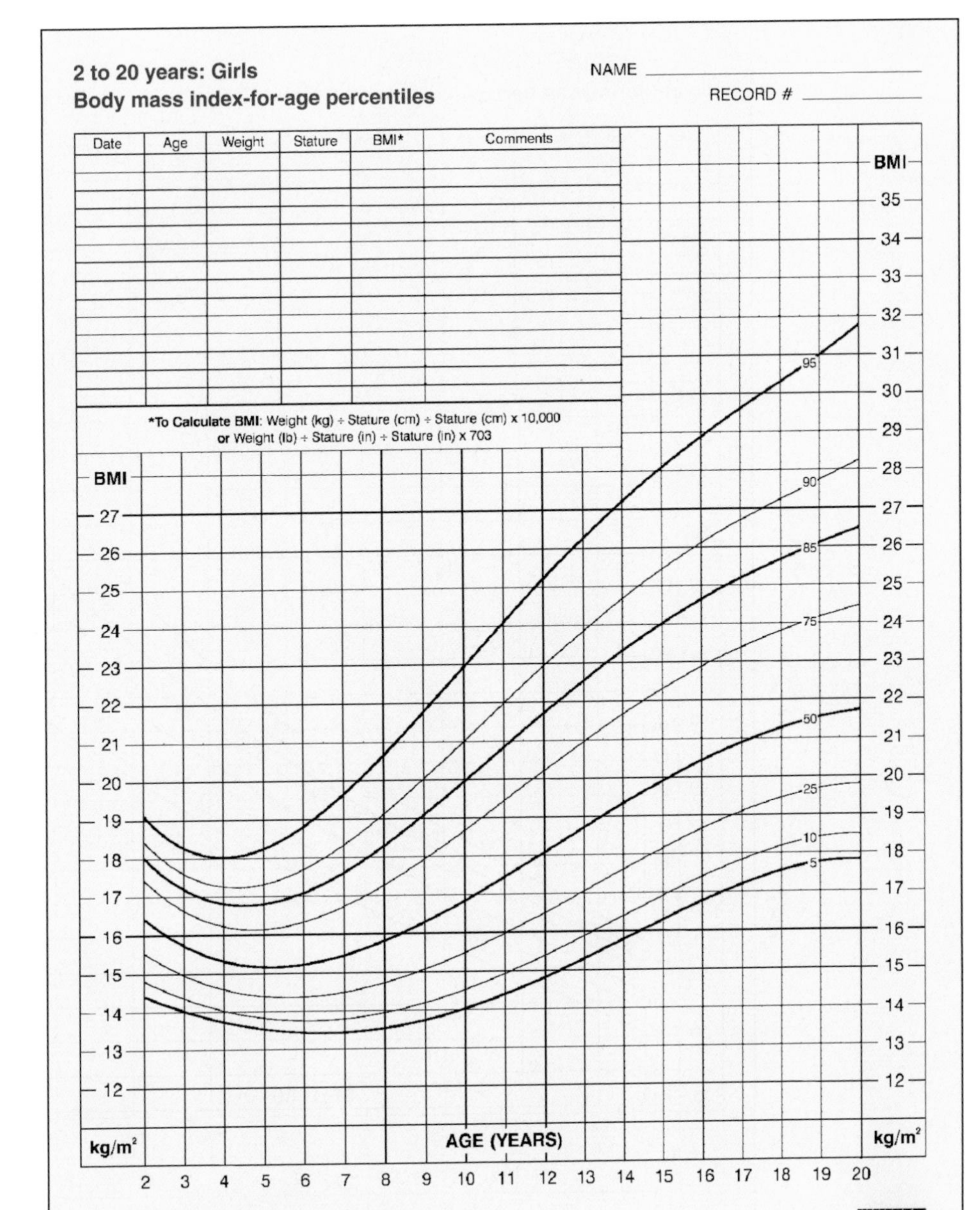
2 to 20 years: Girls
Body mass index-for-age percentiles
NAME
RECORD #
Date
Age
Weight
Stature
BMI*
Comments
*To Calculate BMI: Weight (kg) ÷ Stature (cm) ÷ Stature (cm) x 10,000
or Weight (lb) ÷ Stature (in) ÷ Stature (in) x 703
BMI
35
34
33
32
31
30
29
28
27
26
25
24
23
22
21
20
19
18
17
16
15
14
13
12
95
90
85
75
50
25
10
5
kg/m²
AGE (YEARS)
2 3 4 5 6 7 8 9 10 11 12 13 14 15 16 17 18 19 20
Published May 30, 2000 (modified 10/16/00).
SOURCE: Developed by the National Center for Health Statistics in collaboration with
the National Center for Chronic Disease Prevention and Health Promotion (2000).
http://www.cdc.gov/growthcharts

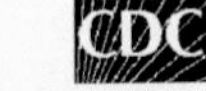
CDC
SAFER·HEALTHIER·PEOPLE™

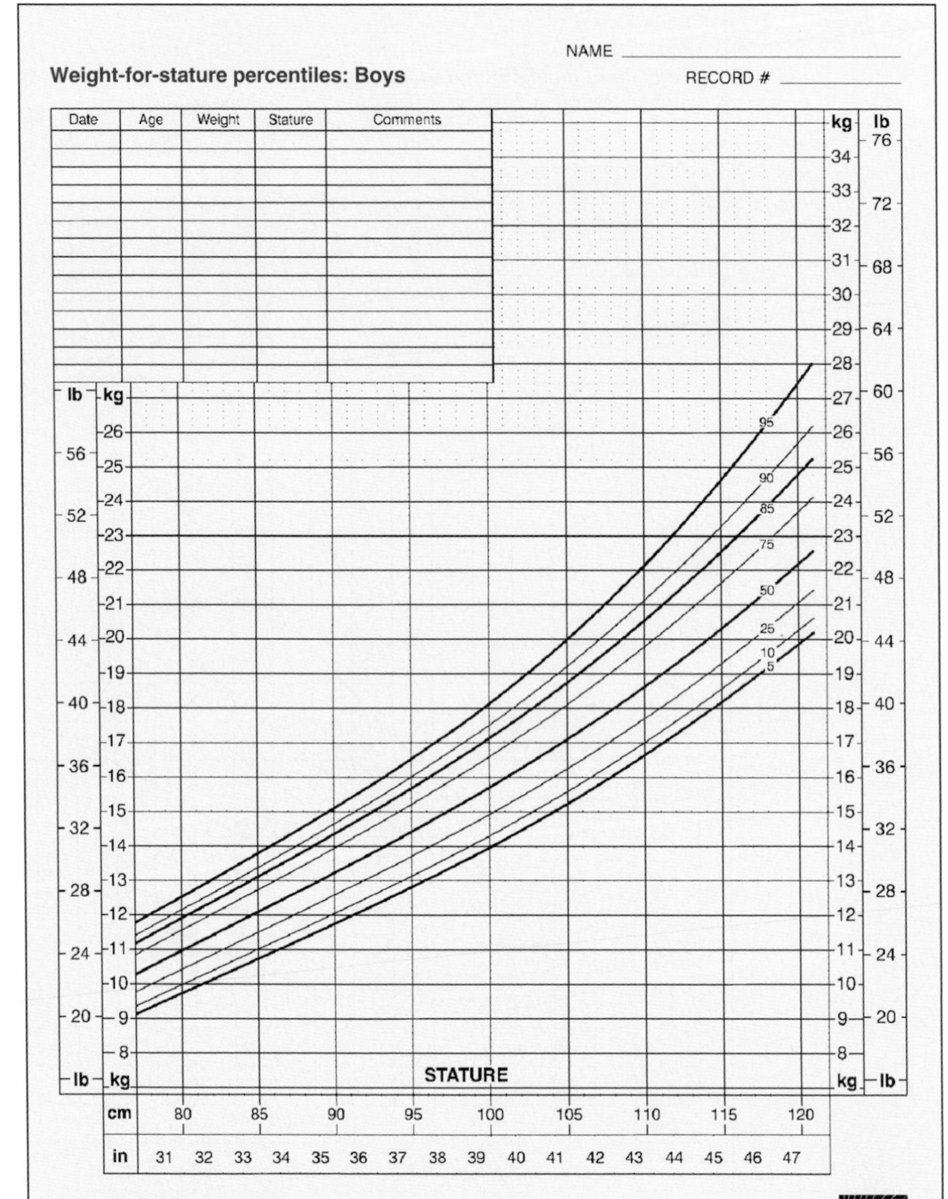

Published May 30, 2000 (modified 10/16/00).
SOURCE: Developed by the National Center for Health Statistics in collaboration with the National Center for Chronic Disease Prevention and Health Promotion (2000).
http://www.cdc.gov/growthcharts

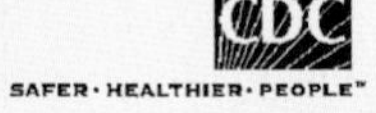

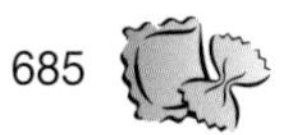

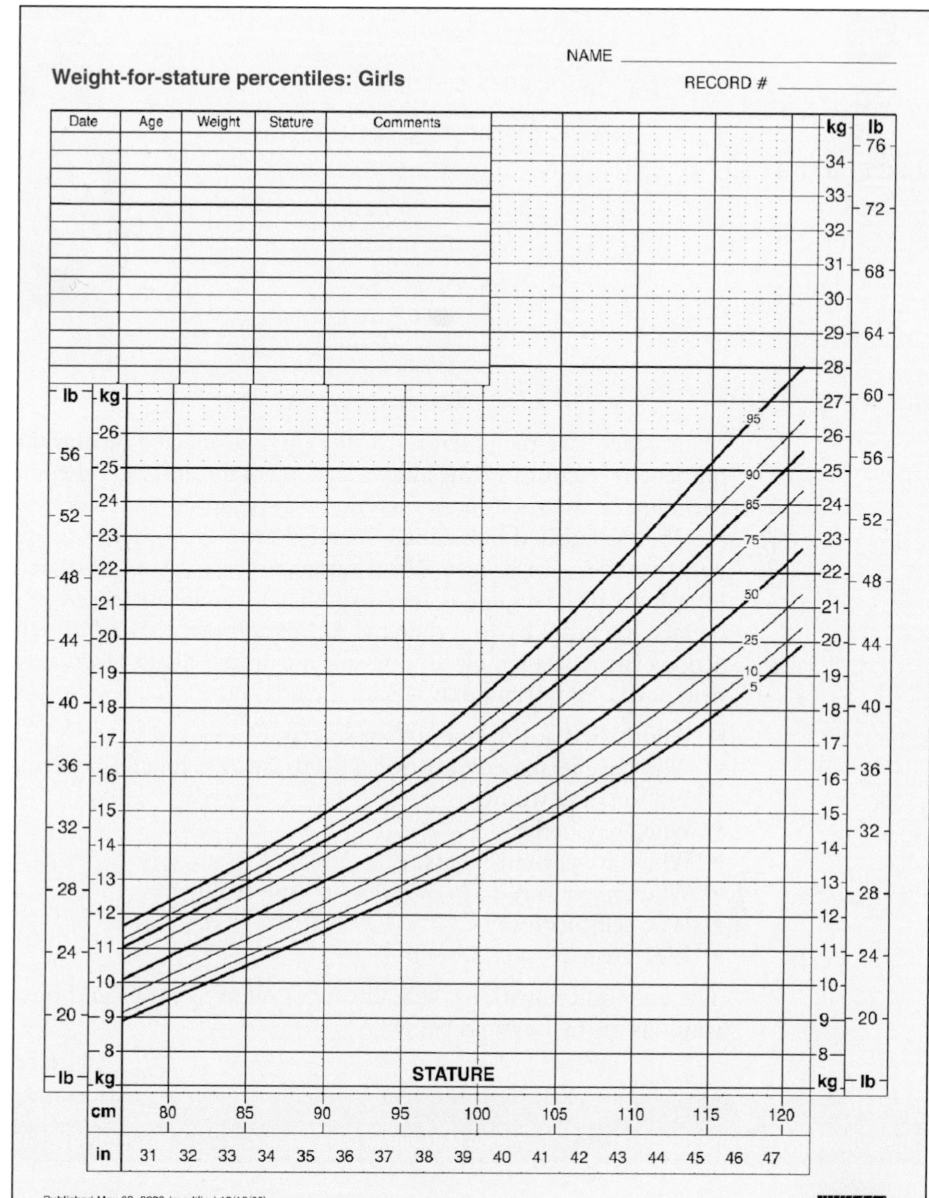

Published May 30, 2000 (modified 10/16/00).
SOURCE: Developed by the National Center for Health Statistics in collaboration with the National Center for Chronic Disease Prevention and Health Promotion (2000).
http://www.cdc.gov/growthcharts

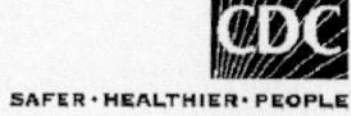

6

Diet and Drugs

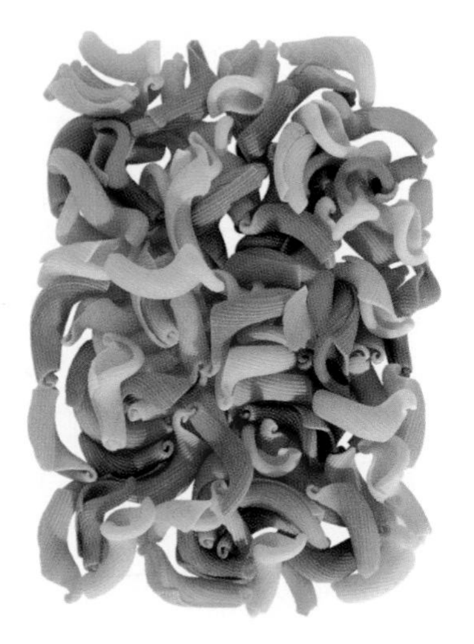

Many drugs have the potential to affect and be affected by nutrition. Sometimes, drug-nutrient interactions are the intended action of the drug. At other times, alterations in nutrient intake, metabolism, or excretion may be unfortunate side effects of drug therapy.

Well-nourished individuals on short-term drug therapy may easily withstand the negative effects of drug-nutrient interactions. Patients who are malnourished or on long-term drug regimens may experience significant nutrient deficiencies and decreased tolerance to drug therapy. Although potential and actual drug-nutrient interactions vary considerably among specific drugs, clients at greatest risk for developing drug-induced nutrient deficiencies include those

- Whose diets are chronically inadequate
- Who have increased nutritional needs, such as infants, adolescents, and pregnant and lactating women
- Who are elderly
- Who have chronic illnesses
- Who are on long-term or multiple drug regimens
- Who self-medicate
- Who are substance abusers

The common nutritional side effects of selected drugs and possible nutrition interventions are highlighted below.

(*text continues on page 696*)

Drug Classification and Examples	Common Nutritional Side Effects	Possible Nutrition Interventions/ Food Interactions
Analgesics		
Narcotic: codeine, meperidine, morphine sulfate	N/V, gastrointestinal upset, constipation, lethargy	May need increased fiber and fluids. Avoid alcohol.
Nonnarcotic: aspirin, ibuprofen, naproxen	N/V, gastrointestinal upset, gastrointestinal bleeding, constipation	Avoid gastrointestinal irritants with long-term use, such as pepper, caffeine, and alcohol. Increase intake of foods rich in folic acid, vitamin C, and iron.

Drug Classification and Examples	Common Nutritional Side Effects	Possible Nutrition Interventions/ Food Interactions
Antacids		
Aluminum hydroxide	Constipation	May need folic acid supplement with long-term use. May need ↑ phosphorus diet if used as ulcer treatment.
Calcium carbonate	Constipation, chalky taste	Maintain adequate hydration.
Magnesium hydroxide	N/V, gastrointestinal distress, diarrhea	Increase fiber and fluids. Separate from oral meds/ supplements by ≥2 h.
Antianemic		
Epoetin Alpha	Edema, N/V, diarrhea, ↑blood pressure, weakness	Follow ↓Na, ↓K diet; may need folic acid, B_{12}, and Fe supplement.
Antianxiety agents		
Alprazolam	N/V, diarrhea, constipation, drowsiness, dry mouth	Take with food. Avoid alcohol. Limit caffeine.
Buspirone hydrochloride	Dry mouth, drowsiness	Avoid alcohol. Limit caffeine. Caution with grapefruit juice. Take with food to ↓GI distress.
Lorazepam	Drowsiness	Limit caffeine to <500 mg/d.
Antiarrhythmic		
Sotalol	N/V, gastrointestinal distress, diarrhea, dry mouth, altered taste, edema, drowsiness	Food decreases absorption. Avoid alcohol. Avoid natural licorice. Limit caffeine.
Antibiotics		
Amoxicillin	N/V, diarrhea, drowsiness	Take with food. Avoid GI irritants. Consider MVI supplement.
Ampicillin	N/V, diarrhea	Take on empty stomach 1 hr before or 2 hr after meals.
Azithromycin	N/V, gastrointestinal distress, diarrhea	Take 1 h before or 2 h after full meal. Consider MVI supplement.
Ciprofloxacin	N/V, diarrhea	Maintain adequate hydration. Do not take with antacids or supplements containing magnesium, aluminum, or calcium. Do not take with iron, zinc, Mg, Al, Ca, or multivitamin supplements containing minerals. Avoid natural licorice.

(table continues on page 688)

Drug Classification and Examples	Common Nutritional Side Effects	Possible Nutrition Interventions/ Food Interactions
Clarithromycin	N/V, gastrointestinal distress, diarrhea, altered taste	Avoid alcohol. Limit caffeine. Consider MVI.
Dirithromycin	N/V, gastrointestinal distress, diarrhea	Take with food. May need low-potassium diet.
Erythromycin	N/V, gastrointestinal distress	Take with 8 oz water on empty stomach 1 hr before or 2 h after meals. Do not take with fruit juice.
Lomefloxacin	N/V, gastrointestinal distress, diarrhea, constipation, altered taste, dry mouth	Avoid caffeine. Increase fluids. May need high-fiber, low-potassium, low-sodium diet.
Penicillin	GI distress, N/V	Maintain hydration. Take with food to ↓distress.
Piperacillin/tazobactam	N/V, gastrointestinal distress, diarrhea, constipation, edema	May need low-sodium diet. Limit caffeine. Consider MVI.
Trimethoprim with sulfamethoxazole	N/V, diarrhea, gastrointestinal distress, drowsiness, anorexia	Maintain adequate hydration. May need folacin supplement. Take on an empty stomach.
Anticoagulants		
Ticlopidine	N/V, gastrointestinal upset, diarrhea	Take with or immediately after food. Avoid GI irritants.
Warfarin	Diarrhea	Maintain consistent vitamin K intake.
Anticonvulsants		
Carbamazepine	N/V, drowsiness	Take with food. Avoid alcohol. May deplete sodium. Limit caffeine. Caution with grapefruit juice.
Clonazepam	Drowsiness	Take with food. Avoid alcohol.
Ethosuximide	N/V, gastrointestinal distress, diarrhea, drowsiness	Avoid alcohol. Take with food to ↓GI distress.
Felbamate	N/V, gastrointestinal distress, diarrhea, constipation, drowsiness, edema, altered taste	May need low-sodium diet, high potassium. Do not crush or chew. Limit caffeine.
Phenobarbital	Drowsiness, taste changes	Causes vitamin D deficiency, low calcium absorption. May need vitamin D, B_{12}, B_6, C, calcium, and folacin supplements with long-term use. Limit caffeine.
Phenytoin	N/V, constipation, drowsiness	Increase foods rich in vitamin D, vitamin K, B_{12} and folacin. Limit caffeine.
Valproic acid	N/V, gastrointestinal distress, drowsiness, diarrhea	Avoid alcohol. Take with food to ↓GI distress. Limit caffeine.

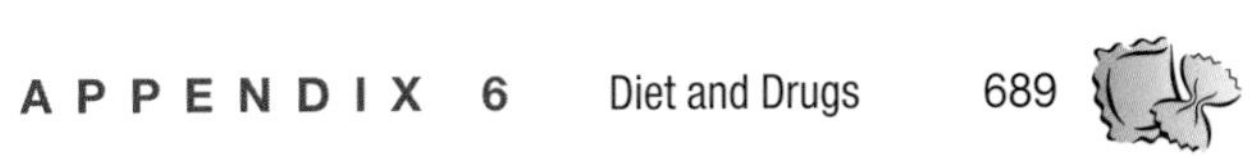

Drug Classification and Examples	Common Nutritional Side Effects	Possible Nutrition Interventions/ Food Interactions
Antidepressants		
Amitriptyline	Constipation, drowsiness, dry mouth	Avoid caffeine and alcohol. Take with food to ↓GI distress.
Bupropion HCl	Constipation, dry mouth	Take with food. Avoid alcohol. Avoid GI irritants with long-term use. Limit caffeine.
Clomipramine HCl	N/V, gastrointestinal distress, constipation, dry mouth	Take with food. May need high fiber, high fluids.
Escitalopram	Drowsiness, fatigue, N/V, diarrhea, dry mouth, anorexia, constipation, taste changes, flatulence, GI distress	Avoid alcohol. Take with food to ↓GI distress.
Fluoxetine HCl	N/V, diarrhea, dry mouth, drowsiness	Tryptophan supplements increase side effects. Limit caffeine.
Imipramine	N/V, constipation, dry mouth, drowsiness	Take with food. Avoid caffeine and alcohol. High fiber may decrease drug effectiveness. Causes increased urinary losses of riboflavin.
Mirtazapine	Constipation, dry mouth, ↑appetite, ↑weight, drowsiness	Take at bedtime. Avoid alcohol. May need ↓Na diet.
Nefazodone	Dry mouth, N/V, constipation	Avoid alcohol.
Paroxetine	N/V, diarrhea, constipation, drowsiness, thirst, dry mouth	No tryptophan supplements. Avoid alcohol. Limit caffeine.
Phenelzine	Drowsiness, anorexia	Avoid caffeine, alcohol, and foods high in tyramine. May need vitamin B_6 supplement.
Sertraline HCl	N/V, gastrointestinal distress, diarrhea, altered taste, dry mouth, drowsiness	Take with food. Avoid alcohol. Limit caffeine.
Antidiabetics		
Acarbose	GI distress, diarrhea, flatulence	Take 3 times daily with the first bite of each meal. Limit caffeine.
Chlorpropamide	S/E rare	Avoid alcohol. May need ↓Na diet.
Glipizide	S/E rare	Diet important. Avoid alcohol. Take 30 min before eating. Limit caffeine.
Glyburide	S/E rare	Diet important. Avoid alcohol. Limit caffeine.
Metformin	GI distress, N/V, diarrhea	Diabetic diet important. Limit caffeine. May need B_{12} supplement.

(table continues on page 690)

Drug Classification and Examples	Common Nutritional Side Effects	Possible Nutrition Interventions/ Food Interactions
Miglitol	GI distress, diarrhea	Diabetic diet important. May need iron supplement with long-term use.
Pioglitazone	Edema	Diabetic diet important. Alcohol with MD approval only.
Repaglinide	Diarrhea	Diabetic diet important. Take ≤30 min before meals. Limit caffeine.
Rosiglitazone	Weight gain	Diabetic diet important. Limit caffeine.
Antidiarrheals		
Diphenoxylate HCl with atropine sulfate	Gastrointestinal distress, constipation, dry mouth	Take with food. Avoid alcohol.
Octreotide acetate	N/V, gastrointestinal distress, diarrhea	Maintain adequate hydration. Limit caffeine.
Antifungals		
Amphotericin	N/V, anorexia, gastrointestinal distress	Maintain adequate hydration. Increase potassium and magnesium intake. Limit caffeine.
Fluconazole	N/V	May need high-potassium diet.
Ketoconazole	N/V	Separate from antacids and histamine blockers by 2 hours. Limit caffeine.
Antigout		
Allopurinol	N/V, diarrhea	High fluid intake to prevent renal stones. No high doses of vitamin C.
Colchicine	N/V, gastrointestinal distress, diarrhea	Avoid alcohol. May decrease absorption of protein, fat, vitamin A, carotene, iron, calcium, sodium, and potassium. High fluid intake to prevent renal stones.
Antihypertensives		
ACE inhibitors: benazepril, captopril, fosinopril	Hyperkalemia, altered taste, dry mouth	No licorice. May need low-sodium, low-calorie diet. No potassium supplement, avoid ↑K foods.
Aldactazide	Dry mouth	Take with food. Avoid alcohol. May need low-sodium, low-calorie diet. No licorice. Avoid high-potassium foods. Limit caffeine.

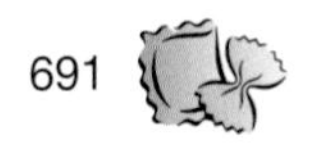

Drug Classification and Examples	Common Nutritional Side Effects	Possible Nutrition Interventions/ Food Interactions
Amlodipine	N/V, edema	Take with food. May need low-sodium, low-calorie diet. ↓K^+ No ↑K^+ salt substitute. No licorice or grapefruit juice.
Atenolol	N/V, diarrhea, dry mouth, drowsiness	Take separately from calcium supplements and antacids. No licorice.
Bisoprolol fumarate	Drowsiness	May need low-sodium, low-potassium, low-calorie, low-fat, high-fiber diet. Avoid natural licorice.
Clonidine	N/V, dry mouth, constipation, drowsiness	May need low-sodium, low-calorie, ↑fiber diet. No licorice. Avoid alcohol.
Doxazosin mesylate	Drowsiness	May need low-sodium diet. Avoid natural licorice.
Eplerenone	No side effects common	Grapefruit juice increases drug level by 25%. No potassium-containing salt substitutes without MD approval.
Guanfacine	Drowsiness, dry mouth, constipation	Take with food. May need high-fiber, high-fluid diet. Avoid natural licorice.
Hydralazine HCl	N/V, edema, diarrhea, ↓appetite	Take consistently either with or without food. May need low-sodium, low-calorie diet. No licorice. May need vitamin B_6 supplement to avoid nerve damage in hands and feet.
Isradipine	N/V, gastrointestinal distress, diarrhea, constipation	Take with food. May need low sodium, high fiber, high fluids. Limit caffeine.
Methyldopa	Edema, dry mouth, drowsiness	May need low-sodium, low-calorie diet. No licorice. Increase B_{12}. Take iron supplement 2 h before or after drug. Avoid natural licorice.
Metoprolol tartrate	Drowsiness, diarrhea	Take with food. May need low-sodium, low-calorie diet. No licorice. Limit caffeine.
Minoxidil	Edema	May need low-sodium, low-calorie diet. No licorice. Limit caffeine.

(table continues on page 692)

Drug Classification and Examples	Common Nutritional Side Effects	Possible Nutrition Interventions/ Food Interactions
Nifedipine	N/V, gastrointestinal distress, diarrhea, constipation, drowsiness, edema	May need low-sodium, low-calorie diet. No licorice. ↑K^+ Take on empty stomach or with ↓fat snack, not with grapefruit juice.
Prazosin HCL	N/V, drowsiness	May need low-sodium, low-calorie diet. No licorice. Avoid alcohol. Limit caffeine.
Antinausea		
Chlorpromazine HCl	Constipation, dry mouth, drowsiness	Take with food. Avoid caffeine and alcohol. Separate B_{12} and magnesium supplements by 2 hours.
Dronabinol	Dry mouth, N/V, gastrointestinal distress, drowsiness	Avoid alcohol.
Granisetron HCl	N/V, constipation, altered taste	May need high-fiber, high-fluid diet.
Ondansetron HCl	Constipation, gastrointestinal distress, diarrhea, drowsiness	Limit caffeine.
Antineoplastic		
Anastrozole	N/V, gastrointestinal distress, diarrhea, constipation, edema, dry mouth	May need low-sodium diet. Consider MVI.
Busulfan	N/V	Limit alcohol and caffeine. Consider MVI.
Carboplatin	N/V, gastrointestinal distress, diarrhea, constipation, weakness	May need high-fiber, high-fluid, adequate potassium, magnesium, calcium diet.
Carmustine	N/V	Avoid alcohol. Increase fluid. Consider MVI.
Cisplatin	N/V, diarrhea, altered taste, weakness	Maintain adequate hydration. May need mineral supplement due to increased urinary excretion of magnesium, potassium, calcium, zinc, and copper. Limit caffeine.
Cyclophosphamide	N/V	Increase fluid to ≥3 L/d. Consider MVI.
Cytarabine	N/V, diarrhea	Increase fluid. Consider MVI.
Dacarbazine	N/V	Increase fluid. Restrict food 4–6 h before treatment. Consider MVI.
Dactinomycin	N/V, gastrointestinal distress, diarrhea, weakness	Increase fluid. Consider MVI.

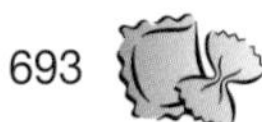

Drug Classification and Examples	Common Nutritional Side Effects	Possible Nutrition Interventions/ Food Interactions
Docetaxel	N/V, diarrhea, edema	May need ↓Na. Consider MVI.
Doxorubicin	Gastrointestinal distress, N/V	May need ↑fluid. Consider MVI.
Estramustine phosphate sodium	N/V, gastrointestinal distress, diarrhea, weakness, edema, decreased appetite	Take separately from dairy products and sources of calcium. May need ↑fluid, ↓Na, ↓concentrated carbohydrates diet.
Etoposide	N/V, diarrhea	May need vitamin B_6 supplement.
Fluorouracil	N/V, gastrointestinal distress, diarrhea, taste changes	May need vitamin B_6 supplement.
Irinotecan HCl	N/V, severe diarrhea	Electrolyte imbalances may occur from severe diarrhea.
Melphalan	N/V, gastrointestinal distress, diarrhea	Take on empty stomach.
Methotrexate	N/V, diarrhea, drowsiness, anorexia, GI distress, weakness	Folate antagonist. Folate deficiency may increase drug toxicity. May decrease absorption of fat, vitamin B_{12}, and calcium. Goal fluid: 2–3 L/d.
Paclitaxel	N/V, diarrhea, edema	May need low-sodium diet. May need vitamin B_6 supplement.
Vinblastine sulfate	N/V, anorexia, stomatitis	Increase fluid to 2–3 L/d.
Vinorelbine	N/V, stomatitis, anorexia	
Antiparkinson		
Benztropine mesylate	Constipation, dry mouth	Take with food. Avoid alcohol.
Bromocriptine mesylate	N/V, gastrointestinal distress, constipation, drowsiness	Take with food. May need high fiber, high fluids. Avoid alcohol. Limit caffeine.
Levodopa	N/V, gastrointestinal distress, dry mouth, anorexia, dysphagia	Do not take with high-protein foods, amino acids, or protein hydrolysates. Do not take with high-fiber meals. Limit vitamin B_6 to <5 mg/d.
Selegiline	N/V	If >10 mg drug/d, avoid high-tyramine foods. Limit caffeine.
Antiprotozoan		
Atovaquone	N/V, gastrointestinal distress, diarrhea	Take with high-fat meal or snack. Limit caffeine.
Metronidazole	N/V, gastrointestinal distress, altered taste, anorexia, diarrhea	May need fluid and electrolyte replacement if stools are liquid. Take with food to ↓GI distress.

(table continues on page 694)

Drug Classification and Examples	Common Nutritional Side Effects	Possible Nutrition Interventions/ Food Interactions
Antipsychotic		
Haloperidol	N/V, gastrointestinal distress, diarrhea, constipation, drowsiness, dry mouth	Do not mix concentrate with coffee, tea, or fruit juice (drug may precipitate). Take with food. Avoid caffeine and alcohol.
Thioridazine HCl	Constipation, drowsiness, dry mouth, edema	Take with food. Avoid caffeine and alcohol. May need ↓Na diet.
Antivirals		
Acyclovir	N/V	Maintain adequate hydration. Limit caffeine and alcohol. Consider MVI supplement.
Didanosine (DDI)	N/V, gastrointestinal distress, diarrhea, thirst, edema	Take on empty stomach. Do not mix with acidic beverage; mix powder form with 4 oz water.
Famciclovir	N/V	May need high-fiber, high-fluid ↑calorie diet.
Foscarnet sodium	N/V, gastrointestinal distress, diarrhea, ↓appetite	Maintain adequate hydration. May need ↓Na, ↑K.
Indinavir sulfate	N/V	Take on empty stomach. Need adequate fluid to avoid renal stones. Limit caffeine. Not with grapefruit juice.
Lamivudine	N/V, diarrhea, drowsiness	Maintain adequate hydration. Limit caffeine.
Nelfinvir mesylate	N/V, diarrhea	Mix with water, milk, or formula. Limit caffeine.
Ritonavir	N/V, gastrointestinal distress, diarrhea, altered taste	Mix with chocolate milk, Ensure, or Advera to improve taste. Provide MVI. May need ↓K^+, ↓fat diet.
Saquinavir mesylate	N/V, gastrointestinal distress, diarrhea	Take with grapefruit juice to ↑bioavailability. Increase fluid. Limit caffeine.
Stavudine (D_4T)	N/V, gastrointestinal distress, diarrhea, constipation	Maintain adequate hydration. Take on empty stomach. Avoid natural licorice.
Zalcitabine	N/V, diarrhea	Do not take within 2 h of magnesium- or aluminum-containing antacids. Limit caffeine.
Zidovudine (AZT)	N/V, diarrhea	Monitor for anemia. Limit caffeine and alcohol.

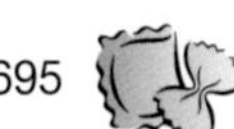

Drug Classification and Examples	Common Nutritional Side Effects	Possible Nutrition Interventions/ Food Interactions
Bronchodilators		
Albuterol sulfate	N/V, gastrointestinal distress, dry mouth, altered taste, hypertension	Take with food. Avoid caffeine. Avoid natural licorice. May need ↓Na^+ diet.
Aminophylline	N/V, anorexia, ↓weight	Avoid caffeine. Maintain consistent intake of protein and carbohydrate for consistent drug levels.
Ipratropium bromide	N/V, gastrointestinal distress, dry mouth	Not appropriate for people with allergies to soy lecithin, soybeans, or peanuts.
Theophylline	GI distress	High-protein, low-carbohydrate diet causes decreased blood levels of drug. Limit caffeine.
Corticosteroid		
Dexamethasone	N/V, gastrointestinal distress, ↑appetite, ↑weight	May need low-sodium, high-protein, ↑K^+ diet. May need increased potassium; calcium; vitamins A, C, D, B_6; and folacin.
Diuretic		
Chlorothiazide	Hypokalemia	Avoid alcohol. May need potassium and magnesium supplement. No licorice. May need ↓Na, ↑K^+ diet.
Spironolactone	N/V, gastrointestinal distress, diarrhea, thirst, dry mouth	Maintain adequate hydration. No licorice. Avoid high-potassium intake. Limit caffeine.
Hypnotic		
Flurazepam HCl	Drowsiness	Take at bedtime. Avoid alcohol.
Zolpidem tartrate	S/E not common	Food decreases and delays drug absorption.
Immunosuppressant		
Azathioprine	N/V, anemia	May need vitamin B_{12} and folic acid supplement. May need ↑ fluid.
Cyclosporine	N/V, gastrointestinal distress, diarrhea, hyperkalemia	May need low-fat, low-potassium, low-calorie diet.
Muromonab	N/V, gastrointestinal distress, diarrhea, edema, weakness	Maintain adequate hydration. Limit caffeine. Consider MVI.

(table continues on page 696)

Drug Classification and Examples	Common Nutritional Side Effects	Possible Nutrition Interventions/ Food Interactions
Lipid Lowering		
Atorvastatin calcium	↑ or ↓appetite, weight gain	Need low-fat diet. May need increased fiber and fluids. Caution with grapefruit juice. Limit caffeine.
Cholestyramine	N/V, gastrointestinal distress, constipation	May need supplements of calcium, magnesium, iron, zinc, folacin, B_{12}, and fat-soluble vitamins due to decreased absorption. Limit caffeine.
Clofibrate	N/V, gastrointestinal distress, diarrhea	Low-fat, low-cholesterol diet important. Limit caffeine.
Colestipol	N/V, gastrointestinal distress, diarrhea, constipation	Low-fat, low-cholesterol diet important. May need multivitamin with mineral supplement.
Ezetimibe	Nausea	Need ↓fat, ↓cholesterol diet.
Fluvastatin	Gastrointestinal distress	Need low-fat, low-cholesterol diet. Limit caffeine.
Lovastatin	N/V, gastrointestinal distress, diarrhea, constipation	May need low-fat, low-cholesterol, low-calorie diet. Do not take fiber, pectin, or oat bran within 3 h of dosage. Caution with grapefruit juice. Limit caffeine.
Niacin	N/V, gastrointestinal distress, diarrhea, constipation	Need low-fat, low-cholesterol, low-calorie diet. Take with food. Limit caffeine.
Simvastatin	Gastrointestinal distress, constipation	Need low-fat, low-cholesterol, low-calorie diet. Avoid alcohol. Limit caffeine.

N/V = nausea and vomiting

MONOAMINE OXIDASE INHIBITORS (MAOIs)

Monoamine oxidase inhibitors (MAOIs) are antidepressants that potentiate the cardiovascular effect of tyramine and other vasoactive amines in food. A hypertensive crisis may occur within several hours after foods containing tyramine are infected with MAOIs. Signs and symptoms include increased blood pressure, headache, pallor, nausea, vomiting, restlessness, dilated pupils, sweating, palpitations, angina, and fever. Death caused by intracranial bleeding occurs rarely. Tyramine-containing foods that are contraindicated during MAOI therapy include the following:

 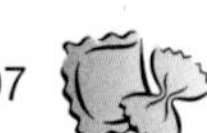

Aged, dried, fermented, salted, smoked, and pickled meat and fish, including processed meats and luncheon meats such as bacon, sausage, liverwurst, hot dogs, corned beef, pepperoni, salami, bologna, and ham
All aged and mature cheese, such as blue, Boursault, brick, Brie, Camembert, cheddar, Emmentaler, gruyere, mozzarella, parmesan, processed American, provolone, Romano, Roquefort, and Stilton
Broad beans and pods
Certain alcoholic beverages, such as beer, Chianti wine, burgundy, sherry, vermouth, and ale
Fermented soybean products including miso and some tofu products
Overripe and spoiled fruit
Sauerkraut
Sourdough and homemade yeast breads
Yeast extracts and meat extracts, which can be found in soups, gravies, stews, and sauces

The following foods should be limited to ½ cup or 4 oz or less per day during MAOI therapy:

Buttermilk
Caviar
Certain fruits, such as bananas, avocados, canned figs, raisins, red plums, raspberries
Chocolate and products containing chocolate
Coffee
Other wines and distilled spirits
Sour cream
Soy sauce, teriyaki sauce
Yogurt

REFERENCES

Burke, P., Roche-Dudek, M., & Roche-Klemma, K. (2003). *Drug-nutrient resource* (5th ed.). Riverside, IL: Roche Dietitians, LLC.
Skidmore-Roth, L. (2004). *Mosby's nursing drug reference.* St. Louis: Mosby.

INDEX

Note: Page numbers followed by *b* indicate a box; those followed by *f*, an illustration; and those followed by *t*, a table.

A

Abacavir (Ziagen, ABC), for HIV infection/AIDS, 661*t*
Abdomen, cancer of, radiation therapy complications in, 640*t*
Abdominal fat, 377, 380*f*
Absorption
  of amino acids, 49
  of calcium, 104, 140
  of carbohydrates, 22
  of fat, 74–75
  impairment of. *See* Malabsorption
  of iron, 133, 146–147
  of magnesium, 142
  of minerals, 133
  of protein, 49
  of sugars, 22
  of vitamins, natural vs. synthetic, 96
  water role in, 128
Acarbose (Precose), for diabetes mellitus, 580, 689*t*
Acceptable Daily Intake (ADI), of artificial sweeteners, 40
Acceptable Macronutrient Distribution Range (AMDR)
  for alpha-linolenic acid, 674*t*
  for carbohydrates, 31, 674*t*
  description of, 182–183
  for fat, 81, 81*t*, 674*t*
  for linoleic acid, 674*t*
  for proteins, 54, 674*t*
Acculturation
  of African Americans, 250–251
  American interest in ethnic foods and, 261–264, 263*b*
  of Asian Americans, 255–257
  assessment of, 257–258
  definition of, 248
  factors influencing, 248–249
  food substitutions in, 249
  of Mexican Americans, 254
  new foods in, 249
  regional food specialty availability and, 264
  rejection of traditional foods in, 249
Accutrim (phenylpropanolamine), for weight loss, 399
Acesulfame K, 39*t*, 41
Acetyl coenzyme A, in tricarboxylic acid cycle, 157, 158
Achlorhydria, nutrition therapy for, 493–494
Acid-base balance
  amino acids in, 46
  chloride in, 135*t*
  minerals in, 132
  potassium in, 135*t*
  sodium in, 134, 135*t*
Acne, chocolate and, 343
Acquired immunodeficiency syndrome. *See* HIV infection/AIDS
Activity. *See* Exercise (physical activity)
Actos (pioglitazone), for diabetes mellitus, 581, 690*t*
Acute renal failure
  nutrition therapy for, 625–627
  pathophysiology of, 625–626
Acyclovir, food interactions with, 693*t*
Adequate Intake (AI). *See also specific nutrients*
  for breast-feeding, 668*t*–669*t*, 671*t*, 673*t*
  for children, 668*t*–669*t*, 671*t*, 673*t*
  description of, 182
  for fat, 81, 81*t*
  for infants, 668*t*–669*t*, 671*t*, 673*t*
  in pregnancy, 668*t*–669*t*, 671*t*, 673*t*
ADI (Acceptable Daily Intake), of artificial sweeteners, 40
Adipex (phentermine), for weight loss, 399
Adipose tissue. *See* Fat (body)
Adolescents
  diabetes mellitus in, 594–595
  eating disorder onset in, 408
  growth charts for, 680*f*–685*f*
  nutrition for, 337–340
    calcium in, 338
    chronic disease risk and, 340
    concerns with, 339–340
    growth rate and, 337–338
    iron in, 338–339
    in pregnancy, 340
    unhealthful dieting and, 339–340
pregnancy in, 295–296, 340
Advanced vitamin supplement formulas, 123
Aerobic exercise, metabolism in, 162
African Americans
  acculturation by, 250–251
  health beliefs of, 251–252
  healthy diet suggestions for, 252, 547*b*
  traditional food practices of, 250, 251*f*
Age
  vs. body mass index
    for adolescents, 681*f*
    for children, 681*f*
  vs. calcium requirements, 328*f*
  as coronary heart disease risk factor, 533
  vs. height, of adolescents, 680*f*, 682*f*
  vs. iron requirements, 329*f*
  vs. target heart rate, 168
  water requirements and, 131*t*
  vs. weight, of infants, 313–314
Agenerase (amprenavir), for HIV infection/AIDS, 661*t*
Aging/older adults, 347–371
  Alzheimer's disease in, 360–361
  basal metabolic rate in, 163
  body system changes in, 351–352
  demographics of, 351
  diabetes mellitus in, 595–597
  healthy diet for, 355–357
  hypertension and, 551
  in long-term care facilities, 362–366, 364*b*, 365*b*
  mineral supplements for, 357
  nursing process for, 366–368
  nutritional assessment in, 357, 358*b*
  nutritional implications of, 351–352
  nutritional needs of, 352–354, 355*t*
  nutritional risk factors in, 357, 358*b*

Aging/older adults (*continued*)
obesity in, 361
osteoarthritis in, 358–359
osteoporosis in, 359–360
social isolation of, 361–362
theories of, 350
vitamin B_2 deficiency in, 111
vitamin D in, 104
vitamin supplements for, 118, 120, 357
Ahimsa (nonviolence applied to foods), 260–261
AI. *See* Adequate Intake (AI)
AIDS. *See* HIV infection/AIDS
Alaska Natives, healthy diet suggestions for, 547*b*
Albumin
in fluid and electrolyte balance maintenance, 46
normal levels of, 9
in nutritional assessment, 9–10, 10*t*
Albuterol
for chronic obstructive pulmonary disease, 470
food interactions with, 695*t*
Alcohol use
birth defects due to, 283
in breast-feeding, 300
for coronary heart disease prevention, 544–545
in diabetes mellitus, 575*t*, 579
in *Dietary Guidelines for Americans 2005*, 185*b*
in eating disorders, 408
folate deficiency in, 112
in Healthy Eating Index, 192*t*
in Healthy Eating Pyramid, 193*f*, 194
in hypertension, 556
in nutritional assessment, 6
in pregnancy, 282–283
vitamin B_1 deficiency in, 110
vitamin B_3 deficiency in, 111
vitamin supplements for, 121
Aldactazide, food interactions with, 690*t*
Aldosterone, release of, in stress, 458, 459*t*
Allergy, food
breast-feeding diet and, 301
to breast milk, 308
foods causing, 343
in nutritional assessment, 6
Allopurinol, food interactions with, 690*t*
Allyl sulfides, sources and effects of, 119*t*
Alpha-glycosidase inhibitors, for diabetes mellitus, 580
Alpha-linolenic acid
in fats, 68*t*
recommendations for
Acceptable Macronutrient Distribution Range, 81, 81*t*, 182, 674
Adequate Intake, 673*t*
in breast-feeding, 673*t*
in children, 673*t*
in coronary heart disease prevention, 540
Dietary Reference Intake, 673*t*
in infants, 673*t*
in pregnancy, 673*t*
sources of, 59
Alpha-tocopherol, 105. *See also* Vitamin E (tocopherols)
Alprazolam, food interactions with, 687*t*
Aluminum hydroxide, food interactions with, 687*t*
Alzheimer's disease
fish intake and, 368–369
nutritional interventions for, 360–361
vitamin E for, 105
AMDR. *See* Acceptable Macronutrient Distribution Range (AMDR)
Amenorrhea, in anorexia nervosa, 407
American Cancer Association, healthy eating guidelines of, 200*b*–201*b*
American Diabetes Association
exchange list of, 389*t*, 581, 584*b*–587*b*, 585, 587–588
recommendations of, 573
American Dietetic Association
exchange list of, 581, 584*b*–587*b*, 585, 587–588
National Renal Diet of, 619–621
American Heart Association, healthy eating guidelines of, 200*b*–201*b*
American Institute for Cancer Research, healthy diet guidelines of, 200*b*–201*b*
Amino acids
adverse effects of, 55
in breast milk, 297
deamination of, 51–52, 158, 160
in DNA synthesis, 51
as energy source, 52, 158
essential, 47
in complete proteins, 52
in incomplete proteins, 53–54
in plants, 57
in fat formation, 52, 156
formation of
glucose in, 26
in protein digestion, 48–49, 48*f*
in protein turnover, 51
glucogenic, 51–52, 158, 458–459
ketogenic, 160
limiting, 53–54
in metabolic pool, 49
metabolism of, 49–52, 51*b*, 158
names of, 47*b*
nonessential, 47, 47*b*
in parenteral nutrition formulas, 450
patterns of, in liver failure, 519
protein synthesis from, 46–49
recommendations for, in critical illness, 462–463
structures of, 46–47, 47*f*
supplements for, 55
transamination of, 47
Aminopeptidase, in protein digestion, 48*f*, 49
Aminophylline, food interactions with, 695*t*
Amitriptyline, food interactions with, 689*t*
Amlodipine, food interactions with, 691*t*
Ammonia, formation of
in amino acid deamination, 52
in liver failure, 520
Amoxicillin, food interactions with, 687*t*
Amphotericin, food interactions with, 690*t*
Ampicillin, food interactions with, 687*t*

Amprenavir (Agenerase, APV), for HIV infection/AIDS, 661*t*
Amylase
  in breast milk, 298
  in starch digestion, 22, 23*f*
Anabolism, 156–157, 157*f*, 158*f*
  definition of, 25
  of fat, 76
Anaerobic metabolism, 158, 161–162
Analgesics, food interactions with, 686*t*
Anastrozole, food interactions with, 692*t*
Androstenedione, as ergogenic acid, 170*t*
Anemia
  hypochromic, 147
  iron-deficiency, 147, 328–329
  macrocytic, in vitamin B_{12} deficiency, 109*t*
  microcytic, 147
  pernicious, in vitamin B_{12} deficiency, 114
Angiotensin-converting enzyme inhibitors, food interactions with, 690*t*
Anorexia
  vs. anorexia nervosa, 479
  appetite stimulants for, 659*t*
  in cancer, 637*f*, 645
  definition of, 479
  management of, 409–411
  nutrition therapy for, 478–479, 645
  in older adults, 363
  teaching points for, 411–412
Anorexia nervosa
  vs. anorexia (lack of appetite), 468
  assessment of, 408–409
  description of, 406–407
  etiology of, 408
Antacids, 493–494, 687*t*
Antianxiety agents, food interactions with, 687*t*
Antiarrhythmics, food interactions with, 687*t*
Antibiotics, food interactions with, 687*t*–688*t*
Antibodies
  in breast milk, 298
  in colostrum, 298
Anticavity strategies, 36
Anticipatory nausea and vomiting, 645
Anticoagulants, food interactions with, 688*t*
Anticonvulsants, food interactions with, 688*t*
Antidepressants, food interactions with, 689*t*
Antidiabetic drugs, 580–581. *See also* Insulin
  food interactions with, 689*t*–690*t*
Antidiuretic hormone, release of, in stress, 458, 459*t*
Antiemetics, food interactions with, 692*t*
Antifungals, food interactions with, 690*t*
Antihypertensive drugs, 552, 690*t*–692*t*
Antineoplastic therapy
  breast-feeding contraindication with, 302
  food interactions with, 692*t*–693*t*
  nutritional effects of, 638–639
  nutrition therapy for, 645–648
Antioxidants
  cancer and, 660
  for coronary heart disease prevention, 544
  definition of, 97
  function of, 97
  phytochemicals as, 118, 119*t*
  for unsaturated fats, 69
  vitamin A as, 101
  vitamin C as, 115
  vitamin E as, 105
  vitamins as, 97
Antipsychotics, food interactions with, 693*t*
Antisecretory drugs, for gastritis, 493–494
Antithymocyte globulin, 622
Anuric phase, of acute renal failure, 625
Anxiety
  in diabetes mellitus, 589
  in enteral nutrition, 443*b*–444*b*
Appetite
  denial of. *See* Anorexia nervosa
  loss of. *See also* Anorexia
    intake promotion in, 468
    vitamin supplements for, 121
  stimulants for, 658, 659*t*
APV (amprenavir), for HIV infection/AIDS, 661*t*
Arginine, for critical illness, 463
Aristolochic acid products, 223*t*
Arroz con leche, 253
Artificial nutrition. *See* Enteral nutrition; Parenteral nutrition
Artificial sweeteners, 38, 39*t*, 40–41
  in diabetes mellitus, 576
  in pregnancy, 283–284
Ascites, nutritional therapy for, 520–522
Ascorbic acid. *See* Vitamin C (ascorbic acid)
Asian Americans
  acculturation by, 256
  health beliefs of, 247, 257
  healthy diet suggestions for, 257, 547*b*
  traditional food practices of, 255, 256*f*
Aspartame, 39*t*
  phenylketonuria and, 274
  safety of, 40
Aspiration, pulmonary, in enteral nutrition, 438
Aspirin, food interactions with, 686*t*
Assessment, 5–10
  appearance in, 8–9, 9*b*
  in breast-feeding, 302–303
  of children, 313
  definition of, 5
  in eating disorders, 408–409
  in enteral nutrition, 439
  gastrointestinal status in, 478
  health history in, 5
  of infants, 320–321
  intake information in, 6
  laboratory values in, 9–10, 10*t*
  medication history in, 8
  of older adults, 357, 358*b*
  in pregnancy, 291–293
  questions for, 194–195
  social history in, 9
  supplement history in, 8
  weight history in, 7–8, 7*t*, 8*b*

Atenolol, food interactions with, 691*t*
Atherogenic diet, as coronary heart disease risk factor, 532, 535
Atherosclerosis
definition of, 530
diet promoting, 535
pathogenesis of, 530, 531*f*, 532*f*
prevention of. *See also* Cholesterol (blood), lowering of
alcohol intake and, 544–545
lifestyle change diet in, 538–542, 539*f*, 543*b*
nutritional supplements in, 542, 543*b*, 545
in renal disease, 606
Athletes
carbohydrate intake and, 25
carbohydrate-loading diet for, 169
eating disorders in, 408
ergogenic acids for, 168, 170*t*
muscle building in, eating for, 61–62
Atkins diet, 391, 391*t*
Atole, 253
Atorvastatin (Lipitor), for cholesterol lowering, 536, 537*t*, 696*t*
Atovaquone, food interactions with, 693*t*
ATP, energy in, 161
Attention-deficit disorder, food additives and, 343
Autism, gluten-free diet for, 525
Avandia (rosiglitazone), for diabetes mellitus, 581, 690*t*
Aversions, food, in cancer, 647
Azathioprine (Imuran)
food interactions with, 695*t*
after renal transplantation, 622
Azithromycin, food interactions with, 687*t*
AZT (zidovudine), for HIV infection/AIDS, 661*t*, 693*t*

B

Bacillus cereus, in foodborne illness, 233*t*
Bacteria
in enteral formulas, 437–438
reduction of, in low-microbial diet, 522, 522*b*
translocation of, in parenteral nutrition, 448
Banding, gastric, for obesity, 400, 400*f*
Basal energy expenditure, 458, 461*b*
Basal metabolic rate, 163–164
of older adults, 352
in pregnancy, 275
Beans, dry. *See* Meat, poultry, fish, dry beans, eggs, and nuts group
BEE (basal energy expenditure), 458, 461*b*
Behavior skills, in diabetes mellitus, 589, 590*f*, 591, 592*b*
Behavior therapy, for weight management, 396, 397*b*–398*b*
Benazepril, food interactions with, 690*t*
Benecol margarine, for coronary heart disease prevention, 544
Benztropine, food interactions with, 693*t*
Beriberi, 108*t*, 110
Beta-carotene
as antioxidant, 97
deficiency of, 99*t*
functions of, 99*t*
as provitamin, 96
sources of, 99*t*, 101
storage of, 103
toxicity of, 99*t*
Beta-hydroxy beta-methylbutyrate (HMB), as ergogenic acid, 170*t*
Beverages
intake of, 129–130, 131*t*, 282
osmolality of, 432, 433
Bifidus factor, in breast milk, 298
Biguanides, for diabetes mellitus, 580
Bile, in fat digestion, 75, 75*f*
Bile acid sequestrants, for cholesterol lowering, 537*t*
Binge eating, in bulimia nervosa, 407
Binge eating disorder, 407
Biotechnology, food, 235–237
Biotin
as coenzyme, 97
deficiency of, 109*t*
functions of, 109*t*, 114
recommendations for
Adequate Intake, 668*t*
in breast-feeding, 279*t*, 668*t*
in children, 668*t*
Dietary Reference Intakes, 668*t*
in infants, 668*t*
in pregnancy, 279*t*, 668*t*
sources of, 109*t*, 114
toxicity of, 109*t*
Birth defects, fruit and vegetable intake and, 116–117
Bisoprolol, food interactions with, 691*t*
Black cohosh, 220*t*, 346*b*
Bleeding, in scurvy, 115
Blenderized (pureed) diet, 423*t*, 434
Blindness, night, in vitamin A deficiency, 99*t*
Bloating, in enteral nutrition, 441*b*
Blood clotting, vitamin K for, 107
Blood pressure, high. *See* Hypertension
Blood urea nitrogen, in renal disease, protein intake and, 607
Blood volume, in pregnancy, 276
BMI. *See* Body mass index
BMR. *See* Basal metabolic rate
Body composition, basal metabolic rate and, 163
Body image alterations, in enteral nutrition, 444*b*
Body mass index
vs. age
for adolescents, 681*f*, 683*f*
for children, 681*f*, 683*f*
in anorexia nervosa, 406
calculation of, 372
definition of, 7, 372
nomograms for, 372, 378*t*–379*t*
normal, 7, 7*t*, 372
for older adults, 361
in obesity, 376–377, 378*t*–379*t*

in pregnancy, 274
vs. waist circumference, 377
Bolus feedings, in enteral nutrition, 436
Bone
calcium in, 138
disorders of. *See also* Osteoporosis
in vitamin A deficiency, 99*t*
peak mass of, 327
Bone marrow transplantation, for cancer, nutritional effects of, 641, 641*b*
Boost nutritional supplement, 644
Boron, 150
Bottle feeding. *See* Formulas, infant
Botulism, 233*t*
Bovine spongiform encephalopathy ("mad cow disease"), 234
Bowel rest, for diarrhea, 481
Brain
cancer of, radiation therapy complications in, 640*t*
glucose as fuel for, 25
nutritional effects of, cancer of, 636*t*
Bran, 28*f*
Bread, cereal, rice and pasta group. *See also* Grains
in breast-feeding, 281*t*
calcium in, 616*t*
carbohydrates in, 27–28, 28*f*
in coronary heart disease prevention diet, 539*f*
in DASH diet, 553*t*
fat in, 77
fiber in, 33, 287
as functional foods, 228*t*
introduction of, to infants, 317, 318*b*, 319
light vs. whole grain, 41
in MyPyramid, 188*f*
for older adults, 355
phosphorus in, 616*t*
in pregnancy, 281*t*
protein in, 616*t*
sodium in, 555, 555*b*, 560*b*
sugar-free, calories in, 395
in Therapeutic Life Change Diet, 553*t*
Breakfast
cereal for. *See* Bread, cereal, rice and pasta group
skipping of, 334
Breast cancer, prevention of, fiber in, 33
Breast-feeding, 296–305. *See also* Breast milk
benefits of, 296–297, 296*b*, 304, 314
contraindications to, 302
failure to establish, 303*b*
infant colic and, 323*b*
information sources for, 305
mechanics of, instruction on, 304–305
nutritional needs during, 299–300, 305
Adequate Intake, 668*t*–669*t*, 671*t*, 673*t*
assessment of, 302–303
calories, 299
in diabetes mellitus, 301
Dietary Reference Intakes, 668*t*–669*t*, 671*t*, 673*t*
guidelines for, 300–301
macronutrients, 673*t*
minerals, 281*t*, 671*t*
Recommended Dietary Allowance, 668*t*–669*t*, 671*t*, 673*t*
vitamins, 281*t*, 668*t*–669*t*
water, 299–300
problems with, 303*b*
promotion of, 303–305, 303*b*
recommendations for, 314
solid food introduction with, 316–319, 318*b*
statistics on, 304, 314
Breast milk
allergy to, 308
colostrum and, 298
composition of, 297–299
duration of feeding and, 299
vs. infant formula, 315*t*
maternal diet effects on, 299
vs. stage of lactation, 298
pump for, 305
renal solute load of, 298
Bromocriptine, food interactions with, 693*t*
Bronchodilators, food interactions with, 695*t*
Buddhism, food practices in, 261
Buffet restaurants, healthy choices from, 266*b*
Bulimia nervosa
assessment of, 408–409
description of, 407
etiology of, 408
management of, 411
teaching points for, 411–412
Bupropion, food interactions with, 689*t*
Burns
nutrition therapy for, 465, 467–468
protein requirements in, 55
Burping, in formula feeding, 317*b*
Buspirone, food interactions with, 687*t*
Busulfan, food interactions with, 692*t*

C

Ca. *See* Calcium
Cachexia
cancer, 636, 637*f*, 638
cardiac, 562
Cadmium, 150
CafÈ con leche, 253
Caffeine
blood pressure and, 566
in breast-feeding, 301
elimination of, in diarrhea, 484*b*
as ergogenic acid, 170*t*
in pregnancy, 282–283
sources of, 283
water balance and, 151
Calcification
in atherosclerosis, 530, 531*f*
in vitamin D toxicity, 100*t*
Calcijex (calcitriol), for renal disease, 618
Calcitonin, in calcium regulation, 138, 140
Calcitriol (Calcijex, Rocatrol), for renal disease, 618

Calcium, 138–140
absorption of, 104, 140
balance of, 138, 140
body distribution of, 138
in bread, cereal, rice and pasta group, 616*t*
in breast milk, 315*t*
deficiency of, 139*t*
in malabsorption, 495*t*
in older adults, 353
in fats, oils, and sweets group, 617*t*
in fruit group, 616*t*
in fruit juices and drinks, 320*f*
functions of, 132, 139*t*
in infant formula, 315*t*
intake of, 140–141
in kidney stones, 628, 630
in meat, poultry, fish, dry beans, eggs, and nuts group, 617*t*
in milk, yogurt, and cheese group, 616*t*
osteoporosis and, 359–360
recommendations for, 139*t*
Adequate Intake, 140, 327–328, 328*f*, 671*t*
in adolescents, 338
vs. age, 328*f*
in breast-feeding, 281*t*, 671*t*
in children, 327–328, 328*f*, 671*t*
Dietary Reference Intakes, 671*t*
in end-stage renal disease, 608*t*, 616*t*–617*t*, 618
in infants, 313*f*, 671*t*
in kidney stones, 630
in older adults, 353, 354*t*
in pre-end stage renal disease, 608*t*
in pregnancy, 280, 281*t*, 671*t*
in weight management, 394–395
sources of, 58, 139*t*, 140, 356, 395, 616*t*–617*t*
supplements of, 140–141
in breast-feeding, 300
for coronary heart disease prevention, 545
for liver transplant candidates, 523
in pregnancy, 286
toxicity of, 139*t*
in vegetable group, 616*t*
in vegetarian diets, 58
Calcium carbonate, food interactions with, 687*t*
Calcium channel blockers, for hypertension, 552
Calories
in artificial sweeteners, 38
in breast milk, 315*t*
counting of, in weight management, 384–385
definition of, 156
dense, foods containing, 363
density of, increasing, 464*b*, 643–644, 644*b*
in dextrose vs. glucose, 450
discretionary, 30, 80
eaten at night, 173
empty, 36
in enteral formulas, 430*t*, 431
in Estimated Energy Requirements, 183
expenditure of
in basal metabolism, 163–164
in Harris-Benedict equations, 458
imbalance of, obesity in, 378–381
increasing, 171, 172
in physical activity, 164–165, 165*b*
in stress, 458
in thermic effect of food, 166
in fat, 73–74, 212*f*, 213–214
food intake patterns and, 189*t*
in fruit juices and drinks, 320*f*
in glucose, 25
in infant formula, 315*t*
intake of, imbalance of, obesity in, 378–381
on labels, 212*f*, 213–214
in milk, 78
in modular supplements, 428
for muscle building, 61, 62
in MyPyramid, 187
in "net carbs," 412–413
in nutritional supplements
clear, 420
commercially prepared, 427
milk-based, 427
one-hundred, food containing, 380
in parenteral nutrition formulas
central, 450–451
peripheral, 448
in protein, 46
protein-free, 610–611
recommendations for
in acute renal failure, 626
in anorexia, 410
in breast-feeding, 299
in burns, 467
in cancer, 643–644, 644*b*
in children, 327
in chronic obstructive pulmonary disease, 468–470
in coronary heart disease prevention, 540
in critical illness, 461–462, 461*b*
in cystic fibrosis, 326*b*
in diabetes mellitus, 575*t*, 578–579, 582*b*–583*b*
in end-stage renal disease, 608*t*, 613–614
estimation of, 461–462, 461*b*
in healing, 466*t*
in HIV infection/AIDS, 657
in kidney transplantation, 621*t*, 622
in liver disease, 520
in liver transplant candidates, 523
in nephrotic syndrome, 628
in older adults, 352–353
in pre-end stage renal disease, 608*t*, 613–614
in pregnancy, 278–279, 279*t*
in pressure ulcers, 362
in renal disease, 608*t*, 613–614
serving sizes based on, 189*t*
in steatorrhea, 494
in stress, 461–462, 461*b*
in therapeutic diets, 420
in toddlers, 321–322
in weight loss, 384–385, 386*b*

in reduced-fat vs. regular cookies, 393
severe restriction of, 385, 386*b*. *See also* Fasting
in sugar alcohols, 412–413
in sugar-free products, 395
total expenditure of, calculation of, 165*b*
for vegetarian diets, 60
Calorimetry, indirect, in critical illness, 461–462
Campylobacter enteritis, 233*t*
Canada, food guide of, 198*f*–199*f*
Cancer, 635–654
antioxidants and, 660
canola oil and, 660
in celiac disease, 508
chlorinated drinking water and, 152
fruit and vegetable intake and, 116–117
nursing process in, 652–654
nutritional effects of
cachexia in, 636, 637*f*, 638
local, 635, 636*t*
systemic, 635–636
treatment-based, 638–641, 639*t*–640*t*, 641*b*
nutrition therapy for, 641–650
anorexia in, 645
calories in, 643–644, 644*b*
diarrhea in, 648
dry mouth in, 647–648
fatigue in, 646
feeding methods for, 648–649, 649*t*
food aversions in, 647
goals of, 642–643
individualized, 643
nausea and vomiting in, 645–646
nutrient needs in, 643
nutritional supplements in, 650–651
palliative, 650
phases of, 641–642
for prevention of secondary cancer, 651–652
protein in, 643–644, 644*b*
psychologic issues in, 642
sore mouth in, 647
taste changes in, 646–647
prevention of
fiber in, 33
functional foods for, 228*t*
healthy eating guidelines for, 197–199, 200*b*, 201*b*, 202*t*
nutrition for, 651–652
phytochemicals in, 119*t*
vitamin E for, 105
treatment of, nutritional effects of, 638–641, 639*t*, 640*t*, 641*b*
in women, 345–346
Canola oil, cancer-causing substances in, 660
Captopril
food interactions with, 690*t*
side effects of, 552
Carbamazepine, food interactions with, 688*t*
Carbohydrates, 19–44. *See also specific types, e.g.,* Fiber; Glucose; Starch; Sucrose
absorption of, 22
in bread, cereal, rice and pasta group, 27–28, 28*f*
in breast milk, 297, 315*t*
classifications of, 20–22
complex, 21–22
counting of, in diabetes mellitus, 588–589
definition of, 21
in *Dietary Guidelines for Americans 2005,* 185*b*
digestion of, 22, 23*f*
for energy, 25–26
in enteral formulas, 430*t*
in exchange list, 581
"fattening" nature of, 41
in fruit group, 29
functions of, 25–26
glycemic index of, 24, 24*t*, 196, 572–573, 575, 595–597
in health promotion, 32–41
fiber and, 32–35
sugar and, 35–41, 38*b*, 39*t*
in Healthy Eating Pyramid, 196
in infant formula, 315*t*
labeling of, 37
in light breads, 41
loading of, for endurance, 169
low-fat, for vomiting, 480
in meat, poultry, fish, dry beans, eggs, and nuts group, 30
metabolism of, 22, 24–25, 24*t*
in milk, yogurt, and cheese group, 29
in modular supplements, 428
net carbs, 412–413
in parenteral nutrition formulas, 450
in pregnancy, for nausea and vomiting, 287
recommendations for, 31, 31*t*, 36–37
Acceptable Macronutrient Distribution Range, 182, 674*t*
Adequate Intake, 673*t*
in breast-feeding, 673*t*
in children, 673*t*
in coronary heart disease prevention, 541
in diabetes mellitus, 573, 574*t*, 596*b*
Dietary Reference Intake, 673*t*
in hypoglycemia, 593
in infants, 673*t*
in liver disease, 520
in pregnancy, 673*t*
Recommended Dietary Allowance, 673*t*
in weight management, 390–394, 391*t*, 392*t*
restriction of, in COPD, 469
simple, 20–21, 23*f*, 24, 29
sources of, 26–31, 27*f*, 28*f*
storage of, 26
in therapeutic diets, 420, 425
total, 573
in vegetable group, 29
Carboplatin, food interactions with, 692*t*
Carboxypeptidase, in protein digestion, 48*f*, 49
"Carbs," grains as, 27
Cardiac cachexia, 562

Cardiovascular disease. *See also* Atherosclerosis; Coronary heart disease; Hypertension
in anorexia nervosa, 407
epidemiology of, 530
fiber for, 33
fruit and vegetable intake and, 116–117
prevention of, vitamin E for, 105
sugar consumption and, 35
trans fats and, 71–72, 540–541
in women, 345–346, 346*b*
Caries, dental
from bottle feeding, 317*b*, 319*f*
in bulimia nervosa, 407
in cancer therapy, 647–648
fluoride and, 149–150
sugar and, 36
Carmustine, food interactions with, 692*t*
Carnitine, 114
Carotenoids. *See also* Beta-carotene
sources of, 101
Casein hydrolysate infant formulas, 315
Catabolism, 157–160
in cancer, 636, 638
definition of, 25
fat, 76
glucose, 157–158
protein, 458–459
in stress, 458–459
Catechins, sources and effects of, 119*t*
Catecholamines, release of, in stress, 458, 459*t*
Catheters, for parenteral nutrition, complications with, 449*b*
Celebrations, foods used in, 246–247
Celiac disease, 508, 509*b*–513*b*, 513
Cell(s), water in, 128
Central adiposity, 377, 380*f*
Central nervous system, cancer of
nutritional effects of, 636*t*
radiation therapy complications in, 640*t*
Central total parenteral nutrition. *See* Total parenteral nutrition
Cereal. *See also* Bread, cereal, rice and pasta group
for breakfast, 334
Cerivastatin, for cholesterol lowering, 537*t*
Chaparral, 223*t*
CHD. *See* Coronary heart disease
Cheese. *See* Milk, yogurt, and cheese group
Chelated minerals, 152
Chemotherapy
breast-feeding contraindication with, 302
food interactions with, 692*t*–693*t*
nutritional effects of, 638–639
nutrition therapy for, 645–648
Chest, cancer of, radiation therapy complications in, 640*t*
Chewing
dysphagia diet for, 490*t*
of fiber, 470
of fruit, 356
of vegetables, 356
Chewing gum, sugar alcohols in, 36, 38
Childhood nutrition, 326–340
artificial sweeteners in, 41
assessment of, 313
breakfast in, 334
concerns about, 332–337, 334*f*
food refusal in, 333
growth charts for, 676*f*–685*f*
growth rate and, 326–327
healthy diet for, 329–330, 331*f*, 332*b*
healthy eating habits for, 330, 332
healthy lifestyles and, 336–337
meal-time pitfalls in, 333
obesity prevention in, 336–337
overweight and, 335–336
problems with, 332–337
recommendations for, 327–329, 328*f*, 329*f*
Acceptable Macronutrient Distribution Range, 674*t*
Adequate Intake, 668*t*–669*t*, 671*t*, 673*t*
calcium, 327–328, 328*f*
in diabetes mellitus, 594–595
Dietary Reference Intakes, 668*t*–669*t*, 671*t*, 673*t*
iron, 328–329, 329*f*
macronutrients, 673*t*
minerals, 671*t*
MyPyramid, 330, 331*f*
Recommended Dietary Allowance, 668*t*–669*t*, 671*t*, 673*t*
vitamins, 104, 327, 668*t*–669*t*
sample menu for, 332*b*
snacks in, 333
soft drinks and, 334–335
Chinese restaurants, healthy choices from, 266*b*–267*b*
Chloride
body distribution of, 138
deficiency of, 135*t*, 138
functions of, 135*t*, 138
recommendations for, 135*t*
sources of, 135*t*, 138
toxicity of, 135*t*
Chlorine, in drinking water, 152
Chlorothiazide, food interactions with, 695*t*
Chlorpromazine, food interactions with, 692*t*
Chlorpropamide, food interactions with, 689*t*
Chocolate, acne and, 343
Choking, foods causing, 330
Cholecalciferol, recommendations for, 104
Cholecystitis, 524–525
Cholelithiasis, 524–525
Cholesterol (blood), 534. *See also* Lipoprotein(s)
in atherosclerosis, 530
in coronary heart disease, 530
diet effects on, 535
lowering of
counseling on, 545–546, 547*b*–548*b*
diet for, 538–542, 538*t*, 539*f*
drugs for, 536, 537*t*
fiber for, 33
food interactions and, 696*t*
functional foods for, 228*t*

lifestyle changes for, 73
nicotinic acid for, 111
nursing process for, 548–550
nutritional supplements for, 542, 543*b*, 545
vitamin E for, 105
in metabolic syndrome, 534, 534*t*
in older adults, 366
physical activity and, 535
saturated fats effects on, 70
synthesis of, 73
total, 531, 532*t*
trans fats effects on, 71, 540–541
Cholesterol (dietary), 68*t*, 72–73
in breast milk, 298
in milk, yogurt, and cheese group, 78
recommendations for, 86–87
in coronary heart disease prevention, 540
in diabetes mellitus, 574*t*, 578
in nephrotic syndrome, 628
sources of, 72–73, 542, 578
Cholestyramine, for cholesterol lowering, 537*t*, 696*t*
Choline, 114
recommendations for
Adequate Intake, 668*t*
in breast-feeding, 281*t*, 668*t*
in children, 668*t*
Dietary Reference Intakes, 668*t*
in infants, 668*t*
in pregnancy, 281*t*, 668*t*
Chondroitin sulfate, for osteoarthritis, 359
Christianity, food practices in, 259
Chromium, 150
deficiency of, 145*t*
functions of, 145*t*, 150
recommendations for, 145*t*
Adequate Intake, 671*t*
in breast-feeding, 671*t*
in children, 671*t*
Dietary Reference Intakes, 671*t*
in infants, 671*t*
in pregnancy, 671*t*
sources of, 145*t*, 150
supplements of, for coronary heart disease prevention, 543*b*
toxicity of, 145*t*
Chronic obstructive pulmonary disease, nutrition therapy for, 468–470
Chylomicrons, 75–76
Chymotrypsin, in protein digestion, 48*f*, 49
Cimetidine (Tagamet), for gastritis, 493
Ciprofloxacin, food interactions with, 687*t*
Cirrhosis, 519
Cis-fats, 71, 71*f*
Cisplatin, food interactions with, 692*t*
Cl. *See* Chloride
Clarithromycin, food interactions with, 688*t*
Clear liquid diets, 420, 421*t*, 480
Cleft palate, nutrition in, 323*b*
Clock-focused orientation, as cultural value, 248
Clofibrate, for cholesterol lowering, 537*t*, 696*t*
Clomipramine, food interactions with, 689*t*
Clonazepam, food interactions with, 688*t*
Clonidine, food interactions with, 691*t*
Closed feeding, in enteral nutrition, 437
Clostridium botulinum toxin, 233*t*
Clostridium perfringens, in food poisoning, 233*t*
Cobalamin. *See* Vitamin B_{12} (cobalamin)
Cobalt, 133, 150
Codeine, food interactions with, 686*t*
Coenzymes
biotin as, 114
definition of, 97
folate as, 112
non-B vitamins as, 114
pantothenic acid as, 114
vitamin B_1 as, 110
vitamin B_2 as, 110–111
vitamin B_6 as, 111–112
vitamin B_{12} as, 113–114
vitamins as, 97
Coffee, blood pressure and, 566
Colchicine, food interactions with, 690*t*
Colesevelam, for cholesterol lowering, 537*t*
Colestipol, for cholesterol lowering, 537*t*, 696*t*
Colic, 323*b*
Colitis, hemorrhagic, foodborne, 230, 231*t*
Collagen, synthesis of, vitamin C for, 115
Colon cancer
nutritional effects of, 636*t*
prevention of, fiber in, 33
surgical complications in, 639*t*
Colostomy
complications of, 639*t*
nutrition therapy for, 514–515, 515*b*
pathophysiology of, 514
Colostrum, 298
Coma, hepatic, 519–520
Combivir (zidovudine-lamivudine), for HIV infection/AIDS, 661*t*
Comfort foods, 13, 247
Comfrey, 223*t*
Complementary proteins, 53–54
Complete proteins, 52–54
Complete vitamin supplement formulas, 123
Complex carbohydrates, 21–22. *See also specific type, e.g.,* Fiber; Starch
Conception, nutrition before, 272–273
Congestive heart failure, 556–565
definition of, 556
medical treatment of, 556
nursing process for, 564–565
nutrition therapy for, 558, 559*b*–561*b*, 562, 563*t*
Congregate meal programs, for older adults, 361–362
Consistency, of diet, modified, 420, 421*t*–423*t*
Constipation
definition of, 481
in diverticular disease, 518
in enteral nutrition, 442*b*
fiber for, 32
nutrition therapy for, 481, 484, 485*b*–486*b*
in pregnancy, 287–288

Consumer issues, 208–242
biotechnology, 235–237
food irradiation, 237, 237*f*
food quality, 227*b*, 228*t*
food safety. *See* Safety
information and misinformation, 209–217, 210*b*, 212*f*, 215*b*, 217*b*
supplements. *See* Herbal supplements; Mineral supplements; Supplement(s); Vitamin supplements
Contaminated food. *See* Foodborne illness
Continuous drip method, for enteral nutrition, 436
Convenience foods, 262, 263*b*
obesity and, 380–381
sodium in, 555, 555*b*
COPD (chronic obstructive pulmonary disease), nutrition therapy for, 468–470
Copper
body distribution of, 149
deficiency of, 145*t*
functions of, 145*t*, 149
recommendations for, 145*t*
Adequate Intake, 671*t*
in breast-feeding, 671*t*
in children, 671*t*
Dietary Reference Intakes, 671*t*
in infants, 671*t*
in pregnancy, 286, 671*t*
Recommended Dietary Allowance, 671*t*
sources of, 145*t*
toxicity of, 145*t*, 149
Core foods, 245–246
Coronary heart disease, 529–556
alcohol intake and, 544–545
causes of, 530, 531*f*, 532*f*
genetic factors in, 533
nursing process for, 548–550
premature, 533
prevention of, 536, 537*b*, 537*t*, 538. *See also* Cholesterol (blood), lowering of
risk assessment for, 530–536
cholesterol type and, 530–533, 532*t*, 533*t*
diet in, 535
homocysteine in, 535–536
inactivity in, 535
metabolic syndrome in, 534, 534*t*
proinflammatory factors in, 536
triglyceride level in, 534
treatment of
cholesterol-lowering drugs in, 536, 537*b*, 537*t*, 538
cultural considerations in, 547*b*–548*b*
lifestyle change diet in, 538–542, 538*t*, 539*f*
nutritional supplements in, 542–545, 543*b*
patient education on, 545–548, 547*b*–548*b*
Corticosteroids
food interactions with, 695*t*
nutritional effects of, 505
after renal transplantation, 622
Cortisol, release of, in stress, 458, 459*t*
Counseling, nutritional. *See* Nutrition counseling; Nutrition education
Cow's milk, for infants, 320
Cracking, of parenteral nutrition formulas, 452
Cranberry, as supplement, 220*t*
Cranberry juice, urinary tract infections and, 631
Cravings, in pregnancy, 294, 294*b*
C-reactive protein, as coronary heart disease risk factor, 536
Creatine, as ergogenic acid, 170*t*
Creatine phosphate, energy from, 161
Creutzfeldt-Jakob disease, variant, 234
Critical illness, metabolic changes in, 458–464
complications of, 459–460
hormonal, 458, 459*t*
nursing process for, 471–473
nutrition therapy for, 460–464, 461*b*, 464*b*
protein catabolism, 458–459
Crixivan (indinavir), for HIV infection/AIDS, 661*t*, 693*t*
Crohn's disease
nursing process for, 506–507
nutrition therapy for, 504–505
pathophysiology of, 504
Culture
adaptation in (acculturation), 248–249, 257–258
definition of, 242
foodways of
celebrations, 4–5
comfort foods, 5
core foods, 245–246
eating techniques, 247
edibility, 242–243, 243*f*
ethnic restaurants, 264, 265*b*–267*b*
food preparation methods, 4
food roles, 245–246
food selection and, 244–245, 245*f*
food substitutions, 249
food uses, 4–5
health beliefs, 247
impacting mainstream foodways, 261–263, 263*b*
meal timing, 247
new foods, 249
occasional foods, 246
regional specialties, 264
secondary foods, 246
health promotion and, 257–259
nutrition counseling based on, 258–259
religious practices and, 259–261
subgroups in, 242, 249
traditional diets and, 249–257, 251*f*
African-American, 250–252, 251*f*, 547*b*
Alaska Native, 547*b*
Asian-American, 255–257, 256*f*, 547*b*
Judaism, 547*b*–548*b*
Mexican-American, 252–255, 253*f*, 547*b*
Native-American, 547*b*
rejection of, 249
values of, 248
weight gain and, 381
Cyclic total parenteral nutrition, 452
Cyclophosphamide, food interactions with, 692*t*

Cyclosporine (Neoral, Sandimmune)
for cholesterol lowering, 537*t*
food interactions with, 695*t*
after renal transplantation, 622
Cystic fibrosis, 325*b*–326*b*
Cytarabine, food interactions with, 692*t*
Cytokine production, in HIV infection/AIDS, 656

D

Dacarbazine, food interactions with, 692*t*
Dactinomycin, food interactions with, 692*t*
Daidzein, sources and effects of, 119*t*
Daily Reference Value (DRV), on labels, 212, 212*f*, 213
Daily Value (DV)
on labels, 212, 212*f*, 213
for sodium, 136
Dairy products. *See* Milk, yogurt, and cheese group; *specific products*
DASH (Dietary Approaches to Stop Hypertension) diet, 545, 551–552, 553*t*–554*t*, 555*b*, 556*b*, 557*t*–558*t*
ddC (zalcitabine), for HIV infection/AIDS, 661*t*, 693*t*
ddI (didanosine), for HIV infection/AIDS, 661*t*, 693*t*
Deamination, of amino acids, 51–52, 158, 160
Decubitus ulcers. *See* Pressure ulcers
Dehydration
in enteral nutrition, 441*b*
of infants, in hot weather, 314
of older adults, 362
in short-bowel syndrome, 516
Delavirdine (Rescriptor, DLV), for HIV infection/AIDS, 661*t*
Dementia, Alzheimer's
nutritional interventions for, 360–361
vitamin E for, 105
Density, nutrient, in pregnancy, 282
Dental caries. *See* Caries, dental
Dexamethasone, food interactions with, 695*t*
Dexatrim (phenylpropanolamine), for weight loss, 399
Dextrose. *See also* Glucose
vs. glucose, 450
Diabetes mellitus, 570–604
in adolescents, 340, 594–595
in African Americans, 251–252
artificial sweeteners in, 40
breast-feeding in, 301
in children, 594–595
complications of
long-term, 572–573
management of, 591, 593, 594*b*
definition of, 571
enteral nutrition in, 597
epidemiology of, 571
exchange list for, 389*t*, 581, 584*b*–587*b*, 585, 587–588
gestational, 290–291, 595, 596*b*
in hospitalized patients, 597
hyperglycemia in, 593
hypoglycemia in, 593, 594*b*
illness in, 593
life cycle considerations in, 594–597, 596*b*
management of, 593–597. *See also* Diabetes mellitus, nutrition recommendations for
behavioral changes in, 589, 590*f*, 591, 592*b*
in complications, 591, 592*b*, 593, 594*b*
drugs in, 580–581
exercise in, 591
type 1, 579
type 2, 581
in Mexican Americans, 254
mortality in, 572
nursing process for, 598–600
nutrition recommendations for, 573–589, 574*t*–571*t*
alcohol use, 579
calories, 578–579
carbohydrate counting in, 588–589
cholesterol, 578
eating out, 592*b*
exchange list for, 389*t*, 581, 584*b*–587*b*, 585, 587–588
fat, 576–578
fiber, 576
"free" foods in, 585
label reading in, 592*b*
liberal diet in, 366
meals in, 581–589, 582*b*–588*b*
mineral supplements, 579
MyPyramid in, 588*b*, 589
protein, 576
sweeteners, 575–576
total carbohydrates in, 573
type 1, 579
type 2, 581
vitamin supplements, 579
in older adults, 366, 595–597
in pregnancy, 290–291, 595, 596*b*
sugar consumption and, 35
sweet tooth and, 601
type 1
description of, 571
management of, 579
pregnancy in, 595, 596*b*
type 2
description of, 571–572, 572*b*
fiber for, 33
management of, 581
oral hypoglycemics for, 572
pregnancy in, 595, 596*b*
risk factors for, 571–572
Diagnosis, nursing, in nutritional care process, 10, 11*b*
Dialysate, definition of, 614
Dialysis
in acute renal failure, 626
in end-stage renal disease. *See* End-stage renal disease
nutrient recommendations for, 608*t*
omega-3 fish oil supplements in, 631

Diarrhea
in cancer, 648
in diverticular disease, 518
fatty (steatorrhea), 494–495, 495*t*, 496*b*–498*b*
in HIV infection/AIDS, 655–656
in lactose intolerance, 502
nutrition therapy for, 480–481, 482*b*–484*b*, 648
in short-bowel syndrome, 516
Didanosine (Videx EC, ddI), for HIV infection/AIDS, 661*t*, 693*t*
Diet(s)
acculturation of. *See* Acculturation
atherogenic, as coronary heart disease risk factor, 532, 535
Atkins, 391, 391*t*
blenderized (pureed), 423*t*, 434
carbohydrate-loading, 169
cholesterol-lowering, 538–542, 538*t*, 539*f*
clear liquid, 420, 421*t*, 480
definition of, 385
diabetic, sweeteners in, 40
easy to chew, 490*t*
Feingold, 343
gluten-free, 508, 509*b*–513*b*, 513, 525
ground, for dysphagia, 490*t*
healthy. *See* Healthy diet
high-fat, 81
high-fiber, 481, 484, 485*b*–486*b*
high-protein, 61, 499*b*
hospital, 420–425
house, in hospital, 420
lactose-restricted, 503*b*
liquid, 420, 421*t*–423*t*
low-calorie, 385, 386*b*
low-carbohydrate, 390–394, 391*t*, 392*t*, 412
low-fat. *See* Low-fat diets
low-fiber
for diarrhea, 481, 482*b*–484*b*
for diverticular disease, 518
low-microbial, in liver transplant candidates, 522, 522*b*
low-phenylalanine, 274–275, 324*b*–325*b*
low-phosphorus, 612, 614, 616*t*–617*t*
low-protein. *See* Protein (dietary), restriction of
modified consistency, 420, 421*t*–423*t*
normal, in hospital, 420
Ornish, 391*t*, 541
potassium-enriched, 562, 563*t*
Pritikin, 541
pureed, for dysphagia, 490*t*
regular, in hospital, 420
rigid, 16
sodium-restricted. *See* Sodium, restriction of
soft (bland, low fiber), 420, 423*t*–424*t*, 490*t*
texture-modified, for liver disease, 522
therapeutic, 420, 425
Therapeutic Lifestyle Change, 538–542, 538*t*, 539*f*, 552, 553*t*–554*t*
as tolerated, in hospital, 420
total diet approach to, 83
unhealthful, in adolescents, 339–340
very low-calorie, 385, 386*b*
"yo-yo," 413
Zone, 391*t*
Dietary Approaches to Stop Hypertension (DASH) diet, 545, 551–552, 553*t*–554*t*, 555*b*, 556*b*, 557*t*–558*t*
Dietary fiber. *See* Fiber
Dietary folate equivalents, 112, 273
Dietary Guidelines for Americans, 183, 184*b*–186*b*
on carbohydrate intake, 36–37
for children, 329–330
on hospital food, 418
on sugar intake, 36–37
Dietary Reference Intakes, 181–183, 181*f*. *See also specific components*
in breast-feeding, 668*t*–669*t*, 671*t*, 673*t*
for calcium, 280
for children, 327, 668*t*–669*t*, 671*t*, 673*t*
for infants, 668*t*–669*t*, 671*t*, 673*t*
in pregnancy, 668*t*–669*t*, 671*t*, 673*t*
Dietary supplements. *See* Herbal supplements; Mineral supplements; Supplement(s); Vitamin supplements
Diethylpropion (Tenuate), for weight loss, 399
Dietitian, counseling by, 13–14
Digestion
of carbohydrates, 22, 23*f*
of fat, 74, 75*f*
of proteins, 48–49, 48*f*
water in, 128
Dihydrofolate, 112
1,25-Dihydroxycholecalciferol, 606
Dipeptidase, in protein digestion, 48*f*, 49
Dipeptides, definition of, 49
Diphenoxylate, food interactions with, 690*t*
Dirithromycin, food interactions with, 688*t*
Disaccharides, 20–21, 23*f*
Discretionary calories, 30, 80, 189*t*
Distention, in enteral nutrition, 441*b*
Diuretic(s)
for congestive heart failure, 556, 562
food interactions with, 695*t*
potassium-wasting, for hypertension, 552
Diuretic phase, of acute renal failure, 625
Diverticular disease, 32, 518
Diverticulitis, definition of, 518
Diverticulosis, definition of, 518
DLV (delavirdine), for HIV infection/AIDS, 661*t*
DNA
carbohydrates in, 26
synthesis of
folate in, 112
vitamin B_{12} in, 113
Docetaxel, food interactions with, 693*t*
Docosahexanoic acid, 69–70
in breast milk, 298
in fish, Alzheimer's disease and, 368–369
sources of, 59
Doxazosin, food interactions with, 691*t*
Doxorubicin, food interactions with, 693*t*
DRIs. *See* Dietary Reference Intakes

Dronabinol (Marinol)
  for appetite stimulation, in HIV infection/AIDS, 659*t*
  food interactions with, 692*t*
Drugs/medications. *See also specific drugs*
  basal metabolic rate and, 164
  breast-feeding contraindication with, 302
  in enteral nutrition, 438–439
  for gastroesophageal reflux disease, 492
  gastrointestinal distress due to, 478
  for hypertension, 552
  for inflammatory bowel disease, 505
  interactions of
    with food, 686*t*–697*t*
    with herbal supplements, 220*t*–222*t*
  malabsorption of, in stress, 460
  in nutritional assessment, 8
  in parenteral nutrition, 451
  vs. supplements, 219, 222–224, 223*t*
  vitamin B_3 as, 111
  vitamin B_6 as, 112
  vitamin C as, 115
  vitamin E as, 105–106
  vitamins as, 98
  weight gain due to, 381
  for weight management, 396, 398–399, 399*t*
DRV (Daily Reference Value), on labels, 212, 212*f*, 213
Dry mouth, in enteral nutrition, 445*b*
d4T (stavudine), for HIV infection/AIDS, 661*t*, 693*t*
Dumping syndrome
  causes of, 495
  in enteral nutrition, 436
  nutrition therapy for, 500, 501*b*, 502
  pathophysiology of, 499–500
Duodenal ulcer, nutrition therapy for, 492, 493*b*
DV (Daily Value), on labels, 212, 212*f*, 213
Dysphagia
  definition of, 488
  nursing process for, 487–488
  nutrition therapy for, 489, 490*t*, 491
  pathophysiology of, 488–489

E

EAR (Estimated Average Requirement), 182
Eastern Orthodox Christianity, food practices in, 259
Eating behaviors and habits
  in anorexia nervosa, 406–407
  in bulimia nervosa, 407
  in children, 330, 332, 334*f*
  cultural variation in, 247
  disorders of. *See* Eating disorders
  mindful vs. mindless, weight management and, 388
  self-monitoring of, 396
  in weight management, 396, 397*b*
Eating disorders, 406–412
  in adolescents, 339–340
  assessment of, 408–409
  description of, 406–407
  etiology of, 408
  management of, 409–412
  teaching points for, 411–412
Eating Disorders Not Otherwise Specified, 407
Eating out. *See* Restaurant meals
Echinacea, 220*t*
Eclampsia, pregnancy-induced, 291
Edema, in congestive heart failure, 556
Edibility, cultural determination of, 242–243, 243*f*
EER (Estimated Energy Requirements), 183, 321–322
Efavirenz (Sustiva, EFV), for HIV infection/AIDS, 661*t*
Effluent, from colostomy or ileostomy, 514
Eggs. *See* Meat, poultry, fish, dry beans, eggs, and nuts group
Eicosapentaenoic acid, 59, 69–70
Elderly persons. *See* Aging/older adults
Electrolyte(s). *See also* Fluid and electrolyte balance; *specific electrolytes, e.g.,* Sodium; Potassium
  in parenteral nutrition, 451
Electron transport chain, 158
Elimination, water in, 128
Ellagic acid, sources and effects of, 119*t*
Empty calories, 36
Emulsifiers, phospholipids as, 72
Encephalopathy, hepatic, 519–520
Endosperm, 28*f*
End-stage renal disease
  drug treatment of, 618
  nutrition therapy for, 613–621
    calcium in, 608*t*, 616*t*–617*t*, 618
    calories in, 608*t*, 613–614
    enteral formulas in, 620
    fluid in, 608*t*, 615, 617–618
    meals in, 619–621
    menus for, 609*b*
    minerals in, 608*t*, 619
    omega-3 fish oil supplements in, 631
    phosphorus in, 608*t*, 615, 616*t*–617*t*
    potassium in, 608*t*, 615
    protein in, 608*t*, 613, 616*t*–617*t*
    sodium in, 608*t*, 615
    vitamins in, 608*t*, 618–619
Energy. *See also* Calories; Energy metabolism
  amino acids for, 52
  for exercise, 161–162
  extraction from food. *See* Absorption; Digestion; Metabolism
  from fat, 73–74, 158–160
  fuels for, 160–162
  from glucose, 25–26
  in health promotion, 166–172
    aerobic exercise amount, 167–168, 170*t*
    carbohydrate-loading, 169
    increasing activity, 171–172
    physical activity benefits in, 166–167, 167*f*, 167*t*
    strength and stretching exercises, 168, 170
  from protein, 46, 158
  requirements for, 162–166, 165*b*
    in basal metabolism, 163–164
    in older adults, 352
    in physical activity, 164–165, 165*b*
    in thermic effect of food, 166

Energy expenditure. *See also* Calories, expenditure of
basal, 458, 461*b*
in cancer, 636, 638
in HIV infection/AIDS, 655
resting, 163, 458, 461*b*
Energy metabolism, 155–176
anabolism in, 156–157, 157*f*, 158*f*
catabolism in. *See* Catabolism
in fasting, 160–161
fat in, 158–160
glucose in, 157–158
in physical activity, 161–162
protein in, 158
Enriched food, definition of, 95
Ensure nutritional supplement, 644
Enteral nutrition, 428–447
for acute renal failure, 627
advancing feeding in, 437
for anorexia nervosa, 411
aspiration in, 438
bolus feedings in, 436
for burns, 467–468
for cancer, 648–649, 649*t*
for chronic obstructive pulmonary disease, 469
complications of, 441*b*–445*b*
continuous drip method for, 436
for critical illness, 463–464
cyclic feedings in, 436–437
definition of, 428
in diabetes mellitus, 597
equipment for, 434
ethical issues in, 429
formulas for, 429–430
calorie density of, 431
contamination of, 437–438
delivery methods for, 434–437
disease-specific, 433
dye added to, 453
fiber content of, 433–434
high-protein, 432
hydrolyzed, 430, 430*t*, 431
immunonutrition, 464
osmolality of, 432, 433
protein density of, 432
in renal disease, 620
routine vs. stress, 473
selection of, 431–434
standard, 429–430
for stress, 473
water content of, 431–432
for HIV infection/AIDS, 658
indications for, 428–429
initiating feeding in, 437
intermittent feedings in, 436
for liver disease, 519, 522
medication administration with, 438–439
monitoring of, 439
nursing process for, 440–447, 441*b*–445*b*
for pancreatitis, 523
vs. parenteral nutrition, 429
for renal disease
end-stage, 620
pre-end stage, 607, 609*b*, 610
for respiratory insufficiency, 469
routes for, 434, 435*t*
safety of, 437–439
for short-bowel syndrome, 516
taste detected in, 453
tolerance of, 437–439
transition to oral diet from, 439
trouble-shooting in, 441*b*–445*b*
tube patency in, 438, 443*b*
Enteritis, regional (Crohn's disease)
nursing process for, 506–507
nutrition therapy for, 504–505
Enteropathy, gluten-induced (celiac disease), nutrition therapy for, 508, 509*b*–513*b*, 513
Enzymes. *See also specific enzymes*
in breast milk, 298
functions of, 46
minerals interactions with, 132–133
vitamins as, 97
Ephedra (ma huang), 223
Epinephrine, in glycogen degradation, 25
Epivir (lamivudine), for HIV infection/AIDS, 661*t*, 693*t*
Eplerenone, food interactions with, 691*t*
Epoetin alfa (Procrit, Epogen), for renal disease, 618, 687*t*
Equal. *See* Aspartame
Ergogenic aids, in exercise, 168, 170*t*
Erythromycin, food interactions with, 688*t*
Erythropoietin, function of, 606
Escherichia coli, in foodborne illness, 230, 231*t*
Escitalopram, food interactions with, 689*t*
Esophageal phase, of swallowing, 489
Esophagus
cancer of
nutritional effects of, 636*t*
surgical complications in, 639*t*
reflux into, nutrition therapy for, 491–492
Essential amino acids, 47, 47*b*, 52–54, 57
Essential fatty acids, 69–70, 81
Essential vitamins, 96
Estimated Average Requirement (EAR), 182
Estimated Energy Requirements (EER), 183, 321–322
Estramustine, food interactions with, 693*t*
Ethical issues, in enteral nutrition, 429
Ethnic factors. *See* Culture
Ethnic food, 261, 266*b*–267*b*
Ethnocentrism, 248
Ethosuximide, food interactions with, 688*t*
Etoposide, food interactions with, 693*t*
Evaluation, in nutritional nursing care, 15–16
Event-focused orientation, as cultural value, 248
Exchange lists, for diabetes mellitus, 389*t*, 581, 584*b*–587*b*, 585, 587–588
Excretion, of minerals, 133
Exercise (physical activity)
benefits of, 166–167, 167*f*, 167*t*, 395–396
breathless feeling during, 162
for children, 330
definition of, 166

in diabetes mellitus, 591
in *Dietary Guidelines for Americans 2005,* 184*b*
energy requirements for, 161–162, 164–165, 165*b*
fuels for, 161–162
in Healthy Eating Pyramid, 193, 193*f*
for hypertension, 555
increasing, 171
insufficient
as coronary heart disease risk factor, 535
weight gain in, 381, 382*f*
in MyPyramid, 188*f,* 190–191
for older adults, 359–360
recommendations for, 167–168, 170*t,* 199, 200*b*–201*b,* 396
timing of, 173
water loss in, 129
for weight management, 395–396
Ezetimibe, food interactions and, 696*t*

F

Failure to thrive, 322*b*–323*b*
Famciclovir, food interactions with, 693*t*
Fast food restaurants
exchange list applied to, 587
healthy choices from, 266*b*
obesity and, 380–381
Fastin (phentermine), for weight loss, 399
Fasting, 160–161
basal metabolic rate and, 164
in Christianity, 259
in Hinduism, 260
in Islam, 260
in Judaism, 260
in pregnancy, 282
for weight management, 385, 386*b*
Fat (body). *See also* Body mass index; Obesity
abdominal, 377, 380*f*
in adolescents, 337
anabolism of, 76
in apple-shaped people, 377, 380*f*
calories in, 73
catabolism of, 76, 160
central, 377, 380*f*
energy storage in, 73–74, 76
as fuel, in pregnancy, 275
metabolism of, in exercise, 161–162
in pear-shaped people, 377, 380*f*
redistribution of, in HIV infection/AIDS, 659–660
synthesis of, 76, 156–157, 158*f*
from amino acids, 52
from glucose, 26
Fat (dietary). *See also* Fat(s), oils, and sweets group
absorption of, 74–75
Acceptable Macronutrient Distribution Range for, 182–183, 674*t*
in bread, cereal, rice, and pasta group, 77
in breast milk, 297, 299, 315*t*
calories in, 73–74
catabolism of, 76
cholesterol, 68*t,* 72–73, 86–87
digestion of, 74, 75*f*
energy from, 73, 158–160
in enteral formulas, 430, 430*t*
essential fatty acids in, 69–70, 81
in exchange list, 583
fat gram counting and, 89–90
in fats, oils, and sweets group, 80
fatty acid mixtures in, 68, 68*t*
in fruit group, 78
functions of, 73–74
in health promotion, 86–89, 87*f*
in Healthy Eating Index, 192*t*
hidden in foods, 265*b*
hydrogenated, 68, 68*t,* 70–71, 83*b*
for increased calorie density
in cancer, 643–644, 644*b*
in critical illness, 464*b*
in infant formula, 315*t*
insulating function of, 74
lowering of, 81–86, 83*b*–84*b*
low-fat substitutes for, 83*b*
malabsorption of, steatorrhea in, 494–495, 495*t,* 496*b*–498*b*
marbling of, 80
in meat, poultry, fish, dry beans, eggs, and nuts group, 79–80
in Mediterranean diet, 86–87, 87*f*
metabolism of, 76, 158–160
in milk, yogurt, and cheese group, 78
monounsaturated, 67–68, 68*t*
in coronary heart disease, 540
in diabetes mellitus, 574*t,* 578
in MyPyramid, 76–80
oxidation of, glucose role in, 26
in parenteral nutrition formulas, 450–451
percentage of calories from, on labels, 212*f,* 213–214
phospholipids as, 72
polyunsaturated, 68, 68*t,* 69
in breast milk, 297
for coronary heart disease prevention, 540
in diabetes mellitus, 574*t,* 577
portion sizes of, 496*b*
recommendations for, 80–86, 81*t*
Adequate Intake, 673*t*
in breast-feeding, 673*t*
in cancer, 643–644, 644*b*
cholesterol, 86–87
in critical illness, 464*b*
in diabetes mellitus, 576–577
Dietary Reference Intake, 673*t*
in infants, 673*t*
in kidney transplantation, 621*t,* 622
in liver disease, 520
in nephrotic syndrome, 628
omega-3, 85
Recommended Dietary Allowance, 673*t*
after renal transplantation, 622
saturated, 84–85, 85*t*
total fat, 82–83, 83*b*–84*b,* 85*t,* 577–578
trans, 84–85, 85*t,* 540–541
unsaturated, 85
in weight management, 390–394, 391*t,* 392*t*

Fat (dietary) (*continued*)
- replacers for, 87–89
- restriction of. *See* Low-fat diets
- saturated ("bad"), 67–68, 68*t*, 70–72, 71*f*
  - cholesterol levels and, 538, 540
  - in diabetes mellitus, 574*t*, 577
  - reduction of, 84–85
  - in vegetarian diets, 61
- selection of, 89
- structures of, 67–68
- trans, 71–72, 71*f*
  - coronary heart disease and, 540–541
  - diabetes mellitus and, 574*t*, 577
  - recommendations for, 84–85, 85*t*, 540–541
  - sources of, 394, 577
- triglycerides. *See* Triglycerides
- unsaturated ("good"), 67–70, 68*t*, 85
  - recommendations for, 85
  - in weight management diet, 394
- in vegetable group, 77–80, 77*f*
- in vegetarian products, 61

Fat(s), oils, and sweets group
- calcium in, 617*t*
- in coronary heart disease prevention diet, 538–540, 539*f*
- in DASH diet, 554*t*
- in diabetes mellitus, 574*t*, 575–576
- in *Dietary Guidelines for Americans 2005*, 184*b*–185*b*
- fat content of, 80
- nutrients in, 30
- for older adults, 356
- phosphorus in, 617*t*
- protein in, 617*t*
- sodium in, 560*b*
- in Therapeutic Life Change Diet, 554*t*
- in weight management diet, 394

Fate, acceptance of, as cultural value, 248

Fatigue, in cancer, nutrition therapy for, 646

Fat redistribution syndrome (lipodystrophy), in HIV infection/AIDS, 659–660

Fat-soluble vitamins, 98–105, 99*t*–101*t*. *See also specific vitamins*

Fatty acids. *See also* Omega-3 fatty acids
- absorption of, 74–75
- in breast milk, 297
- carbon chain length of, 67
- catabolism of, 76
- cis-, 71, 71*f*
- definition of, 69
- essential, 69–70, 81, 297
- in fat formation, 156–157, 158*f*
- formation of, in digestion, 74, 75*f*
- hydrogenated, 68, 68*t*, 70–71, 83*b*
- metabolism of, 76
- monounsaturated, 68, 68*t*
  - in coronary heart disease, 540
  - in diabetes mellitus, 574*t*, 578
- in phospholipids, 72
- polyunsaturated, 68, 68*t*, 69–70
  - for coronary heart disease prevention, 540
  - in diabetes mellitus, 574*t*, 577
- trans, 71–72, 71*f*, 84–85, 85*t*, 540–541
- unsaturated ("good"), 67–70, 68*t*, 84*b*, 85

Fatty streaks, in atherosclerosis, 530, 531*f*

Fear, in enteral nutrition, 444*b*

Feeding Infants and Toddlers Study (FITS), 321–322

Feeding tubes. *See* Enteral nutrition

Feingold diet, 343

Felbamate, food interactions with, 688*t*

Fenofibrate, for cholesterol lowering, 537*t*

Fetal alcohol syndrome, 283

Fever, basal metabolic rate in, 164

Fiber, 21–22
- benefits of, 32–35
- in bread, cereal, rice and pasta group, 33, 287
- digestion of, 22, 23*f*
- easily chewed, 470
- in enteral formulas, 430*t*, 433–434
- in flaxseed, 89
- in fruit group, 29
- in fruit juices and drinks, 320*f*
- functional, 22
- in Healthy Eating Index, 192*t*
- insoluble, 21–22
- lack of, in low-carbohydrate diets, 391, 393
- in meat, poultry, fish, dry beans, eggs, and nuts group, 30
- in pills, 525
- recommendations for, 31, 31*t*, 33–35, 34*t*
  - Adequate Intake, 481, 673*t*
  - in breast-feeding, 673*t*
  - in bulimia nervosa, 411
  - in cancer protection, 33
  - in cardiovascular disease, 33, 541–542
  - in children, 673*t*
  - in chronic obstructive pulmonary disease, 470
  - in constipation, 32, 481, 484, 485*b*–486*b*
  - Daily Recommended Intake, 673*t*
  - in diabetes mellitus, 33, 574*t*, 576
  - in diverticular disease, 32, 518
  - in infants, 673*t*
  - in obesity, 32
  - in pregnancy, 287, 673*t*
  - in toddlers, 322
- in refined grains, 28
- vs. residue, 433
- restriction of, for diarrhea, 481, 482*b*–484*b*
- retaining in storage and processing, 226, 227*b*
- soluble, 21–22, 543*b*
- sources of, 21–22, 287
- teaching on, 483*b*
- total, 22
- in vegetable group, 29
- in whole grain products, 27

Fibric acids, for cholesterol lowering, 537*t*

Fifty-plus vitamin supplement formulas, 123

Fight BAC! Campaign, for food safety, 230, 234, 235*f*

Fish. *See also* Meat, poultry, fish, dry beans, eggs, and nuts group
- Alzheimer's disease and, 368–369
- contaminated, breast-feeding and, 300
- as functional food, 228*t*

Fish oils, 69–70, 71
Alzheimer's disease and, 368–369
for cancer, 650
Fitness, definition of, 166
FITS (Feeding Infants and Toddlers Study), 321–322
Flan, 253
Flavin adenine dinucleotide, vitamin B_2 interactions with, 111
Flavin mononucleotide, vitamin B_2 interactions with, 111
Flaxseed, 89
Flours, refined vs. whole grain, 27–28
Fluconazole, food interactions with, 690*t*
Fluid(s). *See also* Water
overload of, in enteral nutrition, 442*b*
recommendations for
in acute renal failure, 626
in colostomy, 514
in critical illness, 463
in diarrhea, 481
in end-stage renal disease, 608*t*, 615, 617–618
in ileostomy, 514
in kidney stones, 630
in kidney transplantation, 621*t*, 622
in nephrotic syndrome, 627–628
in older adults, 352–353, 356
in pre-end stage renal disease, 608*t*
in steatorrhea, 495
in vomiting, 480
restriction of
in congestive heart failure, 562
in liver disease, 521
in renal disease, 615, 617–618
sources of, 618
in therapeutic diets, 425
Fluid and electrolyte balance
chloride in, 135*t*
minerals in, 132
in parenteral nutrition, 450
potassium in, 135*t*
proteins in, 46
in refeeding syndrome, 410
sodium in, 134, 135*t*
Fluoride, 149–150
deficiency of, 145*t*, 150
functions of, 132, 145*t*, 149
recommendations for, 145*t*
Adequate Intake, 671*t*
in breast-feeding, 671*t*
in children, 671*t*
Dietary Reference Intakes, 671*t*
in infants, 671*t*
in pregnancy, 671*t*
sources of, 145*t*, 149–150
toxicity of, 145*t*, 150
Fluorouracil, food interactions with, 693*t*
Fluoxetine, food interactions with, 689*t*
Flurazepam, food interactions with, 695*t*
Fluvastatin, for cholesterol lowering, 537*t*, 696*t*
Folacin, as coenzyme, 97
Folate
deficiency of, 109*t*, 113
in malabsorption, 495*t*
in older adults, 353
definition of, 272
vs. folic acid (synthetic), 272
food preparation effects on, 96
in fruit juices and drinks, 320*f*
functions of, 109*t*, 112
for hyperhomocysteinemia, 535
metabolism of, 112–113
preconception, 273
recommendations for, 101*t*, 113, 273
Adequate Intake, 668*t*
in breast-feeding, 281*t*, 668*t*
in children, 668*t*
Dietary Reference Intakes, 668*t*
in healing, 466*t*
in infants, 313*f*, 668*t*
in pregnancy, 113, 118, 272–273, 281*t*, 286, 668*t*
Recommended Dietary Allowance, 668*t*
sources of, 109*t*, 112, 273
tolerable upper intake levels for, 101*t*
toxicity of, 109*t*, 113
vitamin B_{12} interactions with, 113
Folic acid. *See also* Folate
definition of, 272
Food
allergy to. *See* Allergy, food
aversions to, in cancer, 647
as basic necessity, 5
drug interactions with, 686*t*–697*t*
functional, 226–229, 228*t*, 544
illness borne by. *See* Food poisoning; Foodborne illness
intake of. *See* Intake
organically grown, 229–230
preparation of
by African Americans, 250
by Asian Americans, 255
convenience foods and, 262, 263*b*
for coronary heart disease prevention, 545–548, 547*b*
cultural factors in, 246
for fat content reduction, 498*b*
at home vs. restaurants, 264, 265*b*–267*b*
in Judaism, 260
by Mexican Americans, 252–253
trends in, 261–264, 263*b*
vitamin fate in, 96
solid, introduction of, to infants, 316–319, 318*b*
supplemental, 427–428
thermic effect of, 166
Food additives
attention-deficit disorder and, 343
vitamins as, 97–98
Foodborne illness, 230–234
in bone marrow transplantation, 641, 641*b*
in enteral nutrition, 437–438

Foodborne illness (*continued*)
epidemiology of, 230
in HIV infection/AIDS, 660
"mad cow disease" as, 234
in pregnancy, 284
prevention of, 230, 231*t*–233*t*, 234, 235*f*
symptoms of, 230, 231*t*–233*t*
vehicles for, 231*t*–233*t*
Food group approach, to weight management, 388, 390*t*
Food Guide Pyramid, replaced by MyPyramid, 186
Food lists, in National Renal Diet, 620
Food Nutrition and the Prevention of Cancer, 197
Food poisoning. *See also* Foodborne illness
in enteral nutrition, 437–438
perfringens, 233*t*
staphylococcal, 232*t*
Food pyramids. *See also* MyPyramid
Asian-American, 255, 256*f*
Food Guide Pyramid, 186
Healthy Eating Pyramid, 191, 193–196, 193*f*
Latin American, 253, 253*f*
Foodways. *See also* Culture, foodways of
definition of, 243
Foremilk, composition of, 299
Formulas
enteral nutrition. *See* Enteral nutrition, formulas for
infant, 314–316
in cleft palate, 323*b*
composition of, vs. breast milk, 314, 315*t*
examples of, 314
growth rate with, 320–321
overfeeding with, 316
parameters for feeding, 316*t*
for phenylketonuria, 324*b*–325*b*
preparation of, 316
solid food introduction with, 316–319, 318*b*
specialized, 315
teaching points for, 317*b*
types of, 315–316
Fortified food
calcium in, 140
definition of, 95
vs. non-fortified food, 123
Fortovase (saquinavir), for HIV infection/AIDS, 661*t*, 693*t*
Foscarnet, food interactions with, 693*t*
Fosinopril, food interactions with, 690*t*
"Free," definition of, in nutrient claims, 215*b*
"Free" foods, in exchange list, 585
Free radicals, antioxidants and, 97
Fructose, 20
absorption of, 22
metabolism of, 22, 24–25
restriction of, in diabetes mellitus, 575–576
in sucrose, 20
Fruit group
in breast-feeding, 281*t*
calcium in, 616*t*
for cancer prevention, 197–198
carbohydrates in, 29
for children, 331*f*
for chronic obstructive pulmonary disease, 470
for coronary heart disease prevention, 539*f*
in DASH diet, 553*t*
in *Dietary Guidelines for Americans 2005,* 184*b*–185*b*
easy chewing, 356
fat in, 78
fiber in, 29
food intake patterns and, 189*t*
as functional foods, 228*t*
in Healthy Eating Index, 192*t*
in Healthy Eating Pyramid, 193*f*, 195
intake of, 117
irradiation of, 237
low-potassium, 619
in MyPyramid, 188*f*
nutrient value of, retaining in storage and processing, 226, 227*b*
for older adults, 355–356
organically grown, 229–230
phosphorus in, 616*t*
potassium in, 562, 563*t*
in pregnancy, 281*t*
vs. processed sweets, 37
protein in, 616*t*
sodium in, 560*b*
in Therapeutic Life Change Diet, 553*t*
for toddlers, 322
vitamins in, 116–118, 117*b*, 119*t*
water in, 130
Fruit sugar. *See* Fructose
Full liquid diet, 421*t*–422*t*
Functional fiber, definition of, 22
Functional foods, 226–229, 228*t*, 544

G

Galactose, 20
absorption of, 22
metabolism of, 22, 24–25
Gallbladder disease, 524–525
Garlic
as functional food, 228*t*
as supplement, 220*t*
"Gassy" foods, 410, 514, 515*b*
Gastric acid
in protein digestion, 48–49, 48*f*
secretion of, stimulation of, 493*b*
Gastric bypass, for obesity, 400, 401*f*
Gastric lipase, in fat digestion, 75*f*
Gastric residuals, in enteral nutrition, 436
Gastric restriction surgery, for obesity, 400, 400*f*
Gastritis, nutrition therapy for, 493–494
Gastroesophageal reflux disease, nutrition therapy for, 491–492
Gastrointestinal system
assessment of, 478
cancer of
nutritional effects of, 636*t*
surgical complications in, 639*t*

disorders of. *See also specific disorders, e.g.,* Anorexia; Constipation
nutrition for
in common problems, 478–479
in gallbladder disease, 524–525
intestinal, 494–518
in liver disease, 519–523
in pancreatitis, 523–524
upper tract, 488–494
HIV infection/AIDS effects on, 655–656
in pregnancy, 275
stress effects on, 460
Gastroparesis, in diabetes mellitus, 572
Gastrostomy, for enteral nutrition, 435*t,* 436
Gemfibrozil, for cholesterol lowering, 537*t*
Gender differences, in adolescent growth, 337–338
Genes, for protein synthesis, 49
Genetic engineering, in food production, 235–237
Genetic factors
in coronary heart disease, 533
in hypercholesterolemia, 542
in obesity, 380
Genistein, sources and effects of, 119*t*
Germ, wheat, 28*f*
Gestational diabetes, 290–291, 595, 596*b*
Gingko biloba, 221*t,* 368
Ginseng, 221*t*
Glipizide, food interactions with, 689*t*
Glomerular filtration rate, in end-stage renal disease, 613
Glucagon
in insulin release, 25
release of, in stress, 458, 459*t*
Glucogenic amino acids, 51–52, 158, 458–459
Glucophage (metformin), for diabetes mellitus, 580, 689*t*
Glucosamine sulfate, for osteoarthritis, 359
Glucose, 20
absorption of, 22
amino acid formation from, 26
availability of, in stress, 458
blood levels of. *See also* Hyperglycemia; Hypoglycemia
in postprandial state, 24–25
in renal disease, 612
calories of, 25
compounds formed from, 26
vs. dextrose, 450
for energy, 25–26
fat synthesized from, 26, 76
formation of, from amino acids, 51–52
glycogen formation from, 26, 156
intolerance of
in diabetes mellitus, 571
in liver disease, 519, 520
in metabolic syndrome, 534, 534*t*
in ketosis prevention, 26
metabolism of, 22, 24–25
disorders of. *See* Diabetes mellitus
in exercise, 161–162
in pregnancy, 275
protein-sparing function of, 25, 52
release of, from glycogen, 25
in sucrose, 20
synthesis of, 158
Glutamine
for critical illness, 463
as ergogenic acid, 170*t*
Gluten-induced enteropathy (celiac disease)
nutrition therapy for, 508, 509*b*–513*b,* 513
pathophysiology of, 508
Glyburide, food interactions with, 689*t*
Glycemic control, in diabetes mellitus
complications and, 572–573
in older adults, 595–597
Glycemic index, 24, 24*t,* 595–597
in diabetes mellitus management, 572–573, 575
factors affecting, 196
Glycemic response, definition of, 24
Glycerol
formation of, in fat digestion and metabolism, 74, 75*f,* 76
metabolism of, 76, 159
in phospholipid structure, 72
in triglyceride structure, 69
Glycogen, 21
degradation of, 25
energy from, in fasting, 160
for exercise, 161–162
formation of, 26, 156
Glycolysis, 157–158
anaerobic, in exercise, 161–162
Glycosuria, in enteral nutrition, 442*b*
Glyset (miglitol), for diabetes mellitus, 580, 690*t*
Goals, in nutritional care process, 11–12
Goitrogens, 148
Grains. *See also* Bread, cereal, rice and pasta group
carbohydrates in, 27–28, 28*f*
for children, 331*f*
fiber in, 34, 34*t*
food intake patterns and, 189*t*
gluten in, 508, 509*b*–513*b,* 514
in Healthy Eating Pyramid, 193, 193*f,* 195
for older adults, 355
refined, 28
sodium in, 560*b*
in Therapeutic Life Change Diet, 553*t*
in vegetarian diets, 60
whole, 27–28, 28*f,* 34, 34*t*
Granisetron, food interactions with, 692*t*
Grape juice, as functional food, 228*t*
Great Britain, food guide of, 196, 197*f*
Greek restaurants, healthy choices from, 267*b*
Green tea extract, for coronary heart disease prevention, 543*b*
Ground diet, for dysphagia, 490*t*
Group welfare, as cultural value, 248
Growth
of adolescents, 337–338
basal metabolic rate in, 164
charts for, 676*f*–685*f*
of children, 326–327, 676*f*–685*f*

Growth (*continued*)
failure to thrive and, 322*b*–323*b*
of infants, 313–314, 313*f*
assessment of, 320–321
formula-fed vs. breast-fed, 320–321
Growth hormone, for appetite stimulation, in HIV infection/AIDS, 659*t*
Guanfacine, food interactions with, 691*t*
Gynecological age, nutritional needs and, 295–296

H

Halal (Islamic dietary laws), 260
Haloperidol, food interactions with, 693*t*
Hamwi method, weight-height analysis, 7, 7*t*
Haram (Islamic prohibited foods), 260
Harris-Benedict equations, 461–462, 461*b*
Hawthorn, for coronary heart disease prevention, 543*b*
HDL. *See* Lipoprotein(s), high-density (HDL, good)
Head and neck cancer
nutritional effects of, 636*t*
radiation therapy complications in, 640*t*
surgical complications in, 639*t*
Head circumference, vs. age, 677*f*–679*f*
Healing
nutrition therapy for
in burns, 465, 467–468
postoperative, 465, 466*t*–467*t*
protein requirements for, 55
Health beliefs
of African Americans, 251–252
of Asian Americans, 257
cultural variation in, 247
of Mexican Americans, 254
Health claims, on labels, 214–215, 216*b*
Health history, in nutrition assessment, 5
Health promotion
for adults and older adults, 347–371
breast-feeding, 303–305, 303*b*
carbohydrates in, 32–41
fiber and, 32–41
sugar and, 35–41, 38*b*, 39*t*
consumer issues in, 208–242
cultural issues in, 243–270
energy, 166–172
aerobic exercise amount, 167–168, 170*t*
carbohydrate-loading, 169
increasing activity, 171–172
physical activity benefits in, 166–167, 167*f*, 167*t*
strength and stretching exercises, 168, 170
fat in, 86–89, 87*f*
healthy eating guidelines for, 180–207
in infancy through adolescence, 312–346
in pregnancy, 271–296
protein in, 56–62, 57*b*, 59*f*
vitamins in, 116–123. *See also* Vitamin supplements
water intake in, 151
Healthy diet, guidelines for, 179–207. *See also specific reference values*
Adequate Intake, 182
in African Americans, 252
American Cancer Association, 200*b*–201*b*
American Heart Association, 200*b*–201*b*
American Institute for Cancer Research, 200*b*–201*b*
in Asian Americans, 257
in children, 329–330
convenience foods in, 263*b*
dietary excess focus of, 180
Dietary Guidelines for Americans, 183, 184*b*–186*b*
Dietary Reference Intakes, 181–182, 181*f*
Estimated Average Requirement, 181*f*, 182
Estimated Energy Requirements, 183
health agency recommendations, 196–204, 200*b*–201*b*, 202*t*, 203*f*
Healthy Eating Index (HEI), 191, 192*t*
Healthy Eating Pyramid, 191, 193–196, 193*f*
in Mexican Americans, 255
MyPyramid. *See* MyPyramid
New American Plate, 197–199, 203*f*
for older adults, 355–357
from other countries, 196
Recommended Dietary Allowance, 181–182, 181*f*
Tolerable Upper Intake Level, 182
for weight management, 394–395
Healthy Eating Index (HEI), 191, 192*t*
for children, 334
Healthy Eating Pyramid, 191, 193–196, 193*f*
Heartburn
nutrition therapy for, 491–492
in pregnancy, 288
Heart disease. *See* Cardiovascular disease; Coronary heart disease
Heart failure, congestive. *See* Congestive heart failure
Heart rate, target, in exercise, 168
HEI (Healthy Eating Index), 191, 192*t*
Height
vs. age, for children and adolescents, 680*f*, 682*f*
basal metabolic rate and, 164
in body mass index calculation, 7, 7*t*, 372, 378*t*–379*t*
in nutritional assessment, 7, 7*t*
vs. weight, 684*f*, 685*f*
in childhood nutritional assessment, 313
Helicobacter pylori infections, peptic ulcer in, 492
Hemochromatosis, 147
Hemodialysis, nutrient recommendations for, 608*t*
Hemolytic uremic syndrome, foodborne, 230, 231*t*
Hemorrhagic colitis, foodborne, 230, 231*t*
Hepatic disorders. *See* Liver, disease of
Hepatitis, 519
Hepatitis A, foodborne, 234*t*
Herbal supplements
banned from sale, 223
for cancer, 650–651
dosages of, 224
vs. drugs, 219, 222–224, 223*t*
education on, 225–226
health problems linked to, 223*t*
in nutritional assessment, 6
in pregnancy, 286–287
self-prescribed, 224
standardization of, 224
top 10 selling, 220*t*–222*t*

"High," definition of, in nutrient claims, 215*b*
High-density lipoprotein. *See* Lipoprotein(s), high-density (HDL, good)
High-fiber diet, for constipation, 481, 484, 485*b*–486*b*
High-potency vitamin supplements, 123
High-quality proteins, 54
Hindmilk, composition of, 299
Hinduism, food practices in, 260–261
Hip fracture, in older adults, 359
Hispanic Americans
  acculturation by, 254
  health beliefs of, 247, 254
  healthy diet suggestions for, 255
  traditional food practices of, 252–253, 253*f*
Histamine receptor antagonists, for gastritis, 493–494
History, in nutrition assessment, 5
  in eating disorders, 408–409
  weight in, 7–8, 7*t*, 8*b*
Hivid (zalcitabine), for HIV infection/AIDS, 661*t*, 693*t*
HIV infection/AIDS, 654–661
  breast-feeding contraindication in, 302
  cytokine production in, 656
  gastrointestinal abnormalities in, 655–656
  metabolic effects of, 655
  nutritional status effects of, 655–656
  nutrition therapy for, 656–660
    counseling on, 657
    for drug efficacy enhancement, 660, 661*t*
    foodborne illness and, 660
    goals of, 656
    symptom-related, 658–660
    in wasting, 656–658, 659*t*
  poor intake in, 656
  selenium deficiency in, 149
HMB (beta-hydroxy beta-methylbutyrate), as ergogenic acid, 170*t*
Holidays, foods used in, 246–247
Homocysteine, 111
  elevated, as coronary heart disease risk factor, 535–536
  folate effects on, 112
  vitamin B_6 and, 112
Hormones
  basal metabolic rate and, 164
  in breast milk, 298
  minerals interactions with, 132
  replacement of, for menopause, 346*b*, 349
  stress, 458, 459*t*
  synthesis of, from amino acids, 46
Hospital food, 418–428
  for diabetes mellitus, 597
  diet types for, 420–425
    house, 420
    modified consistency, 420, 421*t*–423*t*
    normal, 420
    regular, 420
    therapeutic, 420, 425
    as tolerated, 420
  intake of, promotion of, 426
  nutritional supplements in, 425, 427–428
  serving of, 418, 426
  supervision of, 418
Hospitalized patients
  diabetes mellitus in, 597
  enteral nutrition for. *See* Enteral nutrition
  feeding algorithm for, 419*f*
  hospital food for, 418–428, 421*t*–423*t*
  menus for, 16, 426
  parenteral nutrition for. *See* Parenteral nutrition
Hot-cold theory of foods, 247
Hot flashes, 346*b*
House diet, in hospital, 420
Human immunodeficiency virus (HIV) infection. *See* HIV infection/AIDS
Human milk. *See* Breast milk; Breast-feeding
Hunger
  in exercise, 173
  in weight loss diets, 387
Hydralazine, food interactions with, 691*t*
Hydrochloric acid, in protein digestion, 48–49, 48*f*
Hydrogenated fats, 68, 68*t*, 70–71, 83*b*
Hydrolyzed formulas, for enteral nutrition, 430, 430*t*, 431
Hyperactivity, sugar and, 35
Hypercalciuria, kidney stones in, 630
Hypercatabolism, in burns, 465
Hypercholesterolemia. *See also* Cholesterol (blood)
  definition of, 530
  genetic factors in, 542
  in older adults, 366
Hyperglycemia
  in diabetes mellitus, 571
    in acute illness, 593
    routine, 593
  in parenteral nutrition, 450
Hyperinsulinemia
  hypoglycemia in, 601
  in type 2 diabetes mellitus, 571
Hyperkalemia, in acute renal failure, 626
Hypermetabolic conditions
  burns as, 465, 467–468
  complications of, 459–460
  COPD as, 468–470
  definition of, 458
  hormonal changes in, 458, 459*t*
  liver transplantation, 523
  nutrition therapy for, 460–464, 461*b*, 464*b*
  protein catabolism in, 458–459
  surgery as, 465, 466*t*–467*t*
Hyperphosphatemia, in renal disease, 615
Hypertension, 551–556
  in African Americans, 252
  alcohol use and, 556
  in coronary heart disease, 530, 533
  DASH diet for, 545, 551–552, 553*t*–554*t*, 555*b*, 556*b*, 557*t*–558*t*
  definition of, 551
  drugs for, 552
  epidemiology of, 551
  exercise for, 555

Hypertension (*continued*)
in metabolic syndrome, 534, 534*t*
nutrition therapy for, 612
in older adults, 365
pregnancy-induced, 291
in renal disorders, 606, 612
smoking cessation for, 556
sodium intake and, 136, 365
weight loss for, 551
Hyperthyroidism, basal metabolic rate in, 164
Hypertonic enteric formulas, 433
Hypertriglyceridemia
as coronary heart disease risk factor, 534–535
in diabetes mellitus, 578
in metabolic syndrome, 534, 534*t*
nursing process for, 548–550
Hypervitaminosis A, 99*t*, 102–103
Hypoalbuminemia, in nutritional assessment, 9–10, 10*t*
Hypochromic anemia, in iron deficiency, 147
Hypoglycemia
in diabetes mellitus, 591, 593, 594*b*
in dumping syndrome, 500
in exercise, 591
functional, 601
Hypokalemia, in acute renal failure, 626
Hypophosphatemia, in parenteral nutrition, 450
Hypothyroidism, basal metabolic rate in, 164

I

Ibuprofen, food interactions with, 686*t*
"Ideal" body weight, 7, 7*t*
IDV (indinavir), for HIV infection/AIDS, 661*t*, 693*t*
Ileostomy
complications of, 639*t*
nutrition therapy for, 514–515, 515*b*
pathophysiology of, 514
Illness, foodborne. *See* Foodborne illness
Imipramine, food interactions with, 689*t*
Immune system, omega fatty acids effects on, 473
Immunodeficiency. *See specific disorders, e.g.,* HIV infection/AIDS
Immunonutrition formulas, 464
Immunosuppressants
food interactions with, 695*t*
after renal transplantation, 622
Immunotherapy, for cancer, nutritional effects of, 641
Imuran (azathioprine)
food interactions with, 695*t*
after renal transplantation, 622
Inactivity, obesity and, 381, 382*f*
Incomplete proteins, 53–54
Indian restaurants, healthy choices from, 267*b*
Indigestion, nutrition therapy for, 491–492
Indinavir (Crixivan , IDV), for HIV infection/AIDS, 661*t*, 693*t*
Indirect calorimetry, in critical illness, 461–462
Individualism, as cultural value, 248
Inedible food, definition of, 243, 243*f*
Infant(s)
cleft palate in, 323*b*
colic in, 323*b*
cystic fibrosis in, 325*b*–326*b*
growth rate of, 313–314, 313*f*, 676*f*–679*f*
low-birth weight, maternal weight and, 276–277
nutrition for, 313–321
Adequate Intake, 668*t*–669*t*, 671*t*, 673*t*
vs. adult nutrition, 313, 313*f*
breast-feeding. *See* Breast milk; Breast-feeding
Dietary Reference Intakes for, 668*t*–669*t*, 671*t*, 673*t*
formulas, 314–316, 315*t*, 316*t*, 317*b*
intake assessment in, 320–321
macronutrients, 673*t*
minerals, 671*t*
protein requirements in, 55
Recommended Dietary Allowance for, 668*t*–669*t*, 671*t*, 673*t*
solid food introduction in, 316–319, 318*b*
vitamins, 668*t*–669*t*
weight for height standard and, 313
phenylketonuria in, 324*b*–325*b*
premature, formulas for, 315
pyloric stenosis in, 324*b*
weight gain in, 320–321
Infections
in critical illness, 460
foodborne. *See* Foodborne illness
in parenteral nutrition, 449*b*
Inflammatory bowel disease
lactose intolerance in, 502
nursing process for, 506–507
nutrition therapy for, 504–505
pathophysiology of, 504
types of, 502
Information and misinformation, 209–217
client education on, 217
combating misinformation, 211–212
fraudulent, 210, 210*b*
half-life of, 209
labeling. *See* Labels
reliability of, 209–210, 210*b*
sources of, 209
on weight loss diets, 387
Ingredient list, on labels, 214
Inorganic compounds, minerals as, 132
Inositol, 114
Insensible water loss, 129, 129*t*
Insoluble fiber, definition of, 21–22
Insulin
excess of
in diabetes mellitus type 2, 571
hypoglycemia in, 601
replacement of, in diabetes mellitus, 579–580
resistance to
in diabetes mellitus, 571
exercise and, 591
in high-calorie diet, 579
secretion of, 24
absence of, in type 1 diabetes mellitus, 571
in liver failure, 519
in low-carbohydrate diet, 393
in stress, 458, 459*t*

Intake. *See also* Adequate Intake (AI); *specific nutrient*
adequate and appropriate, promotion of, 12–13
in anorexia nervosa, 410
of artificial sweeteners, 41
in breast-feeding, assessment of, 302–303
of calcium, in adolescents, 338
of carbohydrates, 31, 31*t*, 36–37
excessive, obesity in, 380–381
of fat, 80–86, 81*t*
of fiber, 31, 31*t*, 33–35, 34*t*
of hospital food, promotion of, 426
in nutritional assessment, 6
poor, in HIV infection/AIDS, 656
promotion of, in poor appetite, 468
of proteins, 54–56, 55*b*
of vitamins, 101*t*
of water, 129–130, 131*t*
Intermittent feedings, in enteral nutrition, 436
International Units (IU), for vitamin D, 104
Intestinal disorders
cancer, nutritional effects of, 636*t*
nutrition therapy for, 494–518
celiac disease, 508, 509*b*–513*b*, 513
colostomy, 513–515, 515*b*
diverticular disease, 518
dumping syndrome, 495, 500, 501*b*, 502
goals of, 494
ileostomy, 513–515, 515*b*
inflammatory bowel disease, 502, 504–505
lactose intolerance, 502, 503*b*
malabsorption, 494–495, 495*t*, 496*b*–498*b*
nursing process for, 506–507
short-bowel syndrome, 516–517, 517*b*
steatorrhea, 494–495, 495*t*, 496*b*–498*b*
Intrinsic factor, vitamin B_{12} and, 113–114
Invirase (saquinavir), for HIV infection/AIDS, 661*t*, 693*t*
Iodine
body distribution of, 148
deficiency of, 144*t*
functions of, 133, 144*t*
recommendations for, 144*t*, 148
Adequate Intake, 671*t*
in breast-feeding, 671*t*
in children, 671*t*
Dietary Reference Intakes, 671*t*
in infants, 671*t*
in pregnancy, 671*t*
Recommended Dietary Allowance, 671*t*
sources of, 144*t*, 148
toxicity of, 144*t*
Ionamin (phentermine), for weight loss, 399
Ipratropium bromide, food interactions with, 695*t*
Irinotecan, food interactions with, 693*t*
Iron, 146–147
absorption of, 133, 146–147
bioavailability of, 146
body distribution of, 146
in breast milk, 298, 315*t*
in cereals, for infants, 317, 319
deficiency of, 144*t*, 146–147, 328–329
in adolescents, 338–339
in malabsorption, 495*t*
in renal disease, 619
functions of, 132, 144*t*
in infant formulas, 314–315, 315*t*
recommendations for, 144*t*
Adequate Intake, 671*t*
in adolescents, 338–339
vs. age, 329*f*
in breast-feeding, 281*t*, 671*t*
in children, 328–329, 329*f*, 671*t*
Dietary Reference Intakes, 671*t*
in healing, 467*t*
in infants, 671*t*
in older adults, 354*t*
in pregnancy, 280–281, 281*t*, 671*t*
Recommended Dietary Allowance, 328–329, 329*f*, 671*t*
in vegetarian diets, 58
sources of, 57, 58, 144*t*, 146, 328
supplements of, 147
in breast-feeding, 300
in pregnancy, 285–286
in renal disease, 619
toxicity of, 144*t*, 147
Irradiation, food, 237, 237*f*
Islam, food practices in, 260
Isoflavones
sources and effects of, 119*t*
soy, 221*t*
Isothiocyanates, sources and effects of, 119*t*
Isotonic enteric formulas, 433
Isradipine, food interactions with, 691*t*
Italian restaurants, healthy choices from, 267*b*
IU (International Units), for vitamin D, 104

J

Jainism, food practices in, 261
Japanese restaurants, healthy choices from, 267*b*
Jejunostomy, for enteral nutrition, 435*t*, 463–464
Jejunum, dumping syndrome and, 495, 500, 501*b*, 502
Judaism, food practices in, 259–260, 547*b*–548*b*
Juices
as functional foods, 228*t*
for infants, 318*b*, 319–320, 320*f*
nutrients in, 320*f*

K

K. *See* Potassium
Kaletra (lopinavir-ritonavir), for HIV infection/AIDS, 661*t*
Kava products, 223*t*
Ketoacidosis, in pregnancy, 282
Ketoconazole, food interactions with, 690*t*
Ketogenic amino acids, 160
Ketones and ketone bodies
definition of, 26

Ketones and ketone bodies (*continued*)
formation of
in fasting, 160–161
in stress, 458
Ketosis, prevention of, glucose in, 26
Kidney
disorders of. *See* Renal disorders
function of, 606
solute load in, breast milk composition and, 298
stones of, 628–630, 629*b*
transplantation of, 621–623, 621*t*
Kosher foods, 260
Krebs cycle, 157

L

Labels, 212–216. *See also* Nutrition Facts label
carbohydrate content on, 37
fat content on, 546
health claims on, 214–215, 216*b*
ingredient list on, 214
nutrition description on, 214, 215*b*
Nutrition Facts on, 212–213, 212*f*
practical use of, 217
reading of, in diabetes mellitus, 592*b*
structure/function claims on, 215–216, 217*b*
on supplements
claims on, 224
vitamin, 121–123
warnings on, 224
trans fats on, 215–216
Laboratory values, in nutrition assessment, 9–10, 10*t*
Lactaid, 503*b*
Lactase
deficiency of. *See* Lactose, intolerance of
food products treated with, 504
Lactation. *See* Breast milk; Breast-feeding
Lactic acid, accumulation of, in exercise, 162
Lacto-ovo vegetarians, 56
calcium intake of, 58
Seventh-Day Adventists as, 259
vitamin B_{12} intake of, 60
Lactose
in breast milk, 297
calcium absorption and, 140
intolerance of
in African Americans, 250
infant formulas for, 315
nutrition therapy for, 502, 503*b*, 504
pathophysiology of, 502
restriction of
in diarrhea, 484*b*
in inflammatory bowel disease, 499*b*
in steatorrhea, 494
sources of, 503*b*
Lacto-vegetarians, 56, 58
Lactulose, for hepatic encephalopathy, 520
Lamivudine (Epivir, 3TC), for HIV infection/AIDS, 661*t*, 693*t*
Latinos. *See* Hispanic Americans
Laxatives, in bulimia nervosa, 411
LDL. *See* Lipoprotein(s), low-density (LDL, bad)
"Lean," definition of, in nutrient claims, 215*b*
Lecithin, 72
Length, of infants, charts for, 676*f*–678*f*
Levodopa, food interactions with, 693*t*
Liberal diet approach, in long-term care, 365–366, 365*b*
Lifestyle changes
for cancer prevention, 202*t*
for cholesterol lowering, 73
for diabetes mellitus, 591, 592*b*
for weight management, 386, 388, 389*t*, 390*t*, 398*b*
"Light," definition of, in nutrient claims, 215*b*
Lighter Bake fat replacer, 88
Lignans, sources and effects of, 119*t*
Limiting amino acids, 53–54
Limonene, sources and effects of, 119*t*
Lingual lipase, in fat digestion, 75*f*
Linoleic acid
in breast milk, 297, 315*t*
as essential fatty acid, 69
in infant formula, 315*t*
recomendations for
in coronary heart disease prevention, 540
recommendations for
Acceptable Macronutrient Distribution Range, 81, 81*t*, 182, 674*t*
Adequate Intake, 673*t*
in breast-feeding, 673*t*
in children, 673*t*
Dietary Reference Intake, 673*t*
in infants, 673*t*
in pregnancy, 673*t*
Linolenic acid. *See also* Alpha-linolenic acid
as essential fatty acid, 69
in fats, 68*t*
Lipases, in fat digestion and metabolism, 74, 75*f*, 76
Lipid(s)
cholesterol. *See* Cholesterol
definition of, 67
emulsions of, in parenteral nutrition, 450–451
phospholipids, 72
triglycerides as. *See* Triglycerides
types of, 67–68. *See also* Fat (dietary)
Lipitor (atorvastatin), for cholesterol lowering, 536, 537*t*, 696*t*
Lipodystrophy, in HIV infection/AIDS, 659–660
Lipogenesis, 76
amino acids in, 52
glucose in, 26
Lipoprotein(s)
classification of, 531–532, 532*t*
high-density (HDL, good)
activity effects on, 535
drugs affecting, 536, 537*t*
functions of, 531, 532*t*
low, as coronary heart disease risk factor, 533
in metabolic syndrome, 534
methods for elevating, 566
low-density (LDL, bad)
activity effects on, 535
diet and, 535

functions of, 532, 532*t*
goals of, 533, 533*t*
lowering of. *See* Cholesterol (blood), lowering of
in metabolic syndrome, 534
nursing process for, 548–550
nutritional supplements for, 542–545, 543*b*
variations in, 532
Lipoprotein lipase, in fat digestion and metabolism, 76
Liquid diets, 420, 421*t*–423*t*, 425
for colostomy, 514
for ileostomy, 514
Liquid nutritional supplements, 425, 427–428
Listeria monocytogenes, in foodborne illness, 231*t*, 284
"Lite," definition of, in nutrient claims, 215*b*
Lithium, 150
Liver
amino acid metabolism in, 49
cancer of, nutritional effects of, 636*t*
disease of
nutrition therapy for, 520–522, 521*b*
pathophysiology of, 519–520
transplantation in, 522–523, 522*b*
failure of, 519–520
functions of, 519
protein synthesis in, 49
vitamin A storage in, 101–103
Lomefloxacin, food interactions with, 688*t*
Long-term care, 362–366
commercial supplements in, 362
intake assessment and promotion in, 363, 364*b*
liberal diets in, 365–366, 365*b*
nutrient-dense foods in, 363
pressure ulcers in, 362
restrictive diets in, 364–365
weight changes in, 364
Lopinavir-ritonavir (Kaletra), for HIV infection/AIDS, 661*t*
Lorazepam, food interactions with, 687*t*
Lovastatin, for cholesterol lowering, 537*t*, 696*t*
"Low," definition of, in nutrient claims, 215*b*
Low-birth weight infants
formulas for, 315
maternal weight and, 276–277
Low-carbohydrate diets, 392–394, 392*t*
Low-density lipoprotein. *See* Lipoprotein(s), low-density (LDL, bad)
Low-fat diets
desserts in, 546
fat substitutes in, 83*b*
food preparation for, 545–548, 547*b*–548*b*
for inflammatory bowel disease, 499*b*
for steatorrhea, 494–495, 496*b*–498*b*
vegetable preparation for, 198
for vomiting, 480
for weight management, 391–393, 391*t*, 392*t*
Low-fiber diet, for diverticular disease, 518
Low-microbial diet, in liver transplant candidates, 522, 522*b*
Low-sodium diet. *See* Sodium, restriction of
Lutein, sources and effects of, 101, 119*t*
Lycopene, sources and effects of, 101, 119*t*

M

Macrocytic anemia, in vitamin B_{12} deficiency, 109*t*
Macrolides, for cholesterol lowering, 537*t*
"Mad cow disease," 234
Magnesium
absorption of, 142
body distribution of, 142
deficiency of, 139*t*, 142
in malabsorption, 495*t*
in older adults, 354
in fruit juices and drinks, 320*f*
functions of, 132, 139*t*
recommendations for, 139*t*
Adequate Intake, 671*t*
in breast-feeding, 281*t*, 671*t*
in children, 671*t*
Dietary Reference Intakes, 671*t*
in infants, 671*t*
in pregnancy, 281*t*, 671*t*
Recommended Dietary Allowance, 671*t*
sources of, 139*t*, 354
supplements of, 142, 523
toxicity of, 139*t*
Magnesium hydroxide, food interactions with, 687*t*
Ma huang (ephedra), 223
Malabsorption
in cancer cachexia, 636, 638
in celiac disease, 508
of drugs, in stress, 460
in dumping syndrome, 500
in HIV infection/AIDS, 655–656, 659
in inflammatory bowel disease, 504
of lactose. *See* Lactose, intolerance of
in renal disease, 606
in short-bowel syndrome, 516
Malignancy. *See* Cancer
Malnutrition
in anorexia nervosa, 407
appearance of, in nutritional assessment, 8–9, 9*b*
basal metabolic rate and, 164
in bulimia nervosa, 407
in burns, 465, 467
in chronic obstructive pulmonary disease, 468–470
in congestive heart failure, 562
drug malabsorption in, 460
in dumping syndrome, 500
in end-stage renal disease, 613
gastrointestinal effects of, 460
infections in, 460
in inflammatory bowel disease, 504
in intestinal disorders, 494
in liver disease, 520, 522
in older adults, 362
in pancreatitis, 523
in pregnancy, 291, 292*b*
prevention of, in hospitalized patients, 418
in short-bowel syndrome, 516
signs and symptoms of, 9, 9*b*
skin breakdown in, 459
in surgical patients, 465

Manganese, 149
Adequate Intake for, 671*t*
deficiency of, 145*t*
functions of, 145*t*
recommendations for, 145*t*, 671*t*
sources of, 145*t*
toxicity of, 145*t*
Mannitol, as sugar alternative, 38, 576
Marbling, of meat, 80
Margarine, sterol-rich, for coronary heart disease prevention, 544
Marinol (dronabinol)
for appetite stimulation, in HIV infection/AIDS, 659*t*
food interactions with, 692*t*
Mature vitamin supplement formulas, 123
Meals
for anorexia nervosa, 410
for bulimia nervosa, 411
exchange lists for, 389*t*, 581, 583, 584*b*–587*b*, 585, 587–588
frequency and timing of
for children, 332
cultural variation in, 247
in nutritional assessment, 6
in pregnancy, 282
in transition from enteral to oral diet, 439
for renal disease, end-stage, 619–621
restaurant. *See* Restaurant meals
skipping, weight management and, 388
vitamin supplement timing and, 123
Meals on Wheels, 361–362
Meat. *See also* Meat, poultry, fish, dry beans, eggs, and nuts group
irradiation of, 237
"mad cow disease" from, 234
organically produced, 229
Meat, poultry, fish, dry beans, eggs, and nuts group
in breast-feeding, 281*t*
calcium in, 617*t*
carbohydrates in, 30
for children, 330, 331*f*
in coronary heart disease prevention diet, 539*f*
in DASH diet, 554*t*
in exchange list, 581, 583
fat in, 79–80, 83*b*, 538, 538*t*, 540
fiber in, 30
food intake patterns and, 189*t*
in Healthy Eating Index, 192*t*
in Healthy Eating Pyramid, 193*f*, 195
imitation, 62
for infants, 319
kosher, 260
mercury in, 284
in MyPyramid, 188*f*
in New American Plate, 199
for older adults, 356
phosphorus in, 617*t*
in pregnancy, 281*t*
proteins in, 53–54, 53*f*, 617*t*
in renal disease, 612
sodium in, 555, 555*b*, 560*b*
taste changes in, 647
in Therapeutic Life Change Diet, 554*t*
in vegetarian diets, 56, 59*f*
Mechanical soft diet, 424*t*, 490*t*
Medications. *See* Drugs/medications
Mediterranean diet, 86–87, 87*f*
Medium-chain triglycerides, for steatorrhea, 494
Megace (megestrol), for appetite stimulation, in HIV infection/AIDS, 659*t*
Megadoses, of vitamins, 98
Megestrol acetate (Megace), for appetite stimulation, in HIV infection/AIDS, 659*t*
Meglitinides, for diabetes mellitus, 580
Melphalan, food interactions with, 693*t*
Memory, gingko biloba and, 368
Menaquinones, 106
Menopause
bone loss after, 359
symptom relief for, 346*b*, 349
Men's health issues, 349–350, 351*b*
Menus
for celiac disease, 512*b*
for children, 332*b*
for constipation, 485*b*–486*b*
for DASH diet, 558*t*
for diabetes mellitus, 588*b*
for diarrhea, 483*b*, 484*b*
for dumping syndrome, 501*b*
for inflammatory bowel disease, 499*b*
for liver disease, 521*b*
for low-carbohydrate diet, 392*t*
for low-fat diet, 392*t*, 497*b*
for malabsorption, 497*b*
for older adults, 365*b*
patient selection of, 426
for renal disease, 609*b*
for short-bowel syndrome, 517*b*
for steatorrhea, 497*b*
for weight loss, 387, 389*t*
Meperidine, food interactions with, 686*t*
Mercury, in fish, in pregnancy, 284
Meridia (sibutramine), for weight loss, 399*t*
Metabolic pool, for amino acids, 49
Metabolic syndrome (syndrome X)
coronary heart disease risk in, 534
in diabetes mellitus, 572
Metabolism
adaptation of, to fasting, 160
of amino acids, 158
anaerobic, 158, 161–162
basal, 163–164. *See also* Basal metabolic rate
in burns, 465, 467–468
cancer effects on, 635–636, 637*f*
of carbohydrates, 22, 24–25
changes of, in weight management, 385
in chronic obstructive pulmonary disease, 468–470
definition of, 156
disorders of, in parenteral nutrition, 449*b*, 450

elevated. *See* Hypermetabolic conditions
energy. *See* Energy metabolism
of fat, 76, 158–160
of folate, 112–113
HIV infection/AIDS effects on, 655
in liver disease, 520
in pregnancy, 275
of protein, 49–52, 458–459
in stress, 458–459
in surgical patients, 465, 466*t*–467*t*
water in, 128
Metformin (Glucophage), for diabetes mellitus, 580, 689*t*
Methionine, 111
Methotrexate, food interactions with, 693*t*
Methyldopa, food interactions with, 691*t*
Metoprolol, food interactions with, 691*t*
Metronidazole, food interactions with, 693*t*
Mexican Americans
acculturation by, 254
health beliefs of, 247
healthy diet suggestions for, 255, 547*b*
traditional food practices of, 252–253, 253*f*
Mexican restaurants, healthy choices from, 266*b*
Mg. *See* Magnesium
Micelles, 75
Microcytic anemia, in iron deficiency, 147
Micronutrients
in therapeutic diets, 426
trace minerals as. *See* Mineral(s), trace; *specific minerals*
vitamins as, 95
Miglitol (Glyset), for diabetes mellitus, 580, 690*t*
Milk. *See* Breast milk; Milk, yogurt, and cheese group
Milk, yogurt, and cheese group
in breast-feeding, 281*t*
calcium in, 140, 616*t*
calories of, 395
carbohydrates in, 29
for children, 327–328, 331*f*
consumption of, by adolescents, 338
in coronary heart disease prevention diet, 539*f*
in DASH diet, 553*t*
fat in, 78–79, 83*b*
food intake patterns and, 189*t*
as functional foods, 228*t*
in Healthy Eating Pyramid, 193*f*, 195, 196
for increasing nutrient density, 644*b*
for infants, 313–314, 320
lactose in, 504
in liquid diets, 421*t*–423*t*
for Mexican Americans, 253
in MyPyramid, 188*f*
in nutritional supplements, 427
for older adults, 356
phosphorus in, 616*t*
in pregnancy, 281*t*
protein in, 616*t*
for renal disease, pre-end stage, 612–613
sodium in, 560*b*
in Therapeutic Life Change Diet, 553*t*
in vegetarian diets, 56, 59*f*
vitamin D in, 59
Milk thistle, for cancer, 650–651
Mineral(s), 131–150. *See also* Mineral supplements; *specific minerals*
absorption of, 133
balance of, 133
body distribution of, 131–132
in breast milk, 297–298, 315*t*
chelated, 152
chemistry of, 132
deficiencies of, 139*t*, 144*t*–145*t*
excretion of, 133
functions of, 132–133, 139*t*, 144*t*–145*t*
in infant formula, 315*t*
interactions among, 133
major, 132, 138–142, 139*t*
in parenteral nutrition, 451
recommendations for
Adequate Intake, 671*t*
in breast-feeding, 300, 671*t*
in children, 671*t*
in critical illness, 463
Dietary Reference Intakes, 671*t*
in end-stage renal disease, 608*t*, 619
in HIV infection/AIDS, 658
in infants, 671*t*
in older adults, 353, 354*t*, 355*t*
in pregnancy, 281*t*, 671*t*
Recommended Dietary Allowance, 671*t*
in renal disease, 608*t*, 619
retaining in storage and processing, 226, 227*b*
sources of, 134, 139*t*
storage of, release from, 133
toxicities of, 133, 139*t*, 144*t*–145*t*
trace, 132, 142–150
bioavailability of, 143
deficiencies of, 144*t*–145*t*
functions of, 144*t*–145*t*
health effects of, 142–143, 143*f*
in parenteral nutrition, 451
for renal disease, 619
sources of, 142–150, 144*t*–145*t*
supplements of, 142
toxicities of, 144*t*–145*t*
Mineral supplements
in breast-feeding, 300
calcium, 140–141
for diabetes mellitus, 575*t*, 579
iron, 148
for kidney transplantation, 621*t*, 622
for liver disease, 521
magnesium, 142
in nutritional assessment, 6
for older adults, 357
in pregnancy, 284–286
for pregnancy-induced hypertension, 291
for steatorrhea, 494
toxicity of, 286
zinc, 148

Minoxidil, food interactions with, 691*t*
Mirtazapine, food interactions with, 689*t*
Mobility, limited, in enteral nutrition, 444*b*
Modular products, for nutritional supplementation, 428
Molybdenum, 145*t*, 150
  recommendations for
    Adequate Intake, 671*t*
    in children, 671*t*
    Dietary Reference Intakes, 671*t*
    in infants, 671*t*
    in pregnancy, 671*t*
    Recommended Dietary Allowance, 671*t*
Monitoring, of nutritional status, 14–15
Monoamine oxidase inhibitors, food interactions and, 696–697
Monoglycerides, absorption of, 74–75
Monosaccharides, 20, 22, 23*f*, 24–25. *See also* Fructose; Glucose
Monounsaturated fat, 67–68, 68*t*
  in coronary heart disease, 540
  in diabetes mellitus, 574*t*, 578
Morbid obesity, surgery for, 399–400, 400*f*, 401*f*
"More," definition of, in nutrient claims, 215*b*
Mormons, food practices of, 259, 349–350
Morphine, food interactions with, 686*t*
Mortality
  in anorexia nervosa, 407
  causes of, 180
    in men, 349–350, 351*b*
    in women, 345
Mouth
  digestion in, 22, 23*f*
  dry
    in cancer, 647–648
    in enteral nutrition, 445*b*
  sore, in cancer, 647
Mucus, water in, 128
Multiple organ failure, 460
Multivitamins. *See* Vitamin supplements
Muromonab-CD3
  food interactions with, 695*t*
  after renal transplantation, 622
Muscle(s)
  building of, eating for, 61–62
  function of, minerals in, 132
  protein in, 46
    turnover of, 51
Muslims, food practices of, 260
MyPyramid, 187–191, 188*f*. *See also specific groups*
  for African Americans, 250, 251*f*
  for breast-feeding, 281*t*
  carbohydrates in, 26–27, 27*f*, 36
  for children, 330, 331*f*
  for cholesterol lowering, 538, 539*f*
  for coronary heart disease prevention, 539*f*, 540
  for diabetes mellitus, 588*b*, 589
  fats in, 76–80, 77*f*
  food intake patterns in, 189*t*
  moderation in, 187
  for muscle building, 62
  personalization of, 190
  physical activity in, 188*f*, 190–191
  for pregnancy, 281, 281*t*
  proportion sizes in, 187, 190
  protein in, 52, 53*f*
  Therapeutic Lifestyle Change Diet, 538, 539*f*
  variety in, 187
  web site of, 191
  for weight management, 388, 390*t*
MyPyramid for Kids, 330, 331*f*

N

Na. *See* Sodium
Naproxen, food interactions with, 686*t*
Narcotics, food interactions with, 686*t*
Nasogastric tube, for enteral nutrition, 435*t*
Nasointestinal tube, for enteral nutrition, 435*t*
National Organic Program, 229
National Renal Diet, 619–621
Native Americans, healthy diet suggestions for, 547*b*
Nausea and vomiting
  anticipatory, 645
  in bulimia nervosa, 407
  in cancer, 645–646
  in enteral nutrition, 441*b*
  nutrition therapy for, 479–480
  in pregnancy, 287
Nefazodone, food interactions with, 689*t*
Negative nitrogen balance, definition of, 50, 51*b*
Nelfinavir (Viracept, NLF), for HIV infection/AIDS, 661*t*, 693*t*
Neoral (cyclosporine), after renal transplantation, 622
Neotame, 39*t*
Nephrotic syndrome, nutrition therapy for, 627–628
Nerve function, minerals in, 132
"Net carbs," 412–413
Neural tube defects, prevention of, folate in, 273
Neurologic disorders
  in vitamin B_{12} deficiency, 109*t*, 113
  vitamin B_6 for, 112
Neutral nitrogen balance, definition of, 50, 51*b*
Nevirapine (Viramune, NVP), for HIV infection/AIDS, 661*t*
New American Plate, 197–199, 203*f*
Newborns
  vitamin E deficiency in, 106
  vitamin K deficiency in, 107
New dietary ingredients, 222
Niacin. *See* Vitamin B_3 (niacin)
Niacin equivalents, 111
Niaspan (nicotinic acid), for cholesterol lowering, 537*t*
Nickel, 150
Nicotinamide, 111. *See also* vitamin B_3 (niacin)
Nicotinamide adenine dinucleotide (NAD), vitamin B_3 in, 111
Nicotinamide adenine dinucleotide phosphate (NADP), vitamin B_3 in, 111
Nicotinic acid, 111. *See also* vitamin B_3 (niacin)
  for cholesterol lowering, 111, 537*t*
Nifedipine, food interactions with, 692*t*

Night blindness, in vitamin A deficiency, 99*t*
Nitrogen balance, 50, 51*b*
Nitrogenous wastes, excretion of, 606
NLF (nelfinavir), for HIV infection/AIDS, 661*t*, 693*t*
Non-B vitamins, 114
Nondiet approach, to weight management, 388, 390
Nonessential amino acids, 47, 47*b*
Nonnucleoside reverse transcriptase inhibitors, for HIV infection/AIDS, 661*t*
Nonnutritive sweeteners. *See* Artificial sweeteners
Nontropical sprue (celiac disease), nutrition therapy for, 508, 509*b*–513*b*, 514
Norwalk virus infections, foodborne, 234*t*
Nose, enteral nutrition through, 434, 435*t*
Novir (ritonavir), for HIV infection/AIDS, 661*t*, 693*t*
Nucleoside reverse transcriptase inhibitors, for HIV infection/AIDS, 661*t*
Nursing diagnosis, in nutritional care process, 10, 11*b*
Nursing homes. *See* Long-term care
Nursing process. *See also* Nutritional care process
  for cancer, 652–654
  for congestive heart failure, 564–565
  for diabetes mellitus, 598–600
  for dysphagia, 487–488
  for enteral nutrition, 440–447, 441*b*–445*b*
  for high cholesterol and triglycerides, 548–550
  for inflammatory bowel disease, 506–507
  for multiple trauma, 471–473
  for obesity, 401–406
  for older adults, 366–368
  for pregnancy, 306–308
  for renal disease, 623–625
  for toddler nutritional assessment, 340–343
Nutraceuticals, 226–229, 228*t*
Nutrasweet. *See* Aspartame
Nutrients. *See also specific type*
  absorption of. *See* Absorption
  density of
    in critical illness, 464*b*
    in enteral formulas, 431, 432
    increasing, 464*b*, 643–644, 644*b*
    in modular supplements, 428
    in pregnancy, 282
  retaining in storage and processing, 226, 227*b*
Nutritional assessment. *See* Assessment
Nutritional care process, 4–16
  assessment in, 4–16, 7*t*, 8*b*, 9*b*, 10*t*, 11*b*
  evaluation in, 15–16
  goal setting in, 11–12
  implementation in, 10–16
  nursing diagnosis in, 10, 11*b*
  planning in, 10–16
  priority setting in, 11
Nutritional information. *See* Information and misinformation
Nutritional screen, definition of, 14
Nutrition counseling. *See also* Nutrition education
  culturally sensitive, 258–259
  on diabetes mellitus, 596
  by dietitians, 13–14
  on HIV infection/AIDS, 657
  by nurses, 13–14
  in pregnancy, 278, 288–289, 293–295, 294*b*
  on weight management, in pregnancy, 278, 288–289
Nutrition descriptions, on labels, 214, 215*b*
Nutrition education, 13–14. *See also* Nutrition counseling
  for African Americans, 252
  for Asian Americans, 257
  on beverages, 130
  on breast-feeding, 303–305, 303*b*
  on bulimia nervosa, 411–412
  on calorie content of fat-free foods, 31
  on celiac disease, 513*b*
  on cholesterol lowering, 545–546, 547*b*–548*b*
  on constipation, 486*b*
  on dietary fat reduction, 82, 83*b*–84*b*
  on eating disorders, 411–412
  facilitation of, 14
  on fiber, 483*b*
  on formula feeding, 317*b*
  on healthier lifestyle, 203
  on healthy diet concept, 192*t*
  on healthy eating for children, 335
  on high-protein diets, 50
  increasing physical activity, 171, 172
  on low-fat diets, 498*b*
  for Mexican Americans, 255
  on nutrition information and misinformation, 211–212
  on parenteral nutrition, 453
  on phenylketonuria, 275
  questions for, 194–195
  on sodium-restricted diets, 560*b*–557*b*
  on supplements, 225–226
  on vitamin intake, 102, 120
Nutrition Facts label, 212–213, 212*f*
  products requiring, 237–238
  sodium on, 136
  for vitamin supplements, 121–123
Nutrition status
  cancer effects on, 635–638, 636*t*, 637*f*
  cancer therapy effects on, 638–641, 639*t*, 640*t*, 641*b*
  definition of, 4
  HIV infection/AIDS effects on, 655–656
Nutrition supplements, 425
  for anorexia, 478
  for cancer, 650–651
  clear liquid, 425
  commercially prepared, 427
  for coronary heart disease prevention, 542–545, 543*b*
  foods, 427–428
  gastrointestinal distress due to, 479*b*
  for increasing nutrient density, 644
  milk-based, 427
  modular products as, 428
  in nutritional assessment, 8
  for renal disease, 620

Nutrition therapy
for anorexia, 478–479
for burns, 465, 467–468
for celiac disease, 508, 509*b*–513*b*, 513
for chronic obstructive pulmonary disease, 468–470
for colostomy, 514–515, 515*b*
for congestive heart failure, 558, 559*b*–561*b*, 562, 563*t*
for constipation, 481, 484, 485*b*–486*b*
for coronary heart disease
lifestyle change diet in, 538–542, 538*t*, 539*f*
nutritional supplements in, 542–545, 543*b*
for critical illness, 460–464, 461*b*, 464*b*
for diarrhea, 480–481, 482*b*–484*b*
for diverticular disease, 518
for dumping syndrome, 500, 501*b*
for gallbladder disease, 524–525
for gastritis, 493–494
for gastroesophageal reflux disease, 491–492
for healing, 465, 466*t*–467*t*, 467–468
for hypermetabolic conditions, 460–464, 461*b*, 464*b*
for hypertension, 545, 551–552, 553*t*–554*t*, 555*b*, 556*b*, 557*t*–558*t*, 612
for ileostomy, 514–515, 515*b*
for inflammatory bowel disease, 504–505
for lactose intolerance, 502, 503*b*, 504
for liver disease, 520–522, 521*b*
for malabsorption, 494–495, 495*t*, 496*b*–498*b*
for nausea and vomiting, 479–480
for pancreatitis, 523–524
for peptic ulcers, 492, 493*b*
for renal disease
acute failure, 625–627
end-stage, 608*t*, 609*b*, 613–621, 616*t*–617*t*
kidney stones, 630
kidney transplantation, 621–623, 621*t*
nephrotic syndrome, 627–628
pre-end stage, 607–613, 609*b*, 611*b*
for short-bowel syndrome, 516–517, 517*b*
for steatorrhea, 494–495, 495*t*, 496*b*–498*b*
Nuts. *See also* Meat, poultry, fish, dry beans, eggs, and nuts group
in Healthy Eating Index, 192*t*
in Healthy Eating Pyramid, 194, 193*f*

O

Obesity
in African Americans, 251
assessment of, in children, 336
body mass index in, 378*t*–379*t*
in children, 335–337
complications of, 377, 382–383
cultural views of, 247
definition of, 377
diabetes mellitus in, 571
etiology of, 378–381, 382*f*
extreme, 379*t*
fiber for, 32
genetic factors in, 380
in high-fat diets, 81
hypertension in, 551
in metabolic syndrome, 534, 534*t*
in Mexican Americans, 254
morbid, surgery for, 399–400, 400*f*, 401*f*
nursing process for, 401–406
in older adults, 361
osteoarthritis in, 358
vs. overweight, 377
in pregnancy, 274
prevalence of, 381–382
renal disease in, calorie calculation for, 614
sugar consumption and, 35
treatment of. *See also* Weight management
behavior therapy in, 396, 397*b*–398*b*
benefits of, 383
goals of, 384
motivation for, 383–384
nutritional therapy in, 384–395, 386*b*, 389*t*–391*t*
pharmacotherapy in, 396, 398–399, 399*t*
physical activity in, 395–396
surgical, 399–400, 400*f*, 401*f*
Occasional foods, 246
Octreotide, food interactions with, 690*t*
Oils. *See also* Fat (dietary); Fat(s), oils, and sweets group
for children, 330, 331*f*
food intake patterns and, 189*t*
in Healthy Eating Pyramid, 193, 193*f*, 195
Olestra fat replacer, 88
Oliguric phase, of acute renal failure, 625
Omega-3 fatty acids
for coronary heart disease prevention, 540
for end-stage renal disease, 631
in fish oils, 69–70
immune system effects of, 473
recommendations for, 85
sources of, 59
in unsaturated fats, 69
in vegetarian diets, 59
Omega-6 fatty acids, 70
for coronary heart disease prevention, 540
excess of, immune system effects of, 473
Omeprazole (Prilosec), for gastritis, 493
Ondansetron, food interactions with, 692*t*
Open feeding, in enteral nutrition, 438
Oral hygiene, for sore mouth, 647
Oral hypoglycemic agents, 580–581, 689*t*–690*t*
Oral nutrition
for cancer, 648
for chronic obstructive pulmonary disease, 469
for critical illness, 463, 464*b*
after surgery, 465
Oral phase, of swallowing, 489
Oral preparatory phase, of swallowing, 488–489
Organically grown foods, 229–230
Orlistat (Zenical), for weight loss, 399*t*
Ornish diet, 391*t*, 541
Orthoclone, after renal transplantation, 622
Osmolality, of enteral formulas, 430*t*, 433
Osteoarthritis, in older adults, 358–359

Osteomalacia, in vitamin D deficiency, 104, 327
Osteoporosis
adolescent diet and, 340
in anorexia nervosa, 407
in older adults, 359–360
in vitamin D deficiency, 104
Ostomy, for enteral nutrition, 434, 435*t*
Overfeeding
in critical illness, 461
with infant formulas, 316
in parenteral nutrition, 450
in toddlers, 321–322
Overweight
body mass index in, 378*t*–379*t*
in children, 335–336
definition of, 377
etiology of, 378–381, 382*f*
extreme. *See* Obesity
vs. obesity, 377
prevalence of, 381–382
weight loss in. *See* Weight management
Oxalates
in kidney stones, 629
sources of, 629, 629*b*
Oxidation
definition of, 97
in energy metabolism, 162
Oxidative phosphorylation (electron transport chain), 158
Oxygen, transport of, water in, 128

P

P. *See* Phosphorus
Paclitaxel, food interactions with, 693*t*
Pain, in cancer, nutritional effects of, 635
Palate, cleft, nutrition in, 323*b*
Palliative nutrition therapy, for cancer, 650
Pancreas, cancer of
nutritional effects of, 636*t*
surgical complications in, 639*t*
Pancreatic lipase, in fat digestion, 74, 75*f*
Pancreatitis, 523–524
Pantothenic acid
deficiency of, 109*t*
functions of, 109*t*, 114
recommendations for
Adequate Intake, 668*t*
in breast-feeding, 281*t*, 668*t*
in children, 668*t*
Dietary Reference Intakes, 668*t*
in infants, 668*t*
in pregnancy, 281*t*, 668*t*
sources of, 109*t*, 114
toxicity of, 109*t*
Parathyroid hormone, in calcium regulation, 138
Parenteral nutrition, 447–453
for acute renal failure, 627
administration of, 451–452
for anorexia nervosa, 411
for burns, 468
for cancer, 648–649, 649*t*
central. *See* Total parenteral nutrition
complications of, 449*b*
for critical illness, 463–464
cyclic, 452
definition of, 428
description of, 447
for diarrhea, 481
vs. enteral nutrition, 429
formulas for, composition of, 450–451
for HIV infection/AIDS, 658
indications for, 448
for liver disease, 522
medication administration with, 451
monitoring of, 452–453
nursing management in, 452–453
peripheral, 447–448
teaching on, 453
Pareve foods, 260, 547*b*
Paroxetine, food interactions with, 689*t*
Pasta. *See* Bread, cereal, rice and pasta group
Pasteurization, cold (irradiation), 237, 237*f*
Patency, tube, in enteral nutrition, 438, 443*b*
Pellagra, in vitamin B_3 deficiency, 108*t*, 111
Pelvic cancer, radiation therapy complications in, 640*t*
Penicillin, food interactions with, 688*t*
Pepsin, in protein digestion, 48–49, 48*f*
Peptic ulcers, nutrition therapy for, 492, 493*b*
Percent Daily Value
on labels, 212*f*, 213
for vitamin supplements, 121–122
Percutaneous endoscopic gastrostomy, for enteral nutrition, 436
Perfringens food poisoning, 233*t*
Peripheral foods, 246
Peripheral parenteral nutrition, 447–448
Peritoneal dialysis, nutrient recommendations for, 608*t*
Pernicious anemia, in vitamin B_{12} deficiency, 114
Personal control, as cultural value, 248
Pesticides, for organic farming, 229–230
Pharyngeal phase, of swallowing, 489
Phenelzine, food interactions with, 689*t*
Phenobarbital, food interactions with, 688*t*
Phenolic acids, sources and effects of, 119*t*
Phentermine (Ionamin, Fastin, Adipex), for weight loss, 399
Phenylketonuria
in infants, 324*b*–325*b*
in pregnancy, 274–275
Phenylpropanolamine (Dexatrim, Accutrim), for weight loss, 399
Phenytoin, food interactions with, 688*t*
Phospholipids, 72
Phosphorus
body distribution of, 141
in bread, cereal, rice and pasta group, 616*t*
in breast milk, 315*t*
deficiency of, 139*t*
in fats, oils, and sweets group, 617*t*
in fruit group, 616*t*

Phosphorus (*continued*)
functions of, 132, 139*t*, 141
in infant formula, 315*t*
in meat, poultry, fish, dry beans, eggs, and nuts group, 617*t*
in milk, yogurt, and cheese group, 616*t*
recommendations for, 139*t*
Adequate Intake, 671*t*
in breast-feeding, 671*t*
in children, 671*t*
Dietary Reference Intakes, 671*t*
in infants, 671*t*
in pregnancy, 671*t*
Recommended Dietary Allowance, 671*t*
in renal disease, 608*t*, 612, 615, 616*t*–617*t*
restriction of, in renal disease, 612, 615, 616*t*–617*t*
sources of, 139*t*, 141, 612, 616*t*–617*t*
toxicity of, 139*t*
in vegetable group, 616*t*
Phosphorylation, oxidative (electron transport chain), 158
Phylloquinone, 106
Physical activity. *See* Exercise (physical activity)
Phytic acid, sources and effects of, 119*t*
Phytochemicals, 116–121, 119*t*
lack of, in low-carbohydrate diets, 391, 393–394
Pica, 147, 289
Pioglitazone (Actos), for diabetes mellitus, 581, 690*t*
Piperacillin/tazobactam, food interactions with, 688*t*
Pizza restaurants, healthy choices from, 266*b*
Planning, in nutritional care process, 10–12
Plaques, atherosclerotic, 531, 531*f*, 532*f*
Poisoning, food. *See* Food poisoning; Foodborne illness
Polypeptides, formation of, in protein digestion, 48–49, 48*f*
Polyphenols, sources and effects of, 119*t*
Polysaccharides, 21–22. *See also specific type, e.g.,* Fiber; Starch
Polyunsaturated fat, 68, 68*t*, 69
in breast milk, 297
in coronary heart disease prevention, 540
in diabetes mellitus, 574*t*, 577
Portion sizes
for children, 330
common objects resembling, 190, 265*b*
containing 100 calories, 380
control of, in restaurants, 265*b*
in exchange list, 583
of fat, 496*b*
on labels, 212–213, 212*f*
for meat, 82
in MyPyramid, 187, 190
official, vs. restaurant portions, 381
recommended vs. usual, 190
in restaurant meals, vs. official portion sizes, 381
weight management and, 388
Position
after eating, in gastroesophageal reflux disease, 492
for eating, in dysphagia, 495
Positive nitrogen balance, definition of, 50, 51*b*
Potassium
body distribution of, 137
deficiency of, 135*t*, 137
corticosteroid-induced, 505
in malabsorption, 495*t*
in *Dietary Guidelines for Americans 2005*, 185*b*
excess of, 137
in fruit juices and drinks, 320*f*
fruit low in, 619
functions of, 132, 135*t*
recommendations for, 135*t*, 137
in acute renal failure, 626–627
Adequate Intake of, 137
in diarrhea, 481
in liver transplant candidates, 522
in renal disease, 608*t*, 615
sources of, 135*t*, 481, 562, 563*t*
supplements of
for coronary heart disease prevention, 545
toxicity of, 552
toxicity of, 135*t*, 137, 552
vegetables low in, 615
Poultry. *See* Meat, poultry, fish, dry beans, eggs, and nuts group
Prandin (repaglinide), for diabetes mellitus, 580
Pravastatin, for cholesterol lowering, 537*t*
Prazosin, food interactions with, 692*t*
Prealbumin, in nutritional assessment, 10, 10*t*
Preconception nutrition, 272–273
Precose (acarbose), for diabetes mellitus, 580, 689*t*
Prednisone
for COPD, 470
after renal transplantation, 622
Preeclampsia, pregnancy-induced, 291
Pre-end stage renal disease, 607–613
definition of, 607
nutrition therapy for
calcium in, 608*t*
calories in, 608*t*, 610–611, 611*b*
fluid in, 608*t*
glucose control with, 612
hypertension control with, 612
menus for, 609*b*
minerals in, 608*t*
phosphorus in, 608*t*, 612
potassium in, 608*t*
protein in, 607, 608*t*, 609*b*, 610
recommendations for, 612–613
sodium in, 608*t*
vitamins in, 608*t*
Preformed vitamin A, 101–102
Pregnancy, 271–296
in adolescents, 295–296, 340
alcohol us in, 283
artificial sweeteners in, 41, 283–284
blood volume in, 276
body mass index in, 274
caffeine in, 282–283
constipation in, 287–288
cravings in, 294, 294*b*
diabetes mellitus in, 290–291, 595, 596*b*

foodborne illness avoidance in, 284
gastrointestinal function in, 275
heartburn in, 288
herbal supplements in, 225, 286–287
hypertension in, 291
ideal weight in, 274
meal frequency in, 282
metabolism in, 275
nausea and vomiting in, 287
nursing process applied to, 306–308
nutrient recommendations in, 277–281, 279*t*
Adequate Intake, 668*t*–669*t*, 671*t*, 673*t*
in adolescents, 295–296
assessment of, 291–293, 292*b*
calcium, 280, 281*t*
calories, 278–279, 279*t*
choline, 281*t*
counseling on, 293–295, 294*b*
density, 282
Dietary Reference Intakes, 668*t*–669*t*, 671*t*, 673*t*
fluid, 282
folate, 113, 118, 272–273, 281*t*, 286
iron, 279*t*, 280–281, 285–286
macronutrients, 673*t*
magnesium, 279*t*
minerals, 279*t*, 284–286
MyPyramid in, 281, 281*t*
myths about, 294*b*
protein, 55, 279–280, 279*t*, 280*b*
Recommended Dietary Allowance, 668*t*–669*t*, 671*t*, 673*t*
salt, 282
selenium, 279*t*
in vegetarian diet, 280–281, 285–286
vitamins, 279*t*, 280, 284–286, 668*t*–669*t*
zinc, 279*t*
nutritional assessment in, 291–293, 292*b*
nutrition before, 272–273
obesity in, 274
phenylketonuria in, 274–275
physiologic changes in, 275–277, 276*b*, 279*t*
pica in, 289
vegetarian diets in, 285–286
weight gain in
in adolescents, 295–296
counseling on, 278, 293
distribution of, 276, 276*b*
excessive, 289
inadequate, 276–277, 288–289
pattern of, 277
recommendations for, 276–277
statistics on, 278
Premature infants
formulas for, 315
vitamin E deficiency in, 106
Pressure ulcers
in long-term care, 362
in stress, 459
Prilosec (omeprazole), for gastritis, 493
Primary prevention, definition of, 536
Priorities, in nutritional care process, 11
Pritikin diet program, 541
Procrit (epoetin alfa), for renal disease, 618
Promote nutritional supplement, 644
Protease inhibitors, for HIV infection/AIDS, 661*t*
Protein (body). *See also* Amino acids
catabolism of, in stress, 458–459
degradation of, nitrogen balance in, 50, 51*b*
as energy source, 52
fat formation from, 52
functions of, 46
in metabolic pool, 49
nitrogen balance and, 50, 51*b*
sparing of
glucose in, 25, 52
in pregnancy, 278–279
structures of, 47–48
synthesis of, 49–51, 51*b*
turnover of, 51
Protein (dietary). *See also* Amino acids
absorption of, 49
in bread, cereal, rice and pasta group, 616*t*
in breast milk, 297, 315*t*
complementary, 53–54
complete, 52–54
deficiency of, 56, 495*t*
definition of, 46
density of, increasing, 464*b*, 643–644, 644*b*
digestibility of, 54
digestion of, 48–49, 48*f*
in enteral nutrition, 429–432, 430*t*
as ergogenic acid, 170*t*
in fats, oils, and sweets group, 617*t*
in fruit group, 616*t*
in fruit juices and drinks, 317*f*
in health promotion, 56–62, 57*b*, 59*f*
high-quality, 54, 613
incomplete, 53–54
in infant formula, 315*t*
kidney stones due to, 628
in meat, poultry, fish, dry beans, eggs, and nuts group, 30, 617*t*
metabolism of, 49–52
in milk, yogurt, and cheese group, 616*t*
in modular supplements, 428
in MyPyramid groups, 53*f*
in nutritional supplements
clear, 425
commercially prepared, 427
milk-based, 427
in parenteral nutrition formulas, 450
recommendations for, 54–56, 55*b*
Acceptable Macronutrient Distribution Range, 182, 674*t*
in acute renal failure, 626
Adequate Intake, 673*t*
in body builders, 61–62
in breast-feeding, 279*t*, 673*t*
in burns, 462–463, 467
in cancer, 643–644, 644*b*
in children, 673*t*

Protein (dietary), recommendations for (*continued*)
in chronic obstructive pulmonary disease, 469
in coronary heart disease prevention, 542
in critical illness, 462–463
in cystic fibrosis, 326*b*
in diabetes mellitus, 574*t*, 576
Dietary Reference Intake, 673*t*
in healing, 466*t*
in HIV infection/AIDS, 657
in infants, 673*t*
in inflammatory bowel disease, 499*b*
in kidney transplantation, 621*t*, 622
in liver disease, 520
in liver transplant candidates, 522
in nephrotic syndrome, 627–628
in older adults, 352–353
in phenylketonuria, 274–275
in pregnancy, 55, 279–280, 279*t*, 280*b*, 673*t*
Recommended Dietary Allowance, 673*t*
in renal disease, 607, 608*t*, 609*b*, 610, 613, 616*t*–617*t*, 626
in sepsis, 462–463
in steatorrhea, 494
in stress, 462–463
in surgical patients, 462–463
restriction of, 55
in liver disease, 520
in renal disease, 607, 608*t*, 609*b*, 610, 613, 616*t*–617*t*
sources of, 613, 616*t*–617*t*
soy products, 57, 57*b*
supplements for, 55
in vegetable group, 616*t*
in vegetarian diets, 56–57, 57*b*, 59*f*, 280*b*
in weight loss diet, 50
in weight management diet, 390–394, 391*t*
Protein isolates, for enteral nutrition, 429
Protestantism, food practices in, 259
Provitamin(s), 96
Provitamin A, sources of, 101
Psychiatric disorders, eating disorders as, 406–412
Psychologic issues, in weight change, 381
Pulmonary aspiration, in enteral nutrition, 438
Pureed diet, for dysphagia, 490*t*
Pure vegetarianism (vegans), 56, 58, 114, 285–286
Purging, in bulimia nervosa, 407
Purine, sources of, 630
Purity concept, in Hindu food practices, 260
Pyloric sphincter, alterations of, dumping syndrome in, 495, 500, 502
Pyloric stenosis, 324*b*
Pyridoxal/pyridoxine/pyridoxamine. *See* Vitamin B_6 (pyridoxine, pyridoxal, pyridoxamine)
Pyruvate
in glucose catabolism, 158
metabolism of, 162

Q

Qualified health claims, on labels, 215, 216*b*
Quorn imitation meat, 62

R

Radiation therapy
nutritional effects of, 640, 640*t*
nutrition therapy for, 645–648
Radura symbol, for irradiation, 237, 237*f*
Rancidity, of unsaturated fats, 69
Ranitidine (Zantac), for gastritis, 493
RDA. *See* Recommended Dietary Allowance (RDA)
RDI (Reference Daily Intake), on labels, 212*f*, 213
Recommended Dietary Allowance (RDA). *See also specific nutrients*
in breast-feeding, 668*t*–669*t*, 671*t*, 673*t*
for carbohydrates, 31, 31*t*
for children, 668*t*–669*t*, 671*t*, 673*t*
description of, 181–182, 181*f*
for fat, 673*t*
for fiber, 31, 31*t*, 33–34
for infants, 668*t*–669*t*, 671*t*, 673*t*
for iron, 328, 329*f*
for minerals, 671*t*
in pregnancy, 668*t*–669*t*, 671*t*, 673*t*
for proteins, 54–56, 55*b*
replacement of, 180
for vitamins, 668*t*–669*t*
"Reduced," definition of, in nutrient claims, 215*b*
Red yeast, for coronary heart disease prevention, 543*b*
REE. *See* Resting energy expenditure
Refeeding syndrome
in anorexia nervosa, 410
in critical illness, 461
in parenteral nutrition, 450
Reference Daily Intake (RDI), on labels, 212*f*, 213
Refined grains and flours, definition of, 28
Reflux, gastroesophageal, nutrition therapy for, 491–492
Regional enteritis (Crohn's disease)
nursing process for, 506–507
nutrition therapy for, 504–505
pathophysiology of, 504
Regional food practices, 264
Religions, food practices related to
Buddhism, 261
Christianity, 259
Hinduism, 260–261
Islam, 260
Judaism, 259–260
Sikhism, 261
Renal disorders, 605–633
acute failure, 625–627
kidney function and, 606
nursing process for, 623–625
nutrition therapy for, 606–607, 608*t*
acute failure, 625–627
end-stage, 613–621, 616*t*–617*t*
goals of, 606–607
kidney stones, 630
nephrotic syndrome, 627–628
pre-end stage, 607–613, 609*b*, 611*b*
in transplantation, 621–623, 621*t*
pathophysiology of, 606
secondary, 606
in vitamin D toxicity, 100*t*

Renin, function of, 606
Repaglinide, food interactions with, 690*t*
Rescriptor (delavirdine), for HIV infection/AIDS, 661*t*
Residue. *See also* Fiber
in enteral formulas, 430*t*, 433–434
of gastric contents, after enteral feedings, 436
Respiratory quotient, 469
Restaurant meals
in diabetes mellitus, 592*b*
ethnic food in, 261, 266*b*–267*b*
healthy choices in, 264, 265*b*–267*b*
obesity and, 380–381
portion sizes in, 82
vs. official portion sizes, 381
sodium in, 556*b*
statistics on, 264
Resting energy expenditure, 163
in HIV infection/AIDS, 655
in stress, 458
Restrictive diets, in long-term care, 364–365
Retinaldehyde, 101
Retinoic acid, 101
Retinol, 99*t*, 101, 103
Retinol equivalents, 102
Retrovir (zidovudine), for HIV infection/AIDS, 661*t*, 693*t*
Riboflavin. *See* Vitamin B_2 (riboflavin)
Rice. *See* Bread, cereal, rice and pasta group
Rickets, in vitamin D deficiency, 99*t*–100*t*, 104, 327
Ritonavir (Novir, RTV), for HIV infection/AIDS, 661*t*, 693*t*
RNA, carbohydrates in, 26
Rocaltrol (calcitriol), for renal disease, 618
Roman Catholicism, food practices in, 259
Rosiglitazone (Avandia), for diabetes mellitus, 581, 690*t*
Roux-en Y procedure, for obesity, 400, 401*f*
RTV (ritonavir), for HIV infection/AIDS, 661*t*, 693*t*

S

S. *See* Sulfur
Saccharin, 39*t*, 41
Safety
of artificial sweeteners, 40–41
in *Dietary Guidelines for Americans 2005*, 186*b*
foodborne illness prevention and, 230, 231*t*–233*t*, 234, 235*f*
of supplements, 118, 219, 222
of vitamin supplements, 118
St. John's wort, 221*t*–222*t*
Salad bars, healthy choices from, 266*b*
Saliva, thick, in cancer, 647–648
Salmonellosis, 231*t*
Salt
chloride in, 138
in processed foods, 134, 136*f*
recommendations for, in pregnancy, 282
sensitivity to, 136
sources of, 135*t*
substitutes for, potassium in, 562
Sandimmune (cyclosporine), after renal transplantation, 622
Saquinavir (Fortovase, Invirase), for HIV infection/AIDS, 661*t*, 693*t*
Satiety, 385
Saturated ("bad") fat, 67–68, 68*t*, 70–72, 71*f*
cholesterol levels and, 538, 540
definition of, 69
in diabetes mellitus, 574*t*, 577
reduction of, 84–85, 85*t*
in vegetarian diets, 61
Saw palmetto, 221*t*
Scurvy, 110*t*, 114–115
Seasonings, protein-free, 611*b*
Secondary foods, 246
Secondary prevention, definition of, 536
Seeds, sources of, 518
Selegiline, food interactions with, 693*t*
Selenium, 148–149
deficiency of, 144*t*, 149
functions of, 144*t*, 148
recommendations for, 144*t*
Adequate Intake, 671*t*
in breast-feeding, 279*t*, 671*t*
in children, 671*t*
Dietary Reference Intakes, 671*t*
in infants, 671*t*
in pregnancy, 279*t*, 671*t*
Recommended Dietary Allowance, 671*t*
sources of, 144*t*
toxicity of, 144*t*
Sensible water loss, 129, 129*t*
Sepsis
multiple organ failure in, 460
in parenteral nutrition, 449*b*
Sertraline, food interactions with, 689*t*
Serving sizes. *See* Portion sizes
Set point theory of weight control, 380
Seventh-Day Adventists, food practices of, 259
Shigellosis, 232*t*
Short-bowel syndrome
nutrition therapy for, 516–517, 517*b*
pathophysiology of, 516
Sibutramine (Meridia), for weight loss, 399*t*
Sikhism, food practices in, 261
Silicon, 150
Simple carbohydrates, 20–22, 23*f*, 24, 29. *See also specific types, e.g.,* Glucose
Simplesse fat replacer, 88
Simvastatin, for cholesterol lowering, 537*t*, 696*t*
Skin
breakdown of, in critical illness, 459
disorders of, in vitamin A deficiency, 99*t*
Small intestine
cancer of, 636*t*
fat digestion in, 74, 75*f*
protein digestion in, 48*f*, 49
Smoking
cessation of, for hypertension, 556
as coronary heart disease risk factor, 533
vitamin C intake in, 115

Snacks
for children, 332, 333, 334*f*
in nutritional assessment, 6
obesity and, 380–381
for toddlers, 322
Social factors
in nutritional assessment, 9
in weight gain, 381
Social isolation, in older adults, 361–362
Social support, for weight management, 383, 396
Sodas. *See* Soft drinks
Sodium, 134–136
in bread, cereal, rice and pasta group, 555, 555*b*, 560*b*
in breast milk, 298, 315*t*
deficiency of, 135*t*
in *Dietary Guidelines for Americans 2005,* 185*b*
in fats, oils, and sweets group, 560*b*
in fruit group, 560*b*
functions of, 132, 134–135, 135*t*
in grains, 560*b*
in infant formula, 315*t*
kidney stones due to, 628
on labels, 136, 137*b*
in meat, poultry, fish, dry beans, eggs, and nuts group, 560*b*
in milk, yogurt, and cheese group, 560*b*
in processed foods, 134, 136*f*
recommendations for, 134–136, 135*t*
Adequate Intake, 135–136
in cystic fibrosis, 326*b*
Daily Value, 136
in end-stage renal disease, 608*t*, 615
in hypertension, 365
in kidney transplantation, 621*t*, 622–623
in nephrotic syndrome, 627–628
in older adults, 357
in pre-end stage renal disease, 608*t*
in pregnancy, 282
after renal transplantation, 622–623
regulation of, 134–135
in restaurant meals, 556*b*
restriction of
in congestive heart failure, 558, 559*b*–561*b*, 562
for coronary heart disease prevention, 545
in DASH diet, 545, 551–552, 553*t*–554*t*, 555*b*, 556*b*, 557*t*–558*t*
in hypertension, 545, 551–552, 553*t*–554*t*, 555*b*, 556*b*, 557*t*–558*t*
in liver disease, 520, 521
in salt, 134
sensitivity to, 136
sources of, 134, 135*t*, 555, 555*b*, 560*b*
toxicity of, 135*t*
in vegetable group, 560*b*
Soft (bland, low fiber) diet, 420, 423*t*–424*t*, 490*t*
Soft drinks
calories in, 130
children consuming, 334–335
consumption of, by adolescents, 338
disadvantages of, 130
sugar content of, 37
Solid food, introduction of, to infants, 316–319, 318*b*
Soluble fiber, definition of, 21–22
Solvent, water as, 128
Sorbitol, as sugar alternative, 38, 576
Sore mouth, in cancer, 647
Sotalol, food interactions with, 687*t*
Soul food, 250, 251*f*
Soy products
as complete proteins, 52–53
for coronary heart disease prevention, 544
as functional foods, 228*t*
glossary of, 57*b*
in infant formulas, 315
isoflavones, 221*t*
for menopausal symptoms, 346*b*
oil, 89
Spironolactone, food interactions with, 695*t*
Splenda (sucralose), 39*t*
Spoonful. *See* Aspartame
Sprue, nontropical (celiac disease), nutrition therapy for, 508, 509*b*–513*b*, 514
Standard formulas, for enteral nutrition, 429–430
Standardization, of dietary supplements, 224
Staphylococcus aureus, in food poisoning, 232*t*
Starch, 21
digestion of, 22, 23*f*
sources of, 27–28, 28*f*
in vegetable group, 29
Starvation, 160–161
in anorexia nervosa, 406–407
basal metabolic rate and, 164
for weight management, 386*b*
Stavudine (Zerit, d4T), for HIV infection/AIDS, 661*t*, 693*t*
Steatorrhea, 494–495, 495*t*, 496*b*–498*b*
Sterols, 72. *See also* Cholesterol
in margarines, for coronary heart disease prevention, 544
Stimulus control, in weight management, 396
Stomach
cancer of
nutritional effects of, 636*t*
surgical complications in, 639*t*
dumping syndrome and, 495, 500, 501*b*, 502
gastric acid in
in protein digestion, 48–49, 48*f*
reflux of, 491–492
secretion of, stimulation of, 493*b*
inflammation of, nutrition therapy for, 493–494
protein digestion in, 48–49, 48*f*
residuals in, in enteral nutrition, 436
rupture of, in enteral nutrition, 442*b*
surgery on, for obesity, 399–400, 400*f*, 401*f*
Stomatitis, in cancer, 647
Stones
gallbladder, 524–525
kidney, 629*b*
Strength training, 168, 170
Stress
adaptation to, 458
basal metabolic rate in, 164

enteral formulas for, 473
management of, in weight management, 396
metabolic changes in, 458–464
in burns, 465, 467–468
complications of, 459–460
in COPD, 468–470
hormonal, 458, 459*t*
nursing process for, 471–473
nutrition therapy for, 460–464, 461*b*, 464*b*
protein catabolism, 458–459
in surgery, 465, 466*t*–467*t*
response to, 458
vitamins for, 123
Stretching exercises, 168, 170
Structural function, of minerals, 132
Structure/function claims, on labels, 214–215, 217*b*
Struvite kidney stones, 628
Subclinical nutrient deficiencies, in older adults, 353
Substance abuse, in eating disorders, 408
Subway meals, in weight loss diet, 264
Sucralose, 39*t*
Sucrose, 20–21
Sugar(s), 20–21, 35–41. *See also* Fat(s), oils, and sweets group; *specific sugars, e.g.,* Glucose
absorption of, 22
alternatives to, 37–41
approved list of, 39*t*
in chewing gum, 36
in diabetes mellitus, 40
in pregnancy, 283–284
safety of, 40–41
types of, 37–38
in weight management, 40
dental caries due to, 36
digestion of, 22, 23*f*
disaccharides, 20–21, 23*f*
drawbacks of, 36
as empty-calorie food, 36
energy from, 25–26
on food labels, 37, 214, 238
functions of, 34–35
glycemic index of, 24, 24*t*, 196, 572–573, 575, 595–597
health problems attributed to, 36
metabolism of, 22, 24–25, 24*t*
monosaccharides, 20, 22, 23*f*, 24–25. *See also* Fructose; Glucose
recommendations for, 36–37
sources of, 29, 30, 36–37, 38*b*
Sugar alcohols
calories in, 412–413
in chewing gum, 36
in diabetes mellitus, 576
as sugar alternatives, 37–38
Sulfasalazine, nutritional effects of, 505
Sulfonylureas, for diabetes mellitus, 580
Sulforaphane, sources and effects of, 119*t*
Sulfur
deficiency of, 139*t*
functions of, 132, 139*t*, 142
recommendations for, 139*t*
sources of, 139*t*, 142–143
toxicity of, 139*t*
Sunette (Acesulfame K), 39*t*, 41
Sunlight, vitamin D synthesis and, 103, 104, 327
Supplement(s), 218–226. *See also* Herbal supplements; Mineral supplements; Nutrition supplements; Vitamin supplements; *specific ingredients*
advice on, 225–226
for anorexia, 478
for children, 225
commercial, for older adults, 362
dosages of, 224
vs. drugs, 219, 222–224, 223*t*
gastrointestinal distress due to, 479*b*
health claims of, 224
information on, 225–226
labels for, 218*f*, 225
number of, 219
in pregnancy, 225
purpose of, 218
quality regulation of, 222–223
reasons for using, 219
safety of, 118, 219, 222
self-prescription of, 224
side effects of, 225–226
standardization of, 224
warnings on, 224
Supplement Facts label, for vitamins, 121–122
Surgery
for cancer, nutritional effects of, 638
gallbladder, 525
nutrition therapy for, 465, 466*t*–467*t*
for obesity, 399–400, 400*f*, 401*f*
Sustiva (efavirenz), for HIV infection/AIDS, 661*t*
Swallowing
difficulty with. *See* Dysphagia
physiology of, 488–489
Sweat, sodium lost in, 135–136
Sweet 10. *See* Saccharin
Sweet(s). *See* Fat(s), oils, and sweets group; Sugar
Sweeteners
artificial, 38, 39*t*, 40–41
in diabetes mellitus, 576
in pregnancy, 283–284
in diabetes mellitus, 574*t*, 575–576
equivalent to sugar, 214
Sweet 'n Low. *See* Saccharin
Sweet One (Acesulfame K), 39*t*, 41
"Sweet tooth," in diabetes mellitus, 601
Sweet Twin (saccharin), 39*t*
Syndrome X. *See* Metabolic syndrome

T

Tagamet (cimetidine), for gastritis, 493
Take Control margarine, for coronary heart disease prevention, 544
Target heart rate, in exercise, 168
Taste
changes of, in cancer, nutrition therapy for, 646–647
of enteral nutrition formulas, 453

3TC (lamivudine), for HIV infection/AIDS, 661*t*, 693*t*
Tea, for coronary heart disease prevention, 543*b*
Teaching, client. *See* Nutrition counseling; Nutrition education
Teeth, caries in. *See* Caries, dental
Temperature, environmental, basal metabolic rate and, 164
Temperature regulation
 fat in, 74
 water in, 128
Tenofovir (Viread), for HIV infection/AIDS, 661*t*
Tenuate (diethylpropion), for weight loss, 399
Terminal illness, artificial nutrition in, ethical issues in, 429
Testosterone, for appetite stimulation, in HIV infection/AIDS, 659*t*
Tetrahydrofolate, 112
Theophylline
 for COPD, 470
 food interactions with, 695*t*
Therapeutic Lifestyle Change Diet, 538–542, 538*t*, 539*f*
 vs. DASH diet, 552, 553*t*–554*t*
Thermic effect, of food, 166
Thermoregulation
 fat in, 74
 water in, 128
Thiamin. *See* Vitamin B_1 (thiamin)
Thiazolidinediones, for diabetes mellitus, 580–581
Thioridazine, food interactions with, 693*t*
Thirst, relief for, 617
Thyroid hormones, basal metabolic rate and, 164
Thyroxine, basal metabolic rate and, 164
Thyroxine-binding protein (prealbumin), in nutritional assessment, 9–10, 10*t*
Ticlopidine, food interactions with, 688*t*
Tin, 150
Tocopherols. *See* Vitamin E (tocopherols)
Toddlers, nutrition for, 321–322, 322*b*–323*b*, 340–343
Tolerable Upper Intake Level (UL), 181*f*, 182
Total carbohydrates, in diabetes mellitus, 573, 575
Total diet approach, 82–83
Total fat
 in coronary heart disease, 541
 in diabetes mellitus, 577–578
 recommendations for, 82–83, 83*b*–84*b*, 85*t*
Total fiber, definition of, 22
Total Lifestyle Change Diet, for nephrotic syndrome, 628
Total parenteral nutrition
 administration of, 451–452
 for burns, 468
 for cancer, 648–649, 649*t*
 central, 448
 complications of, 447–448, 449*b*
 cyclic, 452
 description of, 447
 for diarrhea, 481
 formulas for, composition of, 450–451
 for HIV infection/AIDS, 658
 indications for, 447
 for liver disease, 522
 medication administration with, 451
 monitoring of, 452–453
 nursing management in, 452–453
 for short-bowel syndrome, 516
 teaching about, 453
TPN. *See* Total parenteral nutrition
Trace minerals. *See* Mineral(s), trace
Trans fats, 71–72, 71*f*
 coronary heart disease and, 540–541
 diabetes mellitus and, 574*t*, 577
 on labels, 212*f*
 recommendations for, 84–85, 85*t*
 sources of, 394, 577
Transnasal tube feeding, 434, 435*t*
Transplantation
 bone marrow, 641, 641*b*
 kidney, 621–623, 621*t*
 liver, 522–523, 522*b*
Transport proteins, 46
Tretinoin, as drug, 98
Tricarboxylic acid cycle, 157–158
Triglycerides
 absorption of, 74–75
 in body fat. *See* Fat (body)
 carbon chain length of, 67
 definition of, 67
 digestion of, 74, 75*f*
 elevated
  as coronary heart disease risk factor, 534
  in diabetes mellitus, 578
  in metabolic syndrome, 534, 534*t*
  nursing process for, 548–550
 energy from, 73
 essential fatty acids in, 69
 in health promotion, 86–89, 87*f*
 hydrogenated, 68, 68*t*, 70–71, 83*b*
 in Mediterranean diet, 86–87, 87*f*
 metabolism of, 76
 monounsaturated, 67–68, 68*t*
  in coronary heart disease, 540
  in diabetes mellitus, 574*t*, 578
 in MyPyramid, 75–79, 77*f*
 polyunsaturated, 68, 68*t*, 69
  in breast milk, 297
  for coronary heart disease prevention, 540
  in diabetes mellitus, 574*t*, 577
 recommendations for, 80–86, 81*t*
  omega-3, 85
  saturated, 84–85, 85*t*
  total fat, 82–83, 83*b*–84*b*, 85*t*, 577–578
  trans, 84–85, 85*t*
  unsaturated, 67–70, 68*t*, 84*b*, 85
 replacers for, 87–89
 structure of, 67–68
 trans-. *See* Trans fats
 unsaturated ("good"), 67–70, 68*t*, 84*b*, 85
Triiodothyronine, basal metabolic rate and, 164

Trimethoprim-sulfamethoxazole, food interactions with, 688*t*
Tripeptides, definition of, 49
Trizivir (zidovudine-lamivudine-abacavir), for HIV infection/AIDS, 661*t*
Trypsin, in protein digestion, 48*f*, 49
Tryptophan, vitamin B_3 synthesis from, 111
Tube feeding. *See* Enteral nutrition
Tumors. *See* Cancer
Turnover, protein, 51
Tyramine, monoamine oxidase inhibitors interactions with, 696–697

U

UL (Tolerable Upper Intake Level), description of, 181*f*, 182
Ulcers
  peptic, nutrition therapy for, 492, 493*b*
  pressure
    in long-term care, 362
    in stress, 459
United States Pharmacopeia, label of, on vitamin supplements, 122
Unsaturated ("good") fat, 67–70, 68*t*
  definition of, 69
  recommendations for, 85
  in weight management diet, 394
Uremic syndrome, 606–607
Uric acid kidney stones, 630
Urinary tract infections, cranberry juice and, 631
Urine, water loss in, 129
Usnic acid, 223*t*

V

Valerian, 222*t*
Valproic acid, food interactions with, 688*t*
Values, cultural, 248
Vanadium, 150
Vegans, 56
  calcium intake of, 58
  pregnancy in, 285–286
  vitamin B_{12} deficiency in, 114
  vitamins for, 120
Vegetable group
  calcium in, 140, 616*t*
  for cancer prevention, 197
  carbohydrates in, 29
  for children, 331*f*
  for chronic obstructive pulmonary disease, 470
  in coronary heart disease prevention diet, 539*f*
  in DASH diet, 553*t*
  in *Dietary Guidelines for Americans 2005*, 184*b*–185*b*
  easy chewing, 356
  fat in, 78
  fiber in, 29
  food intake patterns and, 189*t*
  as functional foods, 228*t*
  in Healthy Eating Index, 192*t*
  in Healthy Eating Pyramid, 193*f*, 195
  intake of, 117
  irradiation of, 237
  low-fat preparation of, 198
  low-potassium, 615
  in MyPyramid, 187, 188*f*
  nutrient value of, retaining in storage and processing, 226, 227*b*
  for older adults, 355–356
  organically grown, 229–230
  phosphorus in, 616*t*
  potassium in, 562, 563*t*
  in pregnancy, 281*t*
  protein in, 616*t*
  sodium in, 560*b*
  in Therapeutic Life Change Diet, 553*t*
  in toddler diet, 322
  vitamins in, 116–118, 117*b*, 119*t*
  water in, 130
Vegetarian diets, 56–61
  benefits of, 56–57
  breast-feeding and, 298
  calories for, 60
  complementary proteins in, 53–54
  food pyramid for, 59*f*
  nutrients of concern in, 57–60
  poorly planned, 57
  in pregnancy, 280*b*, 285–286
  protein in, 57, 57*b*, 280*b*
  recommendations for, 60–61
  for Seventh-Day Adventists, 259
  types of, 56
  vitamin B_{12} in, 114, 285–286
  zinc deficiency in, 147–148
Vegetarianism, definition of, 56
Vibrio vulnificus, in foodborne illness, 232*t*
Videx EC (didanosine), for HIV infection/AIDS, 661*t*, 693*t*
Vinblastine, food interactions with, 693*t*
Vinorelbine, food interactions with, 693*t*
Viracept (nelfinavir), for HIV infection/AIDS, 661*t*, 693*t*
Viramune (nevirapine), for HIV infection/AIDS, 661*t*
Viread (tenofovir), for HIV infection/AIDS, 661*t*
Viscosity, of enteral formulas, 434
Vitamin(s), 94–126. *See also specific vitamins*
  active forms of, 96
  adequate intake of, assessment of, 120
  as antioxidants, 97
  in breast milk, 298, 299
  chemistry of, 95–96, 95*f*
  as coenzymes, 97
  destruction of, 96
  as drugs, 98
  essential nature of, 96
  fat-soluble, 98–105, 99*t*–101*t*
  as food additives, 97–98
  food preparation effects on, 96
  in health promotion, 116–123, 117*b*, 119*t*. *See also* Vitamin supplements
  megadoses of, 98

Vitamin(s) (*continued*)
in Mexican American diet, 254
minerals interactions with, 132–133
non-B, 114
in parenteral nutrition, 451
precursors of (provitamins), 96
recommendations for, 101*t*
Adequate Intake, 668*t*–669*t*
in breast-feeding, 279*t*, 300, 668*t*–669*t*
in children, 668*t*–669*t*
in critical illness, 463
Dietary Reference Intakes, 668*t*–669*t*
in end-stage renal disease, 608*t*, 618–619
in HIV infection/AIDS, 658
in infants, 313*f*, 668*t*–669*t*
in older adults, 353, 354*t*, 355*t*
optimal dosage, 95
in pre-end stage renal disease, 608*t*
in pregnancy, 279*t*, 280, 668*t*–669*t*
Recommended Dietary Allowance, 668*t*–669*t*
tolerable upper intake levels, 101*t*
retaining in storage and processing, 226, 227*b*
structures of, 95–96, 95*f*
supplements of. *See* Vitamin supplements
synthesis of, in body, 96
toxicity of, 118
water-soluble, 107–115, 108*t*–110*t*, 115*f*
Vitamin A, 101–103
birth defects due to, 286
deficiency of, 99*t*, 102, 495*t*
as drug, 98
forms of, 96
functions of, 99*t*, 101
preformed, 101–102
recommendations for, 101*t*
Adequate Intake, 668*t*
in breast-feeding, 279*t*, 668*t*
in burns, 467
in children, 668*t*
Dietary Reference Intakes, 668*t*
in healing, 466*t*
in infants, 313*f*, 668*t*
in pregnancy, 279*t*, 668*t*
Recommended Dietary Allowance, 102, 668*t*
tolerable upper intake levels, 101*t*
sources of, 99*t*, 101
storage of, 101–103
supplements of, 102
toxicity of, 99*t*, 102–103, 286
Vitamin B_1 (thiamin)
as coenzyme, 97
deficiency of, 108*t*, 110
food preparation effects on, 96
functions of, 108*t*, 110
recommendations for, 101*t*
Adequate Intake, 668*t*
in breast-feeding, 279*t*, 668*t*
in children, 668*t*
Dietary Reference Intakes, 668*t*
in healing, 466*t*
in infants, 668*t*
in pregnancy, 279*t*, 280, 668*t*
Recommended Dietary Allowance, 668*t*
tolerable upper intake levels, 101*t*
sources of, 108*t*, 110
toxicity of, 108*t*
Vitamin B_2 (riboflavin)
as coenzyme, 97
deficiency of, 108*t*, 111, 353
food preparation effects on, 96
functions of, 108*t*, 110–111
recommendations for, 101*t*
Adequate Intake, 668*t*
in breast-feeding, 279*t*, 668*t*
in children, 668*t*
Dietary Reference Intakes, 668*t*
in healing, 466*t*
in infants, 668*t*
in pregnancy, 279*t*, 280, 668*t*
Recommended Dietary Allowance, 668*t*
tolerable upper intake levels, 101*t*
sources of, 108*t*
toxicity of, 108*t*
Vitamin B_3 (niacin)
for cholesterol lowering, 98
as coenzyme, 97
deficiency of, 108*t*, 111
as drug, 111–112
food interactions and, 696*t*
functions of, 108*t*
recommendations for, 101*t*
Adequate Intake, 668*t*
in breast-feeding, 279*t*, 668*t*
in children, 668*t*
Dietary Reference Intakes, 668*t*
in healing, 466*t*
in infants, 668*t*
in pregnancy, 279*t*, 280, 668*t*
Recommended Dietary Allowance, 668*t*
tolerable upper intake levels, 101*t*
sources of, 108*t*, 111
toxicity of, 108*t*, 111
Vitamin B_6 (pyridoxine, pyridoxal, pyridoxamine)
deficiency of, 108*t*, 354
as drug, 112
functions of, 108*t*–109*t*, 111–112
recommendations for, 101*t*
Adequate Intake, 668*t*
in breast-feeding, 279*t*, 668*t*
in cardiovascular disease prevention, 112
in children, 668*t*
Dietary Reference Intakes, 668*t*
in hyperhomocysteinemia, 535
in infants, 668*t*
in older adults, 354, 354*t*
in pregnancy, 279*t*, 280, 668*t*
Recommended Dietary Allowance, 668*t*
tolerable upper intake levels, 101*t*
sources of, 108*t*, 354
toxicity of, 109*t*, 112

Vitamin B_{12} (cobalamin)
in breast milk, 298
deficiency of, 109*t*, 114, 495*t*
folate interactions with, 113
in fortified foods, 95
functions of, 109*t*, 113
intrinsic factor and, 113–114
recommendations for, 101*t*
Adequate Intake, 668*t*
in breast-feeding, 279*t*, 668*t*
in children, 668*t*
in colostomy, 514–515
Dietary Reference Intakes, 668*t*
in hyperhomocysteinemia, 535–536
in ileostomy, 514–515
in infants, 668*t*
in older adults, 354*t*
in pregnancy, 279*t*, 280, 668*t*
Recommended Dietary Allowance, 668*t*
tolerable upper intake levels, 101*t*
sources of, 60, 109*t*, 113, 285–286
supplements of, 60
toxicity of, 109*t*
in vegetarian diets, 60, 285–286
Vitamin C (ascorbic acid)
as antioxidant, 97
deficiency of, 110*t*, 114–115
as drug, 98, 115
as food additive, 97
food preparation effects of, 96
in fruit juices and drinks, 320*f*
functions of, 110*t*, 114–115
for healing, 98
recommendations for, 101*t*
Adequate Intake, 668*t*
in breast-feeding, 279*t*, 668*t*
in burns, 467
in children, 668*t*
Dietary Reference Intake, 668*t*
in healing, 466*t*
in infants, 313*f*, 668*t*
in pregnancy, 279*t*, 668*t*
Recommended Dietary Allowance, 668*t*
tolerable upper intake levels, 101*t*
sources of, 110*t*, 114–115
toxicity of, 110*t*, 115
in vegetarian diets, 60
Vitamin C, crystal structure of, 115*f*
Vitamin D, 103–105
active form of (1,25-dihydroxycholecalciferol), 606
in breast milk, 298
in calcium regulation, 138
deficiency of, 99*t*–100*t*, 104
in malabsorption, 495*t*
in older adults, 354
osteoarthritis in, 358–359
in fortified foods, 95
functions of, 104, 327
as hormone, 104
recommendations for, 104
Adequate Intake, 327, 668*t*
in breast-feeding, 279*t*, 668*t*
in children, 327, 668*t*
Dietary Reference Intakes, 668*t*
in infants, 313*f*, 668*t*
in older adults, 354, 354*t*
in pregnancy, 279*t*, 668*t*
in weight management, 395
sources of, 58–59, 99*t*–100*t*, 103–104, 354
supplements of
in breast-feeding, 300
for end-stage renal disease, 618
for liver transplant candidates, 523
for older adults, 359
in pregnancy, 286
synthesis of, 103–104
toxicity of, 100*t*, 104–105
in vegetarian diets, 58–59
Vitamin E (tocopherols), 105–106
as antioxidant, 97
deficiency of, 100*t*, 106, 321
as drug, 105–106
as food additive, 98
functions of, 100*t*, 105
recommendations for, 101*t*, 106
Adequate Intake, 668*t*
in breast-feeding, 279*t*, 668*t*
in children, 668*t*
in coronary heart disease prevention, 544
Dietary Reference Intakes, 668*t*
in infants, 313*f*, 668*t*
in menopausal symptoms, 346*b*
in pregnancy, 279*t*, 668*t*
tolerable upper intake levels, 101*t*
sources of, 100*t*, 106
toxicity of, 100*t*, 106
Vitamin K, 106–107
deficiency of, 100*t*, 107, 495*t*
functions of, 100*t*, 107
recommendations for
Adequate Intake, 668*t*
in breast-feeding, 279*t*, 668*t*
in children, 668*t*
Dietary Reference Intakes, 668*t*
in healing, 467*t*
in infants, 668*t*
in pregnancy, 279*t*, 668*t*
Recommended Dietary Allowance, 668*t*
sources of, 100*t*, 106–107
toxicity of, 100*t*, 107
Vitamin supplements, 116–123
in alcoholics, 121
assessment for, 120
in breast-feeding, 300
for cancer, 650–651
for colostomy, 514–515
cost of, 122
for diabetes mellitus, 575*t*, 579
for disease prevention, 116–118, 117*b*, 119*t*
for end-stage renal disease, 619

Vitamin supplements (*continued*)
- excess vitamin consumption with, 102
- in finicky eaters, 121
- in fortified foods, 123
- in Healthy Eating Index, 192*t*
- in Healthy Eating Pyramid, 193*f*, 195
- for ileostomy, 514–515
- for kidney transplantation, 621*t*, 622
- labeling of, 121–123
- for liver disease, 521
- megadoses of, 98
- natural vs. synthetic, 122
- necessity of, 116
- in nutritional assessment, 6
- for older adults, 118, 120, 121, 355*t*, 357
- vs. optimal food choices, 121
- Percent Daily Value for, 121–122
- preconception, 273
- in pregnancy, 118, 284–286
- for pregnancy-induced hypertension, 291
- risks of, 118
- safety of, 118
- selection of, 121–123
- for steatorrhea, 494
- for stress, 123
- timing of, 123
- toxicity of, 122, 286
- United States Pharmacopeia standards for, 122
- in vegetarian diets, 60, 61, 120
- in weight loss diets, 121

Vomiting. *See* Nausea and vomiting

W

Waist circumference, in body fat assessment, 377, 380*f*

Warfarin, food interactions with, 688*t*

Wasting
- in cancer, 636, 637*f*, 638
- in cardiac disease, 562
- in HIV infection/AIDS, 655–658, 659*t*

Water, 128–131. *See also* Fluid(s)
- balance of, maintenance of, 129
- bottled vs. tap, 151–152
- chlorine in, 152
- in enteral formulas, 431–432
- fluoridation of, 149–150
- functions of, 128
- in health promotion, 151
- in infant formula preparation, 316
- for infants, 314
- intake of, 129–130, 131*t*
- loss of, 128–129, 129*t*
- for muscle building, 62
- output of, 128–129, 129*t*
- recommendations for, 129–130, 131*t*, 151
  - in breast-feeding, 299–300
  - in burns, 467
  - in COPD, 470
  - in healing, 466*t*
  - in older adults, 352–353, 356
  - in pregnancy, 282
- sources of, 129, 130
- types of, 130

Water-soluble vitamins, 107–115, 108*t*–110*t*, 115*f*. *See also specific vitamins*

Weight
- of adolescents, vs. age, 680*f*, 682*f*
- in basal metabolism calculation, 163
- in body mass index calculation, 7, 7*t*, 372, 378*t*–379*t*
- in breast-feeding, 302
- of children, charts for, 676*f*–678*f*
- cultural views of, 247
- in energy expenditure estimation, 461*b*, 462
- excessive. *See* Obesity; Overweight
- vs. height, 313, 684*f*, 685*f*
- history of, in nutritional assessment, 7–8, 7*t*, 8*b*
- "ideal," 7, 7*t*
- of infants, 313–314, 676*f*–679*f*
- normal, 376–377, 378*t*–379*t*
- in pregnancy, ideal, 274
- water requirements and, 131*t*

Weight change
- in nutritional assessment, 8, 8*b*
- in older adults, 364
- psychologic issues in, 381

Weight gain
- from calories eaten at night, 173
- etiology of, 378–381, 382*f*
- in hypoglycemia treatment, 593
- in infants, 320–321
- in insufficient exercise, 381, 382*f*
- in pregnancy
  - in adolescents, 295–296
  - counseling on, 278, 293
  - distribution of, 276, 276*b*
  - inadequate, 276–277, 288–289
  - pattern of, 277
  - recommendations for, 276–277, 276*b*, 279*t*
  - water in, 276
- prevention of, 384
- promotion of, in anorexia nervosa, 410–411

Weight loss
- intentional. *See* Weight management
- unintentional
  - in breast-feeding, 302
  - in cancer, 636, 637*f*, 638
  - in HIV infection/AIDS, 655–658, 659*t*
  - in long-term care, 364
  - in older adults, 364

Weight management
- in adolescents, 339–340
- artificial sweeteners in, 40
- barriers to, 384
- behavior therapy in, 396, 397*b*–398*b*
- benefits of, 383
- calorie counting in, 74, 384–385, 386*b*
- carbohydrate content and, 390–394, 391*t*, 392*t*
- in children, 329–330
- deceptive diet claims for, 387
- in diabetes mellitus, 571–572, 578–579, 581

in *Dietary Guidelines for Americans 2005,* 184*b*
exercise in, 172
failure of, 385
fat content and, 390–394, 391*t*, 392*t*
food group approach to, 388, 390, 390*t*
goals of, 384
guidelines for, 394–395
high-protein diet in, 49
hunger during, 387
for hypertension, 551
lifestyle changes for, 386, 388, 389*t*, 390, 390*t*
low-carbohydrate diets for, 38*t*, 390–394, 392*t*
low-fat diets for, 391–393, 391*t*, 392*t*
motivation for, evaluation of, 383–384
nondiet approach to, 388, 390
nursing process for, 401–406
nutritional therapy in, 384–395, 386*b*, 389*t*–391*t*
obsession with, 388
in older adults, 361
pharmacotherapy in, 396, 398–399, 399*t*
physical activity in, 395–396
in pregnancy, 277, 288–289
protein content and, 390–394, 391*t*
set point theory of, 380
Subway meals for, 264
surgery in, 399–400, 400*f*, 401*f*
"think thin" in, 397*b*
vitamin supplements for, 121
Wet beriberi, 110
Whey-casein ratio
in breast milk, 315*t*
in infant formula, 315*t*
Whole grains and flours, 27–28, 28*f*
alternates for, 204
sources of, 34, 34*t*
Women's health issues, 345–346, 348–349, 350*b*. *See also* Breast-feeding; Pregnancy
vitamin supplements as, 123
Wound healing, nutrition therapy for
in burns, 465, 467–468
postoperative, 465, 466*t*–467*t*

X

Xylitol, as sugar alternative, 38, 576

Y

Yeast, red, for coronary heart disease prevention, 543*b*
Yogurt. *See* Milk, yogurt, and cheese group
"Yo-yo" dieting, 413

Z

Zalcitabine (Hivid, ddC), for HIV infection/AIDS, 661*t*, 693*t*
Zantac (ranitidine), for gastritis, 493
Zenical (orlistat), for weight loss, 399*t*
Zerit (stavudine), for HIV infection/AIDS, 661*t*, 693*t*
Ziagen (abacavir), for HIV infection/AIDS, 661*t*
Zidovudine (Retrovir, AZT, ZDV), for HIV infection/AIDS, 661*t*, 693*t*
Zinc, 147–148
body distribution of, 147
in breast milk, 298
deficiency of, 144*t*, 147–148, 619
functions of, 133, 144*t*
recommendations for, 144*t*
Adequate Intake, 671*t*
in breast-feeding, 279*t*, 671*t*
in burns, 467
in children, 671*t*
Dietary Reference Intakes, 671*t*
in healing, 467*t*
in infants, 313*f*, 671*t*
in pregnancy, 279*t*, 671*t*
Recommended Dietary Allowance, 671*t*
sources of, 58, 144*t*
supplements of, 148
for liver transplant candidates, 523
in pregnancy, 286
in renal disease, 619
toxicity of, 144*t*
in vegetarian diets, 58
Zolpidem, food interactions with, 695*t*
Zone diet, macronutrients in, 391*t*